IMAGING ANATOMY
Head and Neck

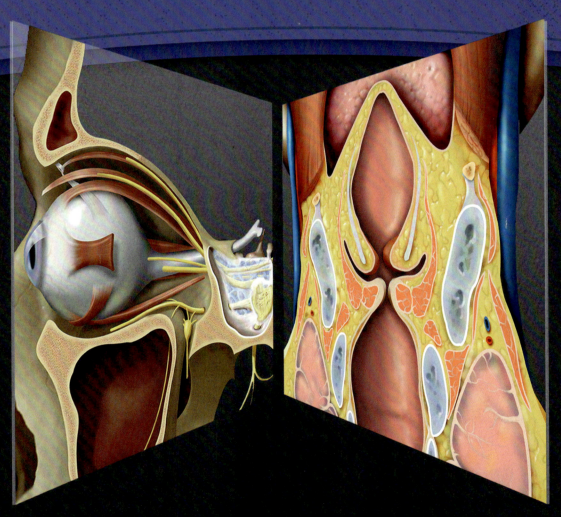

CHAPMAN
HARNSBERGER | VATTOTH

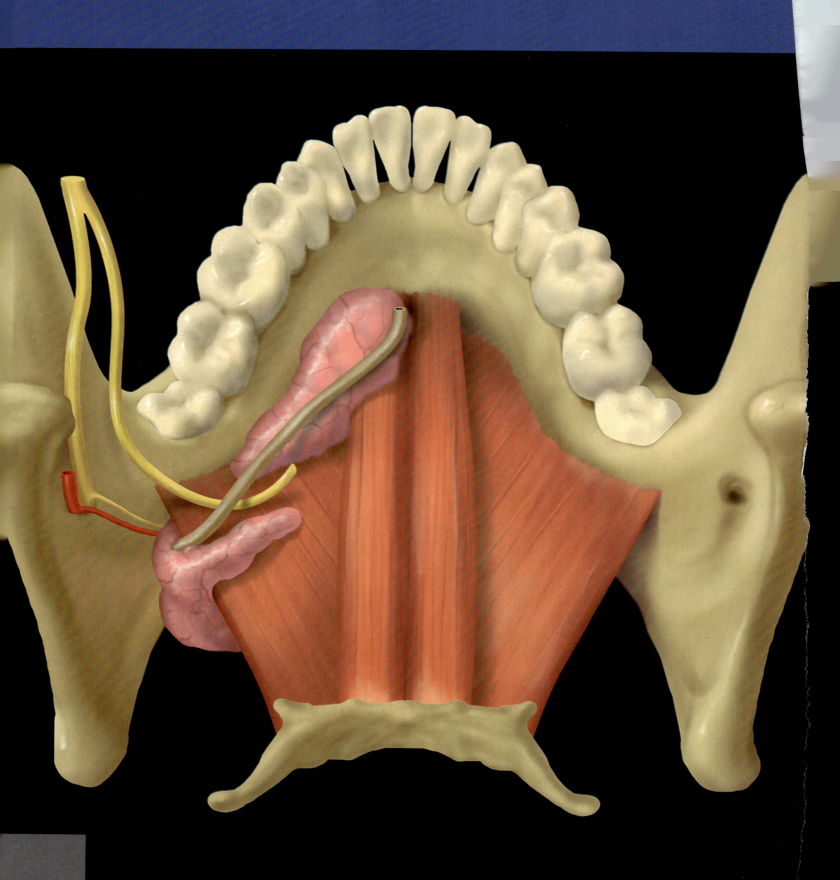

IMAGING ANATOMY

Head and Neck

Philip R. Chapman, MD

Associate Professor
Neuroradiology Section
The University of Alabama at Birmingham
Birmingham, Alabama

H. Ric Harnsberger, MD

Professor of Radiology & Otolaryngology
R. C. Willey Chair in Neuroradiology
University of Utah School of Medicine
Department of Radiology & Imaging Sciences
Salt Lake City, Utah

Surjith Vattoth, MD, FRCR

Associate Professor of Clinical Radiology
Weill Cornell Medicine
Cornell University
New York, New York
Senior Consultant Neuroradiologist
Hamad Medical Corporation
Doha, Qatar

ELSEVIER

1600 John F. Kennedy Blvd.
Ste 1800
Philadelphia, PA 19103-2899

IMAGING ANATOMY: HEAD AND NECK

ISBN: 978-0-323-56872-2

Copyright © 2019 by Elsevier. All rights reserved.

No part of this publication may be reproduced or transmitted in any form or by any means, electronic or mechanical, including photocopying, recording, or any information storage and retrieval system, without permission in writing from the publisher. Details on how to seek permission, further information about the Publisher's permissions policies and our arrangements with organizations such as the Copyright Clearance Center and the Copyright Licensing Agency, can be found at our website: www.elsevier.com/permissions.

This book and the individual contributions contained in it are protected under copyright by the Publisher (other than as may be noted herein).

Notices

Knowledge and best practice in this field are constantly changing. As new research and experience broaden our understanding, changes in research methods, professional practices, or medical treatment may become necessary.

Practitioners and researchers must always rely on their own experience and knowledge in evaluating and using any information, methods, compounds, or experiments described herein. In using such information or methods they should be mindful of their own safety and the safety of others, including parties for whom they have a professional responsibility.

With respect to any drug or pharmaceutical products identified, readers are advised to check the most current information provided (i) on procedures featured or (ii) by the manufacturer of each product to be administered, to verify the recommended dose or formula, the method and duration of administration, and contraindications. It is the responsibility of practitioners, relying on their own experience and knowledge of their patients, to make diagnoses, to determine dosages and the best treatment for each individual patient, and to take all appropriate safety precautions.

To the fullest extent of the law, neither the Publisher nor the authors, contributors, or editors, assume any liability for any injury and/or damage to persons or property as a matter of products liability, negligence or otherwise, or from any use or operation of any methods, products, instructions, or ideas contained in the material herein.

Publisher Cataloging-in-Publication Data

Names: Chapman, Philip R.
Title: Imaging anatomy. Head and neck / [edited by] Philip R. Chapman.
Other titles: Head and neck.
Description: First edition. | Salt Lake City, UT : Elsevier, Inc., [2018] | Includes bibliographical references and index.
Identifiers: ISBN 978-0-323-56872-2
Subjects: LCSH: Head--Anatomy--Handbooks, manuals, etc. | Neck--anatomy--Handbooks, manuals, etc. |
    MESH: Head--anatomy & histology--Atlases. | Neck--anatomy & histology--Atlases. | Diagnostic Imaging--Atlases.
Classification: LCC QM535.I43 2018 | NLM WE 17 | DDC 611.91--dc23

International Standard Book Number: 978-0-323-56872-2

Cover Designer: Tom M. Olson, BA

Printed in Canada by Friesens, Altona, Manitoba, Canada

Last digit is the print number: 9 8 7 6 5 4 3 2 1

Dedication

I would like to especially thank Dr. Ric Harnsberger for inspiring me to tackle this project. I can only hope that the book maintains a tradition of excellence born from the creative and intellectual collaboration of the University of Utah neuroradiology family and many others.

The book is dedicated to my parents, Jerome and Joy, to my wife, April, and our sons, Grayson and Garrison. Without their love and support, this would not have been possible.

PRC

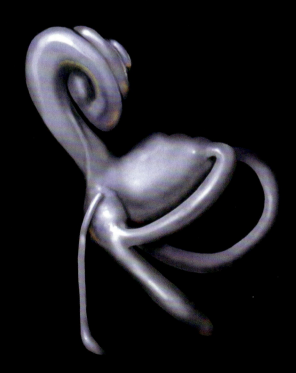

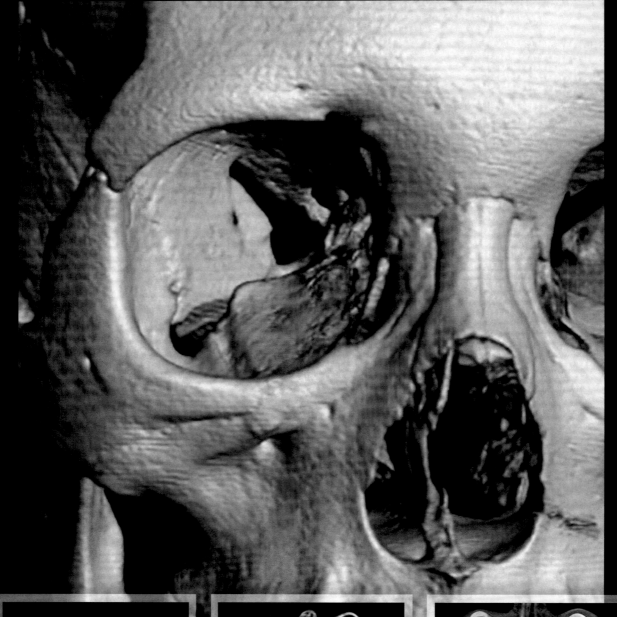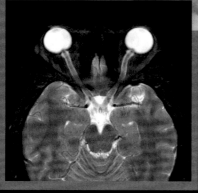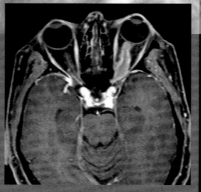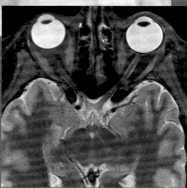

Contributing Authors

Siddhartha Gaddamanugu, MD
Assistant Professor
Department of Radiology
Veterans Affairs Medical Center
The University of Alabama at Birmingham
Birmingham, Alabama

Daniel E. Meltzer, MD
Associate Clinical Professor of Radiology
Icahn School of Medicine at Mount Sinai
New York, New York

Anthony B. Morlandt, MD, DDS
Assistant Professor
Chief, Section of Oral Oncology
Department of Oral and Maxillofacial Surgery
The University of Alabama at Birmingham
Birmingham, Alabama

Aparna Singhal, MD
Program Director, Neuroradiology Fellowship Program
Assistant Professor, Neuroradiology Section
Department of Radiology
The University of Alabama at Birmingham
Birmingham, Alabama

Additional Contributors

Hank Baskin, MD
H. Christian Davidson, MD
Bronwyn E. Hamilton, MD
Kevin R. Moore, MD
Jeffrey S. Ross, MD
Karen L. Salzman, MD
Richard H. Wiggins, III, MD, CIIP, FSIIM

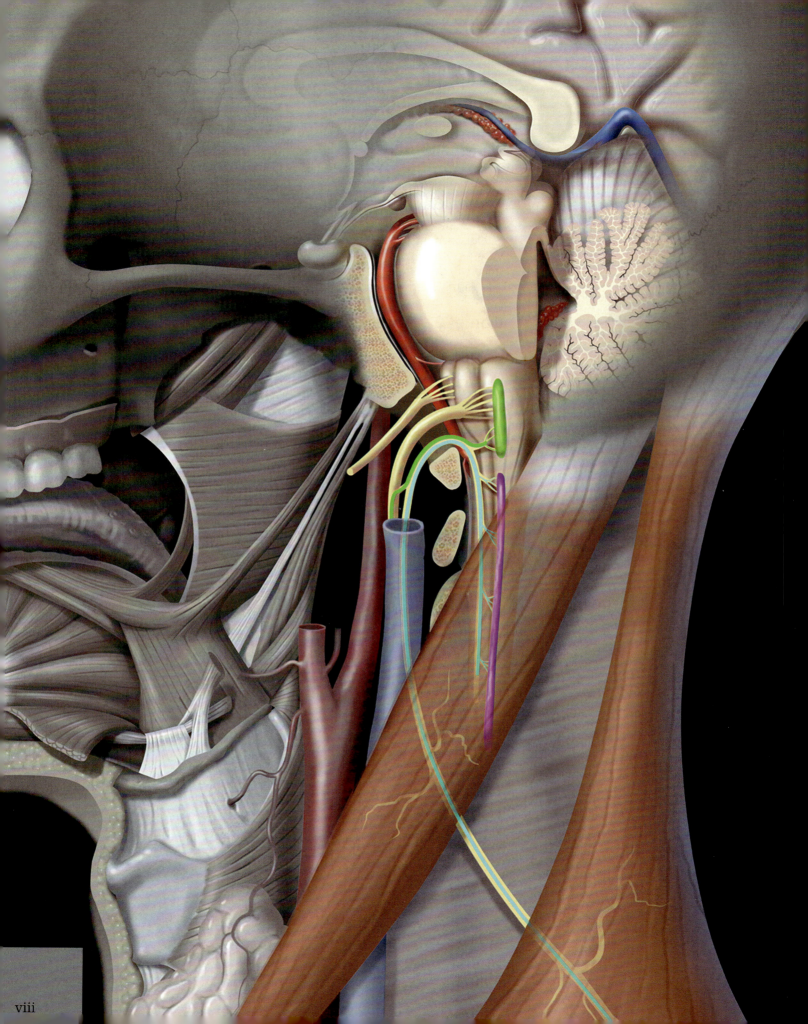

Preface

We are proud to present *Imaging Anatomy: Head and Neck*, which takes its origin from the landmark publication *Diagnostic and Surgical Anatomy: Brain, Head and Neck, Spine*, published in 2006. In this book, head and neck anatomy is approached as a critically important stand-alone subject for radiologists and other professionals who rely on head and neck imaging for patient evaluation and therapy. This concentrated approach was born out of a need to expand the overall content of the original text with new sections, refresh diagnostic images and illustrations, and provide more specific anatomic detail. While the target audience remains the radiologist or radiology resident, this book is intended to provide a comprehensive reference for students, anatomists, and nonradiology professionals, including oncologists, radiation therapists, and head and neck surgeons.

Like *Diagnostic and Surgical Anatomy: Brain, Head and Neck, Spine*, the text is offered in a succinct, bulleted format that provides maximum content in an easy-to-use layout and allows for rapid reference and review. In each section, the critical foundation of normal anatomy is provided along with imaging recommendations and imaging correlations. Radiologic-pathologic correlation is provided when appropriate to emphasize anatomic relationships. The text is accompanied by hundreds of full-color graphic illustrations created by our expert medical illustrators as well as hundreds of high-resolution multiplanar CT, MR, and ultrasound images. Each illustration and image is labeled and comes with its own legend to expedite the learning experience. The result is an organized and readily accessible anatomic atlas of head and neck anatomy.

Purchase of this book comes with an electronic version, Expert Consult, which provides the ultimate in accessibility whether the reader is at home, in the reading room, or in the clinic.

This process of collaboration has been an amazing journey, and I would like to personally thank the many coauthors and the entire staff at Elsevier, especially the medical illustrators. I was truly fortunate to work with and learn from such a fantastic team. We hope you find that *Imaging Anatomy: Head and Neck* will serve as your reference cornerstone for head and neck anatomy in your daily practice.

Philip R. Chapman, MD
Associate Professor
Neuroradiology Section
The University of Alabama at Birmingham
Birmingham, Alabama

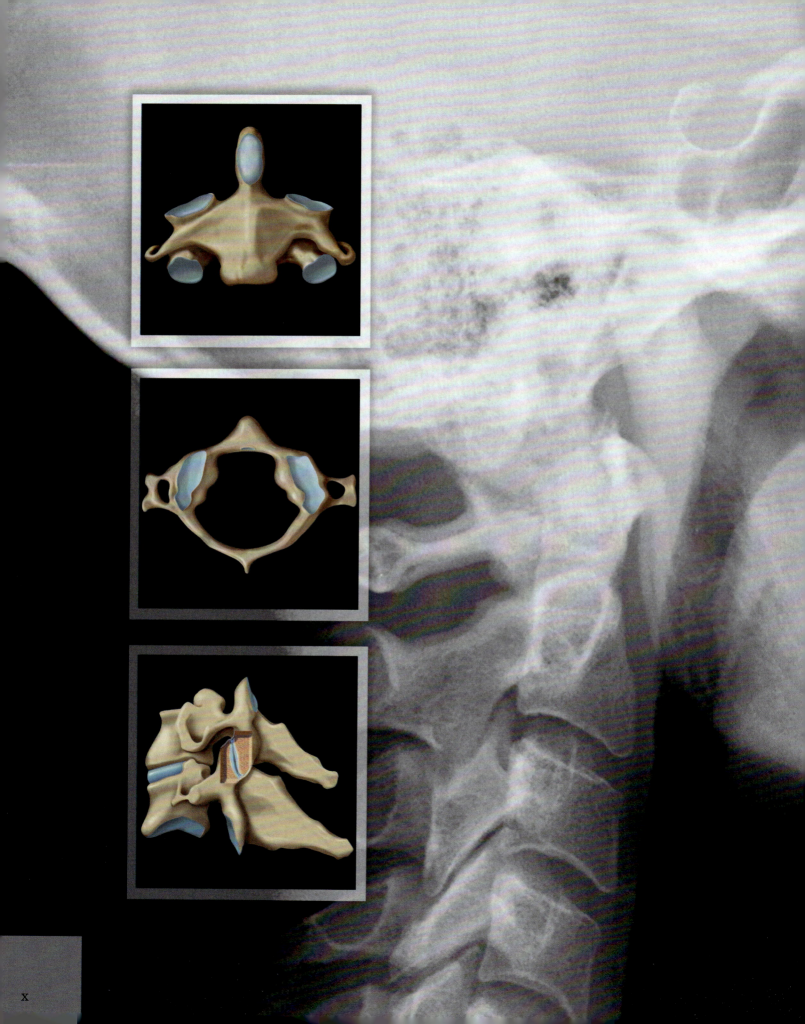

Acknowledgments

Lead Editor

Nina I. Bennett, BA

Text Editors

Arthur G. Gelsinger, MA
Rebecca L. Bluth, BA
Terry W. Ferrell, MS
Matt W. Hoecherl, BS
Megg Morin, BA
Joshua Reynolds, PhD

Image Editors

Jeffrey J. Marmorstone, BS
Lisa A. M. Steadman, BS

Illustrations

Richard Coombs, MS
Lane R. Bennion, MS
Laura C. Wissler, MA

Art Direction and Design

Tom M. Olson, BA
Laura C. Wissler, MA

Production Coordinators

Emily C. Fassett, BA
Angela M. G. Terry, BA
Alexander Eakins, BA

ELSEVIER

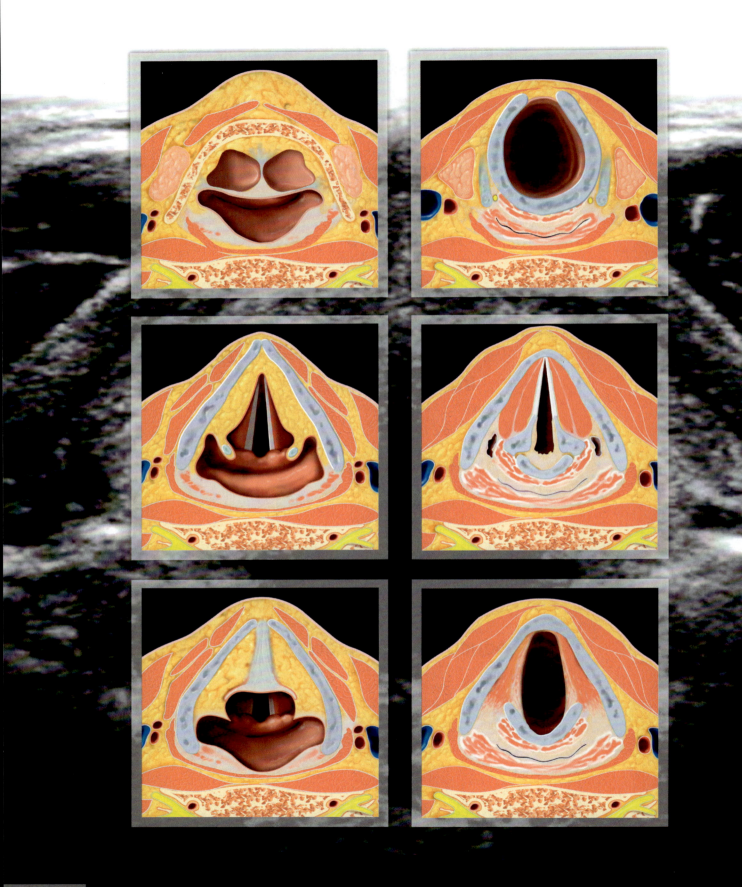

Sections

SECTION 1:
Temporal Bone and Skull Base

SECTION 2:
Cranial Nerves

SECTION 3:
Orbit

SECTION 4:
Nose and Sinuses

SECTION 5:
Suprahyoid and Infrahyoid Neck

SECTION 6:
Oral Cavity

SECTION 7:
Spine

TABLE OF CONTENTS

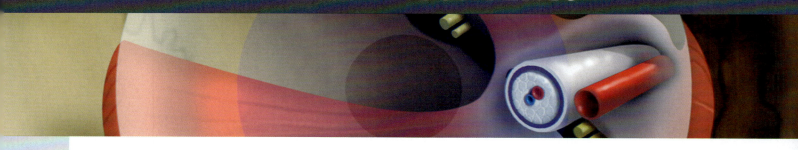

SECTION 1: TEMPORAL BONE AND SKULL BASE

- 4 **Skull Base Overview**
  Philip R. Chapman, MD and Hank Baskin, MD
- 14 **Anterior Skull Base**
  Philip R. Chapman, MD and Hank Baskin, MD
- 30 **Central Skull Base**
  Hank Baskin, MD and Philip R. Chapman, MD
- 40 **Posterior Skull Base**
  Hank Baskin, MD and Philip R. Chapman, MD
- 50 **Temporal Bone Anatomy**
  Philip R. Chapman, MD and H. Ric Harnsberger, MD
- 66 **Temporal Bone Oblique Reformation Anatomy**
  Philip R. Chapman, MD and H. Ric Harnsberger, MD
- 72 **External Auditory Canal Anatomy**
  Philip R. Chapman, MD and H. Ric Harnsberger, MD
- 78 **Middle Ear-Mastoid Anatomy**
  Philip R. Chapman, MD and H. Ric Harnsberger, MD
- 86 **Inner Ear Anatomy**
  Philip R. Chapman, MD and H. Ric Harnsberger, MD
- 94 **Petrous Apex Anatomy**
  Philip R. Chapman, MD and H. Ric Harnsberger, MD
- 102 **CPA-IAC Anatomy**
  H. Ric Harnsberger, MD and Surjith Vattoth, MD, FRCR
- 108 **Temporomandibular Joint**
  Richard H. Wiggins, III, MD, CIIP, FSIIM and Anthony B. Morlandt, MD, DDS

SECTION 2: CRANIAL NERVES

- 116 **Cranial Nerves Overview**
  H. Ric Harnsberger, MD and Philip R. Chapman, MD
- 128 **CNI (Olfactory Nerve)**
  Aparna Singhal, MD and H. Ric Harnsberger, MD
- 132 **CNII (Optic Nerve)**
  Philip R. Chapman, MD and H. Ric Harnsberger, MD
- 140 **CNIII (Oculomotor Nerve)**
  Philip R. Chapman, MD and H. Ric Harnsberger, MD
- 148 **CNIV (Trochlear Nerve)**
  Philip R. Chapman, MD and H. Ric Harnsberger, MD
- 152 **CNV (Trigeminal Nerve)**
  Surjith Vattoth, MD, FRCR
- 164 **CNVI (Abducens Nerve)**
  Philip R. Chapman, MD and H. Ric Harnsberger, MD
- 168 **CNVII (Facial Nerve)**
  Philip R. Chapman, MD and H. Ric Harnsberger, MD
- 176 **CNVIII (Vestibulocochlear Nerve)**
  Philip R. Chapman, MD
- 182 **CNIX (Glossopharyngeal Nerve)**
  Aparna Singhal, MD and H. Ric Harnsberger, MD
- 188 **CNX (Vagus Nerve)**
  Aparna Singhal, MD and H. Ric Harnsberger, MD
- 194 **CNXI (Accessory Nerve)**
  Siddhartha Gaddamanugu, MD and H. Ric Harnsberger, MD
- 198 **CNXII (Hypoglossal Nerve)**
  Aparna Singhal, MD and H. Ric Harnsberger, MD

SECTION 3: ORBIT

- 206 **Orbit Overview**
  Daniel E. Meltzer, MD, Philip R. Chapman, MD, and H. Christian Davidson, MD
- 216 **Bony Orbit and Foramina**
  H. Christian Davidson, MD and Daniel E. Meltzer, MD
- 220 **Optic Nerve/Sheath Complex**
  H. Christian Davidson, MD and Daniel E. Meltzer, MD
- 224 **Globe**
  H. Christian Davidson, MD and Daniel E. Meltzer, MD
- 226 **Cavernous Sinus**
  Philip R. Chapman, MD, Karen L. Salzman, MD, and Bronwyn E. Hamilton, MD

SECTION 4: NOSE AND SINUSES

- 238 **Sinonasal Overview**
  Surjith Vattoth, MD, FRCR
- 248 **Ostiomeatal Unit**
  Surjith Vattoth, MD, FRCR
- 252 **Pterygopalatine Fossa**
  Surjith Vattoth, MD, FRCR and Philip R. Chapman, MD
- 260 **Frontal Recess and Related Air Cells**
  Surjith Vattoth, MD, FRCR

SECTION 5: SUPRAHYOID AND INFRAHYOID NECK

- 272 **Suprahyoid and Infrahyoid Neck Overview**
  Surjith Vattoth, MD, FRCR
- 290 **Parapharyngeal Space**
  Philip R. Chapman, MD and H. Ric Harnsberger, MD
- 298 **Pharyngeal Mucosal Space**
  H. Ric Harnsberger, MD and Daniel E. Meltzer, MD
- 310 **Masticator Space**
  Surjith Vattoth, MD, FRCR and H. Ric Harnsberger, MD
- 320 **Parotid Space**
  Surjith Vattoth, MD, FRCR and H. Ric Harnsberger, MD
- 332 **Carotid Space**
  Surjith Vattoth, MD, FRCR and H. Ric Harnsberger, MD
- 340 **Retropharyngeal Space**
  Surjith Vattoth, MD, FRCR and H. Ric Harnsberger, MD

TABLE OF CONTENTS

348   **Perivertebral Space**
Aparna Singhal, MD and H. Ric Harnsberger, MD

356   **Posterior Cervical Space**
Siddhartha Gaddamanugu, MD and H. Ric Harnsberger, MD

364   **Visceral Space**
Siddhartha Gaddamanugu, MD and Philip R. Chapman, MD

372   **Larynx**
Surjith Vattoth, MD, FRCR

392   **Hypopharynx**
Surjith Vattoth, MD, FRCR

402   **Thyroid and Parathyroid Anatomy**
Surjith Vattoth, MD, FRCR and H. Ric Harnsberger, MD

416   **Cervical Trachea and Esophagus**
Siddhartha Gaddamanugu, MD and H. Ric Harnsberger, MD

426   **Cervical Lymph Nodes**
Surjith Vattoth, MD, FRCR and Philip R. Chapman, MD

440   **Facial Muscles and Superficial Musculoaponeurotic System**
Surjith Vattoth, MD, FRCR

SECTION 6: ORAL CAVITY

452   **Oral Cavity Overview**
H. Ric Harnsberger, MD and Anthony B. Morlandt, MD, DDS

460   **Oral Mucosal Space**
H. Ric Harnsberger, MD and Anthony B. Morlandt, MD, DDS

462   **Sublingual Space**
Surjith Vattoth, MD, FRCR and H. Ric Harnsberger, MD

468   **Submandibular Space**
H. Ric Harnsberger, MD and Surjith Vattoth, MD, FRCR

474   **Buccal Space**
Anthony B. Morlandt, MD, DDS and Philip R. Chapman, MD

480   **Tongue**
Surjith Vattoth, MD, FRCR and H. Ric Harnsberger, MD

486   **Retromolar Trigone**
Surjith Vattoth, MD, FRCR and H. Ric Harnsberger, MD

490   **Mandible and Maxilla**
H. Ric Harnsberger, MD and Daniel E. Meltzer, MD

SECTION 7: SPINE

498   **Craniocervical Junction**
Jeffrey S. Ross, MD and Philip R. Chapman, MD

514   **Cervical Spine**
Jeffrey S. Ross, MD and Philip R. Chapman, MD

532   **Brachial Plexus**
Philip R. Chapman, MD and Kevin R. Moore, MD

IMAGING ANATOMY
Head and Neck

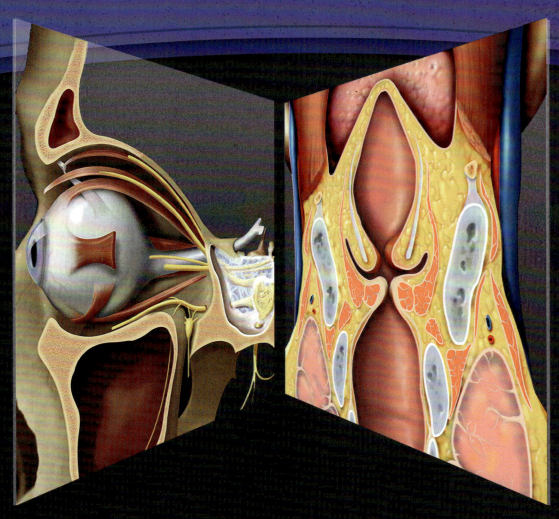

CHAPMAN
HARNSBERGER | VATTOTH

SECTION 1
Temporal Bone and Skull Base

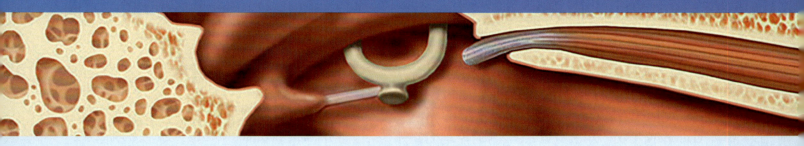

Skull Base Overview	4
Anterior Skull Base	14
Central Skull Base	30
Posterior Skull Base	40
Temporal Bone Anatomy	50
Temporal Bone Oblique Reformation Anatomy	66
External Auditory Canal Anatomy	72
Middle Ear-Mastoid Anatomy	78
Inner Ear Anatomy	86
Petrous Apex Anatomy	94
CPA-IAC Anatomy	102
Temporomandibular Joint	108

Skull Base Overview

TERMINOLOGY

Abbreviations
- Skull base (SB)

Definitions
- SB: Complex osseous foundation of cranial vault, separates intracranial structures from sinuses, orbits, & suprahyoid neck (SHN)
- Transmits critical neurovascular structures between cranial vault & SHN, orbits, sinuses

IMAGING ANATOMY

Overview
- **5 bones** make up base of skull
  - **Paired bones**: Frontal & temporal bones
  - **Unpaired bones**: Ethmoid, sphenoid, & occipital bones
- **2 surfaces**
  - **Endocranial surface**: Brain, pituitary, cisterns, cranial nerves (CN) & intracranial vascular structures, including cavernous sinuses
  - **Exocranial surface**: Extracranial head & neck
    - Anterior portion: Nasal cavity, frontal & ethmoid sinuses, orbits
    - Central portion: Nasopharyngeal mucosal space, masticator, parotid & parapharyngeal spaces
    - Posterior portion: Nasopharyngeal mucosal space, carotid, retropharyngeal, perivertebral spaces
- **3 regions**
  - **Anterior, central, & posterior SB (ASB, CSB, PSB)**
  - **ASB**
    - Anterolateral boundary: Frontal bones
    - Inferior relationships: Nasal vault, ethmoid & frontal sinuses; orbit & orbital canals
    - Superior relationships: Frontal lobes, CNI
    - ASB-CSB boundary: Lesser wing of sphenoid (sphenoid ridge) & planum sphenoidale
  - **CSB**
    - Inferior relationships: Roof of pharyngeal mucosal space, masticator, parotid & parapharyngeal spaces
    - Superior relationships: Temporal lobes, pituitary, cavernous sinus, Meckel cave, CNI-IV, CNVI, CNV1-3
    - CSB-PSB boundary: Dorsum sella & posterior clinoid processes medially, petrous ridges laterally
  - **PSB**
    - Inferior relationships: Posterior pharyngeal mucosal space, carotid, retropharyngeal, perivertebral spaces
    - Superior relationships: Brainstem, cerebellum, CNVII-VIII, CNIX-XII, transverse-sigmoid sinuses
    - Posterior boundary: Occipital bone

Internal Contents
- **ASB**
  - Contents: Frontal, ethmoid bones, lesser wing & planum sphenoidale of sphenoid bone
  - Foramina & structures transmitted
    - **Cribriform plate**: CNI, ethmoid arteries
    - **Optic canal**: CNII, ophthalmic artery
- **CSB**
  - Contents: Body & greater wing of sphenoid bone & anterior temporal bones
  - Foramina & structures transmitted
    - **Superior orbital fissure**: CNIII, CNIV, CNV1, & CNVI & superior ophthalmic vein
    - **Inferior orbital fissure**: Infraorbital artery, vein, nerve
    - **Carotid canal**: Internal carotid artery (ICA), sympathetic plexus
    - **Foramen rotundum**: CNV2, artery of foramen rotundum, & emissary veins
    - **Foramen ovale**: CNV3, lesser petrosal nerve, accessory meningeal branch maxillary artery, & emissary vein
    - **Foramen spinosum**: Middle meningeal artery & vein, meningeal branch of mandibular nerve
    - **Foramen lacerum**: Not true foramen; cartilaginous floor of anteromedial horizontal petrous ICA canal
    - **Vidian canal**: Vidian artery & nerve
- **PSB**
  - Contents: Occipital & posterior temporal bones
  - Foramina & structures transmitted
    - **Internal acoustic meatus**: CNVII, CNVIII, labyrinthine artery
    - **Hypoglossal canal**: CNXII
    - **Foramen magnum**: Spinal portion CNXI, vertebral arteries, & medulla oblongata
    - **Jugular foramen: Pars nervosa**: CNIX, Jacobson nerve, & inferior petrosal sinus
    - **Jugular foramen: Pars vascularis**: CNX, Arnold nerve, CNXI, jugular bulb, & posterior meningeal artery

ANATOMY IMAGING ISSUES

Questions
- Imaging of SB best done as combination of focused MR & bone CT
  - MR requires T1, T2, & T1 C+ with fat saturation for full SB evaluation
  - Bone CT defines bone changes
- SHN spaces/structures abut SB, allowing extracranial tumor to access intracranial area via perineural tumor
  - Masticator space: CNV3
  - Parotid space: CNVII
  - Orbit: CNV1, CNIII, IV, & VI
  - Sinus & nose, pterygopalatine fossa: CNV2

Imaging Recommendations
- **Bone CT**
  - Axial thin slices with coronal reformations
  - Edge-enhancing algorithm & wide window settings (> 2,000 HU) necessary to evaluate bony anatomy
  - Narrow windows (200-400 HU) & smoothing algorithm to inspect regional soft tissues
  - If MR available, contrast unnecessary
- **MR**: Thin slices (≤ 4 mm), axial & coronal, T1, T2, & T1 C+ fat saturated
  - Precontrast T1 images use native fatty marrow for "contrast"
  - Use MRA & MRV for arteries & veins

Imaging Pitfalls
- Prominent foramen cecum, accessory foramina can be normal variants
- MR flow in jugular foramen may mimic mass

Skull Base Overview

GRAPHICS

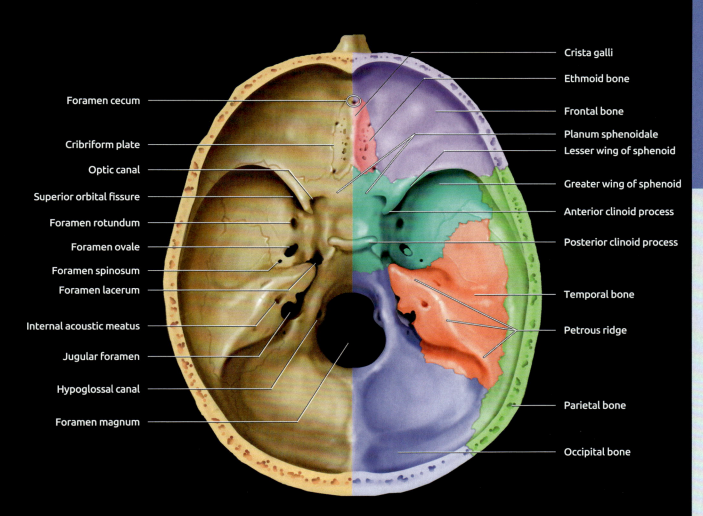

Graphic of endocranial skull base viewed from above with highlighted osseous landmarks labeled on the right is shown. Important foramina are labeled on the left. The skull base is formed by the frontal, ethmoid, sphenoid, temporal, and occipital bones. The frontal, parietal, and occipital bones form the lateral vault of the cranium. The skull base is an undulating surface with grooves formed by the brain above and rough bony structures providing dural attachments. The lesser wing of the sphenoid and planum sphenoidale form the anterior skull base-central skull base border, while the petrous ridge and dorsum sella form the central skull base-posterior skull base boundary. The majority of important foramina are in the central skull base (sphenoid bone).

Skull Base Overview

GRAPHICS

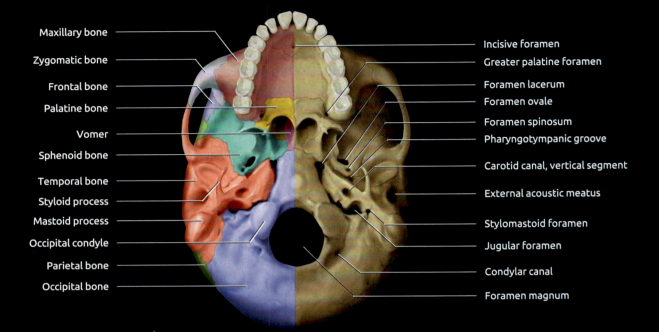

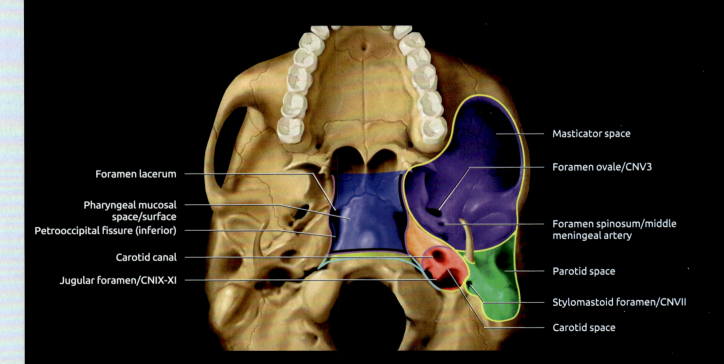

(Top) Graphic of skull base viewed from below shows the complexity of the exocranial skull base with bony landmarks labeled on the left and foramina labeled on the right. Note that in addition to the frontal, sphenoid, temporal, and occipital bones, the undersurface of the skull base is formed by the maxilla, vomer, palatine, and zygomatic bones. The ethmoid bone is not part of the exocranial skull base. **(Bottom)** Graphic of skull base viewed from below shows the relationships to the suprahyoid neck spaces and structures. Four spaces have key interactions with the skull base: Masticator, parotid, carotid, and pharyngeal mucosal spaces. Parotid space (green) malignancy can follow CNVII into the stylomastoid foramen. Masticator space (purple) receives CNV3, while CNIX-XII enter the carotid space (red). The pharyngeal mucosal space abuts the foramen lacerum, which is covered by fibrocartilage in life.

Skull Base Overview

AXIAL BONE CT

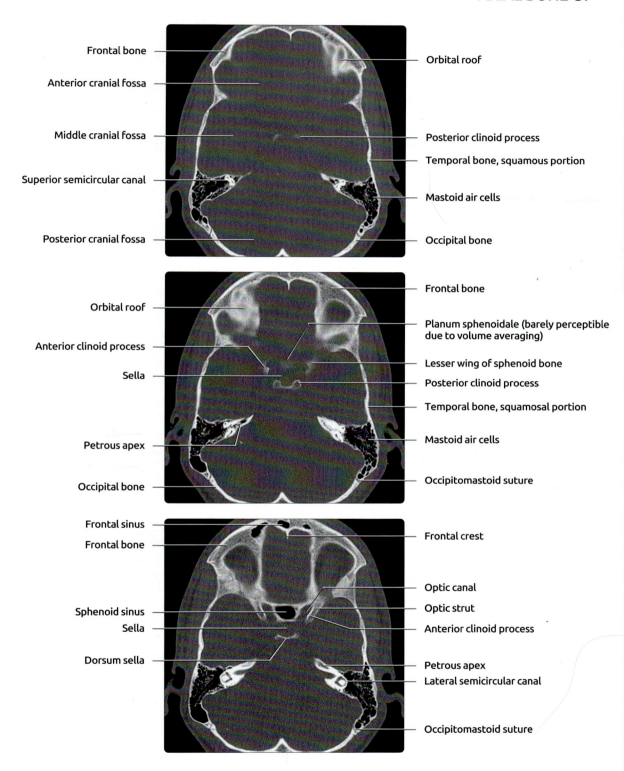

(Top) First of 12 axial bone CT images of the skull base presented from superior to inferior is shown. At level of orbital roof, the brain within the anterior, middle, and posterior fossae is cradled above respective regions of the skull base: Anterior skull base, central skull base, and posterior skull base. (Middle) At level of the upper sella, the lesser wings of the sphenoid and planum sphenoidale, which demarcate the anterior skull base-central skull base border, are barely visible. More posterior, the petrous apices divide the central skull base from the posterior skull base. The posterior skull base houses the cerebellum, covered superiorly by tentorium cerebelli, which attaches to posterior clinoid processes. (Bottom) At the level of the anterior clinoid, the optic canals pass through the sphenoid bone, bounded by the anterior clinoid process laterally and the sphenoid sinus medially. The dorsum sella marks the anteromedial border of the posterior skull base.

Skull Base Overview

AXIAL BONE CT

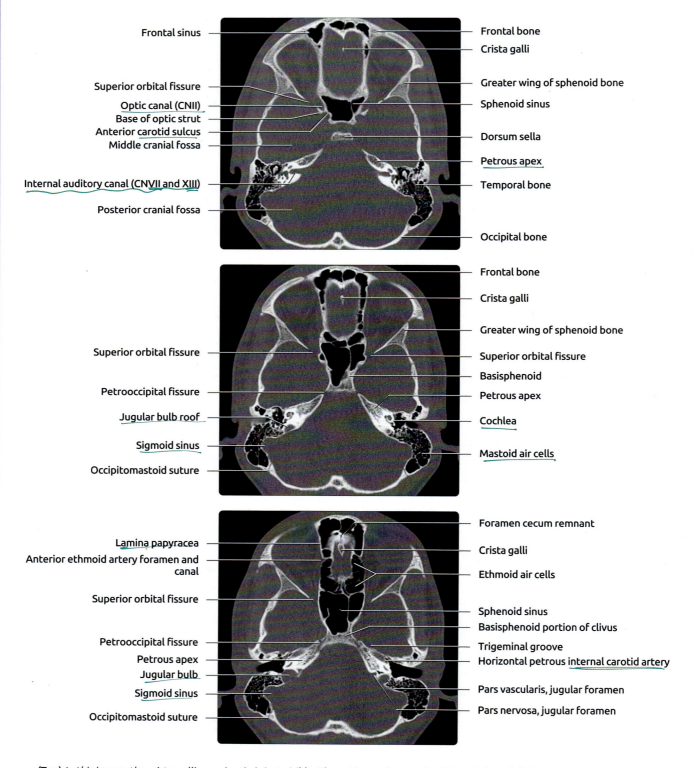

(Top) In this image, the crista galli superior tip is just visible. The optic canal transmits CNII and the ophthalmic artery to the orbit, while the superior orbital fissure transmits CNIII, CNIV, CNV1, CNVI, and the superior ophthalmic vein. Notice the close approximation of the optic canal and superior orbital fissure, separated only by a thin, often pneumatized, optic strut. The internal auditory canal is on the medial wall of the temporal bone. (Middle) Crista galli provides attachment for the falx cerebri and divides the anterior aspect of the anterior skull base into 2 symmetric halves. Note that ethmoid air cells extend superior to the cribriform plate. Sphenoid sinus is immediately below the sella and medial to the superior orbital fissure. The superior margin of petrooccipital fissure is visible at medial tip of petrous apex. It is at this point where the petrosphenoid ligament (Gruber ligament) can be found. This short ligament spans the petrous ridge to the clivus. Below the ligament is the Dorello canal that contains dural venous structures and CNVI. (Bottom) At the anterior base of the crista galli is foramen cecum remnant. The petrooccipital fissure is the most common location for skull base chondrosarcoma.

Skull Base Overview

AXIAL BONE CT

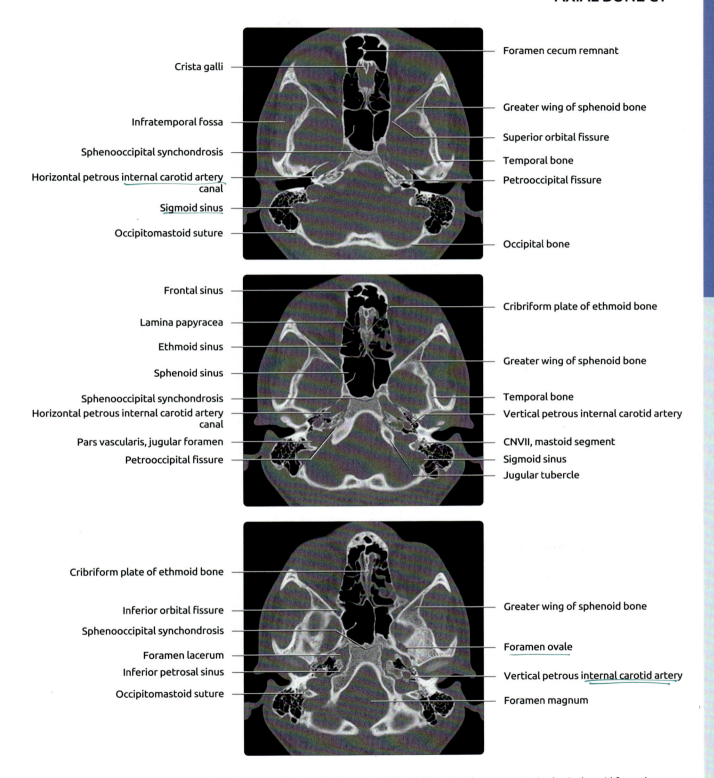

(Top) At the level of the upper clivus, the sphenooccipital synchondrosis is visible, delineating the more anterior basisphenoid from the more posterior basiocciput. Posterolaterally, the petrooccipital fissure is seen separating the more medial occipital bone from the more lateral temporal bone. (Middle) At the level of the cribriform plate of the ethmoid bone, the frontal, ethmoid, and sphenoid sinuses are all visible. Also note the vertical and horizontal segments of the petrous internal carotid arteries. (Bottom) Notice the inferior orbital fissure is bounded by the sphenoid sinus posteromedially and the greater wing of the sphenoid bone laterally. It contains the infraorbital artery, vein, and nerve. The foramen lacerum is occupied by cartilage and is contiguous posteriorly with the petrooccipital fissure. Inferiorly and posteriorly, the petrooccipital fissure contains the inferior petrosal sinus.

Skull Base Overview

AXIAL BONE CT

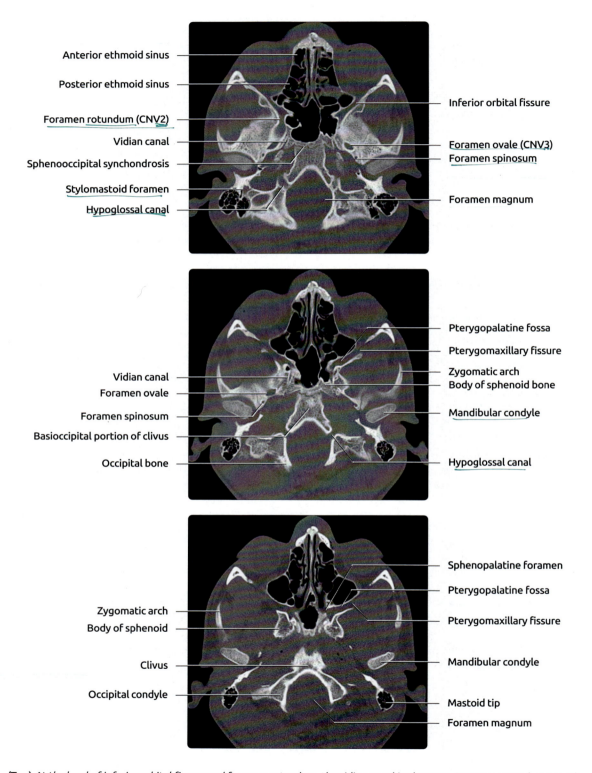

(Top) At the level of inferior orbital fissure and foramen rotundum, the vidian canal is also seen. Foramen rotundum provides a conduit for CNV2 to access the confluence of the medial inferior orbital fissure and the superior pterygopalatine fossa. CNV3 traverses sphenoid bone via the foramen ovale. The hypoglossal canal is seen in the inferior occipital bone. (Middle) This image is at the level of the hypoglossal canal in the low occipital bone. Anteriorly, the pterygomaxillary fissure is the lateral opening of the pterygopalatine fossa. (Bottom) At the inferior margin of the foramen magnum, the mastoid tips are still visible. The pterygopalatine fossa is well seen, connecting medially with the nasal cavity via the sphenopalatine foramen and laterally with the masticator space through the pterygomaxillary fissure. The foramen rotundum and vidian canals also lead into the pterygopalatine fossa.

Skull Base Overview

3D-VRT BONE CT

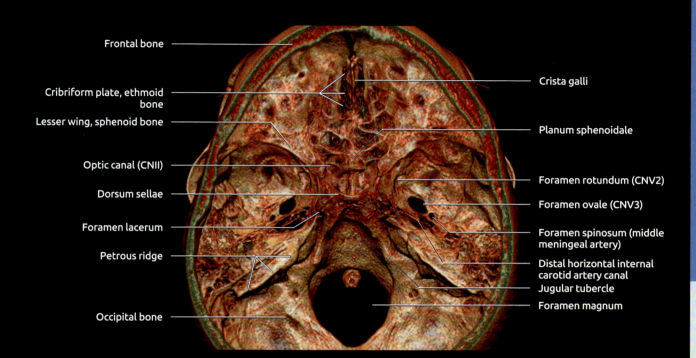

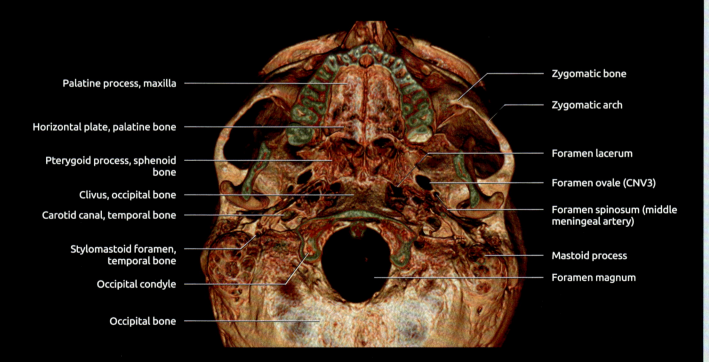

(Top) 3D-VRT image of the osseous skull base from above is shown. Anterior skull base is bounded by frontal bones anteriorly and the lesser wing of the sphenoid and planum sphenoidale posteriorly. Central skull base, with its multitude of fissures and foramina, is made up of sphenoid bone and anterior temporal bone. It is bounded anteriorly by the lesser wing of the sphenoid and posterior planum sphenoidale and posteriorly by the dorsum sellae and petrous ridge. The posterior skull base extends from the dorsum sellae medially and petrous ridges laterally to the occiput posteriorly. **(Bottom)** 3D-VRT image of the osseous skull base from below highlights sphenoid bone with the foramen ovale and spinosum and occipital bone with its occipital condyle. Notice the frontal bone is not seen, but instead, maxillary, palatine, and zygomatic bones are present anteriorly.

Skull Base Overview

SAGITTAL BONE CT & T1 MR

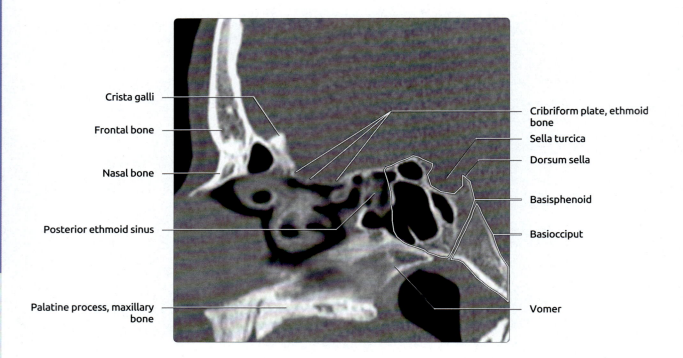

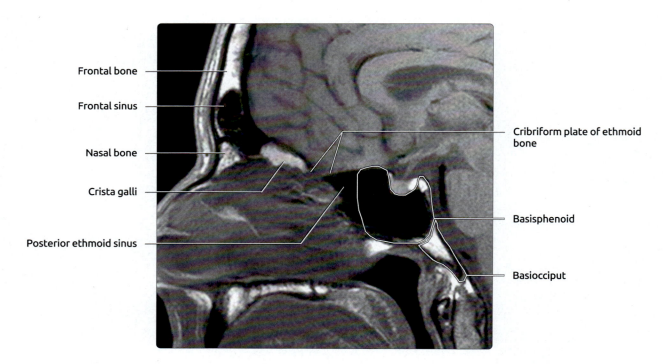

(Top) Paramedian sagittal bone CT through the anterior skull base shows the intimate relationship of the skull base to the paranasal sinuses. From anterior to posterior, note the frontal and nasal bones, crista galli, cribriform plate basisphenoid, and basiocciput. Notice that the sella is entirely embedded in the sphenoid bone. **(Bottom)** Paramedial sagittal T1 MR through the skull base shows the anterior, central, and posterior skull bases. The anterior skull base in this image is made up of the frontal bone, crista galli, and cribriform plate of ethmoid bone. The crista galli is high signal secondary to fatty marrow. The central skull base in the midline is often called the basisphenoid. It is made up of the sphenoid bone-sinus and cradles the pituitary gland. The sphenooccipital synchondrosis separates the basisphenoid from the basiocciput of the posterior skull base.

Skull Base Overview

AXIAL T1 MR

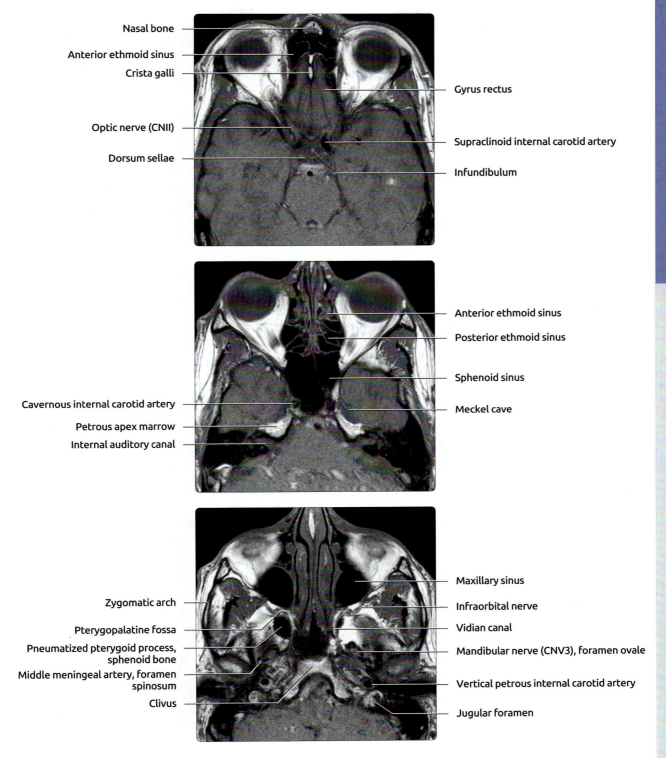

(Top) First of 3 axial T1 MR images through the skull base from superior to inferior shows the high-signal fatty marrow in the crista galli. Adjacent to this are gyri recti of the frontal lobes. *(Middle)* Image through the cavernous sinus reveals the ethmoid sinuses in the ethmoid bones of the anterior skull base and the sphenoid sinus in the sphenoid bone of the central skull base. The petrous apex fatty marrow is high signal with Meckel cave seen on its anterior margin. *(Bottom)* At the level of the pterygopalatine fossa, the infraorbital nerve can be seen exiting anterolaterally. The vidian canal, another sphenoid bone structure, is visible connecting to the medial pterygopalatine fossa. Middle meningeal artery and CNV3 are noted passing through the foramen spinosum and ovale, respectively. More posterolaterally, the carotid canal and jugular foramen can be seen.

Anterior Skull Base

TERMINOLOGY

Definitions

- Anterior skull base (ASB): Skull base anterior to lesser wing of sphenoid (LWS) and planum sphenoidale

IMAGING ANATOMY

Overview

- ASB is floor of anterior cranial fossa and roof of nose, ethmoid sinuses, and orbits
  - Forms broad, relatively flat floor of anterior cranial fossa that predominantly houses frontal lobes of brain
- Bones forming ASB
  - Ethmoid: Cribriform plate and ethmoid sinus roof centrally
  - Frontal: Orbital plate laterally
  - Sphenoid: Planum sphenoidale and lesser wing posteriorly
- Boundaries of ASB
  - Anterolaterally: Frontal bone
  - Posteriorly: LWS and planum sphenoidale
- Relationships of ASB
  - Superior: Frontal lobes, CNI
    - Inferior frontal lobe gyri include gyrus rectus medial to olfactory sulcus, medial orbital gyrus, anterior and posterior orbital gyri, and lateral orbital gyri
  - Inferior: Nasal vault and ethmoid sinus medially, orbit laterally
  - Anterior: Frontal sinuses
  - Posterior: Posterior margins of ASB critically associated with optic nerve canal, superior orbital fissure, and sella

Bony Landmarks of Anterior Skull Base

- **Frontal crest**: Anterior midline ridge between frontal bones; falx cerebri attaches here
- **Crista galli**: Midline upward triangular process of ethmoid bone; anteroinferior falx cerebri attaches here
  - Crista galli is pneumatized (contains mucosal lined air cell) in 10-15% of adults
  - Origin of pneumatization is extension of left or right frontal air cell, not ethmoid sinus
- **Cribriform plate (lamina cribrosa)**: Horizontal perforated bony plate of superomedial ethmoid
  - Forms part of nasal cavity roof
  - Forms floor of olfactory fossa (groove)
  - Shape and depth of olfactory fossa is variable and depends on length of lateral lamella of cribriform plate
    - Keros classification of olfactory fossa depth
      - Type I: < 3 mm
      - Type II: 4-7 mm
      - Type III: 8-16 mm
- **Ethmoid roof (fovea ethmoidalis)**: Horizontal or downward-sloping projection from medial margin of orbital plate
  - Ethmoid roof actually extension of orbital plate of frontal bone
  - Medially, roof fuses with lateral lamella of cribriform plate

- Ethmoid roof forms superior bony margin of ethmoid sinus air cells, separating ethmoid sinuses from anterior cranial fossa
  - Appearance asymmetric > 50% of time
- **Perpendicular plate of ethmoid**: Midline sagittally oriented bony plate that extends below level of cribriform plate and forms superior portion of bony nasal septum
  - Appears contiguous with crista galli above
  - Fuses with vomer by 2 years of age
- **Anterior clinoid process**: Medial aspect of LWS; free edge of tentorium cerebelli attaches here
  - Attaches to body of sphenoid by 2 roots
    - Superior root forms roof of optic canal and merges with planum sphenoidale
    - Inferior root is optic strut and forms lateral and inferior margin of optic canal
    - Variant: Posterior inferior root attaches to sphenoid bone, creating complete bony ring around cavernous internal carotid artery
- **LWS**: Forms sphenoid ridge; separates anterior from central skull base (CSB) forms superior boundary of optic nerve canal
  - Medially, LWS forms superior boundary of optic nerve canal
  - Laterally, LWS forms part of lateral superior margin of superior orbital fissure
- **Planum sphenoidale**: Superomedial plate of sphenoid bone, posterior to cribriform plate, anterior to tuberculum sellae
- **Chiasmatic sulcus (prechiasmatic sulcus)**: Horizontal groove or shelf of variable depth and width just dorsal and slightly inferior to posterior lip (limbus sphenoidale) of planum sphenoidale and just anterior to upper lip of tuberculum sella
  - Some authors would consider part of CSB

Foramina and Fissures of Anterior Skull Base

- **Foramen cecum**
  - Transmits: Variably transmits small emissary vein from nasal mucosa to superior sagittal sinus
  - Location: In margin between posterior aspect of frontal bone and anterior aspect of ethmoid
  - Relationships: Small midline pit found immediately anterior to crista galli
- **Anterior ethmoidal artery foramen, canal, and sulcus**
  - Transmits: Anterior ethmoidal artery, vein, nerve
    - Anterior ethmoidal artery arises from distal ophthalmic artery and passes anteromedially from orbit to olfactory fossa
      - Anterior ethmoidal artery foramen: Small funnel-shaped opening/notch along lamina papyracea of orbit
      - Anterior ethmoidal groove or canal: Small groove/channel through ethmoid sinus roof or sinus proper; connects anterior ethmoid foramen to ethmoid artery sulcus
      - Anterior ethmoidal artery sulcus: Small slit that opens along lateral lamella of olfactory groove, just lateral to cribriform plate
  - Location: Thin passageway between orbit to olfactory groove

Anterior Skull Base

- Relationships: Canal may pass through roof of ethmoid sinus or be "exposed," passing through anterior ethmoid sinus proper
  - If ethmoid artery canal passes through ethmoid sinus proper, it is vulnerable to injury during trauma or surgery
- **Posterior ethmoidal foramen, canal, and sulcus**
  - Transmits: Posterior ethmoidal artery, vein, nerve
  - Location: Passes from posterior orbit, through ethmoid roof, to lateral olfactory groove
  - Relationships: Medial sulcus just posterior to cribriform plate, at seam between cribriform plate and planum sphenoidale
- **Foramina of cribriform plate**
  - Transmits: Afferent fibers from nasal mucosa to olfactory bulbs (CNI)
  - Location: ~ 20 perforations within cephalad ethmoid bone plate
  - Relationships: Medial aspect of ethmoid, supports olfactory bulbs
- **Optic nerve canal**
  - Dural-lined canal through LWS
  - Transmits optic nerve and ophthalmic artery from intracranial compartment to orbital apex
  - Anterior root of lesser wing forms roof of optic nerve canal
  - Inferior root of lesser wing forms optic strut, variably pneumatized pillar that forms inferolateral border of optic nerve canal and separates canal from superior orbital fissure
- **Superior orbital fissure**
  - Oblong defect in posterior orbital apex that provides communication from orbit to cavernous sinus
  - Superior margin formed by LWS
  - Medial margin formed by optic strut
  - Inferior margin formed by greater wing of sphenoid
  - Transmits superior ophthalmic vein and nerves: Nasociliary, frontal, lacrimal, abducens, trochlear, superior and inferior branches of oculomotor

Development of Anterior Skull Base

- **Overview**
  - Skull base originates largely from cartilaginous precursors
    - Minimal contribution from membranous bone
  - > 100 ossification centers in skull base development
  - Ossifies posterior to anterior and lateral to medial
  - Ossification orderly and constant in first 2 years
    - Does not correspond to exact age, however
- **Birth**: ASB develops primarily from cartilage with limited ossification at birth
  - Early ethmoid air cells may be seen, but unossified crista galli is faint
- **1 month**: Ossification begins from ethmoidal labyrinth and turbinates; proceeds medially
- **3 months**: Roof of nasal cavity and tip of crista galli begin to ossify
  - Ethmoid air cells still inferior to cribriform plate
- **6 months**: Nasal roof well ossified; > 90% of infants have partial ossification nasal roof on every coronal CT image
  - Perpendicular plate of ethmoid begins to ossify

- Ethmoid sinus extends above cribriform plate plane
- **12 months**: Crista galli well ossified; > 70% have ossified posterior cribriform plate
- **18 months**: Ethmoid air cells now extend above plane of cribriform plate and orbital plates of frontal bones help form early fovea ethmoidalis
- **24 months**: Fovea ethmoidalis achieves more mature appearance; perpendicular plate of ethmoid begins to fuse with ossified vomer, most patients still have gap between nasal and ethmoid bones
- **> 24 months**
  - ASB nearly completely ossified; small gaps persist in nasal roof until early 3rd year
  - Foramen cecum ossifies as late as 5 years
  - Majority of cribriform plate and at least some of crista galli should be ossified

ANATOMY IMAGING ISSUES

Questions

- Pediatric
  - ASB ossification constant but variable in first 5 years
  - Understanding of normal development will avoid confusion or misdiagnoses
  - Anterior neuropore closes in 4th gestational week
- Adult: Understanding critical relationships to ASB necessary to fully evaluate region
  - Intracranial: Dura, inferior frontal lobe, olfactory bulb, tuberculum sella, cavernous sinus
  - Extracranial: Nasal vault, frontal, ethmoid, sphenoid sinuses, orbit and orbital apex, optic nerve canal, superior orbital fissure

Imaging Recommendations

- MR to search for anterior neuropore anomalies
- MR and CT complimentary in evaluation of ASB abnormalities

Imaging Approaches

- Bone CT viewed at wide windows (> 2,000 HU)
- Reformat at least 2 orthogonal planes
- High-resolution techniques necessary to evaluate microanatomy of ASB

Imaging Pitfalls

- Pediatric
  - Apparent small gaps in ASB under age 3 are normal
  - Do not confuse nonossified foramen cecum for anterior neuropore anomaly
- Adult
  - Beware: Fatty marrow in crista galli or ossified falx cerebri is not pathology

Anterior Skull Base

GRAPHICS

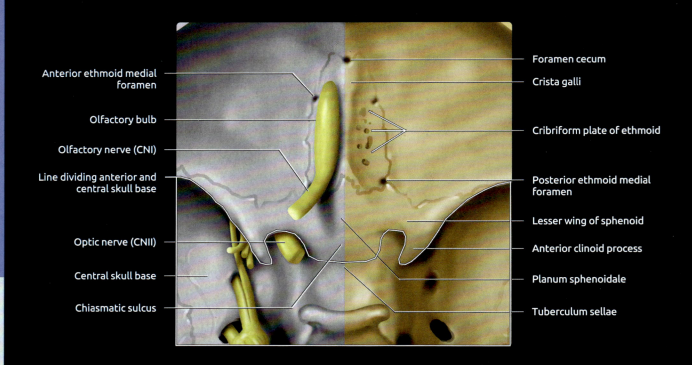

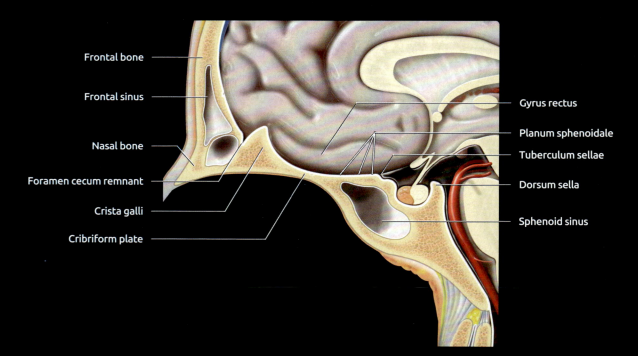

(Top) Graphic of the anterior skull base (ASB) seen from above shows olfactory bulb of CNI lying on the cribriform plate. Neural structures have been removed on the right, allowing visualization of numerous perforations in the cribriform plate, through which afferent fibers from olfactory mucosa pass to form the olfactory bulb. Note the foramen cecum, a small pit anterior to the crista galli, bounded anteriorly by the frontal bone, posteriorly by the ethmoid bone. The posterior margin of the ASB is formed by the lesser wing of sphenoid (LWS) and planum sphenoidale. (Bottom) Sagittal graphic of the ASB shows midline vertical crista galli. Anterior to the crista galli is the foramen cecum remnant, and posterolateral to the crista galli is the horizontal cribriform plate. The planum sphenoidale is the posteromedial ASB.

Anterior Skull Base

GRAPHICS

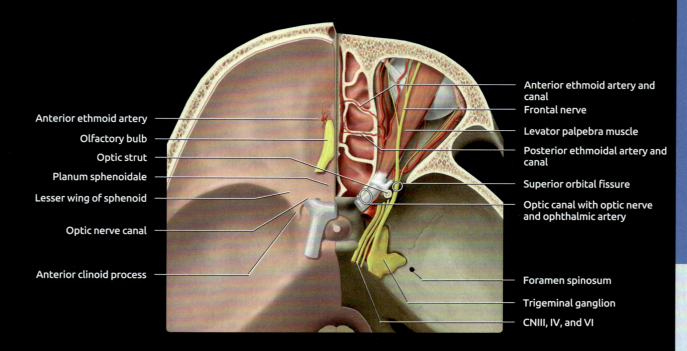

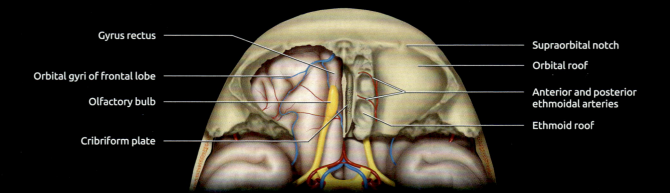

(Top) Graphic shows a partially dissected ASB. Notice the expansive dural covering that can give rise to meningiomas in a variety of anterior locations. On the right side, the cribriform plate, the ethmoid roof, orbital plate of the frontal bone, LWS, and anterior clinoid process have been resected. This exposes the ethmoid air cells, the superior orbit, the optic nerve canal, and the superior orbital fissure. The optic strut, often pneumatized, separates the optic nerve canal medially from the superior orbital fissure laterally. The cavernous sinus has also been dissected, exposing CNIII, IV, and VI. (Bottom) Graphic shows the anatomic relationships of the ASB from below. On the left side, there has been dissection of ASB, revealing the inferior frontal lobe (the orbital gyri), rectus gyrus, and the olfactory nerve. On the right side, the cribriform plate, roof of the ethmoid, and orbital roof are seen from below.

Anterior Skull Base

GRAPHICS

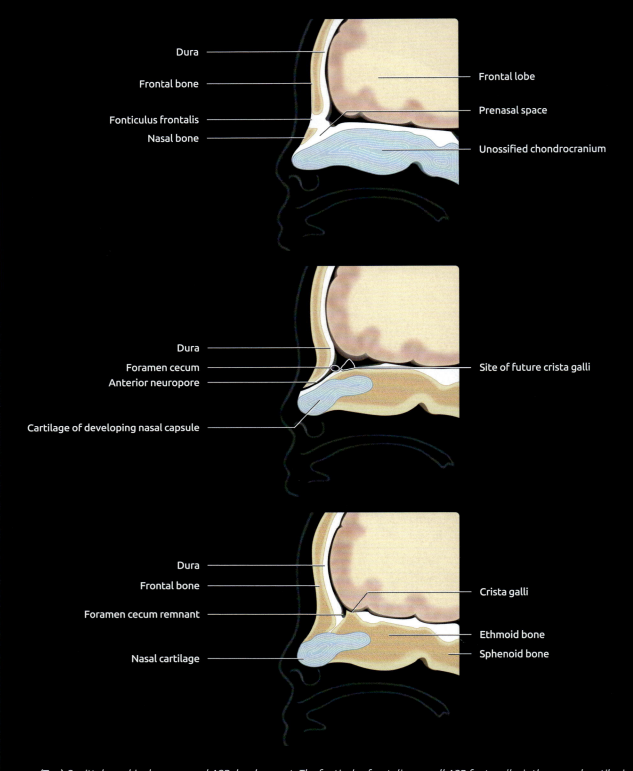

(Top) *Sagittal graphic shows normal ASB development. The fonticulus frontalis, a small ASB fontanelle, is the normal cartilaginous gap between developing, partially ossified frontal and nasal bones. The prenasal space is also present at this time as a dura-filled space between developing nasal bones and cartilage of developing nasal capsule. Both sites can become the location of a cephalocele.* **(Middle)** *Sagittal graphic shows the ASB slightly later in development. The fonticulus frontalis has closed and ossification of the chondrocranium has proceeded from posterior to anterior. The prenasal space is now encased in bone and becomes foramen cecum. A normal stalk of dura extends through foramen cecum to skin (anterior neuropore).* **(Bottom)** *Sagittal graphic shows the ASB even later in development. Anterior neuropore has regressed. Foramen cecum will completely fuse by age 5.*

Anterior Skull Base

AXIAL BONE CT

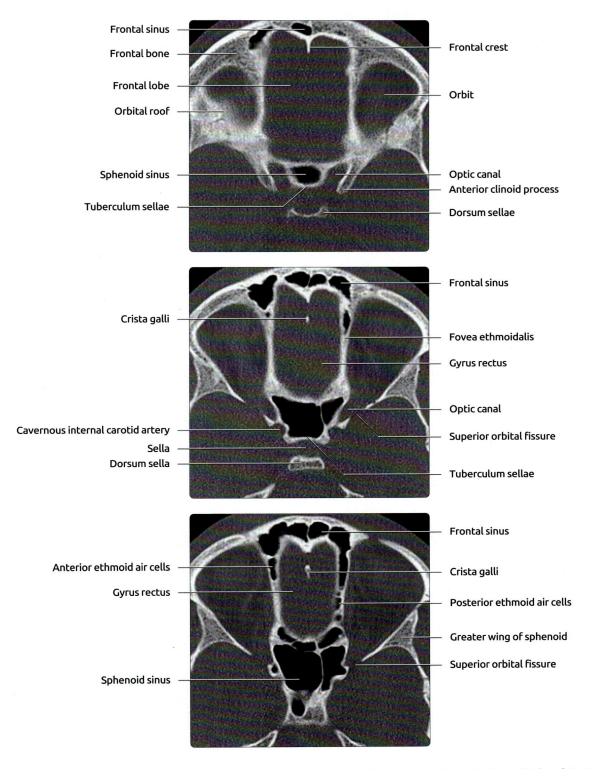

(Top) First of 9 axial bone CT images of the ASB from superior to inferior is shown. This image is at the level of the orbital roof. Notice that the medial aspect of the frontal lobes extend more inferior than the lateral aspect. On this image, the optic canal is seen passing medial to the anterior clinoid process, lateral to the sphenoid sinus. The optic canal is thin and can be obscured by volume-averaging. *(Middle)* More inferiorly, the cephalad tip of the crista galli is seen in the midline, where it and the frontal crest give attachment to the falx cerebri. The superior orbital fissure and optic canal are both visible. *(Bottom)* In this image, the frontal, anterior, and posterior ethmoid and sphenoid sinuses are all seen. Each sinus is named based on the bone in the skull base where it forms.

Anterior Skull Base

AXIAL BONE CT

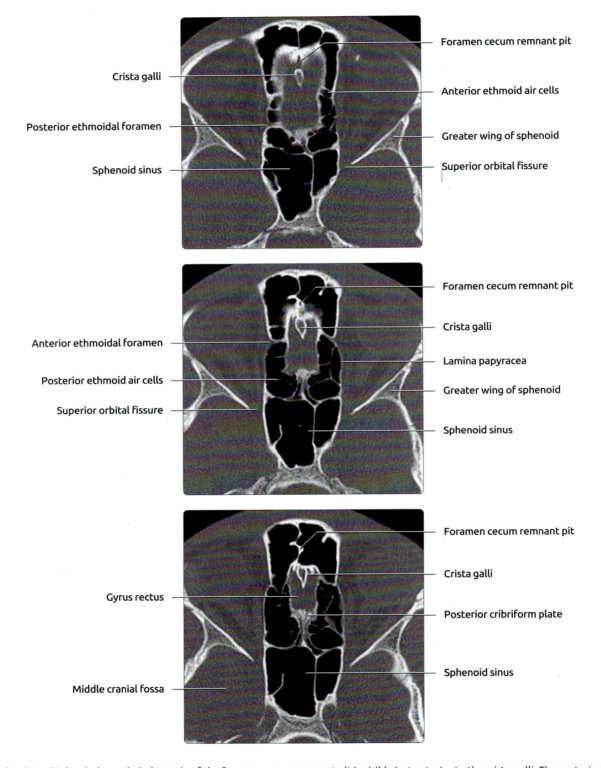

(Top) At this level, the cephalad margin of the foramen cecum remnant pit is visible just anterior to the crista galli. The posterior ethmoidal foramen can be identified at the posterior margin of the cribriform plate (not seen on this image). Although not seen, the olfactory bulb is nestled between the ethmoid sinuses and the crista galli. (Middle) In this image, the ethmoid air cells are laterally bounded by the lamina papyracea, the paper-thin medial wall of the orbit. The anterior ethmoidal foramen can also be seen bilaterally along the lateral wall of the ethmoid sinuses. This foramen contains the anterior ethmoidal artery, vein, and nerve. (Bottom) In this image, the posterior cribriform plate has come into view. Notice the cribriform plate is inferomedial to the ethmoid sinuses themselves.

Anterior Skull Base

AXIAL BONE CT

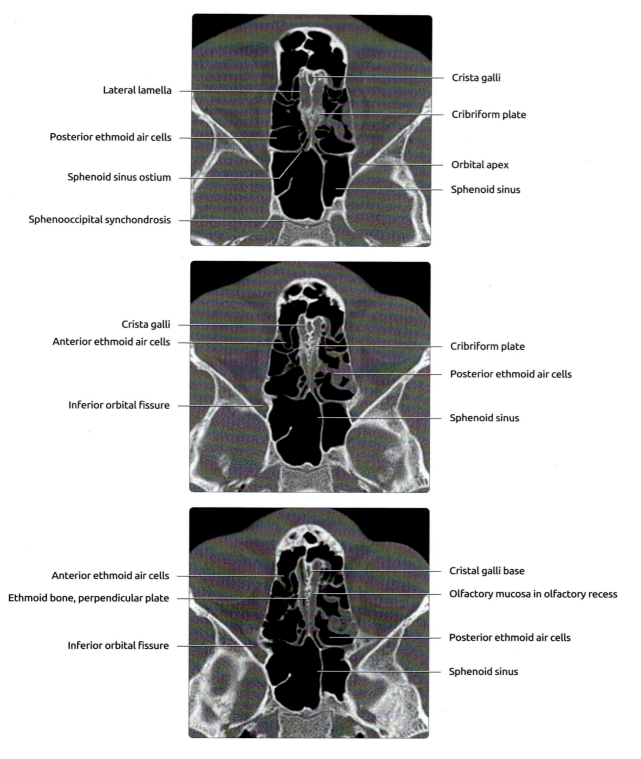

(Top) In this image through the cribriform plate, the perforated bone is visible. Notice the lateral lamella represents the vertical bony wall of the ethmoid sinus that projects inferiorly from the fovea ethmoidalis (ethmoid sinus roof) down to the cribriform plate. This is far better seen on coronal sinus CT. (Middle) The cribriform plate has a variable relationship to the roof of the ethmoid sinuses (fovea ethmoidalis). The more inferior to the fovea ethmoidalis the cribriform plate is found, the larger the dimension of the lateral lamella and the more easily a sinus surgery complication may occur. (Bottom) This image is just below the cribriform plate. The perpendicular plate of the ethmoid bone if visible as is the olfactory mucosa in the olfactory recess of the nasal cavity. The olfactory mucosa is the site of origin of esthesioneuroblastoma.

Anterior Skull Base

CORONAL BONE CT

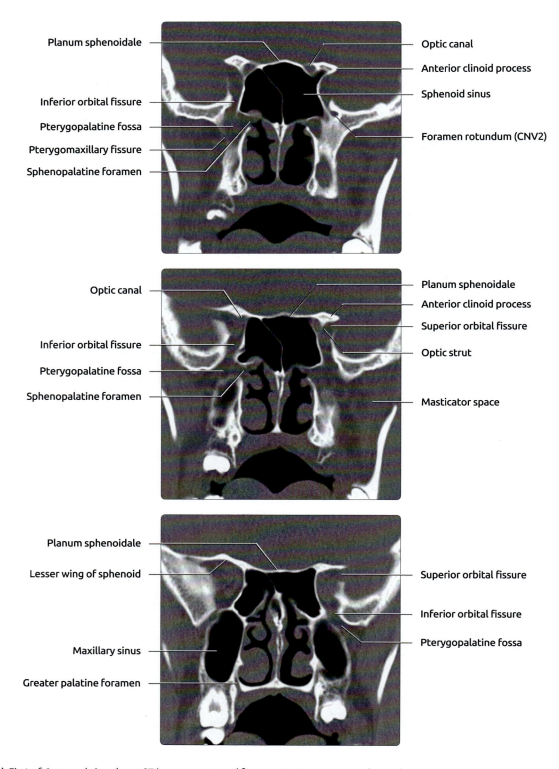

(Top) First of 6 coronal sinus bone CT images presented from posterior to anterior shows the transition from central to anterior skull base. Notice the optic canal medial to the anterior clinoid processes. The inferior orbital fissure is seen inferolateral to the optic canal. The planum sphenoidale is the posterior sphenoid sinus roof. (Middle) Inferior to planum sphenoidale and lateral to the sphenoid sinus is the complex anatomy of the orbital apex. The most superomedial structure of the orbital apex is the optic canal, divided from the superior orbital fissure by a small bony spur called the optic strut. The inferior orbital fissure communicates inferiorly with the pterygopalatine fossa. (Bottom) At the level of orbital apex, the LWS is visible as the posterior orbital roof. The planum sphenoidale is the anterior roof of the sphenoid bone.

Anterior Skull Base

CORONAL BONE CT

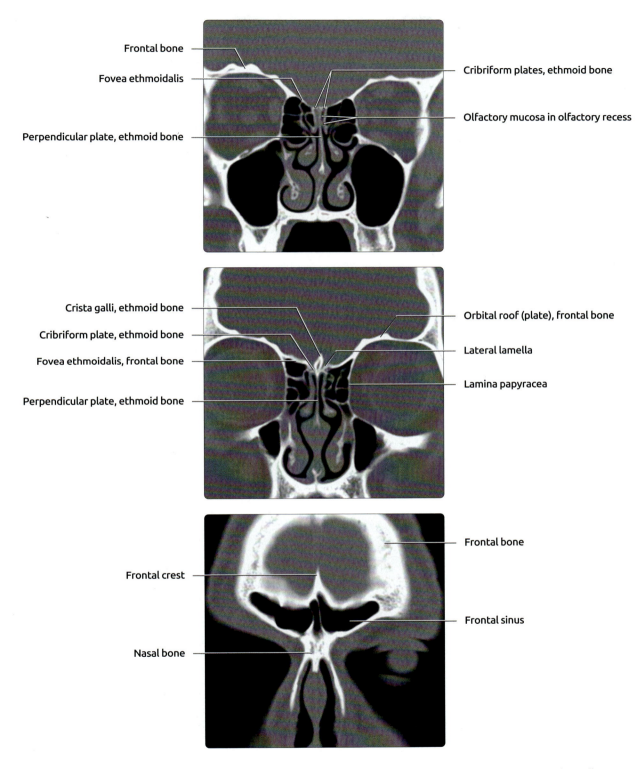

(Top) At the level of the posterior cribriform plate, the fovea ethmoidalis is seen sloping gradually toward the midline. In the midline, the cribriform plates themselves are visible. **(Middle)** At the level of the crista galli, it is possible to see the multiple pieces of the ethmoid bone. The crista galli is the most cephalad portion of the ethmoid bone, extending directly inferiorly into the perpendicular plate of the ethmoid bone. Just lateral to the base of the crista galli are the cribriform plates, lateral lamellae, and fovea ethmoidalis portions of the frontal bone. **(Bottom)** In this image through the frontal bone and sinus, note the anteroinferior nasal bone. Do not confuse the more anterosuperior frontal crest (part of frontal bones) with crista galli (part of ethmoid), not seen on this image.

Anterior Skull Base

AXIAL BONE CT, DEVELOPMENT

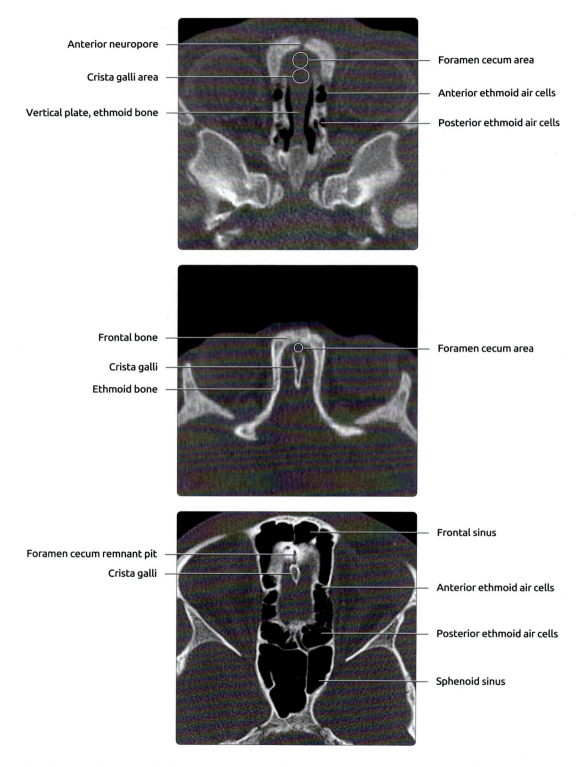

(Top) Axial bone CT through the ASB in a newborn is shown. The unossified gap between the nasal and frontal bones normally contains dura at this age and represents the regressing anterior neuropore. The area of the foramen cecum, crista galli, cribriform plate, and perpendicular plate of the ethmoid bone are all normally unossified in the newborn. (Middle) Axial bone CT through the ASB at 12 months is shown. The crista galli is now well-ossified. The foramen cecum area is still not ossified. The foramen cecum is still open, but the margins cannot be defined. (Bottom) Axial bone CT through the ASB in an adult is shown. The ethmoid air cells now extend far above the horizontal plane of the cribriform plate. The crista galli is thickened and heavily ossified. Although closed, the foramen cecum still demonstrates a small remnant pit.

Anterior Skull Base

CORONAL BONE CT, DEVELOPMENT

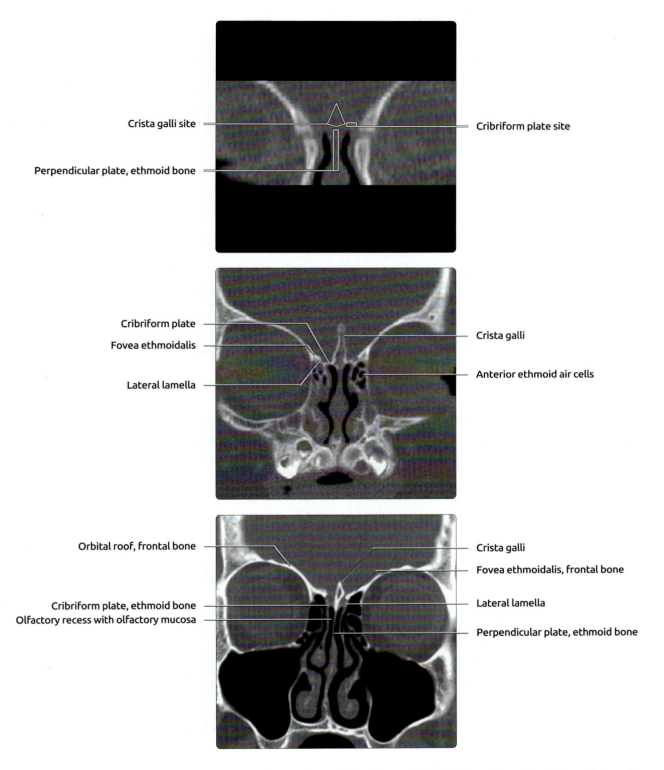

(Top) Coronal bone CT through the ASB in a newborn is shown. The ASB is largely unossified, including crista galli, cribriform plate, and perpendicular plate of ethmoid bone. There is a large gap between the orbital plates of frontal bones. Ethmoid air cells are not yet developed. (Middle) Coronal bone CT through the ASB at 12 months is shown. The ethmoid bone is now mostly ossified, particularly crista galli and posterior cribriform plate. Until 2-3 years of age, unossified gaps in anterior cribriform plate and foramen cecum (not shown) can be normal. Note developing lateral lamella and fovea ethmoidalis are small. (Bottom) Coronal bone CT through the ASB in an adult is shown. The ASB is completely ossified. Ethmoid air cells extend superolateral to plane of the cribriform plate. Fovea ethmoidalis is connected to the cribriform plate by lateral lamella.

CORONAL T2 MR, DEVELOPMENT

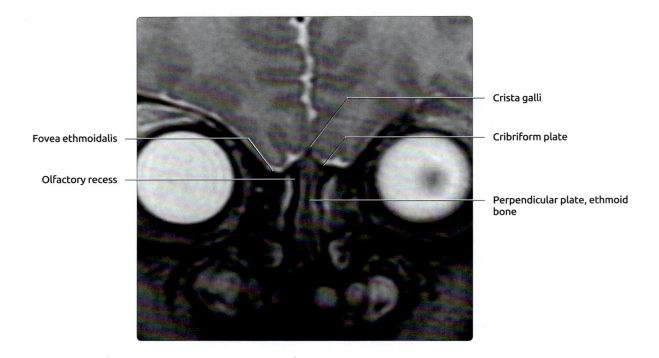

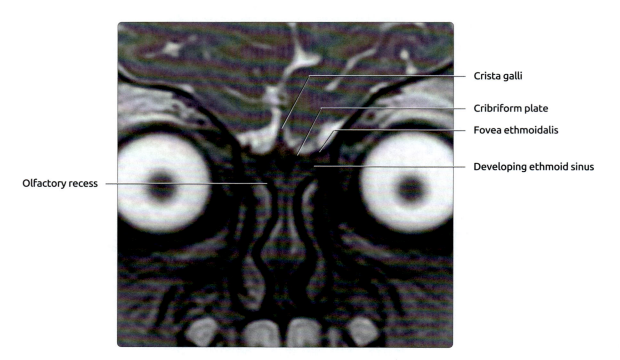

(Top) Coronal T2 MR through the ASB in a newborn is shown. The ASB is poorly ossified at birth. The cartilaginous crista galli and cribriform plate have intermediate signal intensity. (Bottom) Coronal T2 MR through the ASB at 6 months is shown. Notice the distance between the cribriform plate-fovea ethmoidalis and the olfactory recess of the nose is enlarging with the development of ethmoid sinuses.

Anterior Skull Base

CORONAL T2 MR, DEVELOPMENT

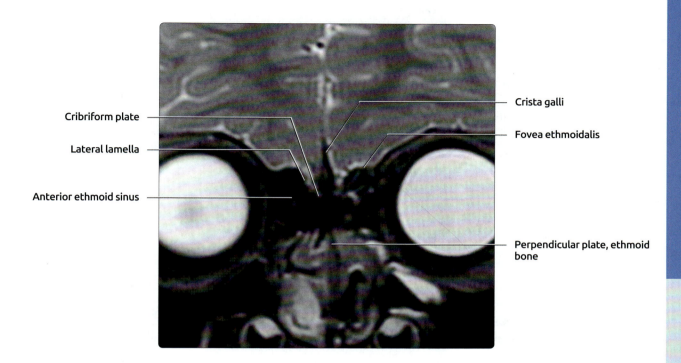

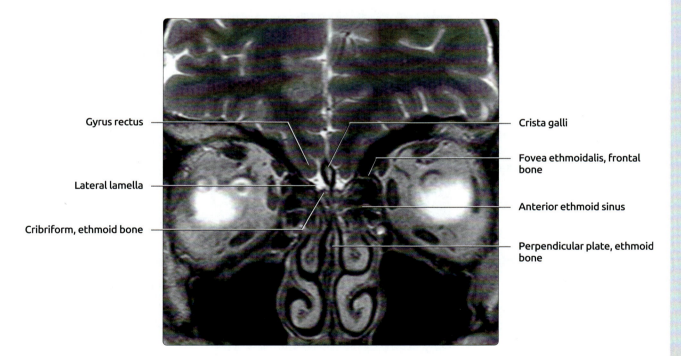

(Top) Coronal T2 MR through the ASB at 12 months is shown. The crista galli, cribriform plate, lateral lamella, and fovea ethmoidalis are largely ossified at this age. As a result, the ASB appears as low signal intensity form cortical bone. Notice the ethmoid sinus aeration now projects cephalad to the level of the crista galli base. The lateral lamella connects the fovea ethmoidalis to the lateral cribriform plate. (Bottom) Coronal T2 MR through the ASB in an adult is shown. By adulthood, there is a significant amount of high-signal fat in the well-ossified crista galli. Gyri recti appear to extend far more inferiorly than in childhood because the ethmoid air cells have enlarged superiorly.

Anterior Skull Base

SAGITTAL T1 MR, DEVELOPMENT

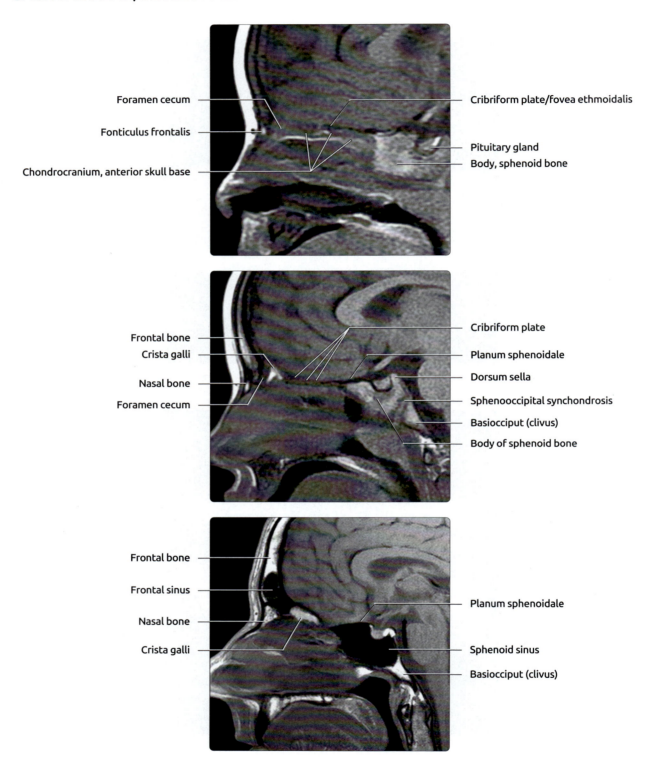

(Top) Sagittal T1 MR of the ASB at 6 months is shown. The area of cribriform plate/fovea ethmoidalis has begun to ossify, hence the low-signal line. Foramen cecum margins are difficult to discern as a result of absent ossification in the area. (Middle) Sagittal T1 MR of the ASB at 18 months is shown. There is rapid ossification of this area in the 1st year of life. Note high-signal fatty marrow in crista galli. Foramen cecum is visible anterior to the crista galli, normally containing a thin dural stalk that will obliterate by 5 years of age. (Bottom) Sagittal T1 MR of the ASB in an adult is shown. Crista galli is readily visible due to its fatty marrow. Foramen cecum is not seen because it is now fused. The frontal bone is distinguishable from the nasal bone anteriorly.

Anterior Skull Base

SAGITTAL T2 MR, DEVELOPMENT

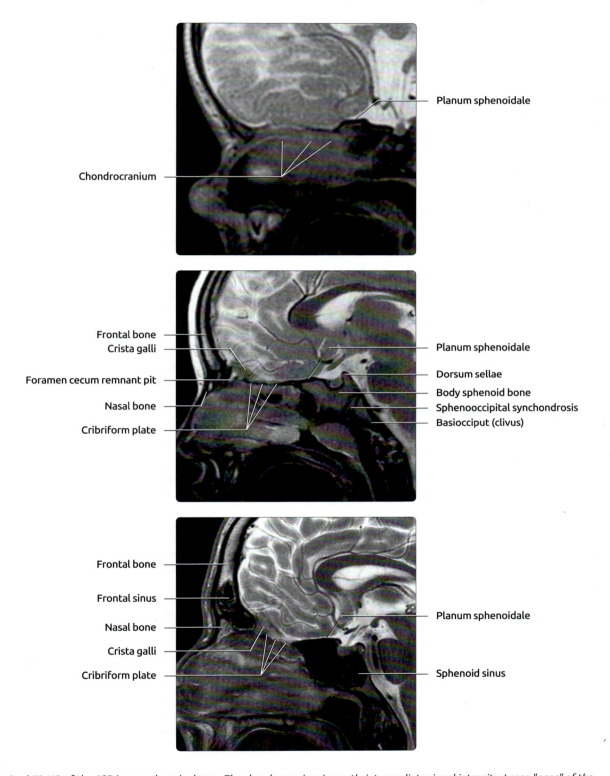

(Top) Sagittal T2 MR of the ASB in a newborn is shown. The chondrocranium is mostly intermediate signal intensity. Large "gaps" of the ASB are seen because there is little ossification, particularly anteriorly. (Middle) Sagittal T2 MR of the ASB at 18 months is shown. As ASB progressively ossifies, crista galli becomes more conspicuous. The frontal and sphenoid bones are higher signal due to fatty marrow. Both the sphenoid and frontal sinuses continue to pneumatize well into the teenage years. Cribriform plate ossification is signaled by a dark line anterior to the planum sphenoidale. (Bottom) Sagittal T2 MR of the ASB in an adult is shown. The crista galli is fully ossified and filled with high-signal fatty marrow. The foramen cecum is fused and therefore not visible. The sphenoid sinus is fully pneumatized.

Central Skull Base

TERMINOLOGY

Abbreviations
- Anterior, central, posterior skull base (ASB, CSB, PSB)
- Greater, lesser wings of sphenoid (GWS), (LWS)

Definitions
- CSB: Skull base posterior to LWS/planum sphenoidale & anterior to petrous ridge/dorsum sella

IMAGING ANATOMY

Overview
- CSB is floor of middle cranial fossa & roof of sphenoid sinus and GWS
- Bones forming CSB
  - Sphenoid bone, basisphenoid, & GWS
  - Temporal bone anterior to petrous ridge
- Boundaries of CSB
  - Anteriorly boundary: Planum sphenoidale posterior margin (limbus sphenoid) medially & LWS laterally
  - Posterior boundary: Dorsum sella medially & petrous ridges laterally
- Relationships of CSB
  - Superior: Pituitary, cavernous sinus, Meckel cave, CNI-IV, CNVI, CNV1-3, temporal lobe
  - Inferior: Anterior roof of pharyngeal mucosal space, masticator, parotid & parapharyngeal spaces

Bony Landmarks of Central Skull Base
- **Sella turcica**: Contains pituitary gland
- **Anterior clinoid processes**: Extend posteromedially off LWS
- **Posterior clinoid processes**: Extend posterolaterally off dorsum sellae; attachment for tentorium cerebelli
- **Chiasmatic sulcus**: Shallow groove between posterior margin of planum sphenoidale and tuberculum sella
- **Tuberculum sellae**: Anterosuperior margin of sella turcica

Foramina and Fissures of Central Skull Base
- **Optic canal**
  - Transmits: CNII with dura, arachnoid & pia, CSF & ophthalmic artery
  - Formed by LWS, superomedial to superior orbital fissure
- **SOF**
  - Transmits: CNIII, CNIV, CNV1, & CNVI, superior ophthalmic vein
  - Formed by cleft between LWS & GWS
- **Inferior orbital fissure**
  - Transmits: Infraorbital artery, vein, & nerve (CNV2)
  - Formed by cleft between body of maxilla & GWS
- **Carotid canal**
  - Transmits: Internal carotid artery & sympathetic plexus
  - Formed by GWS & temporal bone
- **Foramen rotundum**
  - Transmits: CNV2, artery of foramen rotundum, & emissary veins
  - Completely within sphenoid bone; superolateral to vidian canal
  - Provides direct connection to pterygopalatine fossa
- **Foramen ovale**
  - Transmits: CNV3, lesser petrosal nerve, accessory meningeal branch of maxillary artery, & emissary vein
  - Completely within GWS
  - Provides direct connection to masticator space
- **Foramen spinosum**
  - Transmits: Middle meningeal artery & vein, meningeal branch of CNV3
  - Within GWS, posterolateral to foramen ovale
- **Foramen lacerum**
  - Not true foramen
  - Between temporal & sphenoid bones
  - Cartilaginous floor of medial part of horizontal petrous internal carotid artery canal
- **Vidian canal**
  - Transmits: Vidian artery and nerve
  - Formed by sphenoid bone, inferomedial to foramen rotundum

Development of Central Skull Base
- CSB formed by > 25 ossification centers
- Ossification occurs from posterior to anterior
- **Important ossification centers**: Orbitosphenoids, alisphenoids, pre- and postsphenoid, basiocciput
  - **Orbitosphenoids** → LWS, **alisphenoids** → GWS
  - **Presphenoid** and **postsphenoid** fuse at ~ 3 months
  - **Postsphenoid** and **basiocciput** fuse → clivus
- **Sphenooccipital synchondrosis**
  - Between postsphenoid and basiocciput
  - Responsible for most of postnatal skull base growth
  - One of last sutures of skull base to fuse
  - Open until 14 years, fuses by ~ 16 years in girls & ~ 18 years in boys

Variant Anatomy
- **Persistent craniopharyngeal canal**
  - Remnant of Rathke pouch
  - Vertical cleft in sphenoid body at site of fusion of pre- & postsphenoid; just posterior to tuberculum sellae area in adult
  - Extends from sella turcica to nasopharynx
- **Extensive pneumatization of sphenoid sinus**
  - Can cause endosinal vidian canals & foramen rotundum
  - Pneumatized clinoid processes
- **Canaliculus innominatus**
  - Variant canal for lesser superficial petrosal nerve, medial to foramen spinosum
- **Foramen of Vesalius**
  - Transmits emissary vein from cavernous sinus to pterygoid plexus
  - Anterior to foramen ovale

ANATOMY IMAGING ISSUES

Imaging Pitfalls
- Beware sphenoid MR signal changes
  - Sphenoid sinus: Low-signal cartilage until 2 years → high-signal fat until 6 years → low-signal air (adult)
  - Clivus low signal until 25 years, then high-signal fat
- Do not confuse pneumatized clinoid processes with vascular flow voids on MR

Central Skull Base

GRAPHICS

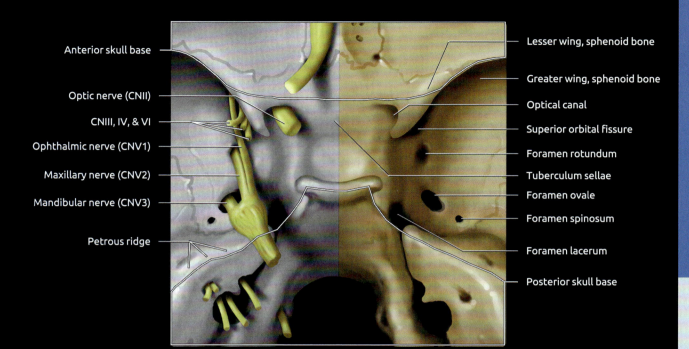

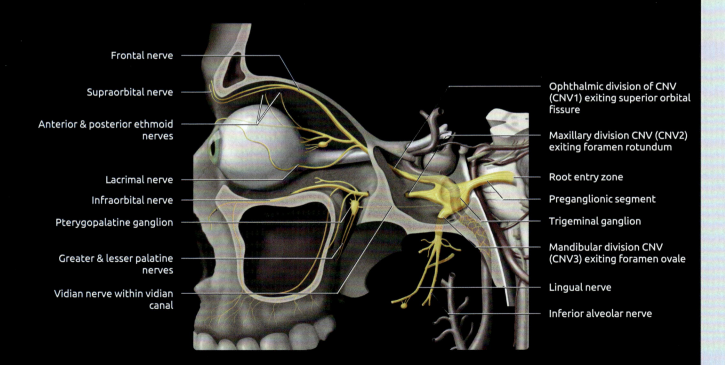

(Top) Graphic of the central skull base (CSB) from above shows important nerves on the left. The numerous fissures & foramina of CSB are shown on the right. Greater wing of sphenoid forms anterior wall of middle cranial fossa. The posterior limit of the CSB is the dorsum sella medially & petrous ridge laterally. *(Bottom)* Sagittal graphic through the central & anterior skull base depicts the trigeminal nerve branches & exiting foramina. Ophthalmic division of CNV exits into orbit via the superior orbital fissure. Maxillary division of CNV exits via foramen rotundum to become infraorbital nerve as well as drop the greater & lesser palatine nerves inferiorly to provide sensation for the hard & soft palates. Mandibular division of CNV exits through foramen ovale, then divides into 2 main trunks, lingual & inferior alveolar nerves. Note the vidian nerve in vidian canal.

Central Skull Base

GRAPHICS

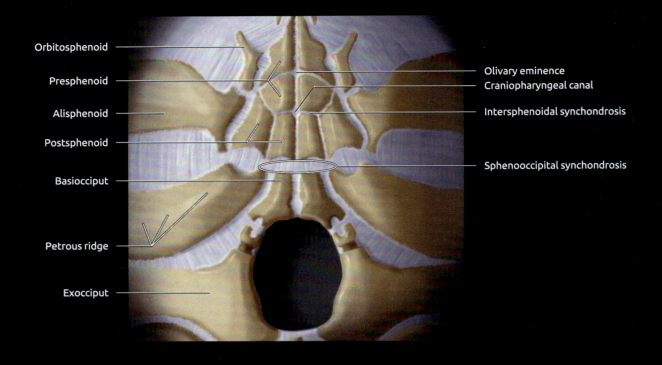

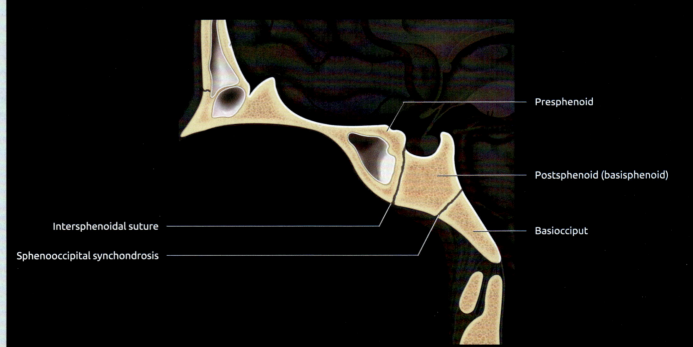

(Top) Graphic of CSB from above shows its many ossification centers. Between the ossification centers of presphenoid is a cartilaginous gap called the olivary eminence, which is obliterated shortly after birth. A persistent cleft, called the craniopharyngeal canal, can also be variably seen in intersphenoid synchondrosis. Do not confuse these variants with pathology. (Bottom) Lateral graphic of CSB shows major ossification centers & the location of sutures. Intersphenoidal suture closes at ~ 3 months age. At about 2 years of age, the presphenoid begins to demineralize & become pneumatized. Pneumatization progresses posteriorly into postsphenoid until ~ age 5-7. Sphenooccipital synchondrosis is one of the last sutures to fuse at ~ age 16. It is the suture most responsible for growth of the skull base.

Central Skull Base

AXIAL BONE CT

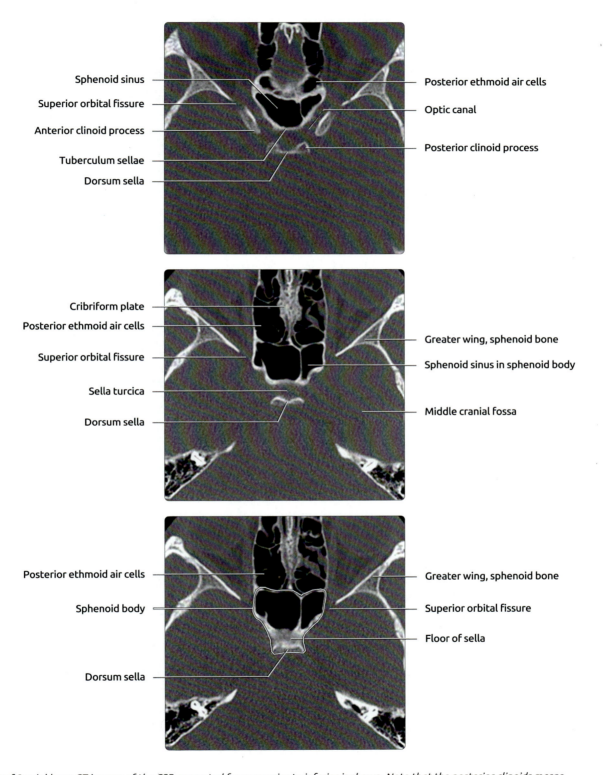

(Top) First of 9 axial bone CT images of the CSB presented from superior to inferior is shown. Note that the posterior clinoids merge with the dorsum sella. The optic canal is bound by the sphenoid sinus medially and the anterior clinoid process laterally. Inferolateral to optic canal is the superior orbital fissure. (Middle) At the level of sella turcica, the superior orbital fissure is seen as the medial opening of the orbit into the middle cranial fossa. It lies below the optic canal, between the greater wing of the sphenoid and the sphenoid sinus. The sella turcica is bound by the dorsum sella posteriorly. (Bottom) In this image, the body of the sphenoid bone is seen to be made up of the sphenoid sinus, sella turcica, and dorsum sella. Anterior to the sphenoid bone is the ethmoid bone.

Central Skull Base

AXIAL BONE CT

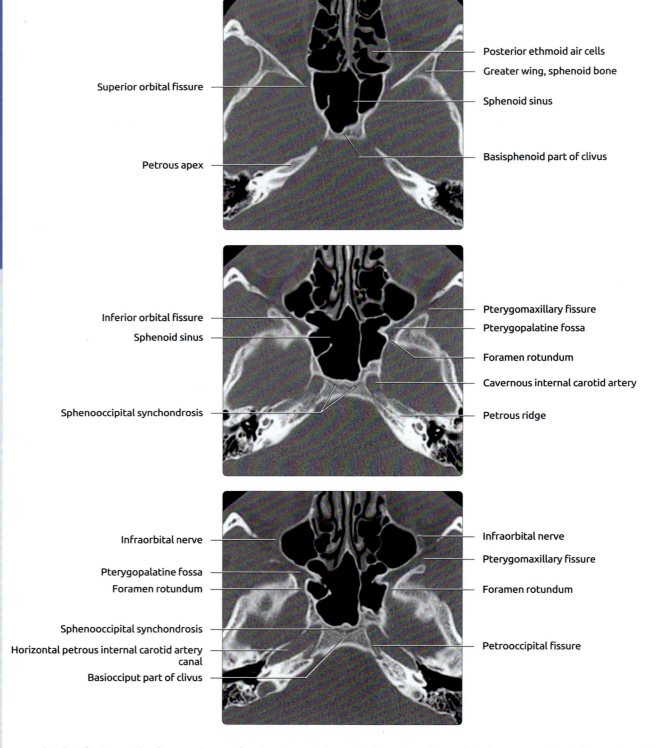

(Top) In this image, the clivus can be seen forming the medial posterior boundary of CSB, while the petrous ridge defines its lateral margin. (Middle) This image shows pneumatization of the sphenoid extending up to the sphenooccipital synchondrosis, which is partly unfused in this young adult. Note the foramen rotundum empties anteriorly into the pterygopalatine fossa, which connects laterally with the masticator space through the pterygomaxillary fissure. (Bottom) At the level of the foramen rotundum, both pterygopalatine fossae are clearly visible. The maxillary division of trigeminal nerve (CNV2) exits the skull base through the foramen rotundum & continues as infraorbital nerve into orbit via inferior orbital fissure. Malignant tumors of the skin of the cheek, orbit, & sinonasal area may all use CNV2 as a perineural route to gain intracranial access.

Central Skull Base

AXIAL BONE CT

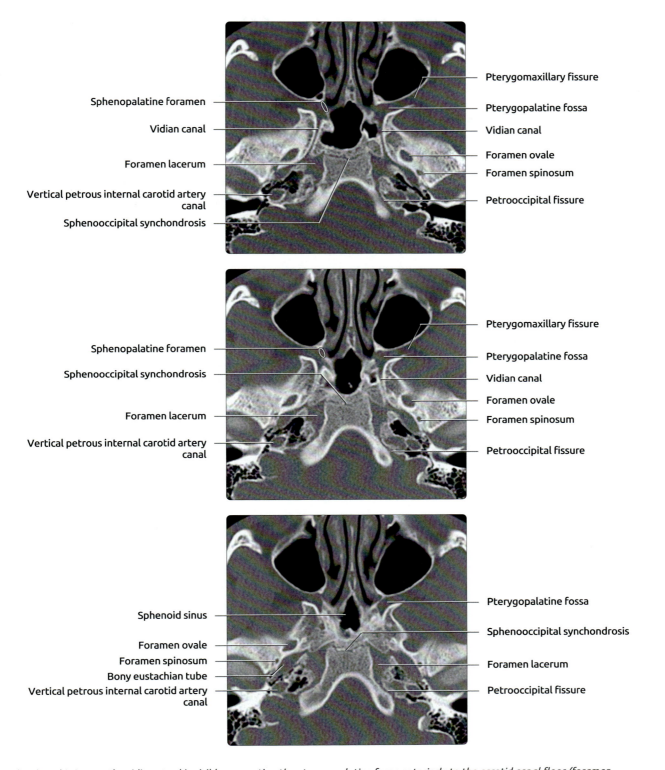

(Top) In this image, the vidian canal is visible connecting the pterygopalatine fossa anteriorly to the carotid canal floor (foramen lacerum) posteriorly. A malignant tumor that has accessed the pterygopalatine fossa may reach the carotid canal of the skull base via perineural spread on the vidian nerve in the vidian canal. There is a medial connection between the pterygopalatine fossa & nose, the sphenopalatine foramen. Juvenile angiofibroma begins along the nasal margin of this foramen. (Middle) In this image, note that the foramen ovale is located in the greater wing of the sphenoid bone. Extracranial perineural malignancy on CNV3 enters the intracranial area via the foramen ovale. (Bottom) In this image, note the foramen spinosum is posterolateral to the foramen ovale in the greater wing of the sphenoid bone. The middle meningeal artery passes intracranially via the foramen spinosum.

Central Skull Base

CORONAL BONE CT

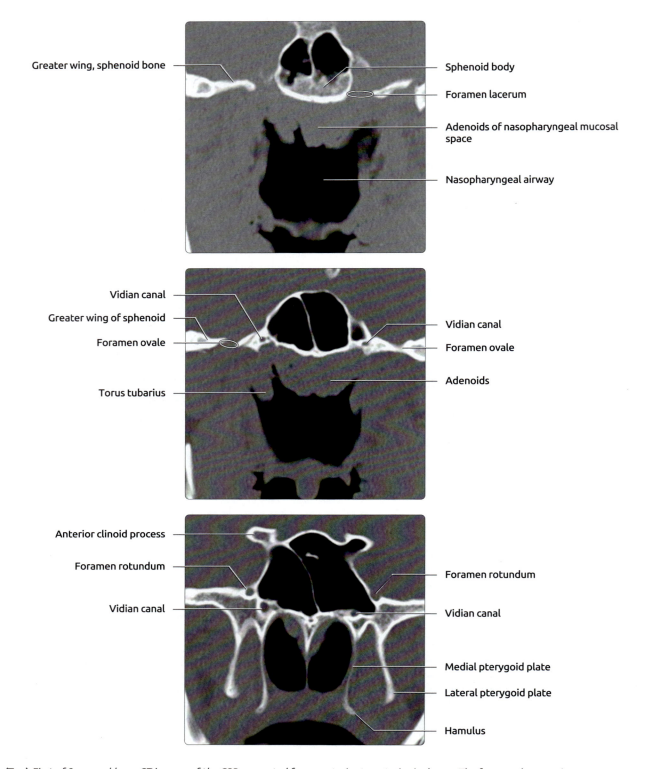

(Top) First of 3 coronal bone CT images of the CSB presented from posterior to anterior is shown. The foramen lacerum is seen as a large defect between the greater wing of the sphenoid bone and the sphenoid body. The foramen lacerum is not a true foramen, it represents the cartilaginous floor of the anteromedial horizontal segment of the petrous internal carotid artery canal. (Middle) In this image, the foramen ovale is evident lateral to the vidian canal and anterolateral to the foramen lacerum. It transmits CNV3 from the middle cranial fossa to the masticator space. (Bottom) More anteriorly, the foramen rotundum and vidian canal are both seen running in the transverse plane. Both the foramen rotundum and vidian canal open into the pterygopalatine fossa. Also note the pterygoid plates inferiorly.

Central Skull Base

AXIAL T1 C+ MR

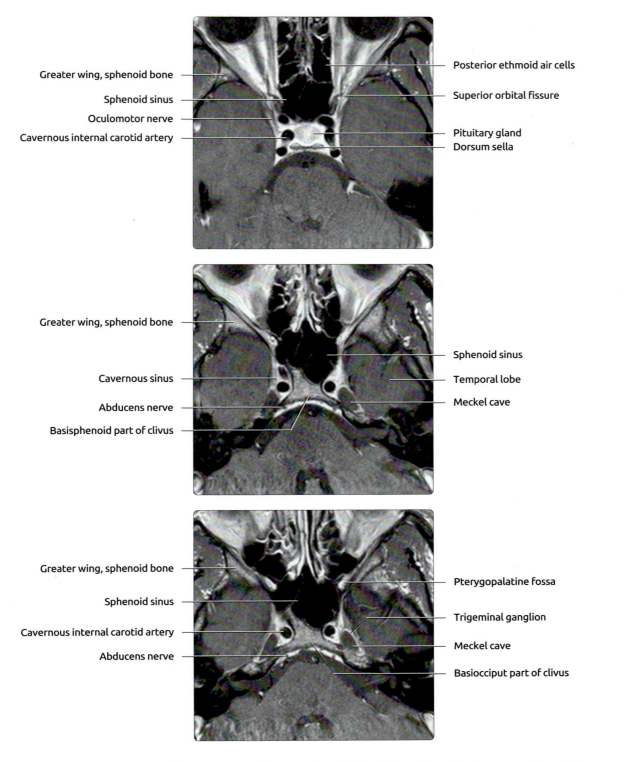

(Top) First of 6 axial T1 C+ MR images of the CSB presented from superior to inferior is shown. The enhancing venous plexus of the cavernous sinus is seen surrounding the cavernous internal carotid artery. Medially, the enhancing pituitary gland in the sella turcica is bound by the dorsum sella posteriorly and the sphenoid sinus anteriorly. *(Middle)* In this image, the upper basisphenoid part of the clivus is seen. Cerebrospinal fluid-filled Meckel cave is seen along the posterior border of the cavernous sinus. *(Bottom)* In this image, the basiocciput part of the clivus is visible. The upper clivus above the fused sphenooccipital synchondrosis is part of the sphenoid bone, while the lower clivus is part of the occipital bone. Notice the marrow space of the clivus enhances.

Central Skull Base

AXIAL T1 C+ MR

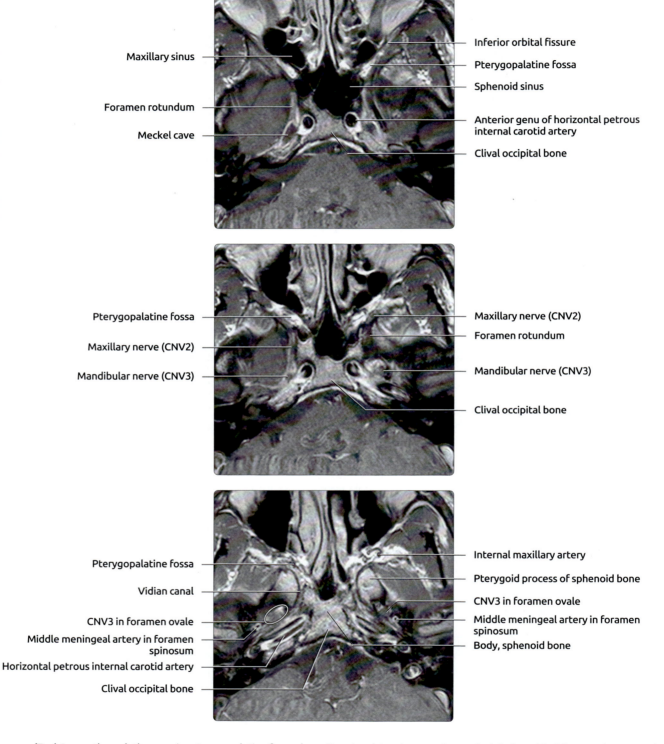

(Top) Image through the superior pterygopalatine fossa shows its anterolateral connection to the inferior orbital fissure. The anteriorly projecting foramen rotundum can also be seen. The sphenoid bone is partially pneumatized (sphenoid sinus). **(Middle)** In this image, the maxillary nerve (CNV2) is seen as a linear low-intensity structure in the foramen rotundum on the right. On the left, this same nerve can be seen exiting the foramen rotundum into the pterygopalatine fossa. **(Bottom)** At the level of the foramen ovale, the mandibular nerve (CNV3) is seen bilaterally. Also note the middle meningeal artery passing through the foramen spinosum. The vidian canal is clearly visible medial to the foramen ovale. The clival occipital bone should be distinguished from the body of the sphenoid bone even though the sphenooccipital fissure cannot be discerned.

Central Skull Base

SAGITTAL T1 & T2 MR, DEVELOPMENT

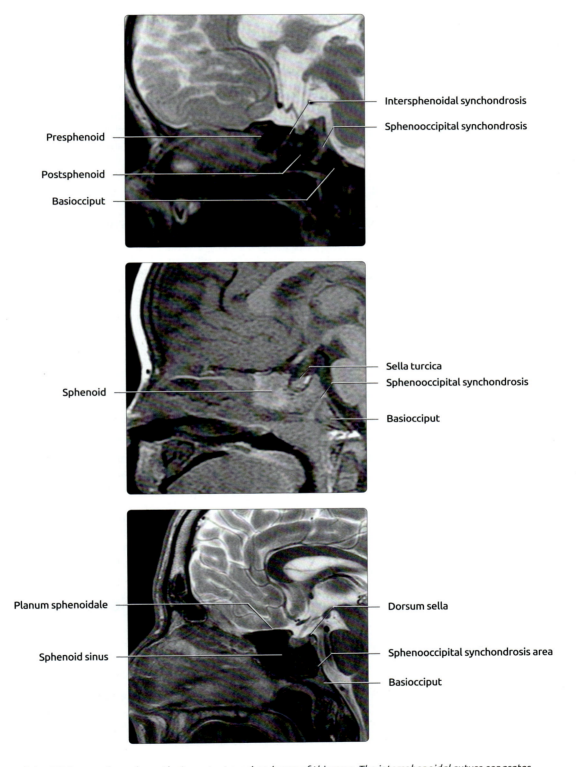

(Top) Sagittal T2 MR of the CSB in a newborn shows the important synchondroses of this area. The intersphenoidal suture separates presphenoid from postsphenoid while the sphenooccipital synchondrosis separates postsphenoid from basiocciput. (Middle) Sagittal T1 MR shows the CSB at 6 months. The intersphenoidal suture closes at ~ 3 months of age, resulting in formation of the sphenoid body from the presphenoid and postsphenoid. There is normal high-signal fat within what used to be presphenoid. The sphenooccipital synchondrosis will remain open until adolescence. (Bottom) Sagittal T2 MR shows the CSB in an adult. Typically, pneumatization extends throughout the entire sphenoid body up to the fused sphenooccipital synchondrosis. The sphenooccipital synchondrosis is one of last sutures of the skull base to close. It fuses completely by ~ 16-18 years of age.

Posterior Skull Base

TERMINOLOGY

Abbreviations
- Posterior skull base (PSB)

Definitions
- Skull base (SB) posterior to dorsum sella and petrous ridges

IMAGING ANATOMY

Overview
- PSB is made up of posterior temporal bones and occipital bone and transmits CNVII-XII, medulla oblongata, and jugular vein
- Bones of PSB
  - Temporal bones posterior to petrous ridges
  - **Occipital bone** (3 parts)
    - **Basilar part** (basiocciput): Quadrilateral part anterior to foramen magnum
    - **Condylar part** (exoccipital): Occipital condyles here; lateral to foramen magnum
    - **Squamous part**: Large bony plate posterosuperior to foramen magnum
- Boundaries of PSB
  - Anterior boundary: Dorsum sella medially and petrous ridges laterally
  - Posterior boundary: Occipital bone
- Relationships of PSB
  - Inferior relationships: Posterior roof of pharyngeal mucosal space, carotid, parotid, retropharyngeal, perivertebral spaces, and cervical spine
  - Superior relationships: Brainstem, cerebellum, CNVII-VIII, CNIX-XII, transverse-sigmoid sinuses

Bony Landmarks of Posterior Skull Base
- **Petrous ridge of temporal bone**
  - Divides central skull base from PSB
  - Attachment for fixed edge of tentorium cerebelli
- **Jugular tubercle**
  - Roof of hypoglossal canal seen well on coronal imaging
  - "Eagle's head" on coronal images is jugular tubercle

Foramina and Fissures of Posterior Skull Base
- **Internal acoustic meatus**
  - Transmits: CNVII-VIII, labyrinthine artery
  - Opening in posterior wall temporal bone superior to jugular foramen
  - Porus acusticus: Internal opening of internal acoustic meatus
- **Jugular foramen**
  - 2 parts: Pars nervosa and pars vascularis partially divided by jugular spine
  - Between temporal and occipital bones
  - Carotid space extends directly up to jugular foramen
  - **Pars nervosa**
    - Transmits CNIX, Jacobson nerve, and inferior petrosal sinus
    - Anteromedial but contiguous with pars vascularis
  - **Pars vascularis**
    - Transmits CNX, Arnold nerve, CNXI, jugular bulb, and posterior meningeal artery
    - Larger than pars nervosa

- **Groove for sigmoid sinus**
  - Groove in medial mastoid temporal bone; cradles sigmoid sinus
- **Hypoglossal canal**
  - Transmits: CNXII
  - Formed in condylar occipital bone
  - Inferomedial to jugular foramen
- **Foramen magnum**
  - Transmits: CNXI (cephalad component), vertebral arteries, and medulla oblongata
  - Formed completely by occipital bone
- **Stylomastoid foramen**
  - Transmits: CNVII
  - Found in exocranial SB surface between mastoid tip and styloid process
  - Extends directly into parotid space

Development of Posterior Skull Base
- Occipital bone has 4 major ossification centers around foramen magnum
  - **Supraoccipital, basioccipital**, and paired **exoccipital**
- PSB is nearly completely ossified by birth
- **Sutures of PSB** remain unfused until 2nd decade
  - Intraoccipital sutures fuses between 8 and 16 years
  - Petrooccipital and occipitomastoid sutures are among last to close (15-17 years)
- **Kerckring ossicle**
  - Small ovoid ossicle at posterior margin of foramen magnum
  - Unfused and separate in 50% of term newborns
  - Kerckring-supraoccipital suture fuses by 1 year

Variant Anatomy of Posterior Skull Base
- **Posterior condylar canal**
  - Inconstant canal for emissary vein and meningeal branch of ascending pharyngeal artery
  - One of largest emissary foramina of SB
- **Asymmetric petrous apices**
  - Can contain high-signal fat or low-signal air
- **Mastoid foramen**
  - Variably transmits emissary vein from sigmoid sinus
- **Persistent Kerckring ossicle**

ANATOMY IMAGING ISSUES

Questions
- PSB is largely ossified at birth but PSB sutures are last in SB to fuse
- PSB is intimately related to carotid and parotid spaces

Imaging Recommendations
- Bone CT with edge enhancement algorithm and wide windows (> 2,000 HU)
- Use coronal imaging to examine normal "double eagles" of hypoglossal canal and jugular foramen area

Imaging Pitfalls
- Watch for asymmetric petrous apex air &/or fat
- Beware of jugular foramen pseudolesion from MR flow phenomenon
- Beware of open synchondroses/suture as pseudofracture

Posterior Skull Base

GRAPHICS

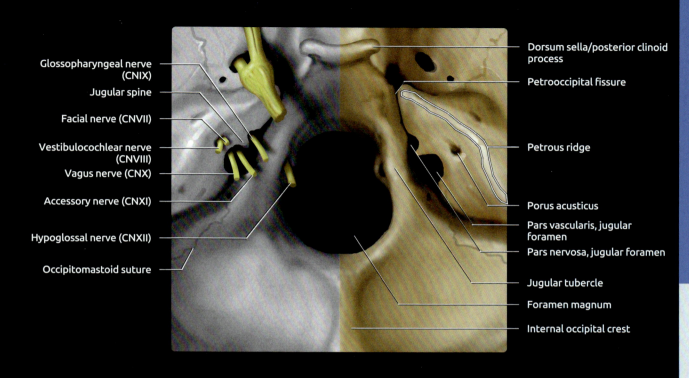

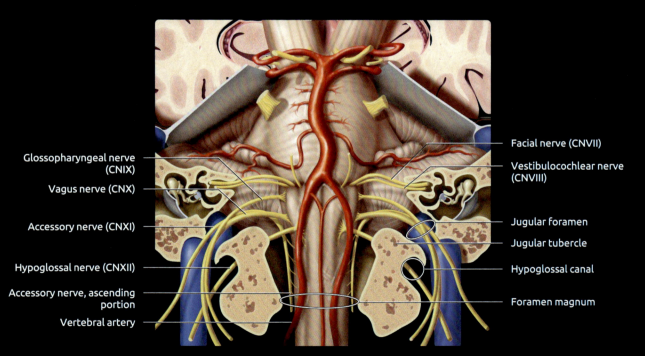

(Top) Graphic of posterior skull base as seen from above is shown. Neural structures are shown on the left, and bony landmarks are shown on the right. Anterior boundary of posterior skull base is clivus medially and petrous ridge laterally. The major foramina are the foramen magnum, porus acusticus, jugular foramen, and hypoglossal canal. Notice that the jugular foramen connects anteriorly with the petrooccipital fissure. *(Bottom)* Coronal graphic of posterior skull base viewed from the front shows the classic double eagle appearance in the area of the hypoglossal canal. The jugular tubercle (eagle's head and beak) separates the inferomedial hypoglossal canal from the jugular foramen. The hypoglossal nerve is found in the hypoglossal canal while CNIX-XI traverse the skull base in the jugular foramen.

Posterior Skull Base

GRAPHIC AND MR VENOGRAM

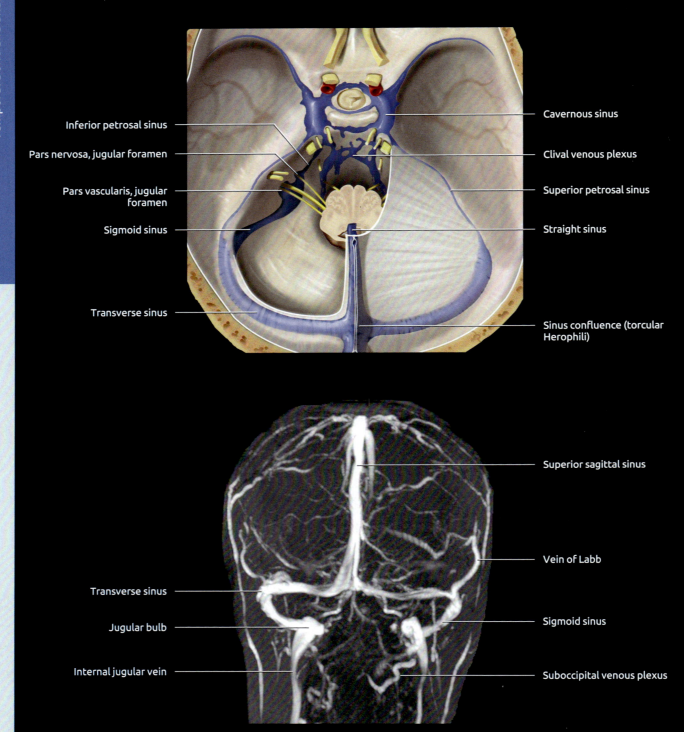

(Top) Graphic shows major dural venous sinuses and jugular foramen from the top down. The midbrain and pons as well as the left 1/2 of the tentorium cerebelli have been removed. Notice the transverse sinus is in the wall of the occipital bone while the sigmoid sinus is in the medial wall of the temporal bone. The 2 portions of the jugular foramen are also visible. The anterior pars nervosa receives the glossopharyngeal nerve (CNIX) while the pars vascularis has the vagus (CNX) and accessory (CNXI) nerves passing through it. (Bottom) Coronal view of MR venogram shows the transverse sinuses feeding through the sigmoid sinuses into the jugular foramen. The jugular bulb connects inferiorly with the internal jugular vein of the carotid space. The slight asymmetry of transverse sinuses is normal.

Posterior Skull Base

AXIAL BONE CT

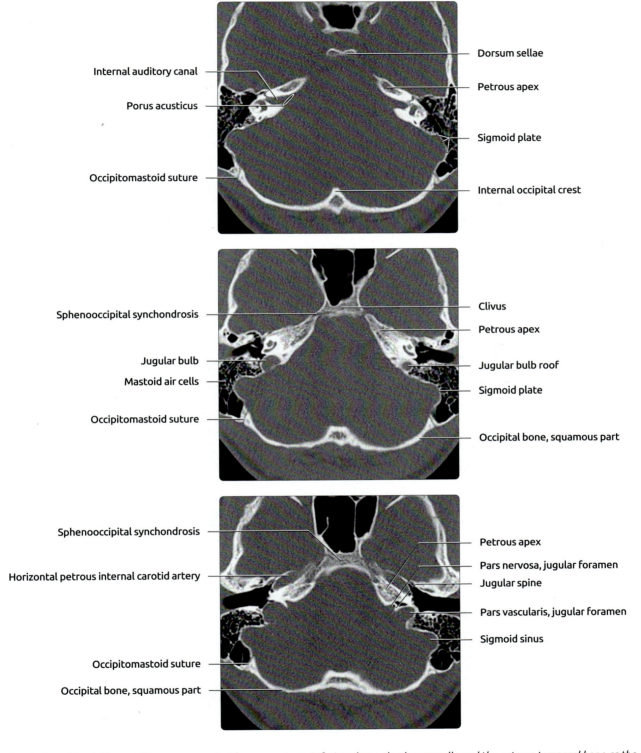

(Top) First of 9 axial bone CT images, presented from superior to inferior, shows the dorsum sella and the petrous temporal bone as the anterior margin of the posterior skull base. Posteriorly, the midline is demarcated by the bony internal occipital crest, which provides attachment for the falx cerebelli. Porus acusticus is the most superior foramen of the posterior skull base and transmits CNVII and CNVIII. (Middle) At the level of the midcochlea, the posterior cranial fossa is completely divided from middle cranial fossa by the clivus and petrous temporal bone. Laterally, the sigmoid plate separates the mastoid air cells from the sigmoid sinus. The jugular bulbs are visible bilaterally. (Bottom) At the level of the midjugular foramen, note smaller anteromedial pars nervosa (CNIX, Jacobsen nerve, inferior petrosal sinus) and larger pars vascularis (jugular bulb, Arnold nerve, CNX, and CNXI).

Posterior Skull Base

AXIAL BONE CT

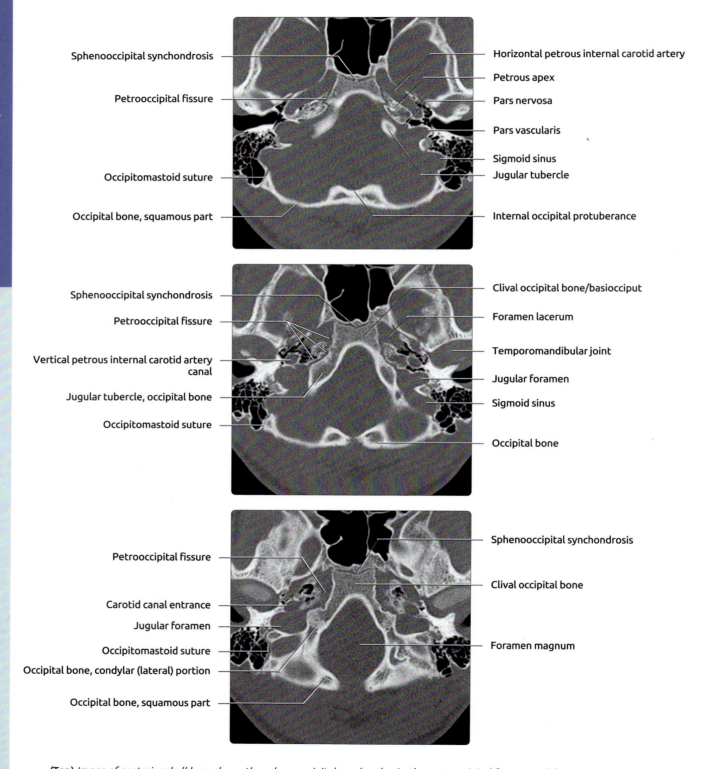

(Top) Image of posterior skull base shows the sphenooccipital synchondrosis, the petrooccipital fissure, and the occipitomastoid suture all in the same plane. The sphenooccipital synchondrosis has not yet fused in this young adolescent. (Middle) Image through the jugular tubercle of the clivus is made up almost completely of anterior occipital bone. The upper 1/3 of the clivus is above the sphenooccipital synchondrosis and is therefore part of the sphenoid bone. (Bottom) In this image, the lower clivus (below the sphenooccipital synchondrosis) is clearly made up of occipital bone. The petrooccipital fissure separates the temporal bone from the occipital bone. The occipitomastoid suture separates the mastoid sinus from the squamosal portion of the occipital bone.

Posterior Skull Base

AXIAL BONE CT

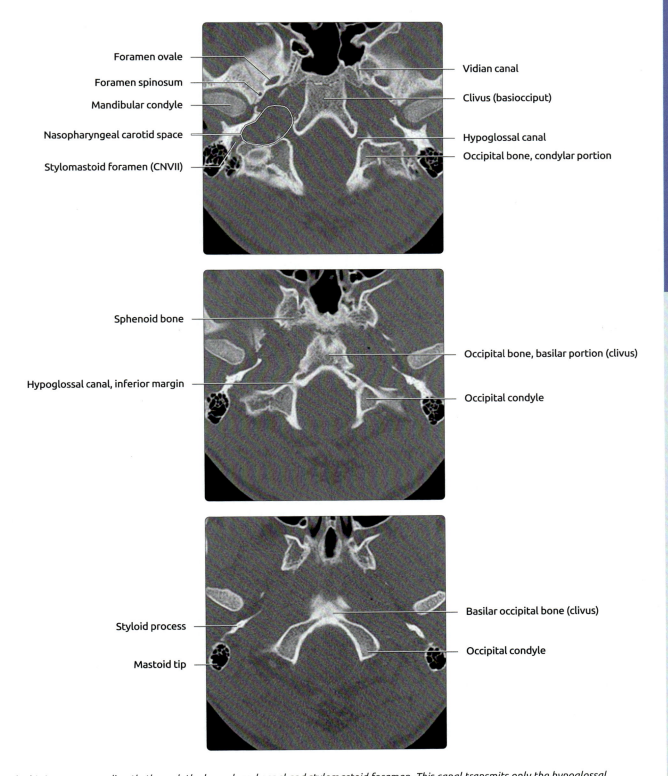

(Top) This image passes directly through the hypoglossal canal and stylomastoid foramen. This canal transmits only the hypoglossal nerve. Notice that as soon as the nerve exits the hypoglossal canal, it immediately enters the nasopharyngeal carotid space to join the glossopharyngeal (CNIX), vagus (CNX), and accessory (CNXI) cranial nerves. (Middle) In this image, the inferior margin of the hypoglossal canal runs within the occipital bone, between the basilar (clival) and condylar portions. The inferior surface of the condylar occipital bone are the occipital condyles. (Bottom) In this image through the occipital condyle, the inferior-most junction of the basilar (clival) occipital bone and the condylar occipital bone is visible. The occipital condyles rest the cranium upon the lateral masses of atlas (C1 vertebral body).

Posterior Skull Base

CORONAL BONE CT

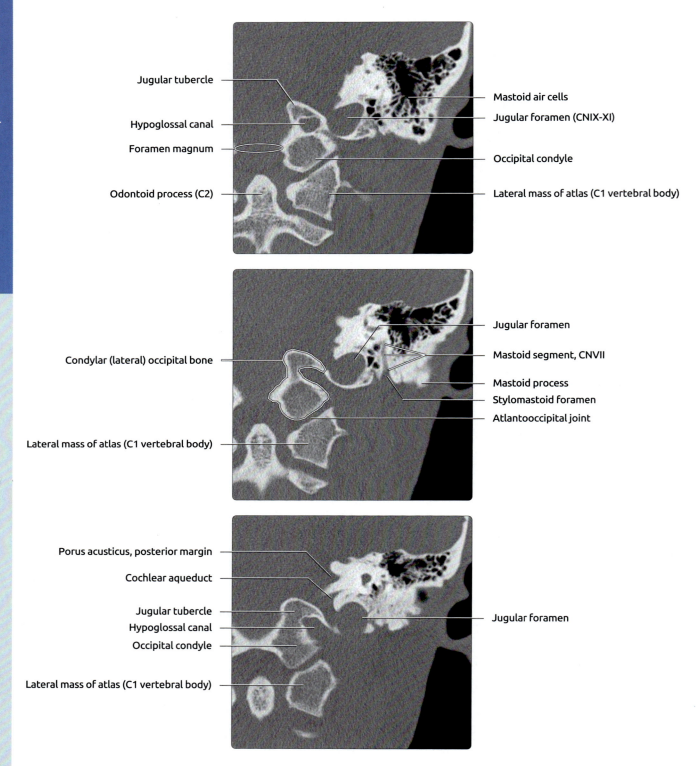

(Top) First of 6 coronal bone CT images of the left posterior skull base, presented from posterior to anterior, is shown. The hypoglossal canal passes through the condylar (lateral) portion of the occipital bone. In the coronal plane with both sides visible, this area has been referred to as the "double eagle." Notice that the eagle's head and beak are the jugular tubercle. (Middle) In this image through the mastoid (descending) portion of intratemporal facial nerve canal, the condylar part of the occipital bone is outlined. (Bottom) This image shows the classic "eagle" of the posterior skull base with the "beak" of the jugular tubercle separating the jugular foramen from the hypoglossal canal. Lesions of the hypoglossal canal affect the undersurface of the "beak" while lesions of the jugular foramen affect the external surface of the "beak."

Posterior Skull Base

CORONAL BONE CT

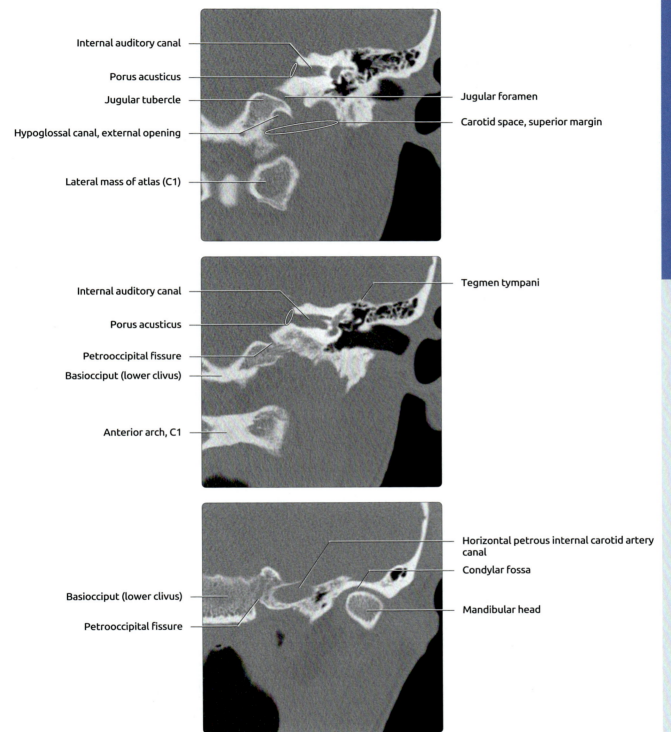

(Top) In this image of the left skull base and temporal bone, notice both the hypoglossal canal and the jugular foramen "empty" into the cephalad carotid space. The upper carotid space therefore contains CNIX-XII as well as the internal jugular vein. (Middle) In this image through the mid internal auditory canal, the petrooccipital fissure is visible, separating the basioccipital portion of the occipital bone from the temporal bone. (Bottom) In this image through the condylar fossa of the temporomandibular joint, the petrooccipital fissure is seen between the basiocciput and the temporal bone. The basiocciput is a large quadrilateral portion of the occipital bone that extends anterosuperiorly from the anterior margin of the foramen magnum to reach the sphenoid bone ~ 2/3 of the way up the clivus.

Posterior Skull Base

AXIAL T1 C+ FS MR

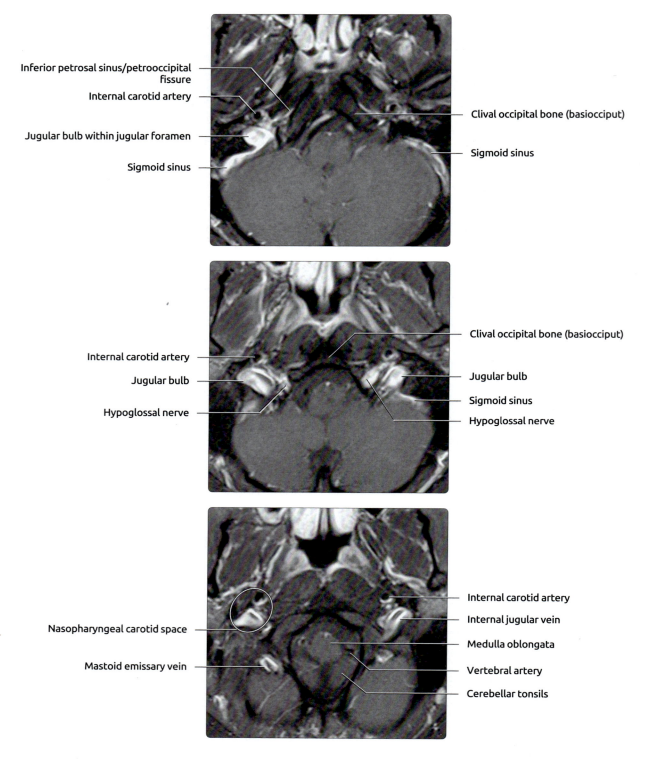

(Top) First of 3 axial T1 C+ FS MR images of the posterior skull base, presented from superior to inferior, is shown. On the patient's right, the high-signal enhancing sigmoid sinus can be seen connecting anteromedially with the jugular bulb. (Middle) At the level of the hypoglossal canals, the hypoglossal nerves can be seen as linear, low-intensity structures surrounded by the enhancing high-signal basiocciput venous plexus. The complex signal seen in both jugular bulbs should not be mistaken for a lesion. (Bottom) At the level of the foramen magnum, the internal jugular vein and internal carotid artery of the carotid space are visible. The vertebral arteries, medulla oblongata, and inferior cerebellar tonsils are normally seen at this level.

Posterior Skull Base

CORONAL T1 C+ MR

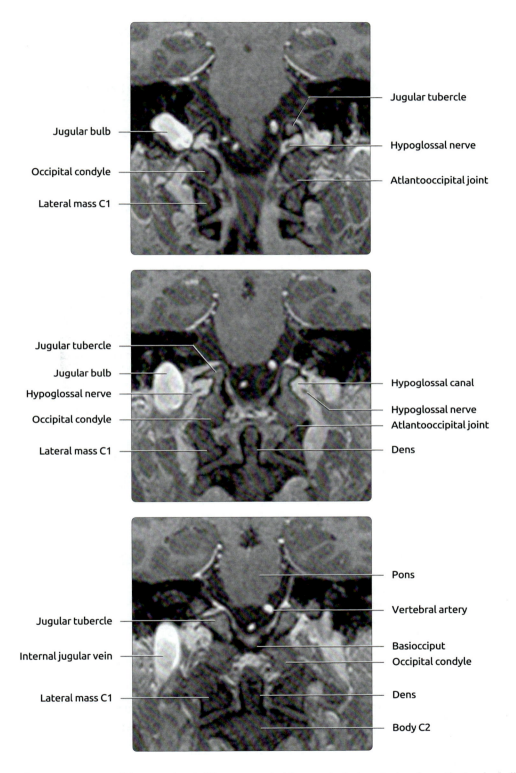

(Top) First of 3 coronal T1 C+ MR images of the posterior skull base, presented from posterior to anterior, shows the jugular bulb within the jugular foramen. The low-signal hypoglossal nerve is seen just below the "eagle's head" in the hypoglossal canal. The high-signal perineural basiocciput venous plexus is visible surrounding the hypoglossal nerve. (Middle) In this image, the classic "double eagle heads" are visible (jugular tubercles) with the hypoglossal nerve seen exiting the inferior hypoglossal canal. As in this case, the jugular bulbs are often asymmetric in size. (Bottom) In this image, the anterior jugular tubercle can be seen meeting the inferior basiocciput. The jugular bulb has connected inferiorly with the internal jugular vein. The internal jugular vein is within the nasopharyngeal carotid space.

Temporal Bone Anatomy

TERMINOLOGY

Abbreviations

- Temporal bone (T-bone)

Definitions

- T-bone: Paired bones located in posterolateral floor of middle & posterior cranial fossae made up of petrous pyramid & mastoid complex

IMAGING ANATOMY

Overview

- 5 bony parts to T-bone
  - **Squamous**: Forms lateral wall of middle cranial fossa
  - **Mastoid**: Aerated posterolateral T-bone
  - **Petrous**: Pyramidal shape medial T-bone containing inner ear (IE), internal auditory canal (IAC), & petrous apex (PA)
  - **Tympanic**: U-shaped bone forming bony external auditory canal (EAC)
  - **Styloid**: Forms styloid process after birth

Internal Contents

- **EAC**
  - Tympanic bone medially, fibrocartilage laterally
  - Medial border is tympanic membrane
  - Nodal drainage to parotid chain
- **Middle ear (ME)-mastoid**
  - **Epitympanum** (attic): ME above line from scutal tip to tympanic CNVII
    - **Tegmen tympani**: Roof of ME cavity
    - **Prussak space** = lateral epitympanic recess
  - **Mesotympanum**: ME proper
    - Posterior wall: 3 key structures = facial nerve recess, pyramidal eminence, sinus tympani
    - Medial wall: Lateral semicircular canal (SCC), tympanic segment CNVII, oval & round window
  - **Hypotympanum**: Shallow trough in floor of ME
  - Mastoid sinus: 4 key structures
    - **Aditus ad antrum**: Connects epitympanum to mastoid antrum
    - **Mastoid antrum**: Large, central mastoid air cell
    - **Körner septum**: Part of petrosquamosal suture running posterolaterally through mastoid air cells
    - **Tegmen mastoideum**: Roof of mastoid air cells
- **IE components**
  - **Bony labyrinth**: Bone that confines cochlea, vestibule, & SCCs
  - **Perilymphatic spaces**
    - Perilymphatic spaces include area in vestibule surrounding utricle & saccule, in SCCs around semicircular ducts, & within scala tympani & vestibuli of cochlea
    - **Perilymph** = fluid within bony labyrinth that "bathes" endolymph-containing membranous labyrinth structures
  - **Membranous labyrinth/endolymphatic spaces**
    - Includes vestibule (utricle & saccule), semicircular ducts, scala media (cochlear duct), & endolymphatic duct & sac

- **Endolymph** = fluid within structures of membranous labyrinth
  - **Cochlea**: ~ 2.5 turns; modiolus; 3 spiral chambers (scala tympani, scala vestibuli, & scala media)
  - SCCs: Superior, lateral, & posterior
    - Superior semicircular canal (SSCC): Projects cephalad; bony ridge over SSCC in roof of petrous pyramid called **arcuate eminence**
    - Lateral SCC: Projects into ME with tympanic CNVII on underside
    - Posterior SCC: Projects posteriorly parallel to petrous ridge
- **PA**
  - Anteromedial to IE
  - Pneumatized or nonpneumatized (marrow)
- **Intratemporal facial nerve**
  - CNVII segments: IAC, labyrinthine, tympanic, mastoid segments
  - **Geniculate ganglion** = anterior genu
  - Posterior genu: Tympanic segment bends inferiorly to become mastoid segment
  - **Stylomastoid foramen**: CNVII exits skull base here
- **Petrous internal carotid artery: C2 segment**
  - ICA: Vertical & horizontal T-bone segments
  - Vertical segment: Rises to genu beneath cochlea
  - Horizontal segment: Projects anteromedially to turn cephalad as precavernous & cavernous ICA
- **Muscles of T-bone**
  - **Tensor tympani muscle**
    - Dampens sound; hyperacusis if injured
    - Innervation: V3 branch
    - Location: Anteromedial wall, mesotympanum
    - Attachment: Tendon inserts on malleus
  - **Stapedius muscle**
    - Dampens sound; hyperacusis if injured
    - Innervation: CNVII
    - Location: Muscle belly in pyramidal eminence
    - Attachment: Tendon attaches on head of stapes

ANATOMY IMAGING ISSUES

Questions

- What is best approach to lesion found in T-bone?
  - Assign lesion to 1 of following T-bone areas: EAC, ME-mastoid, IE, PA, or intratemporal CNVII
    - Construct location-specific DDx; match imaging findings to DDx

EMBRYOLOGY

Embryologic Events

- EAC forms from 1st branchial groove
- Tympanic cavity forms from 1st branchial pouch
- Ossicles form predominantly from 1st & 2nd branchial arches
- Endolymphatic system forms from otocyst
- Perilymphatic space & otic capsule form from surrounding mesenchyme

Practical Implications

- In nonsyndromic EAC atresia, IE spared, as it forms from otocyst migration independent of EAC-ME formation

Temporal Bone Anatomy

GRAPHICS: EXTERNAL EAR AND MIDDLE EAR

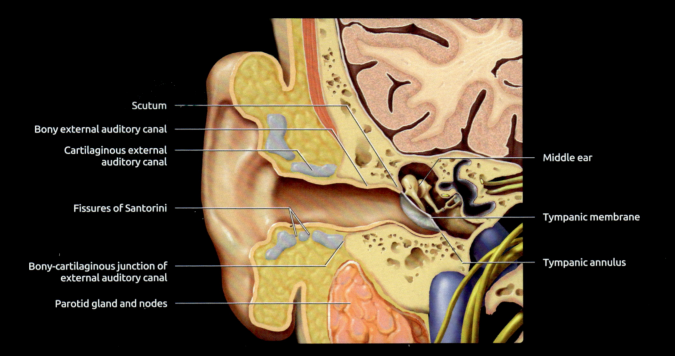

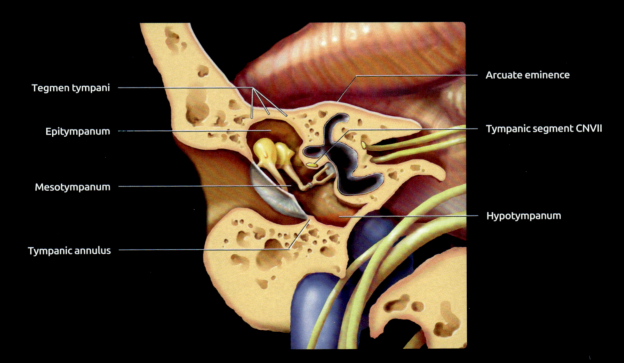

(Top) Coronal graphic shows the external and middle ear. The external auditory canal (EAC) is made up of lateral cartilaginous and medial bony components. Infection of the EAC can penetrate inferomedially to the skull base and associated spaces via the fissures of Santorini (gaps in the EAC cartilage). External ear and EAC lymphatic drainage is to the parotid nodal chain. The medial margin of the EAC is the tympanic membrane, which attaches to the scutum and tympanic annulus. (Bottom) Coronal graphic shows the middle ear, which is divided into 3 components: Epitympanum, mesotympanum, and hypotympanum. The epitympanum (yellow accent) is defined as the middle ear cavity above a line drawn from the scutal tip and tympanic segment of CNVII. Its roof is called the tegmen tympani. The mesotympanum extends from this line inferiorly to a line connecting the tympanic annulus to the base of the cochlear promontory. The hypotympanum (orange accent) lies inferior to this line.

Temporal Bone Anatomy

GRAPHICS: FACIAL NERVE AND CRANIAL NERVE

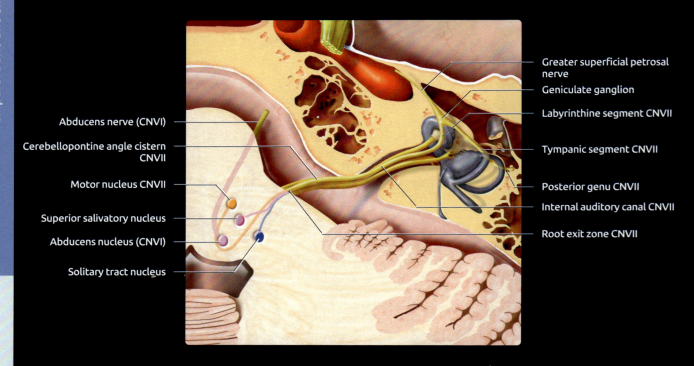

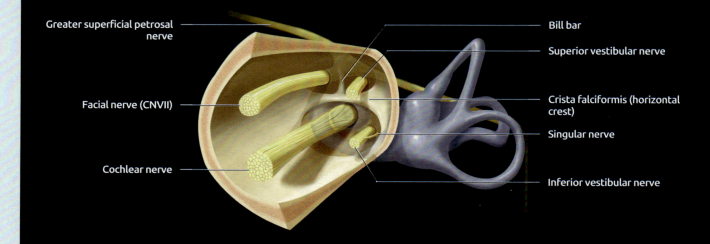

(Top) *Axial graphic shows the facial nerve from the brainstem nuclei to the posterior genu of the temporal bone. The motor nucleus sends out its fibers to circle CNVI nucleus before reaching the root exit zone at the pontomedullary junction. The superior salivatory nucleus sends parasympathetic secretomotor fibers to the lacrimal, submandibular, and sublingual glands. The solitary tract nucleus receives anterior 2/3 tongue taste information.* **(Bottom)** *Graphic depicts cranial nerve relationships in the fundus of the internal auditory canal. Notice that the crista falciformis separates the cochlear nerve and inferior vestibular nerve below from CNVII and the superior vestibular nerve above. Also note Bill bar separating CNVII from the superior vestibular nerve.*

Temporal Bone Anatomy

GRAPHICS: MEMBRANOUS LABYRINTH AND PETROUS INTERNAL CAROTID ARTERY

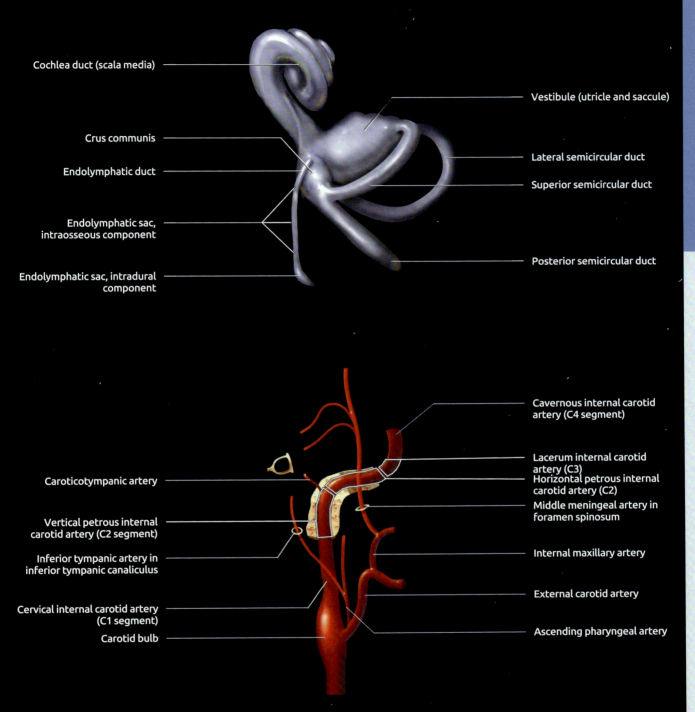

(Top) *Graphic of the membranous labyrinth is shown from above. Key elements of the membranous labyrinth to consider include ~ 2.5 turns of the cochlea, the meeting point of the superior and posterior semicircular ducts (crus communis), and the endolymphatic duct and sac. Note that the endolymphatic duct has intraosseous and intradural components.* (Bottom) *Graphic emphasizes the petrous internal carotid artery (ICA). The cervical ICA enters the carotid canal of the skull base to become the vertical petrous ICA (C2 subsegment ICA). It then turns anteromedially to become the horizontal petrous ICA. The segment of the intracranial ICA just above the foramen lacerum is called the lacerum segment (C3 ICA segment). Note the inferior tympanic artery arising from the ascending pharyngeal artery and passing through the inferior tympanic canaliculus, and the middle meningeal artery arising from the internal maxillary artery and passing through the foramen spinosum.*

Temporal Bone Anatomy

AXIAL BONE CT

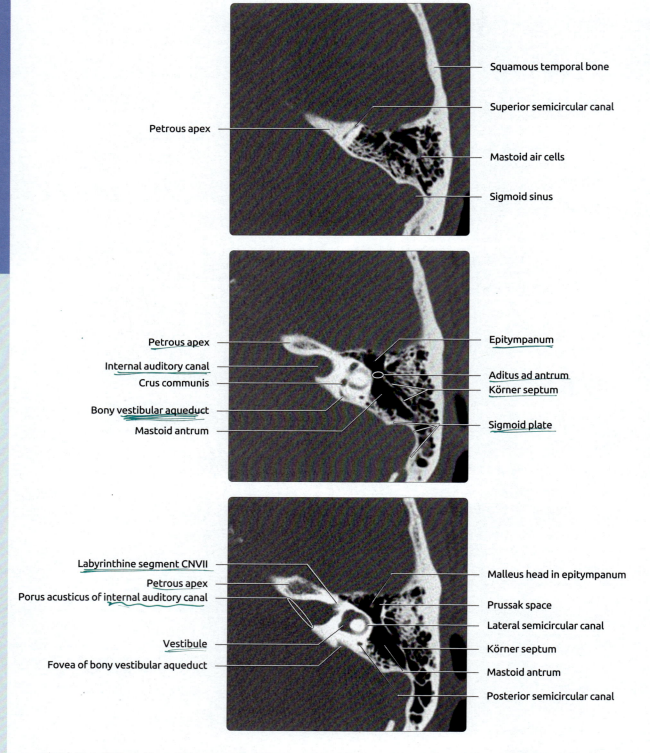

(Top) First of 12 axial bone CT images of the left temporal bone from superior to inferior is shown. The superior semicircular canal projects cephalad from the inner ear. The bony cover over the top of the semicircular canal is called the arcuate eminence. **(Middle)** At the level of the upper internal auditory canal, the aditus ad antrum (L. "entrance to the cave") is seen connecting the epitympanum to the mastoid antrum (L. "cave"). Notice the Körner septum separating the mastoid antrum from the squamous portion of the mastoid air cells. **(Bottom)** At the level of the lateral semicircular canal, the opening to the internal auditory canal, the porus acusticus is particularly well seen. The fovea of the bony vestibular aqueduct along the posterior wall of the temporal bone houses the intradural endolymphatic sac. The Prussak space is visible as the portion of the epitympanum lateral to the ossicles.

Temporal Bone Anatomy

AXIAL BONE CT

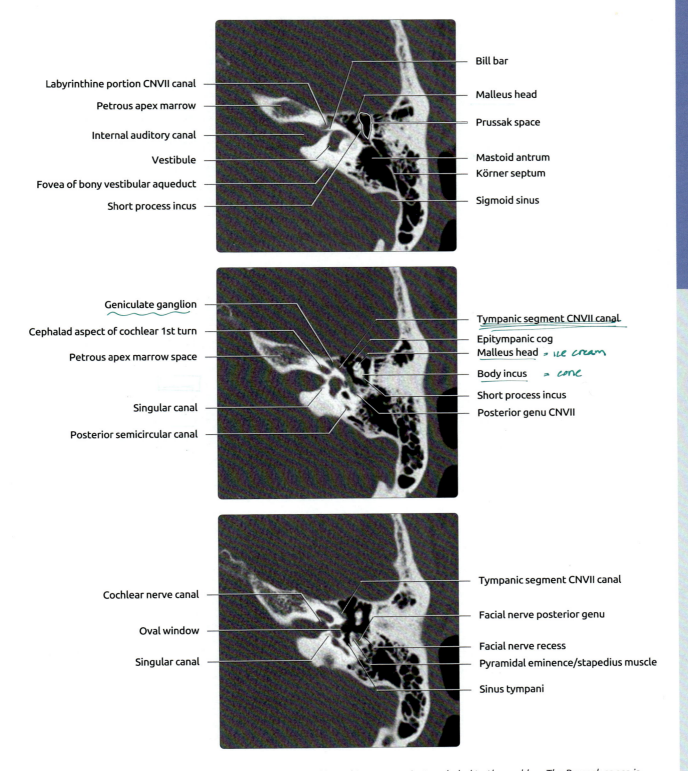

(Top) Image through the labyrinthine segment of the facial nerve shows this structure just cephalad to the cochlea. The Prussak space is now visible as the lateral epitympanic recess. This is the 1st area that the typical pars flaccida cholesteatoma involves in the middle ear. (Middle) The tympanic segment of the facial nerve is seen from the anteromedial geniculate ganglion to the posterior genu, where it changes to become the mastoid segment. The cog is seen crossing the anterior epitympanum. (Bottom) In this image, 3 key structures on the posterior wall of the middle ear cavity are well seen. From medial to lateral, they are the sinus tympani, pyramidal eminence, and facial nerve recess. Also note the oval window along the medial wall of the mesotympanum just anterior to the sinus tympani.

Temporal Bone Anatomy

AXIAL BONE CT

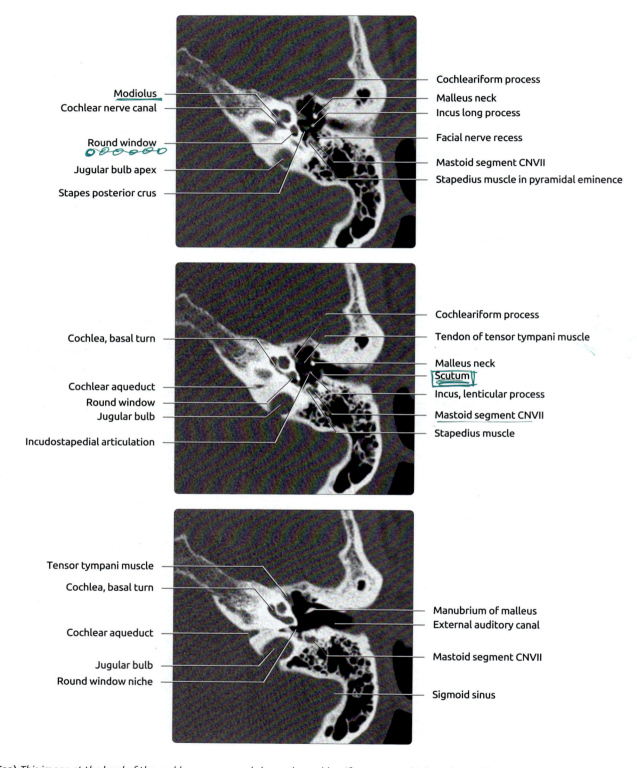

(Top) This image at the level of the cochlear nerve canal shows the cochleariform process high on the cochlear promontory. The cochleariform process is the annulus through which the tendon of the tensor tympani muscle turns toward the more lateral malleus. Stapes crura are visible. The stapedius muscle in the pyramidal eminence is now distinguishable from the mastoid segment of the facial nerve. **(Middle)** Mid cochlear image shows both the cochleariform process and the tendon of the tensor tympani muscle extending over to the malleus. The incudostapedial articulation is visible between the lenticular process of the incus and the stapes head. Also note the round window at the base of the basal turn of the cochlea. **(Bottom)** At the level of the low mesotympanum, note the cochlear aqueduct on the medial wall inferior to the internal auditory canal. The manubrium of the malleus is also visible.

Temporal Bone Anatomy

AXIAL BONE CT

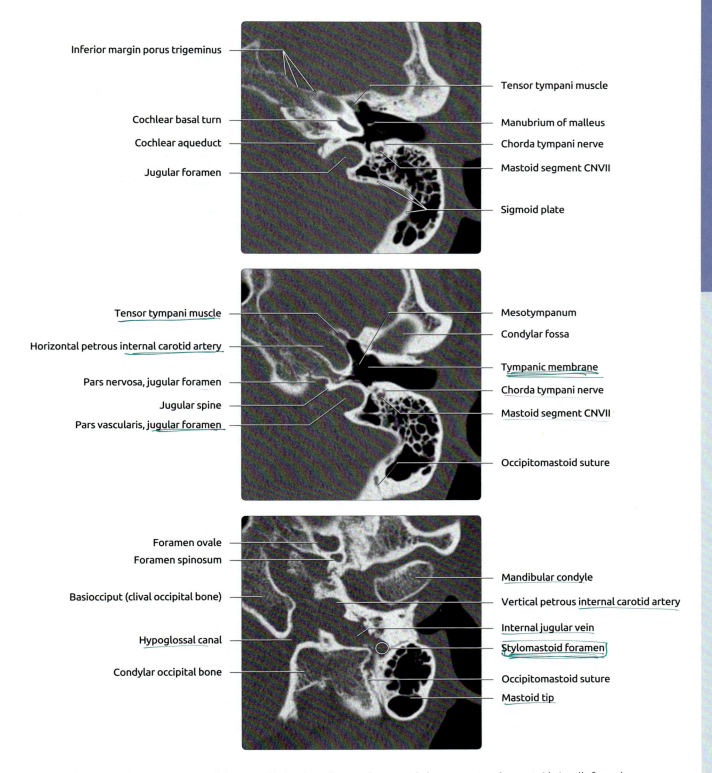

(Top) In this image, the normal cortex of the sigmoid plate is well seen. The sigmoid plate separates the mastoid air cells from the sigmoid sinus. Notice the cochlear aqueduct on the medial temporal bone wall. (Middle) At the level of the mesotympanum, the normal gossamer tympanic membrane is just barely visible. The horizontal petrous ICA canal is seen running anteromedial toward the cavernous sinus. Notice the pars nervosa and pars vascularis of the jugular foramen partially separated by the jugular spine. (Bottom) The mastoid tip is seen in this inferior image. Just anteromedial to the mastoid tip is the stylomastoid foramen where the facial nerve exits the skull base. Notice the entrance to the vertical segment of the petrous ICA canal just medial to the condylar fossa. The occipitomastoid suture should not be mistaken for a fracture line.

Temporal Bone Anatomy

CORONAL BONE CT

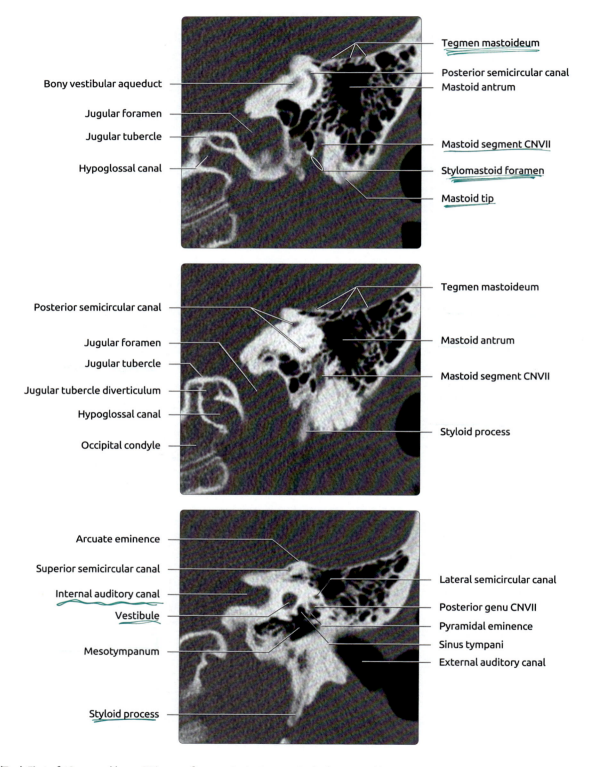

(Top) First of 12 coronal bone CT images from posterior to anterior is shown. In this most posterior image, the stylomastoid foramen and distal mastoid segment of the facial nerve can be seen to be protected by the mastoid tip. The mastoid sinus grows into this protective position in the 1st decade of life. **(Middle)** In this image, the mid mastoid segment of the facial nerve is seen. The jugular foramen and the hypoglossal canal are separated by the "eagle's beak," a portion of the jugular tubercle. **(Bottom)** In this image of the posterior mesotympanum, the 3 critical posterior wall structures are seen. From medial to lateral, these structures are the sinus tympani, the pyramidal eminence, and the facial nerve recess with the posterior genu of CNVII in its depth. Note that it is possible to see the stapedius muscle as a small, round soft tissue density within pyramidal eminence.

Temporal Bone Anatomy

CORONAL BONE CT

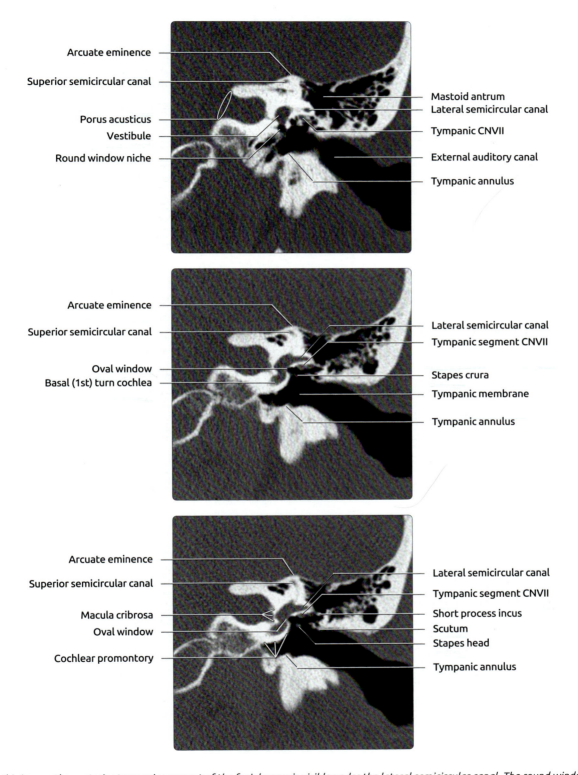

(Top) In this image, the posterior tympanic segment of the facial nerve is visible under the lateral semicircular canal. The round window niche is a small, air-filled area off the medial mesotympanum that leads to the round window membrane. (Middle) At the level of the oval window niche, the basal turn of the cochlea becomes visible. Notice the tympanic membrane is barely seen when it is normal. Its inferior attachment, the tympanic annulus, is a useful landmark separating the middle ear from the medial external ear. (Bottom) In this image, the short process of the incus is seen projecting posteriorly into the aditus ad antrum. Both the tympanic membrane attachments can be seen: The superior scutum and the inferior tympanic annulus. Notice that the cochlear promontory projects out into the mesotympanum. Glomus tympanicum paragangliomas occur here.

Temporal Bone Anatomy

CORONAL BONE CT

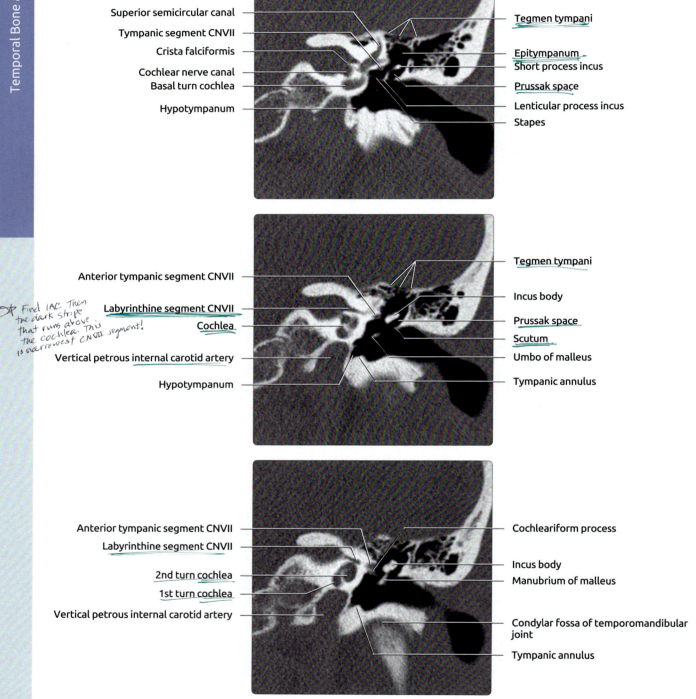

(Top) Image through the mid mesotympanum shows the more superior epitympanum with the long and short processes of the incus forming the medial margin and the lateral epitympanic wall forming the lateral margin of Prussak space. Pars flaccida cholesteatoma involves the middle ear cavity, initially in Prussak space. (Middle) In this image, the tegmen tympani (L. "roof of the cave") can be seen as the superior wall of the epitympanum. Note its normal variable thickness. Just above the cochlea, the facial nerve canal is seen emerging from the fundus of the internal auditory canal to become the labyrinthine segment CNVII. (Bottom) Three key structures are seen together in this image: The labyrinthine segment CNVII, anterior tympanic CNVII, and the cochleariform process. Note the tendon of the tensor tympani muscles projecting from the cochleariform process to attach to the malleus.

Temporal Bone Anatomy

CORONAL BONE CT

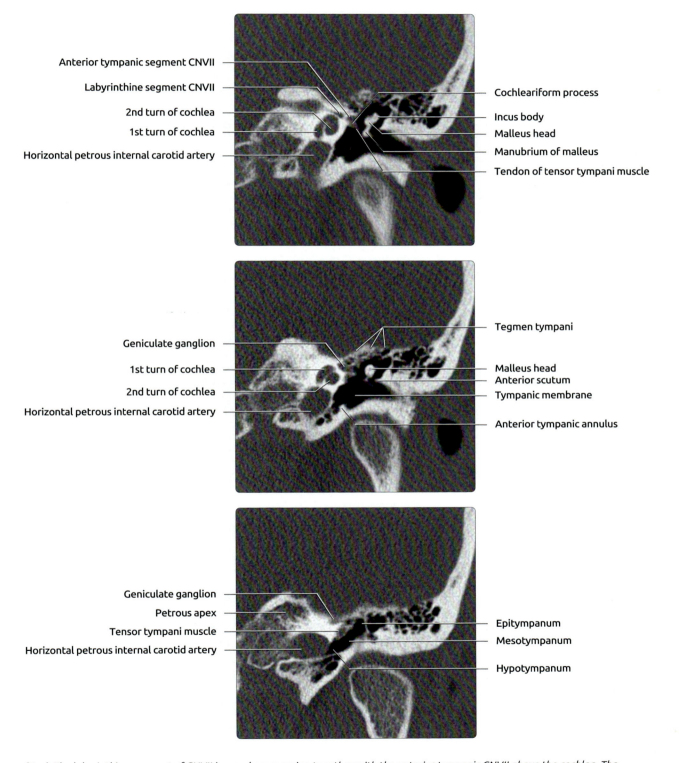

(Top) The labyrinthine segment of CNVII is seen here merging together with the anterior tympanic CNVII above the cochlea. The cochleariform process and tendon of the tensor tympani muscle are both visible. The petrous internal carotid horizontal segment can be seen below the cochlea. *(Middle)* In this image, the tegmen tympani is thick and well defined. The geniculate ganglion in the geniculate fossa is seen on the superolateral cochlea with the horizontal petrous ICA below the cochlea. Both the scutum and tympanic annulus are visible between the gossamer tympanic membrane. *(Bottom)* In the most anterior middle ear cavity, the ossicles are not seen. The geniculate ganglion in the geniculate fossa, along with the tensor tympani muscle, are visible. The horizontal petrous ICA is now projecting anteromedially.

Temporal Bone Anatomy

SAGITTAL T2 MR

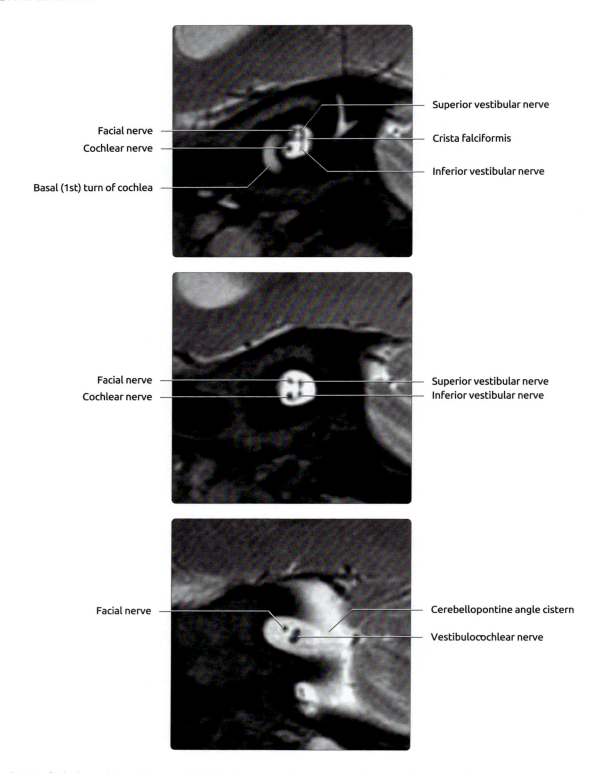

(Top) First of 3 high-resolution oblique sagittal T2 MR images of the internal auditory canal, presented from lateral to medial, shows the facial nerve to be anterosuperior and the cochlear nerve to be anteroinferior. This fundal view reveals the crista falciformis, seen as a vague, low-signal line dividing CNVII and the superior vestibular nerve from the cochlear and inferior vestibular nerves. (Middle) In the mid internal auditory canal, 4 discrete nerves are visible. Notice that the anterosuperior facial nerve is normally slightly smaller than the anteroinferior cochlear nerve. The superior and inferior vestibular nerves are often joined by connecting fibers, as in this example. (Bottom) At the level of the porus acusticus, the vestibulocochlear nerve has the appearance of a "catcher's mitt" with the facial nerve looking like the "ball in the mitt."

Temporal Bone Anatomy

AXIAL T2 MR

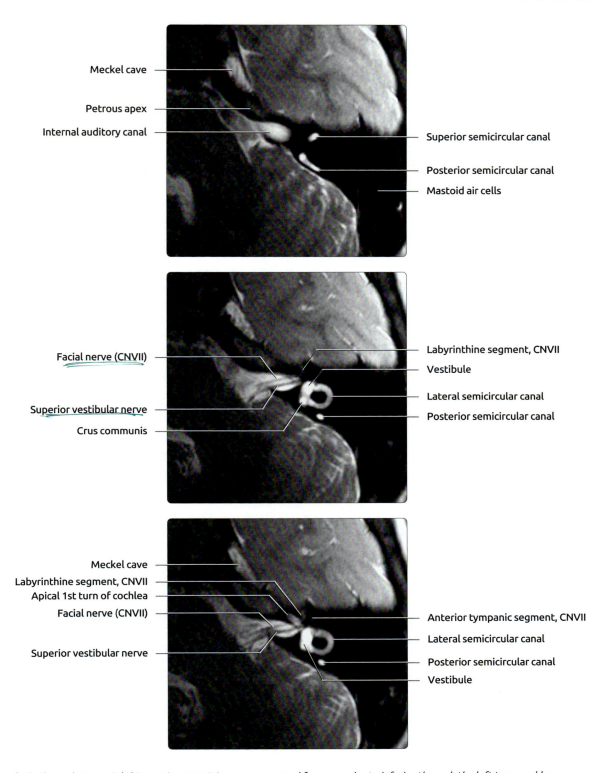

(Top) First of 6 high-resolution axial thin-section T2 MR images, presented from superior to inferior through the left temporal bone, shows the superior internal auditory canal and semicircular canals. (Middle) In this image, the facial nerve is visible anterior and parallel to the superior vestibular nerve in the superior aspect of the internal auditory canal. The fluid spaces of the membranous labyrinth are high signal within the dark signal of the bony labyrinth. (Bottom) In this image, the labyrinthine and anterior tympanic segments of the facial nerve are visible. As they are not surrounded by cerebrospinal fluid, as is CNVII in the internal auditory canal, they are more difficult to see.

Temporal Bone Anatomy

AXIAL T2 MR

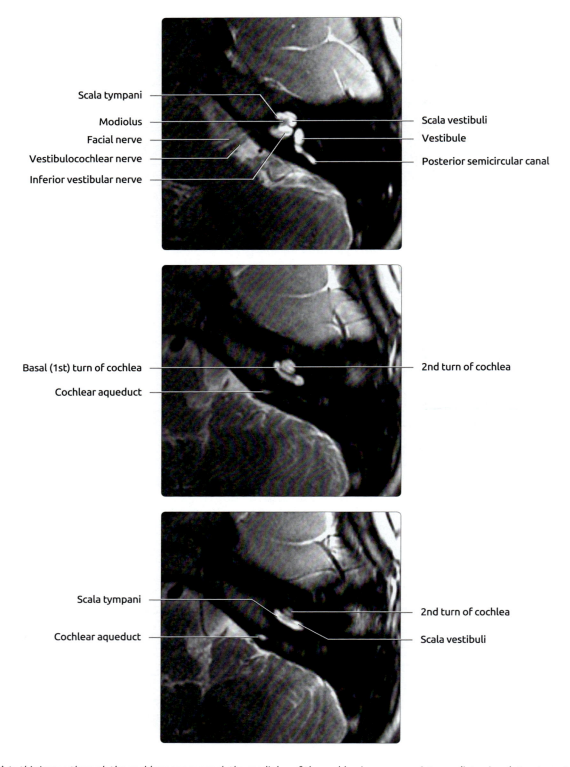

(Top) In this image through the cochlear nerve canal, the modiolus of the cochlea is seen as an intermediate-signal structure at the hub of the cochlea. The 2 larger cochlear chambers are visible. The anterior chamber is the scala vestibuli, and the posterior chamber is the scala tympani. The scala media is not routinely resolvable. *(Middle)* In this image, both the 1st and 2nd turns of the cochlea are visible. The osseous spiral lamina within the cochlea is seen as a fine, low-signal line within the fluid of the cochlear membranous labyrinth. *(Bottom)* The cochlear aqueduct is a tubular-shaped structure on the medial wall of the temporal bone inferior to the internal auditory canal. No definite function can be assigned to this structure.

Temporal Bone Anatomy

CORONAL T2 MR

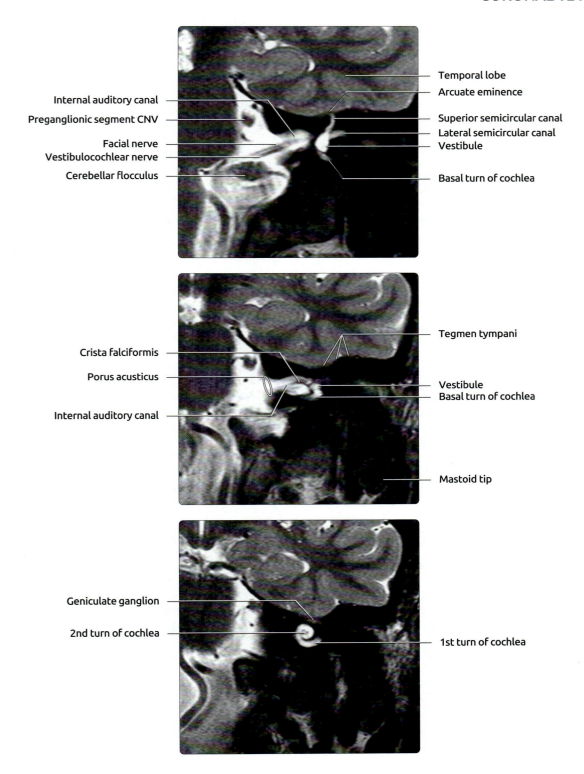

(Top) First of 3 coronal T2 MR images of the left ear from posterior to anterior is shown. The membranous labyrinth of the inner ear is visible as high-signal fluid. Notice the superior and lateral semicircular canals adjacent to the vestibule. (Middle) In this image through the internal auditory canal, an unusually long crista falciformis is seen in the fundus. The area of the tegmen tympani is marked, but no landmarks in the middle ear are visible because both air and bone are low signal on MR imaging. (Bottom) At the level of the cochlea, the snail shape is particularly obvious, displaying both the 1st and 2nd turns. The geniculate ganglion is barely visible above and lateral to the cochlea. Again, note the lack of middle ear definable structures.

Temporal Bone Oblique Reformation Anatomy

TERMINOLOGY

Abbreviations
- Longitudinal oblique view (LOV)
- Transverse oblique view (TOV)

Synonyms
- Stenver view (LOV)
- Pöschl view (TOV)

Definitions
- LOV: Image reformation series parallel to long axis of petrous pyramid
  - Perpendicular to line drawn between vertical components of superior semicircular canal arch
- TOV: Image reformation series perpendicular to LOV
  - Parallel to line drawn between vertical components of superior semicircular canal arch

IMAGING ANATOMY

Overview
- Standard temporal bone CT imaging on multislice CT produces axial data set
  - Coronal reformation data set is standard additional plane in temporal bone imaging
  - LOV and TOV reformations are variably created as additional planes available for viewing
- Many normal temporal bone structures are **not** well seen in either axial or coronal imaging planes
  - Best examples of such structures include facial nerve canal, cochlea, round window, bony vestibular aqueduct (VA), superior and posterior semicircular canals, and cochlear nerve canal
  - Adding longitudinal and transverse oblique reformation to axial and coronal plane as 4-plane standard offering adds considerably to visibility of these structures
    - LOV and TOV CT reformations provide rich set of additional images that may profile some of these structures in unique and helpful ways

Microanatomy Optimized in Longitudinal Oblique View
- 1st cochlear turn plus round window niche/membrane
  - Very useful view for cochlear implant planning as it shows adequate access through round window/basal turn of cochlea
    - Important if labyrinthine ossificans present
- Facial nerve canal view: Geniculate fossa, tympanic segment, posterior genu, and mastoid segment
  - Useful in assessing where along course of tympanic segment facial nerve injury may have occurred
    - Traumatic injury or injury from cholesteatoma

Microanatomy Optimized in Transverse Oblique View
- Bony VA view
  - Normal VA should not be > dimension of normal posterior semicircular canal
    - Enlarged VA on axial CT: > 1-mm diameter halfway between external aperture and crus communis; > 2 mm at opercular margin
    - Enlarged VA has potential syndromic implications

- Transverse oblique axis much more easily profiles VA from external aperture to crus communis than axial plane CT images
- "2-window" view of oval and round windows
  - Shows oval and round window membranes clearly
  - When oval or round window atresia is under consideration, this view is very helpful in confirming either diagnosis
  - Round window access assessment for cochlear implantation is also assisted by this view
- Superior semicircular canal/arcuate eminence view
  - Coronal CT can make diagnosis of dehiscence in most cases
  - Profile of superior semicircular canal in TOV may help make diagnosis and guide type of surgical procedure

ANATOMY IMAGING ISSUES

Imaging Recommendations
- Oblique view checklist
  - Structures best seen with LOV
    - Cochlear turn views
    - Facial nerve canal view: Tympanic segment, posterior genu, and mastoid segment
    - Malleoincudal joint profile
    - Stapes crura 2-dot view
    - Mastoid drainage profile
  - Structures best seen with TOV
    - Bony VA view
    - Oval and round window, "2-window" view
    - Superior semicircular canal and arcuate eminence profile
    - Labyrinthine segment CNVII view
    - Cochlear nerve canal view

Imaging Approaches
- LOV and TOV image reconstruction easily learned and performed by CT technologist
  - Step 1: After axial acquisition, place line parallel to superior semicircular canal
  - Step 2: Reformat 0.75-mm images in **TOV plane** ~ 20 mm on either side of this line
  - Step 3: Place line perpendicular to initial TOV plane to create **LOV plane**
  - Step 4: Reformat 0.75-mm images in LOV plane to sufficiently cover petrous pyramid

Imaging Pitfalls
- Superior semicircular canal anatomy is complex in 3 dimensions, and unfamiliarity can lead to confusion when viewing additional imaging planes, such as LOV and TOV

Temporal Bone Oblique Reformation Anatomy

LONGITUDINAL & TRANSVERSE OBLIQUE REFORMATIONS

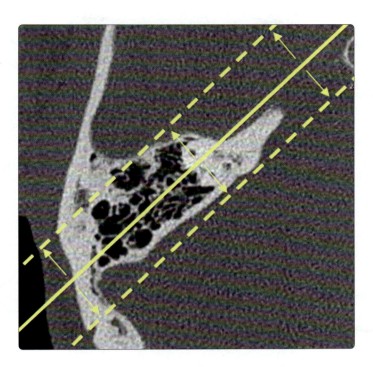

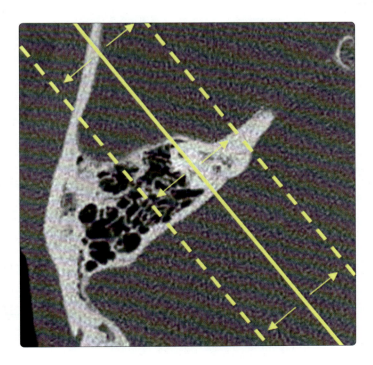

(Top) *The creation of reproducible longitudinal oblique (Stenvers) T-bone reformations can be a challenge for those unfamiliar with T-bone anatomy. Scroll through the axial image data set to the level of the superior semicircular canal. The longitudinal oblique reformation image set is made in a plane perpendicular to the axis created by the line through the superior semicircular canal. Be sure to cover the majority of the petrous pyramid as shown.* **(Bottom)** *Creation of transverse oblique (Pöschl) T-bone reformations can be a challenge for those unfamiliar with T-bone anatomy. Scroll through the axial image data set to the level of the superior semicircular canal. The transverse oblique reformation image set is made in a plane parallel to the axis created by the line through the superior semicircular canal. Be sure the data set extends laterally to cover the middle ear structures.*

Temporal Bone Oblique Reformation Anatomy

LONGITUDINAL OBLIQUE REFORMATIONS

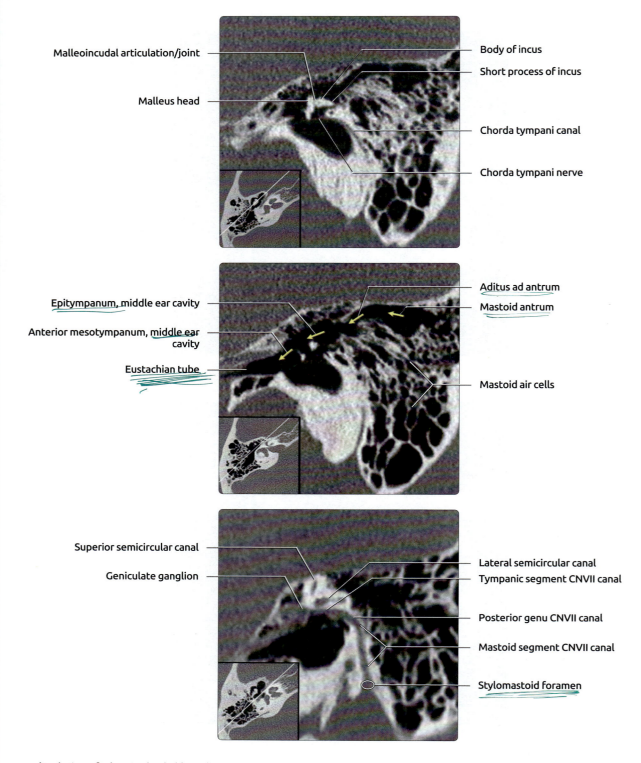

(Top) First of 6 longitudinal oblique bone CT images of the right ear presented from lateral to medial profiles the malleoincudal articulation between the head of the malleus and the body of the incus. Note the chorda tympani nerve canal (rising anteriorly and superiorly from the mastoid segment of facial nerve) as well as the nerve itself in the middle ear cavity. *(Middle)* Moving medially, the 2nd of 6 images highlights the normal mastoid drainage route (arrows). Fluid normally made by mastoid mucosal surfaces passes into the mastoid antrum, and from there, it reaches the middle ear cavity via the aditus ad antrum. The final common pathway exiting the middle ear cavity is the eustachian tube. *(Bottom)* The tympanic segment of CNVII is usually seen entirely on a carefully placed longitudinal oblique reformation. Note the geniculate ganglion, tympanic segment, posterior genu, mastoid segment, and stylomastoid foramen, all seen on this single view. The tympanic segment passes beneath the lateral semicircular canal.

Temporal Bone Oblique Reformation Anatomy

LONGITUDINAL OBLIQUE REFORMATIONS

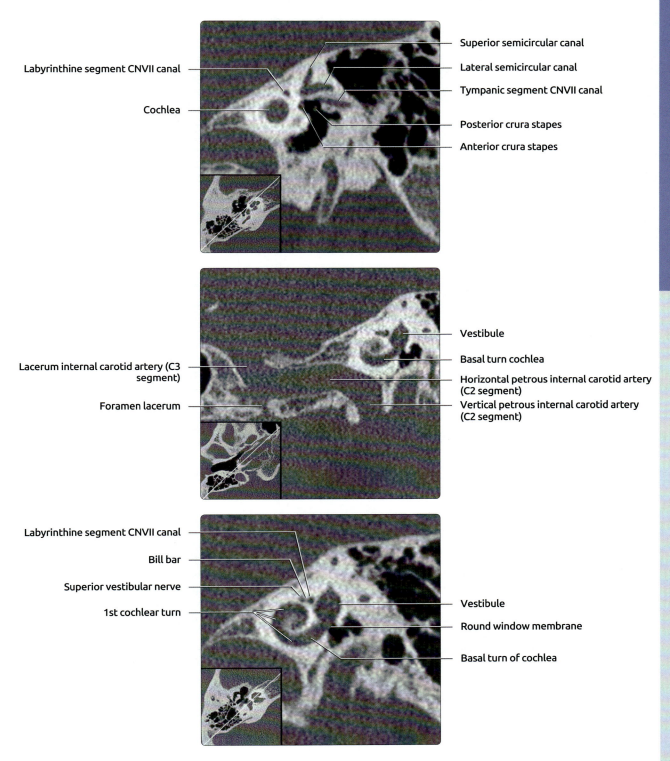

(Top) Fourth of 6 longitudinal oblique CT images of the right ear presented from most lateral to most medial shows the crura of the stapes just before they meet the footplate of the stapes at the oval window. In patients with ossicular anomalies, this level of anatomic information about the stapes can be of great help. (Middle) More medially, the longitudinal oblique reformation through the horizontal petrous internal carotid artery (ICA) lays out the vertical and horizontal petrous ICA segments (C2 segment ICA) as well as the lacerum segment (proximal C3 segment ICA). Note this same reformation also profiles the basal turn of the cochlea. (Bottom) Most medial image of the 6 longitudinal oblique reformats profiles the entire 1st turn of the cochlea. In the notch between the vestibule and apical aspect of the 1st cochlear turn, note the superior vestibular nerve canal and the labyrinthine segment of the CNVII canal. Such a view could be helpful in evaluating cochlear implants.

Temporal Bone Oblique Reformation Anatomy

TRANSVERSE OBLIQUE REFORMATIONS

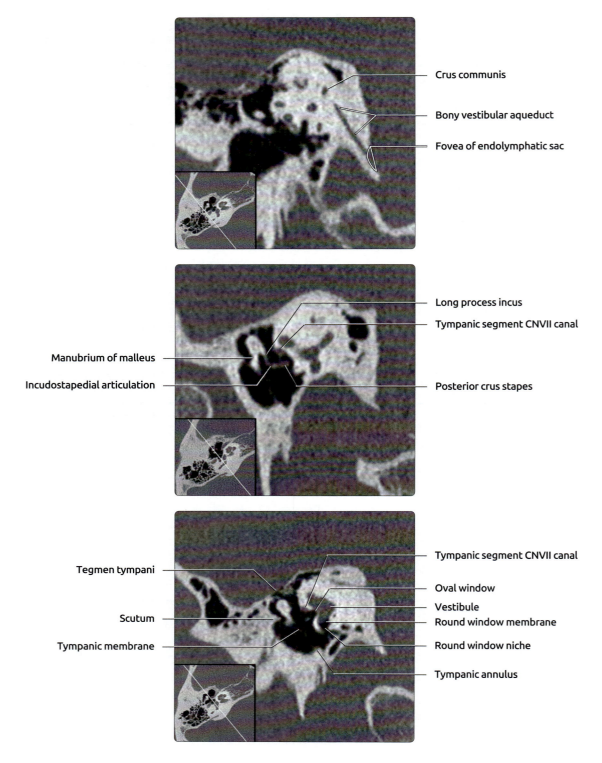

(Top) First of 6 transverse oblique bone CT images of the right ear presented from posterolateral to anteromedial, toward the petrous apex, is shown. This reconstruction profiles the bony vestibular aqueduct as it progresses from the fovea of the endolymphatic sac toward the crus communis of the inner ear. (Middle) Transverse oblique reconstruction along the line of the posterior crus of the stapes permits identification of the incudostapedial articulation. The long process of the incus and manubrium of the malleus are also particularly well seen. (Bottom) The "2-window" view is created by obtaining a transverse oblique reconstruction that passes through the axial view of the oval window (see inset). In this view, the oval window and round window niche and membrane are seen simultaneously. When cochlear implantation is anticipated, this view allows surgeons great confidence that they can access the basal turn of the cochlea through the round window niche with their cochlear implant.

Temporal Bone Oblique Reformation Anatomy

TRANSVERSE OBLIQUE REFORMATIONS

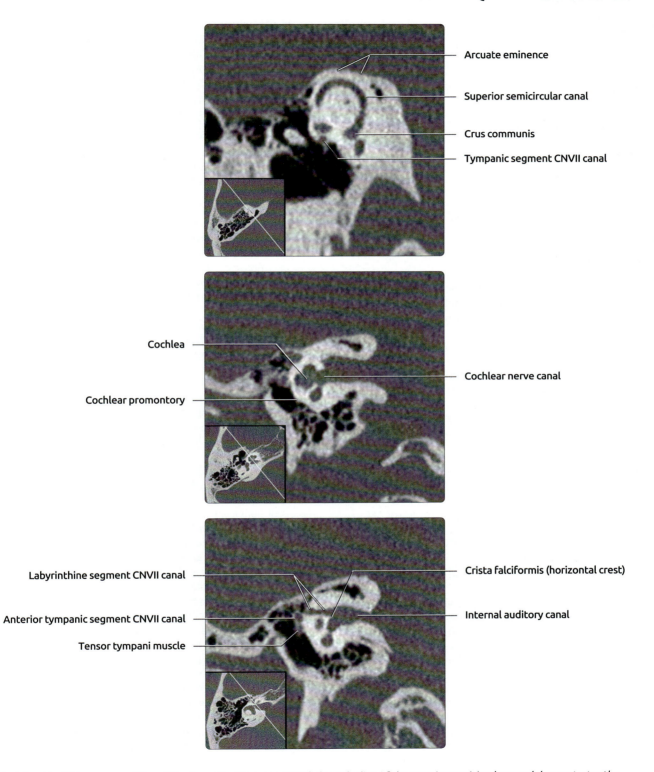

(Top) Fourth of 6 transverse oblique CT reformatted images created along the line of the superior semicircular canal demonstrates the entire span of this canal with the bony ridge above it (arcuate eminence). This view can be very helpful in delineating the extent of superior semicircular canal dehiscence when present. (Middle) This transverse oblique reformation along the line of the cochlear axis clearly delineates the length and dimension of the cochlear nerve canal as it connects the fundus of the internal auditory canal (IAC) to the cochlea. In congenital inner ear lesions where a "trapped cochlea" (cochlea and IAC have no connection, and, therefore, there is no cochlear nerve) is suspected, this view can help verify this imaging impression. (Bottom) In this most anteromedial of the 6 transverse oblique reformation series, the reformation is created along the axis of the labyrinthine segment of CNVII. When CNVII pathology is present, it is very helpful to have multiple different views of its canal.

External Auditory Canal Anatomy

TERMINOLOGY

Abbreviations
- External auditory canal (**EAC**)
- Temporomandibular joint (**TMJ**)

Definitions
- External ear: Made up of pinna (auricle) and cartilaginous and bony EAC

IMAGING ANATOMY

Overview
- External ear
  - Pinna (auricle)
    - Visible part of external ear
    - Major components: Helix, antihelix, tragus, antitragus, concha, lobule, and external meatus of EAC
  - EAC
    - Lateral 1/3 of EAC formed by fibrocartilage
    - Medial 2/3 of EAC is formed by cortical bone
      - □ Anterior, inferior, and lower part of posterior wall formed by tympanic component of temporal bone
      - □ Posterior wall and roof formed by squamous portion
    - Both cartilaginous and bony components are lined by skin
      - □ Skin is continuation of keratinizing stratified squamous epithelium
      - □ Skin in EAC susceptible to common skin pathologies, including infection and neoplasm (squamous cell carcinoma, basal cell neoplasm)

Extent
- EAC extends from meatus of pinna laterally to tympanic membrane (TM)
- Measures 2-3 cm in length, 7-10 mm in diameter
- There are 2 normal sites of relative narrowing of EAC
  - Isthmus (junction of cartilaginous and bony portions)
  - Medial end of EAC, adjacent to TM
- Medial border of bony EAC
  - TM forms medial wall of EAC and separates EAC from middle ear proper
    - Semitransparent membrane with 2 general regions
      - □ Pars tensa region forms most of TM, is relatively tight; central portion (umbo) is tented inward where tip of malleus attaches
      - □ Pars flaccida small upper region that attaches to scutum
  - Scutum is relatively sharp bony spur that is continuation of medial roof of EAC and forms at junction of roof of EAC and lateral wall of middle ear cavity
    - Just medial to scutum is Prussak space (small space that is technically within middle ear)
    - Pars flaccida component of TM attaches to scutum superiorly
    - Scutum is commonly eroded in cases of acquired cholesteatoma that are initiated from pars flaccida
  - Tympanic annulus is fibrocartilaginous ring that attaches to tympanic sulcus (narrow bony rise along floor of EAC) along medial margin of EAC; serves as anchor for TM; ring is incomplete anteriorly and superiorly

Anatomy Relationships
- EAC relationships
  - Anterior: temporomandibular joint (TMJ)
    - Anterior wall of bony ECA also serves as posterior wall of temporomandibular fossa
  - Posterior: Mastoid air cells
  - Superior: Superolateral mastoid air cells
  - Inferior: Parotid space
  - Medial: Middle ear cavity

Internal Contents
- **Lateral cartilaginous component of EAC**
  - Laterally, in cartilaginous component, skin is thicker and contains sebaceous glands, ceruminous glands, and hair follicles
  - Circumferential fibrocartilage is extension of cartilage of concha; supports and maintains patency of EAC
  - Fissures of Santorini
    - Multiple small vertical gaps in anterior fibrocartilaginous wall of EAC provide increased flexibility to canal
    - Fissures are not identified on routine CT or MR imaging
    - Fissures may represent gateway for infection from EAC into parotid space and other proximal deep spaces of neck
    - Malignant otitis externa is thought to utilize this pathway in some cases to spread to adjacent infratemporal regions and to skull base
- **Medial bony component of EAC**
  - U-shaped tympanic bone forms bony EAC
  - Posterior wall shared with mastoid complex
  - Anterior wall shared with TMJ fossa
  - Medial margin defined by TM, which attaches superiorly to scutum and inferiorly to tympanic annulus
  - Medially, within bony EAC, skin is relatively thin, devoid of significant subcutaneous tissue, and tightly adherent to underlying bone
  - Skin in medial canal is continuous with outer layer of TM
- **Sensory innervation to external ear**
  - 4 cranial nerves and 2 upper cervical nerves contribute to sensory innervation
    - Considerable overlap and ambiguity in sensory distribution of these nerves
  - CNV3 supplies tragus, helical crus, anterosuperior wall of EAC, adjacent TM, and TMJ
  - CNVII: Supplies posterior-inferior portion of EAC and adjacent TM
  - CNIX: Supplies inner ear and inner surface of TM
  - CNX: Supplies inner ear, inner surface of TM, and concha (hollow next to ear canal)
  - C2 and C3: Innervate skin in front of and behind ear
    - Also skin of medial and lateral pinna and lobule
- **Arterial supply to external ear**
  - Posterior auricular artery gives off auricular branch
    - Auricular artery ascends behind ear to supply pinna cartilage
  - Superficial temporal artery gives off anterior auricular artery branch
    - Anterior auricular artery supplies anterior portion of pinna, lobule, and part of EAC

External Auditory Canal Anatomy

- o Occipital artery gives off auricular branch
  - – Auricular artery branch supplies back of concha
- **External ear nodal drainage**
  - o Pre- and postauricular nodal groups
  - o Parotid nodal group

ANATOMY IMAGING ISSUES

Questions

- What 2 bony structures help radiologists identify medial border of EAC?
  - o 2 bony structures that mark medial wall of EAC are scutum and tympanic annulus
    - – On coronal CT imaging of temporal bone, normal TM is barely visible
    - – Bony attachments of TMs are always visible
    - – Superior point of TM attachment is scutum
    - – Inferior point of TM attachment is tympanic annulus
- What is it about cartilaginous EAC that permits EAC infection to spread into subjacent deep facial space?
  - o Fissures of Santorini (multiple cartilaginous gaps in floor of lateral EAC) permit EAC infection to readily spread into adjacent deep facial spaces
    - – These fissures are responsible for increased EAC flexibility but have this unwelcome side effect
- If skin malignancy (squamous cell carcinoma, melanoma) affects external ear or adjacent scalp, where do nodal metastases 1st appear?
  - o Pre- and postauricular nodes (clinically apparent) along with intraparotid nodes (may be subclinical)
  - o Remember, bone CT of EAC will not show parotid nodes when present
    - – Acquire soft tissue algorithm image sequences for review of parotid and adjacent soft tissues
- What are most common causes of primary otalgia (origin of pain arises from ear itself)?
  - o Otomastoiditis, cholesteatoma, and foreign bodies lodged within ear canal
- Define term "referred otalgia" (ear pain)
  - o In referred otalgia, source of ear pain does not reside within ear but originates from sources distant from ear
    - – 50% of otalgia cases are referred
    - – In referred otalgia (convergence of common sensory pathways between complex sensory innervation supplying both ear and cranial nerves innervating head and neck), CNS is unable to correctly pinpoint location of pathology
- What are most common causes of referred otalgia?
  - o Any pathology residing within sensory net of CNV, CNVII, CNIX, CNX, and upper cervical nerves C2 and C3 can potentially cause pain (referred otalgia)
  - o Major areas include nose and sinus, pharynx, and oral cavity, including mandible and maxilla

Imaging Recommendations

- Axial high-resolution bone CT with coronal and sagittal reformations best study to evaluate bony integrity of temporal bone, including medial bony component of EAC
- High-resolution multiplanar MR to include T1 without fat saturation, T1 + gadolinium with fat saturation, and STIR images most comprehensive approach for evaluation of temporal bone/skull base pathology

- o Images should include TMJ, parotid gland, nasopharyngeal carotid space, clivus and preclival region

Imaging Approaches

- High-resolution CT with reformations provides preoperative mapping in cases of congenital external ear malformation (auricle/EAC atresia)
- For presumed mass in EAC or lateral temporal bone
  - o CT and MR are complimentary for evaluation of invasive neoplasm (skin or parotid) of temporal bone and surrounding structures
  - o T1 MR + gadolinium with fat saturation best to demonstrate entire extent of tumor
    - – Mastoid invasion
    - – TMJ involvement
    - – Marrow space invasion
    - – Perineural tumor spread of CNVII
  - o CT soft tissue neck completes evaluation for local adenopathy
- Malignant otitis externa and skull base osteomyelitis
  - o Infection may spread well beyond EAC in soft tissues of suprahyoid neck, extending to preclival soft tissues
  - o MR required to evaluate marrow of petrous apex and clivus
- Referred otalgia
  - o CECT best for evaluation of mucosal lesion of pharynx
  - o Scan needs to extend from skull base through hypopharynx

Imaging Pitfalls

- Clinical and imaging findings of neoplasm and invasive infection of EAC can overlap
  - o Biopsy and culture often necessary to confirm diagnosis of invasive process in region
- On CT, fibrocartilage and soft tissues near EAC (including parotid tissue) are difficult to differentiate from adjacent invasive neoplasm and extent of tumor may be overestimated

Temporal Bone and Skull Base

External Auditory Canal Anatomy

AURICLE AND EXTERNAL AUDITORY CANAL NORMAL ANATOMY

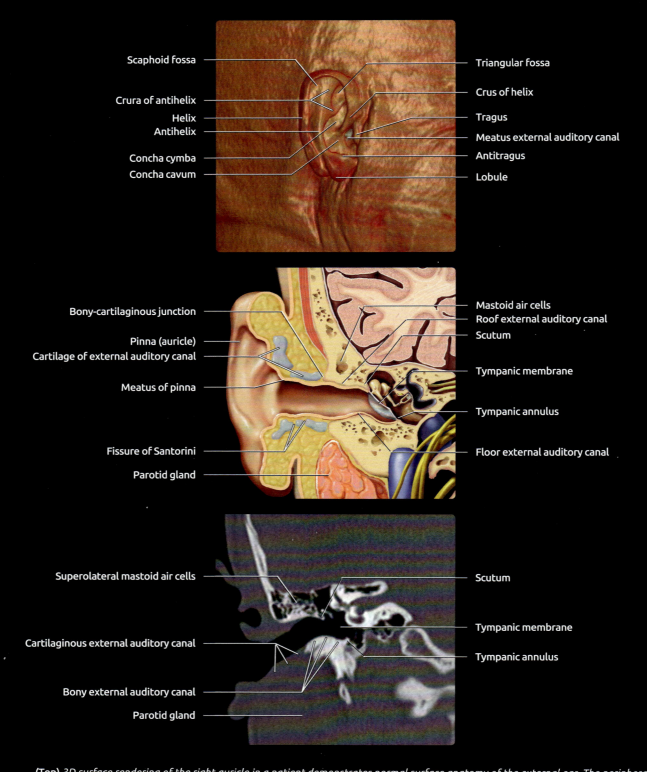

(Top) 3D surface rendering of the right auricle in a patient demonstrates normal surface anatomy of the external ear. The peripheral fold is called the helix, and the inner smaller fold is called the antihelix. Named depressions include triangular fossa, scaphoid fossa, and the concha composed of the cymba and the cavum. (Middle) Coronal graphic shows external and middle ear. The external auditory canal (EAC) is made up of lateral cartilaginous and medial bony components. Infection of the EAC can penetrate inferomedially to the skull base and associated spaces via the fissures of Santorini (gaps in the EAC cartilage). External ear and EAC lymphatic drainage is generally to the parotid nodal chain. The medial margin of the EAC is the tympanic membrane, which attaches to the scutum and tympanic annulus. (Bottom) Coronal bone CT through the right external ear reveals the medial wall of the EAC with its barely visible tympanic membrane attached to the scutum superiorly and to the tympanic annulus inferiorly. Notice that the inferior cartilaginous EAC abuts the parotid space. The superior bony EAC abuts the superolateral mastoid air cells. A large cholesteatoma may break into the roof of the bony EAC if it accesses these superolateral mastoid air cells.

External Auditory Canal Anatomy

NORMAL EXTERNAL AUDITORY CANAL AXIAL CT

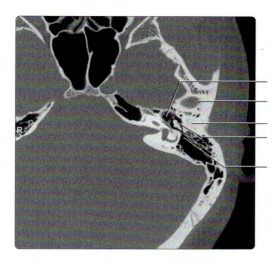

- Anterior epitympanic recess
- Mandibular fossa
- Roof external auditory canal
- Prussak space
- Aditus ad antrum

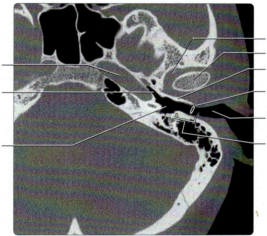

- Carotid canal
- Entrance to eustachian tube
- Tympanic membrane (barely perceptible)
- Temporomandibular joint
- Mandibular condyle
- Anterior wall external auditory canal
- Isthmus
- External auditory canal cartilaginous component
- External auditory canal bony component

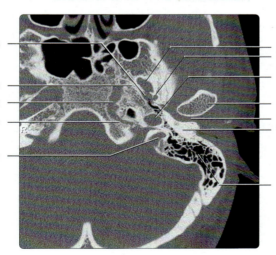

- Eustachian tube cartilaginous
- Petrosphenoid suture
- Foramen lacerum
- Petrooccipital fissure
- Jugular foramen
- Foramen ovale
- Foramen spinosum
- Proximal carotid canal
- Mandibular condyle
- Temporomandibular joint
- Floor of external auditory canal
- Mastoid air cells

(Top) Axial bone CT through the same plane as the roof of the EAC demonstrates dense cortical bone of the roof derived from the squamous portion of the temporal bone. The medial margin of the roof, along with the scutum, forms part of the lateral wall of the middle ear cavity. Prussak space is identified as a small lateral recess between the ossicles and the lateral wall of middle ear. Notice at this level, despite being at the upper margin of the EAC, the mandibular fossa begins to come into view. (Middle) Axial bone CT through the EAC is shown. The cartilaginous EAC represents the lateral 1/3 of the canal, and the bony component represents the medial 2/3. There is mild narrowing of the canal at the bony-cartilaginous junction, called the isthmus. The curvature in the axial plane is obvious in this case. The tympanic membrane (barely perceptible in this case) separates the EAC from the middle ear. The anterior wall of the EAC is relatively thin cortical bone and forms the posterior wall of the mandibular fossa. (Bottom) Axial cone CT demonstrates the relationship of the floor of the EAC (formed by cortical bone derived from tympanic component of the temporal bone) and the inferior structures of the temporal bone and temporomandibular joint (TMJ).

EXTERNAL AUDITORY CANAL SAGITTAL CT

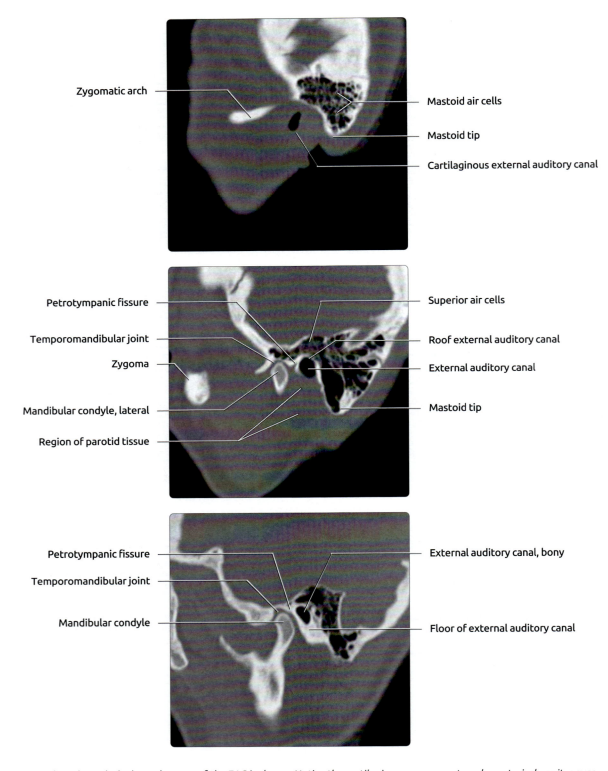

(Top) Sagittal CT through the lateral aspect of the EAC is shown. Notice the cartilaginous component angles anteriorly as it moves laterally. With bone windows, it is difficult to appreciate the relationship of the parotid gland to the inferior margin of the cartilaginous EAC. (Middle) Sagittal bone CT through the EAC and TMJ is obtained near the junction of the cartilaginous and bony components of the EAC. (Bottom) Sagittal bone CT through the EAC and TMJ demonstrates the U-shaped tympanic bone bordered posteriorly by the tympanomastoid suture/mastoid air cells and anteriorly by the petrotympanic fissure and TMJ. A blow to the mandible may readily fracture the bony EAC.

External Auditory Canal Anatomy

EXTERNAL AUDITORY CANAL SAGITTAL MR

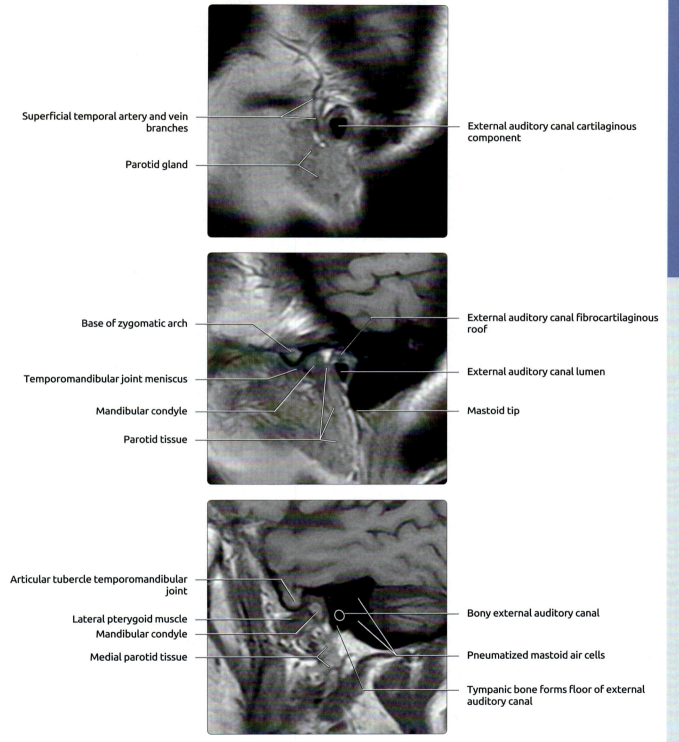

(Top) Sagittal T1 MR though the lateral aspect of the EAC shows the ring of fibrocartilaginous tissue surrounding the EAC that is patent and contains air. Notice the proximity of the EAC with the superior margin of the parotid gland. It may be difficult to differentiate an invasive skin malignancy of the EAC from invasive parotid malignancy. (Middle) Sagittal T1 MR through the TMJ near the junction of the cartilaginous and bony EAC shows the intimate relationship of the EAC to the TMJ, the mastoid air cells, and the superior medial parotid tissue. (Bottom) Sagittal T1 MR obtained through the TMJ is shown. The EAC is difficult to separate from the surrounding hypointensity created by pneumatized air cells and surrounding cortical bone of the tympanic bone. Some minimal parotid tissue can still be observed along the bony floor of the EAC.

Middle Ear-Mastoid Anatomy

TERMINOLOGY

Abbreviations

- Middle ear (ME)
- Temporal bone (T-bone)
- Tympanic membrane (TM)
- Facial nerve (CNVII)

Definitions

- ME
  - 6-sided cavity between external ear and inner ear, containing 3 ossicles and 2 muscles and opening to eustachian tube
- Ossicles
  - 3 smallest bones in human body (malleus, incus, and stapes) in ME that amplify sound vibrations, conveying them from TM to oval window

IMAGING ANATOMY

Anatomy Relationships

- ME (tympanic cavity) sits in T-bone between external and inner ears

Internal Contents

- **ME subdivisions**
  - **Epitympanum** (attic): Upper component of ME
    - **Tegmen tympani** ("roof of cavity"): Thin, bony roof between epitympanum and middle cranial fossa dura
    - **Prussak space**: Inferior-most aspect of lateral epitympanic recess
    - **Anterior epitympanic recess**: Epitympanic recess anteromedial to epitympanic cog; medial wall is anterior tympanic segment of CNVII
    - **Aditus ad antrum** ("entrance to cave"): Connects epitympanum of ME to mastoid antrum
    - Separated from mesotympanum by horizontal line drawn from tip of scutum to tympanic segment of CNVII
  - **Mesotympanum**: Middle component
    - Medial wall includes tympanic segment of CNVII, oval and round windows, and cochlear promontory
    - Separated from hypotympanum by horizontal line connecting tympanic annulus and base of cochlear promontory below
    - Posterior wall and adjacent space referred to as **retrotympanum**
  - **Hypotympanum**: Lower component
    - Shallow trough in floor of ME cavity
  - **Retrotympanum and posterior wall**
    - Includes 3 conspicuous structures from medial to lateral
      - Sinus tympani, pyramidal eminence, and CNVII recess
    - Sinus tympani
      - Posterior outpouching of posterior wall lying medial to pyramidal eminence, stapedius muscle, and FN and lateral to posterior semicircular canal (PSCC) and vestibule
      - Medial to pyramidal eminence, stapedius muscle, and CNVII
      - Lateral to PSSC and vestibule

- Surgical exposure of this medial region of retrotympanum can be difficult due to CNVII and stapedial muscle; can be site of residual disease (cholesteatoma)
    - **Pyramidal eminence**
      - Small, pyramid-shaped mound of bone housing belly of stapedius muscle
      - Base of pyramid is posterior and apex is directed anteriorly
      - Pyramidal eminence is just lateral to sinus tympani and medial to CNVII recess and proximal mastoid segment of CNVII
      - Inferior to pyramidal eminence is tiny subpyramidal space
    - **FN recess**
      - Medial border is posterior genu and proximal mastoid segment of CNVII
      - Lateral border is posterior annulus of TM
- **ME muscles**
  - Tensor tympani and stapedius are striated muscles that operate synergistically to dampen sound vibrations of ossicles
  - **Tensor tympani muscle**
    - Originates from cartilaginous margin of eustachian tube, passes through its own bony canal in wall of anterior ME, and parallels bony eustachian tube
    - On coronal CT, found anteroinferior to anterior tympanic segment of CNVII
    - Tendon passes through cochleariform process and then turns laterally to cross ME to attach to neck of malleus
    - Innervated by branch of mandibular nerve (CNV3) via otic ganglion
    - Measure 2.5 cm in length
  - **Stapedius muscle**
    - Muscle belly found just medial to upper mastoid segment CNVII in base of pyramidal eminence
    - Tendon emerges from apex of pyramidal eminence, then attaches to head or posterior crus of stapes
    - Innervated by CNVII motor branch of mastoid segment
    - Measures ~ 6 mm in length
- **Ossicles of ME**
  - **Malleus** (hammer)
    - Location: Anterior epitympanum and mesotympanum
    - Components: Head, neck, lateral process, anterior process, and manubrium
    - Ligaments and tendons: Superior, anterior, and lateral mallear ligaments; tendon of tensor tympani muscle
  - **Incus** (anvil)
    - Location: Posterior epitympanum and mesotympanum
    - Components: Body; **short, long, and lenticular processes**
    - Ligament: Posterior incudal ligament
  - **Stapes** (stirrup)
    - Location: Medial mesotympanum
    - Components: Head, anterior and posterior crura, and footplate
    - Tendon: Stapedius muscle tendon

Middle Ear-Mastoid Anatomy

- **Stapes superstructure**: Stapes portion derived from 2nd branchial arch = head, crura, tympanic portion of footplate
  - Vestibular portion of footplate of stapes and annular ligament derived from otic capsule
- **TM**
  - Separates external ear from ME
  - Upper 1/3 = **pars flaccida**; lower 2/3 = **pars tensa**
  - Malleus umbo and lateral process embedded in TM
  - 3 layers of TM
    - External layer continuous with skin of external auditory canal (EAC) = ectoderm
    - Inner layer continuous with ME mucosa = endoderm
    - Intermediate fibrous layer = mesoderm
  - Superior attachment: **Scutum** (Latin for "shield")
  - Inferior attachment: **Tympanic annulus**
    - Useful landmark separating hypotympanum medially from inferomedial EAC laterally
- **Medial wall relationships**
  - **Lateral semicircular canal (LSC)**
    - 1 of 3 different bony semicircular canals in each inner ear housing corresponding semicircular ducts
    - Positioned horizontally from vestibule and projects laterally, causing distinct bony ridge along medial wall of epitympanum
    - Susceptible to erosion by ME pathologies (cholesteatoma) and fistula can occur
  - **CNVII nerve canal (tympanic segment)**
    - Tympanic segment of facial nerve canal is tubular bony covering of tympanic segment of nerve itself
    - Begins at geniculate ganglion and runs posteriorly, passing above cochleariform process
    - Runs parallel to and below LSC and above oval window
    - Posterior part lies superolateral to pyramidal eminence and passes into 2nd genu
    - Focal dehiscence of tympanic canal considered normal variant, occurring in as much as 20-25% of adults, and most commonly occurring just above oval window
  - **Cochlear promontory**
    - Rounded, shallow protrusion arising from central aspect of medial wall and projecting into mesotympanum
    - Formed by lateral-most bony covering of basal turn of cochlea
    - Located anterior and inferior to oval window; anterior to round window niche
  - **Oval window niche**
    - Oval window: Opening between ME and vestibule; covered by membrane
    - Stapes footplate occupies window and is circumferentially attached by annular ligament
    - Stapes moves in and out against oval window, causing vibrations of adjacent perilymph, and sound waves are transmitted through scala vestibuli
    - Tympanic facial canal forms roof of oval window niche
    - Includes tiny space surrounding footplate and stapes itself
  - **Round window niche**
    - Round window: Tiny opening of scala tympani of cochlea into posterior aspect of medial wall of ME

- Sits in small, pouch-shaped recess (round window niche) on medial wall, just posterior to promontory
- Scala tympani separated from ME by membrane covering round window
- Sound waves travel from cochlea to round window membrane

ANATOMY IMAGING ISSUES

Questions

- What are 3 important structures across posterior wall of mesotympanum?
  - From medial to lateral: Sinus tympani, pyramidal eminence, and facial recess
  - Sinus tympani may be site of cholesteatoma recurrence; can be blind spot during routine mastoidectomy
  - Pyramidal eminence contains belly of stapedius muscle just medial to mastoid segment of CNVII
  - CNVII recess has mastoid segment of CNVII just posterior to it
- What 2 tendons stabilize ossicle motion during loud noise? Innervation of each muscle? Ossicle attachment point for each?
  - Tensor tympani tendon
    - Tensor tympani muscle innervated by CNV3
    - Tensor tympani tendon attaches to body of malleus
  - Stapedius tendon
    - Stapedius muscle innervated by CNVII motor branch off of mastoid segment
    - Stapedius tendon attaches to hub of stapes or area of incudostapedial articulation

EMBRYOLOGY

Embryologic Events

- EAC forms from 1st branchial groove
- ME forms from 1st branchial pouch
- Ossicles form from 1st & 2nd branchial arches
  - 1st branchial arch: Head and neck of malleus, body and short process of incus
  - 2nd branchial arch: Manubrium of malleus, long and lenticular processes of incus, stapes superstructure

Practical Implications

- EAC atresia is 1st and 2nd branchial apparatus lesion
- Ossicular rotation and deformity part of imaging appearance
- Oval window atresia may or may not be associated with EAC atresia

Temporal Bone and Skull Base

Middle Ear-Mastoid Anatomy

CORONAL GRAPHICS

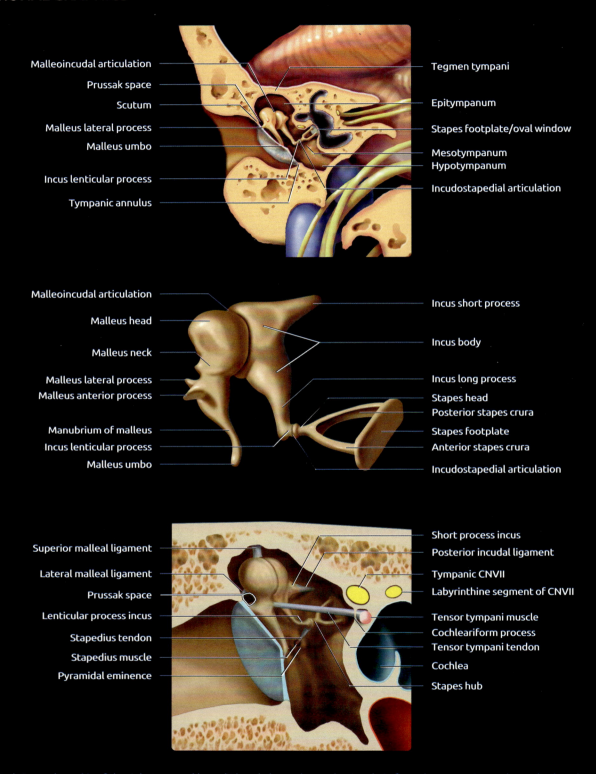

(Top) Coronal graphic of the right temporal bone (T-bone) shows the conductive chain from the tympanic membrane (TM) to the oval window. The TM is attached superiorly to the scutum and inferiorly to the tympanic annulus. The 2 joints between the ossicles are the malleoincudal and incudostapedial articulations. **(Middle)** Graphic of right middle ear (ME) ossicles viewed from the front shows that the anterolateral malleus has a head, neck, and manubrium with lateral and anterior processes. The incus has a large body and short, long, and lenticular processes. The stapes has a head, crura, and footplate. **(Bottom)** Coronal graphic highlights the ME ligaments and tendons. The tensor tympani tendon turns 90° at the cochleariform process to cross the medial ME and attach to the medial body of the malleus. The stapedius tendon emerges from the pyramidal eminence to attach to the stapes hub area. The 4 ossicle ligaments include the superior, lateral, and anterior (not shown) malleal ligaments and the incudal ligament.

Middle Ear-Mastoid Anatomy

MIDDLE EAR: MEDIAL AND LATERAL WALLS

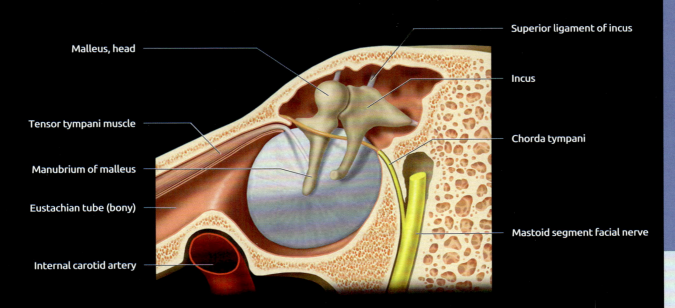

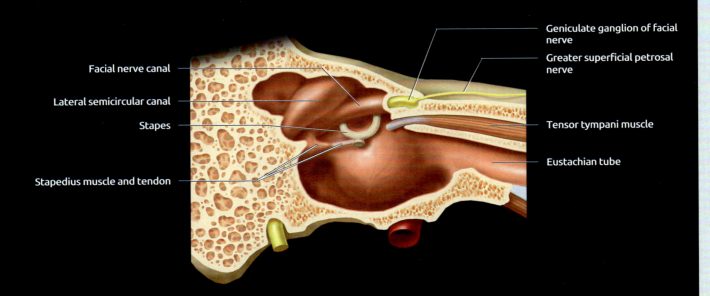

(Top) *Internal view of lateral wall of the ME cavity is shown. The TM represents the dominant structure along the lateral wall of the ME cavity. The central aspect of the membrane is attached to the manubrium of the malleus. Notice the relationship of the chorda tympani nerve as it leaves the mastoid segment of facial nerve, ascends through the T-bone, and then passes along the inner margin of the TM.* **(Bottom)** *In this illustration, the structures of the medial wall are represented. The facial nerve canal is covered by a thin epithelial membrane and bone, passing just superior to the oval window. The stapes attaches to the oval window. The dominant feature of the medial wall is the cochlear promontory that bulges into the ME cavity. The round window niche is identified posterior and inferior to the promontory.*

Middle Ear-Mastoid Anatomy

AXIAL BONE CT

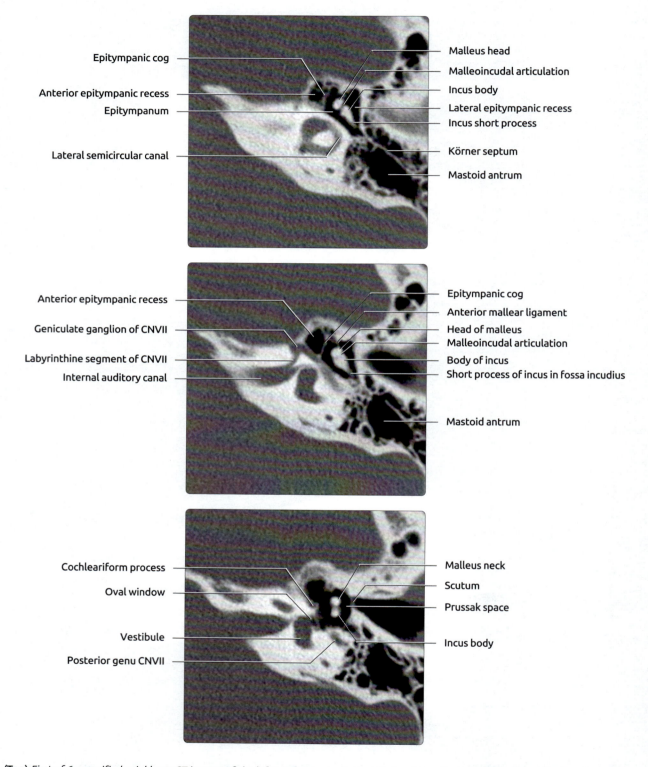

(Top) First of 6 magnified axial bone CT images of the left ear from superior to inferior shows the malleus head articulating with the body of the incus at the malleoincudal articulation. The lateral epitympanic recess is seen lateral to the ossicles. The short process of the incus is pointing into the aditus ad antrum. Notice the Körner septum separating the lateral mastoid air cells from the mastoid antrum. (Middle) In this image through the level of the geniculate ganglion, it is possible to see the anterior epitympanic recess defined by the epitympanic cog laterally and the anterior tympanic segment of the facial nerve. Diseases affecting this area may cause facial nerve paralysis. Surgical removal of the bony cog could also result in facial nerve paralysis. (Bottom) At the level of the oval window, the malleus neck and incus body are seen in the upper mesotympanum. The facial nerve transitions from its tympanic segment to its mastoid segment via the posterior genu.

Middle Ear-Mastoid Anatomy

AXIAL BONE CT

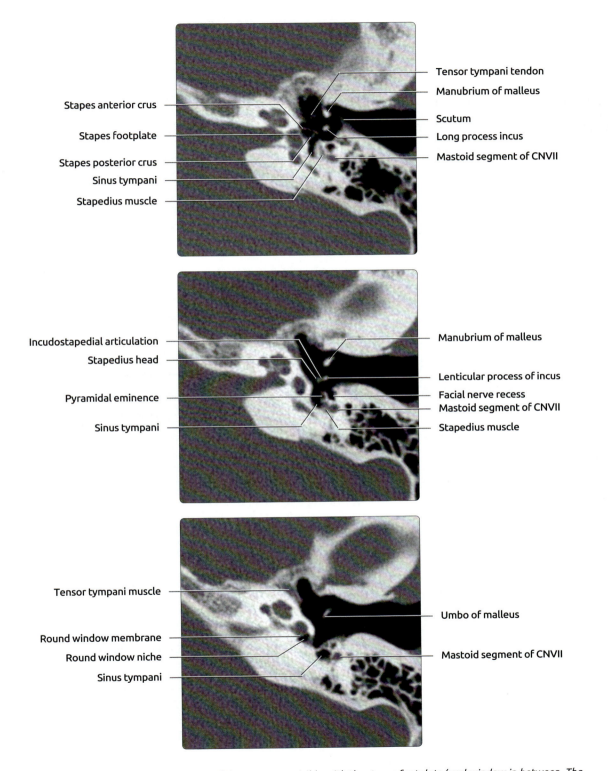

(Top) In this image, the anterior and posterior crura of the stapes are visible with the stapes footplate/oval window in between. The tensor tympani tendon can be seen reaching from the cochleariform process to the manubrium of the malleus. Both the stapedius muscle and the mastoid segment of the facial nerve are seen in the posterior tympanum wall. **(Middle)** In this image, the ridges and recesses of the posterior tympanum are well seen. From medial to lateral, they are the sinus tympani, pyramidal eminence, and facial nerve recess. Behind these structures, observe the stapedius muscle and the mastoid segment of CNVII. Note the incudostapedial articulation connecting the lenticular process of the incus to the head of the stapes. **(Bottom)** The inferior tip of the manubrium is the umbo. At the round window membrane level, the mastoid segment of CNVII is now seen without the stapedius muscle.

Middle Ear-Mastoid Anatomy

CORONAL BONE CT

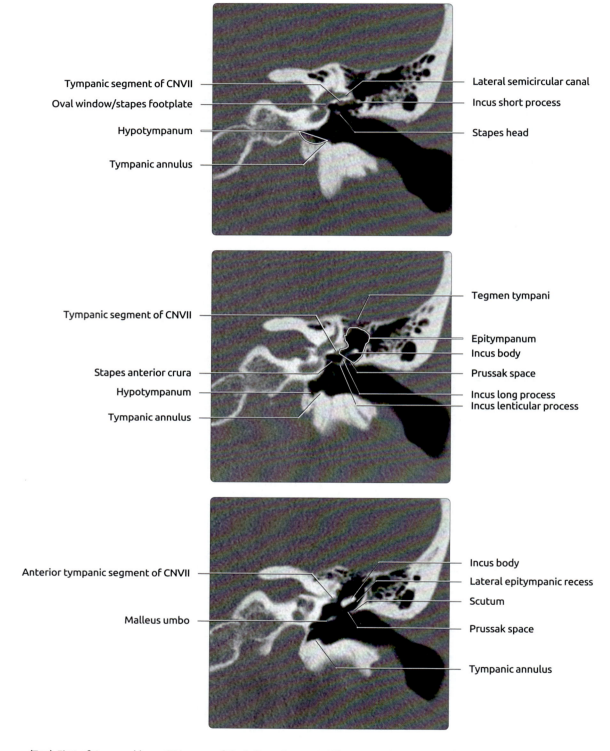

(Top) First of 6 coronal bone CT images of the left ear (presented from posterior to anterior) passes through the oval window. The hypotympanum is the inferior portion of the ME cavity inferior to the line drawn between the base of the cochlear promontory and the tympanic annulus tip. (Middle) At the anterior oval window level, the body, long process, and lenticular process of the incus are seen. The epitympanum is the ME cavity seen above the line between the tympanic portion of CNVII and the scutum. The roof of the epitympanum is the tegmen tympani, whereas the lateral epitympanum is the Prussak space. (Bottom) In this image, the body of the incus is seen at the same level as the umbo of the malleus. The TM is barely visible strung between the superior scutum and inferior tympanic annulus. The epitympanum is the ME cavity area above a line drawn between the tip of the scutum and the tympanic segment of the facial nerve.

Middle Ear-Mastoid Anatomy

CORONAL BONE CT

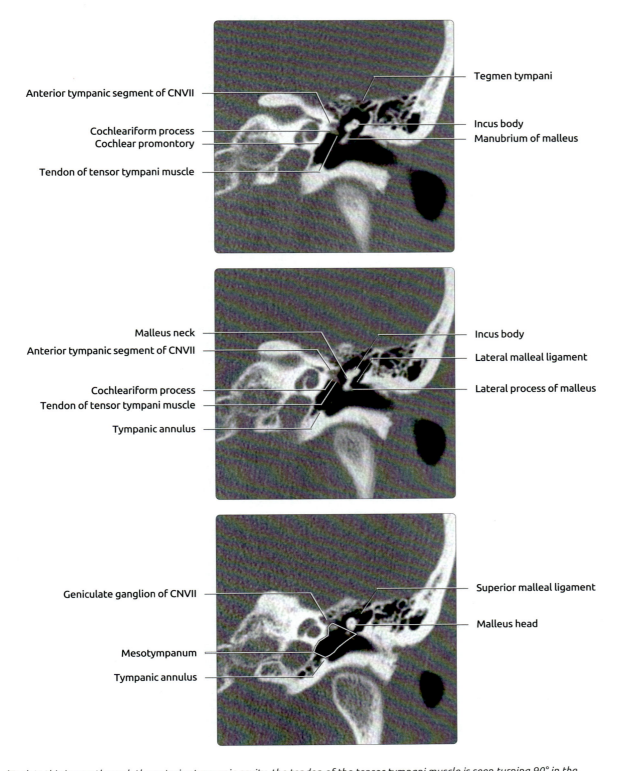

(Top) In this image through the anterior tympanic cavity, the tendon of the tensor tympani muscle is seen turning 90° in the cochleariform process and then projecting over to the manubrium of the malleus. (Middle) The lateral process of the malleus and the umbo are both embedded in the medial surface of the TM. The tendon of the tensor tympani muscle inserts on the medial surface of the manubrium of the malleus. (Bottom) In this image, the head of the malleus can be seen in the anterior epitympanum. The mesotympanum can be defined as the ME cavity below the line connecting the tympanic segment of the facial nerve and the inferior tip of the scutum and above the line connecting the superior tip of the tympanic annulus and the inferior margin of the cochlear promontory.

Inner Ear Anatomy

TERMINOLOGY

Definitions

- Inner ear consists of cochlea, vestibule, semicircular canals (SCCs), associated interconnecting endolymphatic and perilymphatic compartments, and surrounding bony otic capsule
- Inner ear houses sensorineural structures for sound detection (cochlea) and mechanoreceptors for spatial orientation and balance (vestibule and SCCs)

IMAGING ANATOMY

Overview

- **Inner ear**
  - Inner ear also called labyrinth given its complex and intercommunicating internal spaces
  - Inner ear grossly appears as architecturally complex bony compartment (bony labyrinth) that predominantly contains fluid
  - Internal fluid spaces are further organized into distinct functional compartments: Membranous labyrinth and perilymphatic labyrinth
- **Bony labyrinth**
  - Essentially otic capsule and internal osseous architecture
  - Dense enchondral bone that surrounds and defines cochlea, vestibule, and SCCs
  - Hardest bone in body with trilamellar arrangement; contains islands of modified cartilage and high mineral content
- **Membranous labyrinth**
  - Consists of interconnecting, thin-walled, saccular and tubular structures that contain endolymph
  - Is specific site within inner ear for specialized neural receptors for sound (cochlea) and balance (vestibule and SCCs)
  - In cochlea, membranous labyrinth is represented by central tubular canal called scala media (cochlear duct) that contains spiral organ of Corti
  - In vestibule, membranous labyrinth is represented by sac-like components: Utricle and saccule
    - Utricle and saccule each contain focal area (macule) of specialized mechanoreceptors that contain hair cells capable of detecting acceleration and gravitational pull
  - In each SCC, membranous labyrinth consists of tubular compartment called semicircular duct
    - Each semicircular duct contains dilated region (ampulla) that contains crista
    - Cristae are additional mechanoreceptors containing hair cells capable of detecting angular acceleration in multiple directions
  - Endolymphatic duct (ELD) and sac (ELS) represent posterior extensions of membranous labyrinth
    - ELD arises from crus common at junction of posterior and superior SCC and extends posteriorly to ELS interdural structure along posterior petrous ridge
  - **Endolymph** is functional fluid within structures of membranous labyrinth, which bathes and nourishes its sensory epithelium
- **Perilymphatic labyrinth**
  - Fluid-filled space interposed between membranous labyrinth and inner periosteum of bony labyrinth
  - **Perilymph** composed of CSF-like fluid
  - Cochlea contains 2 distinct tubular components of perilymphatic labyrinth: Scala tympani and scala vestibuli
  - Vestibule contains perilymphatic cistern of perilymphatic labyrinth; rounded area containing perilymph surrounds utricle and saccule
  - Thin perilymphatic spaces are also identified in SCCs
  - Perilymphatic labyrinth also includes fissula ante fenestram, fossula post fenestram, and periotic duct

Internal Contents

- **Cochlea**
  - Portion of inner ear responsible for hearing
  - Term is derived from Greek word "kokhlos," meaning land snail
  - Essentially partitioned tube arranged in spiral (snail-like) configuration, making ~ 2.5 turns around central perforated osseous structure called modiolus
  - Basilar turn bulges into medial wall of middle ear cavity, creating promontory
  - Basilar turn merges with vestibule
  - **Modiolus**
    - Conical, central bony axis of cochlea consisting of spongiform bone
    - Modiolus is widest at its base: ~ 4 mm
    - Base is directed toward internal auditory canal and is perforated by branches of cochlear nerve
    - Cochlear nerve fibers traverse modiolus, branching and extending to spiral lamina
  - **Osseous spiral lamina**
    - Thin bony plate projecting outward as it spirals around modiolus from base to apex
    - Provides supportive function and allows organized transmission of cochlear nerve fibers to each cochlear segment
    - Nerve fibers of cochlear nerve (both afferent and efferent) extend through medial aspects of spiral lamina
    - Thin bony plate tapers laterally; lateral margin connects to medial aspect of **basilar membrane**
    - Basilar membrane attaches laterally to spiral ligament at inner margin of otic capsule
    - Basilar membrane together with osseous lamina forms partition between 2 chambers: Scala media and posterior scala tympani
    - Osseous spiral lamina is readily identified on high-resolution CT and MR imaging
  - **Spiral ganglion**
    - Spiral ganglion represents distinct population of primary sensory neurons critical to transmission of sound information to brain
    - Cells are located in modiolus, arranged in spiral configuration, paralleling base of spiral lamina
    - Composed of bipolar cells
    - Each cell body emits peripheral axon extending toward organ of Corti and central axon that projects into auditory nerve
  - **3 spiral chambers of cochlea**
    - **Scala media** (cochlear duct)

Inner Ear Anatomy

- □ Separated from anterior scala vestibuli by vestibular (Reissner) membrane
- □ Separated from posterior scala tympani by basilar membrane
- □ Contains organ of Corti (hearing apparatus) and endolymph
- □ Smallest of 3 chambers and not identified on routine imaging
- **Scala vestibuli**
  - □ Anterior chamber containing perilymph
  - □ Posteriorly and medially within inner ear, scala vestibuli passes through basilar turn into perilymphatic space of vestibule
  - □ Sound vibration of stapes is transmitted to **oval window** and into vestibule
  - □ Sound wave travels through perilymph through scala vestibuli to cochlear apex
  - □ At apex, scala vestibuli is connected to scala tympani by small opening; **helicotrema**
- **Scala tympani**
  - □ Posterior chamber, containing perilymph
  - □ Allows sound waves to travel back from cochlear apex to **round window**
  - □ Round window is opening covered by round window membrane and is 2-3 mm long and ~ 1.5 mm wide
  - □ Scala tympani is intended chamber target for cochlear electrode placement
  - o **Cochlear nerve canal**
    - Opening to base of cochlea from internal auditory canal fundus
- **Vestibule**
  - o Contains perilymph sleeve around vestibular membranous labyrinth
  - o Utricle and saccule are principal vestibular membranous labyrinth components
  - o SCCs arise from superior, posterior, and lateral margins of vestibule
- **SCCs**
  - o Each bony SCC contains outer perilymphatic sleeve and semicircular duct
  - o Superior SCC: Bony covering is **arcuate eminence**
    - Subarcuate artery runs under SCC arch to supply inner ear
    - In child < 5 years old, artery is surrounded by dura and CSF (**subarcuate canaliculus**); involutes by 5 years
    - In adult, artery canal is called **petromastoid canal**
  - o Posterior SCC: Superior SCC meets posterior SCC at **crus communis**
    - Vestibular aqueduct (VA) connects to vestibular inner ear at crus communis
  - o Lateral SCC: Projects laterally into middle ear cavity
- **ELD and ELS**
  - o Found within bony VA
    - VA connects crus communis to fovea (cup-shaped area along posterior temporal bone wall)
    - Bony VA normal dimensions: < 1 mm at midpoint and < 2 mm at operculum (VA opening into fovea)
  - o ELD and ELS project from crus communis of vestibule posterolaterally to fovea along posterior inner ear wall

- ELD transition to ELS is defined by change in wall cell architecture (not visible with imaging)
- ELD is short proximal component connected to crus communis
- ELS is longer with both intraosseous and intradural (fovea area) components

- **Inner ear nerves**
  - o Cochlear nerve: Afferent hearing fibers from bipolar spiral ganglion, which receives afferent information from organ of Corti, coalesce into cochlear nerve
  - o Superior vestibular nerve: Afferent balance fibers from utricle, superior SCC, and lateral SCC coalesce at superior vestibular ganglion into superior vestibular nerve
  - o Inferior vestibular nerve: Afferent balance fibers from saccule and posterior SCC coalesce at inferior vestibular ganglion into inferior vestibular nerve

ANATOMY IMAGING ISSUES

Questions

- Describe process of creating hearing event
  - o Sound focused and amplified by external ear
  - o Tympanic membrane transmits sound to ossicles
  - o Movement of stapes → transmission of fluid waves via oval window through vestibule to cochlear recess
  - o Cochlear recess fluid wave transmitted to scala vestibuli (ascending spiral) of cochlea
  - o Fluid waves (sound waves) enter perilymph of scala vestibuli, then are transmitted via vestibular membrane into scala media endolymph
  - o Displacement of basilar membrane stimulates hair cell receptors in organ of Corti
  - o Hair cell movement generates electronic potentials converted to action potentials in cochlear nerve
    - High-frequency sounds converted at cochlear base
    - Low-frequency sounds converted at cochlear apex

Imaging Recommendations

- Temporal bone CT: Evaluates bony aspects of cochlear diseases
  - o Otosclerosis, labyrinthine ossificans, bony details of complex inner ear dysplasias
- Temporal bone MR: Evaluates membranous labyrinth diseases
  - o T1 C+ MR: Labyrinthitis, intralabyrinthine schwannoma
  - o T2 high-resolution MR: Cochlear nerve size in cochlear implant candidates

CLINICAL IMPLICATIONS

Clinical Importance

- Cochlea responsible for hearing as it transforms fluid motion into electrical energy
- Any disease that affects cochlear nuclei, cochlear nerve, or cochlea can cause sensorineural hearing loss

Temporal Bone and Skull Base

Inner Ear Anatomy

GRAPHICS

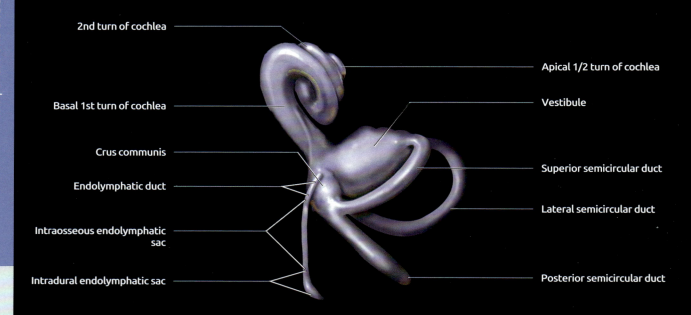

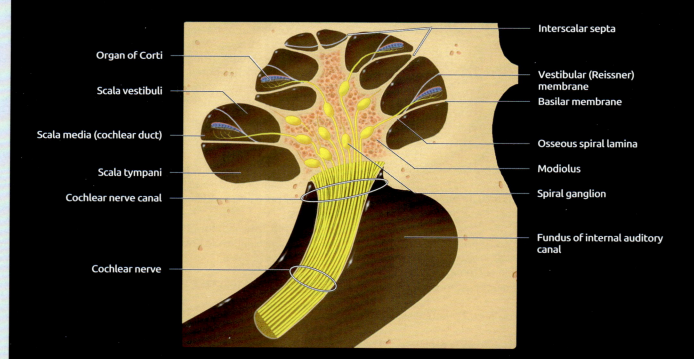

(Top) Graphic shows fluid spaces of inner ear viewed from above. The endolymph-filled structures include the vestibular utricle and saccule, semicircular ducts, scala media of cochlea, and endolymphatic duct and sac. The perilymph-filled areas include the vestibule surrounding the utricle and saccule (between semicircular ducts and walls of the semicircular canals) within the vestibular aqueduct surrounding the endolymphatic duct and within the scala tympani and vestibuli. Notice that the crus communis is the site of endolymphatic duct entry into the more central membranous labyrinth. (Bottom) Graphic of axial view of the cochlea shows the 3 scalar chambers: Scala media, scala vestibuli, and scala tympani. Note that the bipolar cell bodies of the spiral ganglia within the modiolus send distal fibers to the organ of Corti and proximal fibers into the cochlear nerve. The cochlear nerve passes through the cochlear nerve canal into the fundus of the internal auditory canal (IAC).

Inner Ear Anatomy

AXIAL T2 MR

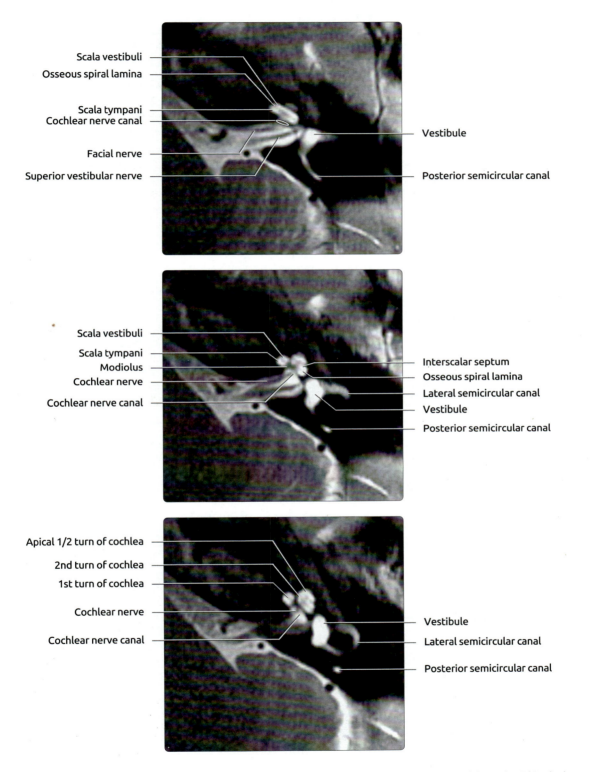

(Top) First of 3 axial T2 MR images of the inner ear from superior to inferior reveals a high-signal membranous labyrinth within the low-signal bony labyrinth. The cochlea is divided by osseous spiral lamina into an anterior scala vestibuli and posterior scala tympani. Note that the scala vestibuli and tympani have equal transverse dimensions. (Middle) In this image through the mid cochlea, the cochlear nerve is visible in the anteroinferior IAC. The cochlear nerve exits the fundus of the IAC to enter the cochlea through the cerebrospinal fluid-filled cochlear nerve canal. The modiolus is visible as an intermediate-intensity structure at the cochlear base. (Bottom) The 1st and 2nd turns and the apical 1/2 turn of the cochlea are all visible on this image. Also notice the cochlear nerve in the cochlear nerve canal on its way to the modiolus.

Inner Ear Anatomy

LONGITUDINAL AND TRANSVERSE CT REFORMATIONS

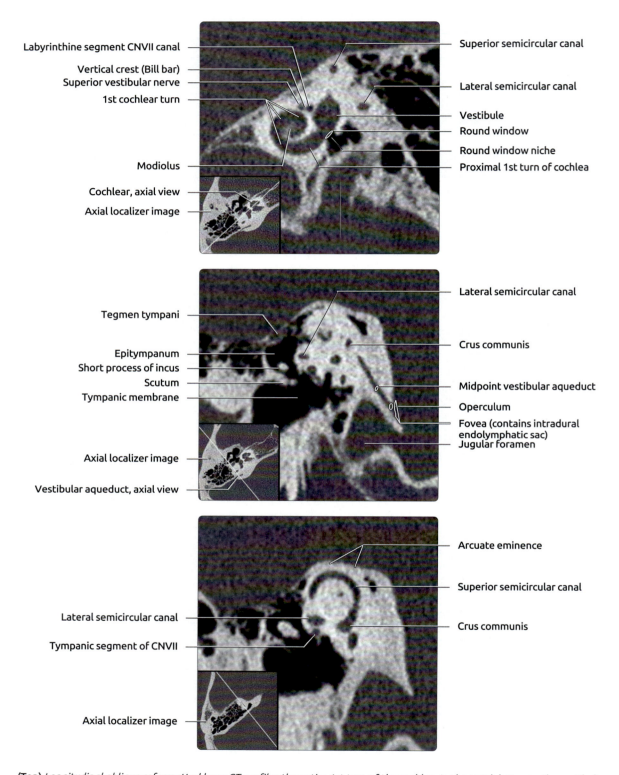

(Top) Longitudinal oblique reformatted bone CT profiles the entire 1st turn of the cochlea. In the notch between the vestibule and the apical aspect of the 1st cochlear turn, notice the superior vestibular nerve canal and the labyrinthine segment of the facial nerve (CNVII) canal. Such a view is helpful in evaluating cochlear implants. **(Middle)** Transverse oblique bone CT of the right ear profiles the bony vestibular aqueduct (VA) as it progresses from the fovea (bony cup in posterior wall where the intradural endolymphatic sac resides) toward the crus communis of the more central inner ear. Normal VA measurements are < 1 mm at the midpoint and < 2 mm at the operculum. **(Bottom)** Transverse oblique bone CT (1 mm) reformat created along the line of the superior semicircular canal demonstrates the entire span of this canal with the bony ridge above it (arcuate eminence). This view can be very helpful in delineating the extent of superior semicircular canal dehiscence when present.

Inner Ear Anatomy

AXIAL BONE CT

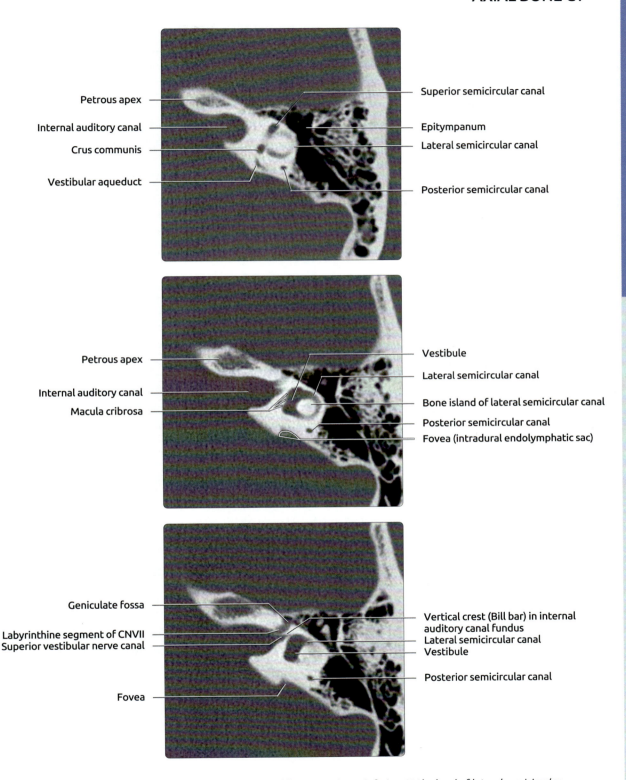

(Top) Series of 6 axial CT images of the left temporal bone is presented from superior to inferior. At the level of lateral semicircular canal, the bony VA is seen turning anteriorly to connect with the more central inner ear at the crus communis. (Middle) At the level of the lateral semicircular canal, the fovea of the bony VA along the posterior wall of the temporal bone houses the intradural endolymphatic sac. Remember that bone CT permits visualization of the bony labyrinth whereas MR shows the radiologist the membranous labyrinth structures. (Bottom) Axial bone CT demonstrates the superior vestibular nerve canal as it pierces the macula cribrosa of the vestibule. Notice that anterior to the superior nerve vestibular canal, the vertical crest in the IAC fundus and the labyrinthine segment of CNVII are visible. This anatomic distinction is the key to differentiate facial nerve schwannoma and superior vestibular nerve schwannoma, an important surgical distinction.

Inner Ear Anatomy

AXIAL BONE CT

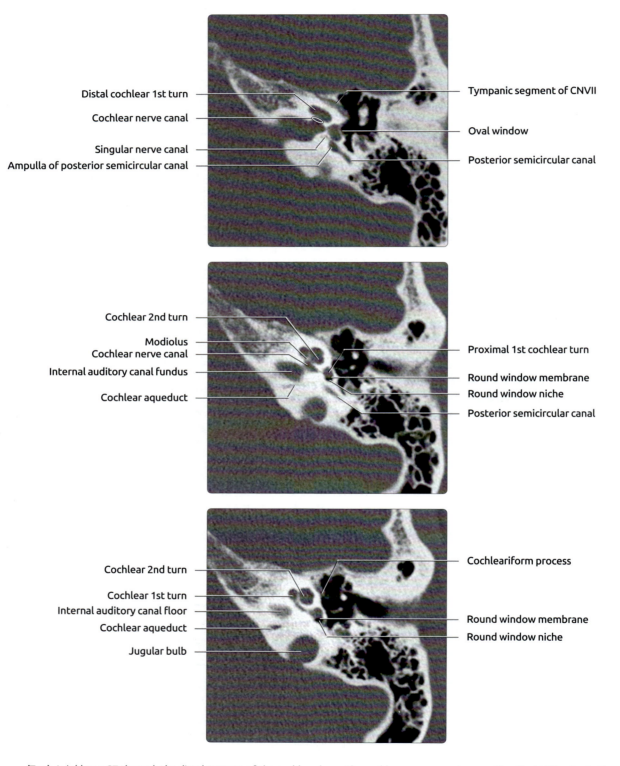

(Top) Axial bone CT through the distal 1st turn of the cochlea shows the cochlear nerve canal connecting the IAC fundus to the cochlea. The singular nerve canal is visible leaving the posterior wall of the IAC and connecting to the ampulla of the posterior semicircular canal. (Middle) Axial bone CT through the round window reveals the proximal cochlear aqueduct on its way to connect to the proximal 1st turn of the cochlea. The cochlear aqueduct contains perilymph. It connects the subarachnoid space and the scala tympani of the cochlea. It is likely vestigial as there is no significant function associated with this structure. (Bottom) Axial bone CT through the floor of the IAC shows the entire proximal 1/2 of the 1st turn of the cochlea. The round window membrane is visible between the 1st turn of the cochlea and the air-filled round window niche. The proximal cochlear aqueduct is seen along the posterior wall of the temporal bone anteromedial to the jugular bulb.

Inner Ear Anatomy

ANATOMIC-PATHOLOGIC CORRELATION

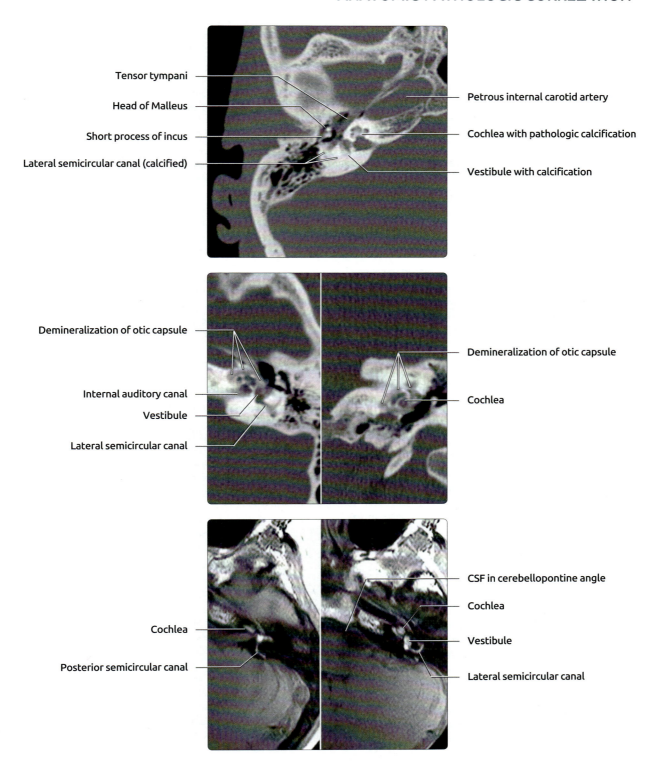

(Top) Axial high-resolution CT scan through the temporal bone with labyrinthitis ossificans in a patient with a previous history of meningitis and subsequent hearing loss demonstrates relative hyperdensity in the cochlea, vestibule, and semicircular canals, compatible with calcification. Severe infection in the inner ear can result in granulation tissue, subsequent fibrosis, and ultimately progressive ossification and profound hearing loss. (Middle) Axial and coronal CT images of retrofenestral otosclerosis in a 50-year-old woman with bilateral mixed hearing loss demonstrates fulminant retrofenestral otosclerosis with extensive demineralization of the otic capsule. The architecture of the inner ear compartments is preserved. (Bottom) Contiguous axial T1-weighted images through the left temporal bone in a patient with sudden loss of hearing in the left ear demonstrates diffuse hyperintensity throughout the membranous labyrinth. The signal characteristics of T1 hyperintensity in the absence of contrast, and the abrupt onset of symptoms, are compatible with labyrinthine hemorrhage. In general, fluid within the membranous labyrinth should follow CSF signal on all sequences.

Petrous Apex Anatomy

TERMINOLOGY

Abbreviations

- Petrous apex (PA), internal carotid artery (ICA), petrooccipital fissure (POF)

Definitions

- Petrous bone: Pyramid-shaped, medial portion of temporal bone (T-bone)
  - Contains inner ear, internal auditory canal (IAC), labyrinthine segment, and anterior genu facial nerve canal and PA
- PA: Portion of petrous bone that is **anteromedial to inner ear and IAC**

IMAGING ANATOMY

Overview

- PA is pyramidal-shaped, medial projection of petrous portion of T-bone
- Given unique location, PA is intimately related to several important anatomic structures, including POF, clivus, Meckel cave, cavernous sinus, and jugular foramen
- Normal imaging appearance on CT or MR is highly dependent on presence of marrow space vs. pneumatized air cells within PA
- **Bone and bone marrow of PA**
  - Most commonly, PA is composed of rim of cortical bone and intrinsic trabecular bone containing bone marrow
  - PA marrow signal on MR characterized by T1 hyperintensity due to marrow fat
  - Abnormal marrow signal can be related to number of causes, ranging from benign (red marrow conversion) to malignant (myeloma, metastatic disease)
- **Pneumatization of PA**
  - Occurs in 9-30% when epithelial-lined air cells develop as medial communications from mastoid air cells
  - Highly variable in extent and can be asymmetric in 5%
  - Air cells of PA are susceptible to similar pathologic processes that occur in mastoid, including obstruction, opacification, inflammation, and infection

Extent

- PA is anatomic subunit of petrous bone, anteromedial to inner ear
- PA is shaped like triangular pyramid with 3 distinct sides, directed medially toward central skull base
- Base is formed at junction with lateral portion of petrous bone and merges with squamous and mastoid segments of T-bone
- Along superior margin of PA, there is narrow ridge (petrous ridge) that extends from apical tip to lateral petrous bone
- Petrous ridge is formed by fusion of 2 sloped surfaces (2 sides of triangular pyramid), ventral slope and dorsal slope
- Ventral slope forms posterior wall of middle cranial fossa
- Posterior slope forms anterior wall of posterior fossa
- 3rd (inferior) side is roughly horizontal, best identified viewing extracranial surface of skull from below, and forms part of skull base

Anatomy Relationships

- **Petrous carotid canal**
  - ICA enters base of petrous bone (becoming petrous segment)
  - ICA travels vertically for ~ 8 mm before turning horizontally (posterior genu) at level of cochlea and then travels anteromedially toward apex through carotid canal
  - ICA emerges from endocranial carotid canal through irregular bony opening, just above horizontal layer of cartilage that bridges foramen lacerum; turns upward (anterior genu), becoming short lacerum segment
  - Sympathetic fibers travel along periphery of ICA through carotid canal
  - Petrous ICA gives rise to 2 small arteries: Caroticotympanic artery and artery of pterygoid (vidian) canal
- **Foramen lacerum**
  - Foramen lacerum represents gap between osseous PA and clivus
  - In dried skull, best identified along extracranial aspect of skull base as irregular quadrangular or triangular space that is continuous superiorly into intracranial compartment, hence term "foramen"
  - In vivo, foramen lacerum is not open; rather, inferior extracranial margin is covered by horizontal plate of fibrocartilage that provides floor to lacerum segment of ICA
  - On axial imaging, foramen lacerum is anteromedial to POF and posterior to vidian canal
  - Important pathway for spread of disease from nasopharynx to central skull base and intracranial compartment
- **Eustachian tube (ET)**
  - Along anterolateral inferior portion of PA and squamous portion of T-bone, there is tubular canal that extends medially from middle ear cavity
  - Tubular canal is double barreled: There are 2 semicanals that parallel each other, one above the other, separated by thin, bony plate (septum canalis musculotubarii or cochleariform process)
  - Upper semicanal transmits tensor tympani muscle
  - Lower one forms posterior bony portion of ET
  - Tensor tympani muscle and ET cross anteriorly and medially from middle ear to nasopharynx, passing through small gap (petrosphenoid fissure) between greater wing of sphenoid and anterior margin of PA
  - As ET passes through this gap, it is medial to foramen spinosum, posterior to foramen ovale, and immediately anterior to horizontal petrous canal
  - At this location, ET transitions from bony canal from middle ear to cartilaginous canal that extends to torus tubarius of nasopharynx
  - Anterior cartilaginous component is often collapsed at imaging and seen only as soft tissue density or signal; occasionally, it contains air or fluid
- **POF**
  - POF is oblique junction between petrous T-bone and basilar occipital bone
  - Joins posterior aspect of foramen lacerum
  - Clinical relevance: Site of origin for majority of skull base chondrosarcomas
- **Trigeminal nerve and Meckel Cave**

Petrous Apex Anatomy

- o **Trigeminal impression**: Shallow groove along petrous ridge superiorly and anteriorly near tip of apex
- o **Porus trigeminus** represents small opening formed by trigeminal impression of PA below and tentorial insertion and superior petrosal sinus along ridge above
- o Trigeminal nerve passes through porus trigeminus into Meckel cave, cistern formed by ventral extension of arachnoid from posterior fossa into medial middle cranial fossa
- o Meckel cave is variable in size, houses trigeminal ganglion
- o Lateral wall is relatively thick, consisting of 2 layers of dura
- o Meckel cave is inferior and posterior to cavernous sinus
- **Dorello canal and CNVI**
  - o Near medial and superior tip of PA, there is small gap that separates PA from clivus
  - o Small ligament, **petrosphenoid ligament of Gruber**, crosses from PA tip to base of posterior clinoid process creating small bridge or roof over gap
  - o This gap or space, called **Dorello canal**, contains venous tissue at confluence of posterior cavernous sinus and petrosal sinuses
  - o CNVI passes from prepontine cistern through Dorello canal to enter cavernous sinus
  - o CNVI palsy and ophthalmoplegia is most common symptom related to PA mass
- **Petrolingual ligament (PLL)**
  - o Extends form PA to lingula of sphenoid bone
  - o PLL invariably surrounds dorsal and lateral walls of lacerum segment of ICA
  - o This ligament is oriented in sagittal plane and is just medial to trigeminal ganglion in Meckel cave
  - o Important surgical landmark that marks point at which ICA lacerum segment transitions to cavernous segment
  - o Also marks inferior and posterior margin of cavernous sinus
- **Cavernous sinus**
  - o Cavernous sinus, superior petrosal sinus, and inferior petrosal sinus converge at petroclival junction
  - o Margins of cavernous sinus roof partially determined by petroclinoid dural folds
    - – **Anterior petroclinoid fold**: Anterior extension of tentorial edge extends from anterior clinoid process to PA and forms lateral margin of roof
    - – **Posterior petroclinoid fold** extends from posterior clinoid process to PA
    - – **Interclinoid fold** extends from anterior to posterior clinoid process
    - – These dural folds form triangle, **oculomotor triangle**, central portion of cavernous sinus roof through which CNIII (oculomotor nerve) and cistern passes
  - o Lateral wall of cavernous sinus extends from superior orbital fissure to PA, just medial to trigeminal impression
    - – Trigeminal segments V1 and V2 are embedded within lateral wall of cavernous sinus
    - – Posteroinferior part of lateral wall of cavernous sinus is contiguous with upper margin of PLL
- **Nasopharynx**
  - o Nasopharyngeal mucosa and superior constrictor muscle are anchored to skull base by pharyngobasilar fascia

- o Pharyngobasilar fascia is attached to clivus, inferior PA, POF, and foramen lacerum
- o ET passes from skull base though gap (foramen Morgagni) in fascia and superior constrictor muscle and terminates in lateral wall of nasopharynx at torus tubarius
- o Levator veli palatini takes origin from undersurface of PA and also passes through foramen Morgagni
- o Tumor and infection can spread from nasopharynx to skull base via ET, foramen Morgagni, foramen ovale, or direct invasion
- o Foramen lacerum also potential pathway of invasion of nasopharyngeal lesion to skull base and cavernous sinus
- **Jugular foramen**
  - o Inferolateral petrous bone forms lateral border of jugular foramen
- **IAC**
  - o Narrow passage along posterior and lateral margin of PA
  - o Transmits CNVII and CNVIII
- **Greater superficial petrosal nerve**
  - o Passes from geniculate ganglion through facial hiatus into epidural space along ventral surface of PA
  - o Parasympathetic fibers join sympathetic fibers from ICA to become vidian nerve within vidian canal

ANATOMY IMAGING ISSUES

Imaging Recommendations

- T-bone CT is excellent for defining osseous destruction and normal-variant asymmetric PA aeration
- CTA is useful for evaluation of petrous ICA
- MR of skull base with T1 noncontrast and nonfat-saturated images combined with contrast-enhanced fat-saturated images allows comprehensive evaluation of soft tissue, marrow space, cavernous sinus, and cranial nerves

Imaging Pitfalls

- Asymmetric marrow and retained secretions in PA air cells may be confused with pathology on MR
  - o CT is helpful in defining asymmetric marrow
  - o CT and MR retained secretions in air cells should not demonstrate trabecular destruction or expansion

Petrous Apex Anatomy

NORMAL PETROUS APEX ANATOMY

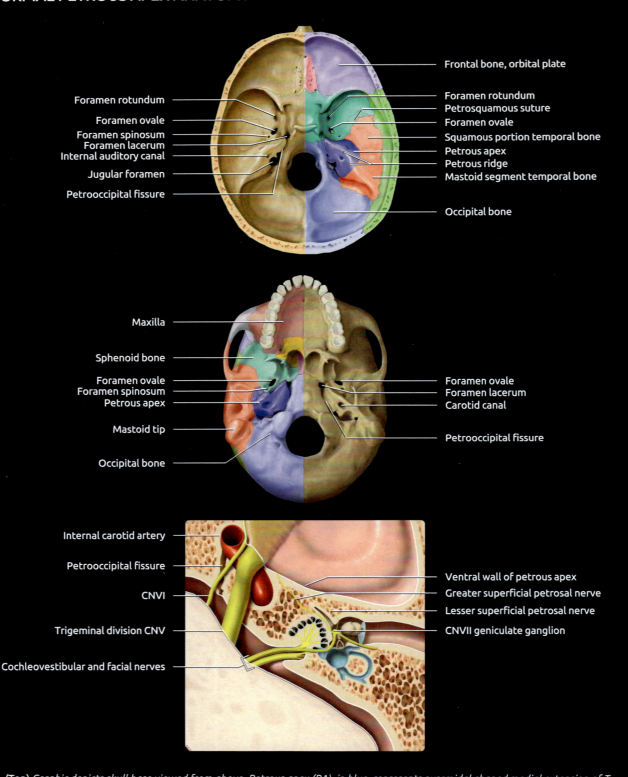

(Top) Graphic depicts skull base viewed from above. Petrous apex (PA), in blue, represents pyramidal-shaped medial extension of T-bone. Petrous ridge is formed by junction of ventral & dorsal slopes. Ventral slope forms posterior margin of middle cranial fossa; dorsal slope forms anterior margin of posterior fossa. Note relationship of PA with sphenoid bone, foramen lacerum, jugular foramen, & clivus. (Middle) External/extracranial view of skull base shows undersurface of PA (blue). Note relationship of PA with irregular, oblique petrooccipital fissure (POF) that separates PA from occipital bone. Foramen lacerum represents a gap between PA & clivus. In a dried skull, this is an opening that communicates with intracranial compartment. In vivo, this opening is covered by fibrocartilage. (Bottom) Axial graphic shows PA below surface of petrous ridge. Petrous carotid is located along anterior margin. CNVI & CNV course over the anterior superior margin near medial tip. Internal auditory canal & inner ear are at posterior margin. Greater superficial petrosal nerve carries parasympathetic fibers from facial nerve geniculate ganglion through facial hiatus along epidural surface of PA to vidian canal.

Petrous Apex Anatomy

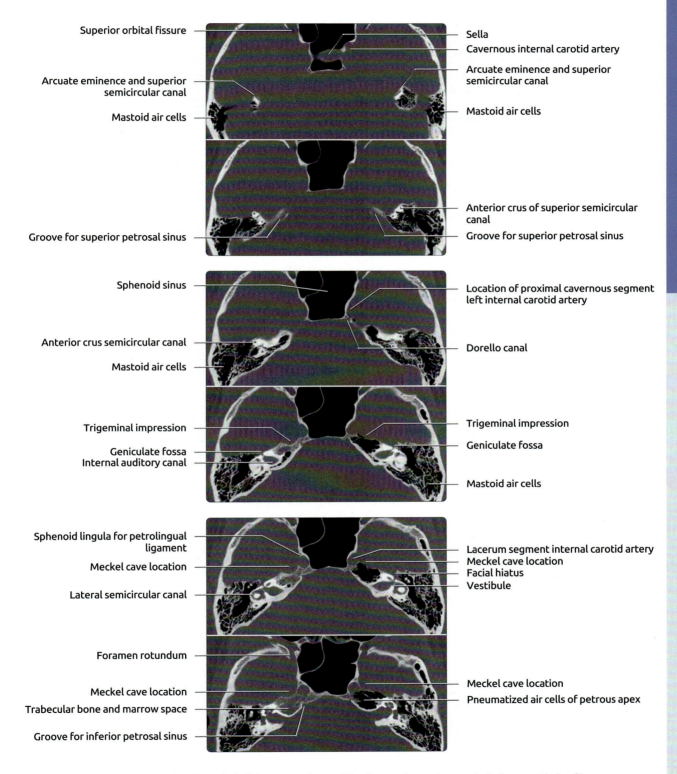

NORMAL ANATOMY OF PETROUS APEX: AXIAL CT

(Top) Axial CT images show petrous ridge through skull base. Superior semicircular canal projects superiorly from vestibule of inner ear, & overlying bone often produces small elevation, arcuate eminence. Superior petrosal sinus lies within groove along attachment of tentorium cerebelli of petrous ridge. (Middle) Axial upper T-bone CT images show extensive pneumatization of mastoid air cells bilaterally. Pneumatization extends into petrous apices bilaterally but asymmetrically. Along superior aspect of petroclival junction, there is a small "canal," Dorello canal, bounded by PA (inferolateral), clivus (inferomedial), & petrosphenoidal ligament of Gruber (superiorly). CNVI passes from prepontine cistern through Dorello canal into cavernous sinus. In lower image, left PA is pneumatized & contains air, while right PA consists mostly of trabecular bone & marrow. (Bottom) Axial CT images through inner ear level show asymmetric pneumatization of PAs. Note relationship of PA to lacerum segment of the internal carotid artery medially as well as its relationship to Meckel cave. Facial hiatus represents a small opening from geniculate ganglion to ventral face of PA & transmits greater superficial petrosal nerve.

NORMAL ANATOMY OF PETROUS APEX: AXIAL CT

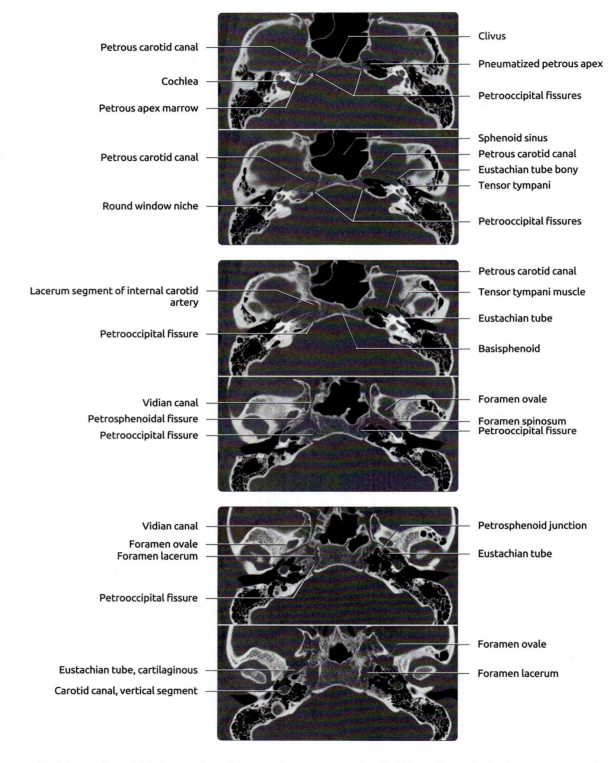

(Top) Descending axial CT images through PAs are shown. POFs are identified bilaterally. At this level, POFs are mostly fused solid with a small groove posteriorly for inferior petrosal sinus. Anterior genu of the petrous ICA turns upward to become lacerum segment. Note the intimate relationship of the anterior genus to the sphenoid sinus. (Middle) Selected descending axial CT images through T-bone again show asymmetry in PAs. The horizontal carotid canal passes obliquely through the petrous bone, from lateral to medial, and the medial opening is just superior to foramen lacerum. (Bottom) Axial CT images through central skull base at level of inferior aspect of PA demonstrate the funnel-shaped vidian canals that transmit vidian nerves through sphenoid bone from Meckel cave to pterygopalatine fossa. Note cartilaginous POF appears to merge anteriorly with the cartilaginous-filled foramen lacerum. The foramen lacerum is a bony gap that is covered by cartilage, and this cartilaginous plate serves as the floor of the medial carotid canal. As the horizontal petrous portion of ICA reaches this point, it turns upward, and the short vertical segment is called the lacerum segment.

Petrous Apex Anatomy

NORMAL PETROUS APEX: CECT

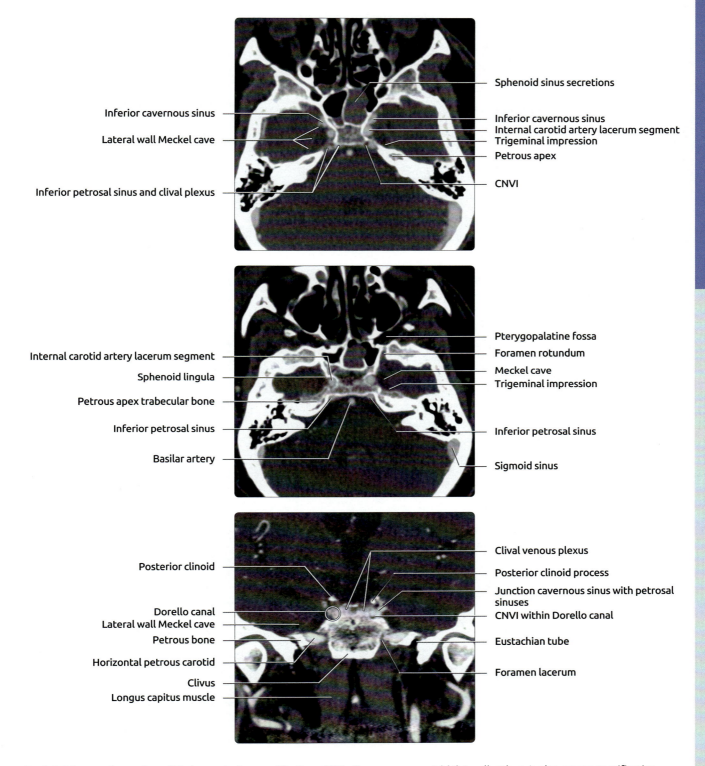

(Top) Axial source image from CTA demonstrates opacification of ICAs (lacerum segments) bilaterally. There is also venous opacification of cavernous sinuses and inferior petrosal sinuses bilaterally. CNVI can be seen passing through venous plexus within Dorello canal bilaterally en route to cavernous sinus. (Middle) Axial CTA through skull base demonstrates relationship of the lacerum segment ICA to trigeminal impression and lower Meckel cave. Intraarterial contrast is identified within the ICAs bilaterally as well as the basilar artery. There is also contrast in inferior petrosal sinuses bilaterally. In this case, there is symmetric lack of pneumatization of PAs. (Bottom) Coronal CECT through clivus demonstrates relationship of Meckel cave to the distal horizontal petrous ICA. CNVI can be visualized passing through the region of the Dorello canal. It is seen as a nonenhancing filling defect within enhancing venous plexus at the junction of cavernous sinus and petrosal sinuses. The foramen lacerum is a triangular opening in the inferior skull base between the inferior tip of the PA and the clivus. Cartilage bridges the gap horizontally and forms floor of the lacerum segment of ICA.

Petrous Apex Anatomy

NORMAL PETROUS APEX: T1 MR

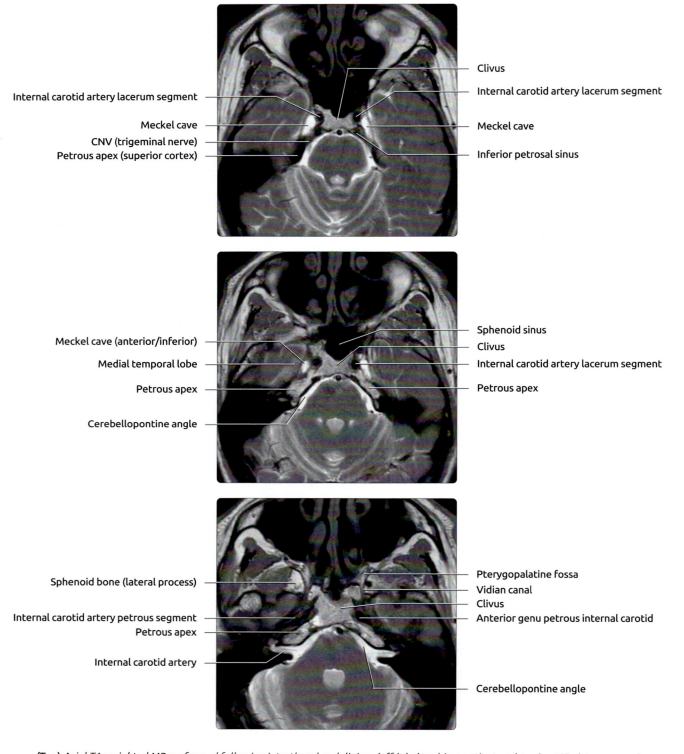

(Top) Axial T1-weighted MR performed following intrathecal gadolinium (off-label use) in a patient undergoing MR cisternogram is shown. Increased signal is identified within the CSF spaces, including prepontine cistern and Meckel cave due to presence of gadolinium. At this axial level, CNV (trigeminal nerve) is passing over the superior cortical rim of the PA, along the trigeminal impression. The upper clivus (basisphenoid) is relatively hyperintense due to marrow fat. With this technique, normal venous structures are relatively hypointense, and do not enhance. (Middle) Axial T1-weighted MR performed following intrathecal gadolinium (off-label use) is shown. This axial slice is below that of image 1. The petrous apices are relatively hyperintense due to presence of marrow fat that is contiguous with marrow fat of the clivus. (Bottom) Axial image through the internal auditory canal demonstrates hyperintensity of the CSF in canals secondary to intrathecal gadolinium. The petrous ICAs are partially visualized as hypointense flow voids. Vidian canal contains fat and the vidian nerve and is contiguous anteriorly with the pterygopalatine fossa.

Petrous Apex Anatomy

ANATOMIC-PATHOLOGIC CORRELATION: POF CHONDROSARCOMA

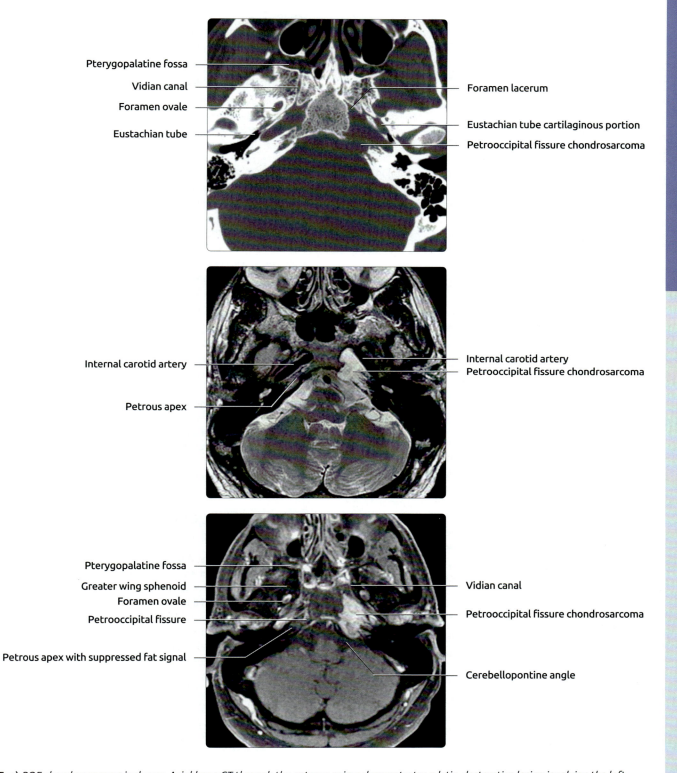

(Top) POF chondrosarcoma is shown. Axial bone CT through the petrous apices demonstrates a lytic, destructive lesion involving the left PA. Note the medial aspect of the lesion involves the POF, a clue to the diagnosis in this case of POF chondrosarcoma. While some chondrosarcomas will demonstrate chondroid calcifications, many lesions in this location are predominantly lytic without calcified matrix. (Middle) Axial T2 MR through the central skull base demonstrates a lobulated hyperintense lesion arising from the POF. This is a path-proven chondrosarcoma. The lesion pushes the petrous ICA anterolaterally. While the lesion appears to have cystic qualities with similar signal to CSF on T2-weighted images, the lesion is actually solid and demonstrates avid enhancement. (Bottom) Axial contrast-enhanced MR with fat-saturated technique allows suppression of any high signal related to fat and allows better detection of enhancing lesions that might occur in bone marrow. This chondrosarcoma demonstrates robust enhancement at the POF and PA. The lesion is expansile, causing bone destruction and marrow replacement.

CPA-IAC Anatomy

TERMINOLOGY

Abbreviations

- Cerebellopontine angle (CPA) & internal auditory canal (IAC)
- Superior vestibular nerve (SVN) & inferior vestibular nerve (IVN)
- Anterior inferior cerebellar artery (AICA)

Definitions

- **CPA-IAC cistern**: Cerebrospinal fluid (CSF) space in CPA & IAC containing CNVII & CNVIII & AICA loop
- **IAC fundus**: Lateral CSF-filled cap of IAC cistern containing distal CNVII, SVN, IVN, & cochlear nerve
- **Cochlear nerve canal**: Bony opening connecting IAC fundus to cochlea
- **Porus acusticus**: Large opening at medial aspect of IAC connecting it to CPA cistern

IMAGING ANATOMY

Internal Contents

- **Vestibulocochlear nerve (CNVIII)**: CPA-IAC cistern
  - Components
    - Vestibular (balance) & cochlear (hearing) portions
  - **Cochlear nerve portion, CNVIII course**
    - Leaves **spiral ganglion** as auditory axons
    - Travels as **cochlear nerve** in anterior-inferior quadrant of IAC
    - Joins SVN & IVN at porus acusticus to become CNVIII bundle in CPA cistern
    - Crosses CPA cistern as posterior nerve bundle to enter brainstem at pontomedullary junction
    - Enters brainstem & bifurcates to synapse with both dorsal & ventral cochlear nuclei
  - **CNVII & CNVIII orientation in IAC cistern**
    - "7up, coke down" useful pneumonic
    - CNVII anterosuperior; cochlear nerve anteroinferior
    - SVN posterosuperior; IVN posteroinferior in IAC; vestibular ganglion in IAC called Scarpa ganglion
- **Facial nerve (CNVII)**: CPA-IAC cistern
  - Root exit zone in pontomedullary junction
  - Travels anterior to CNVIII in CPA cistern
  - Anterosuperior in IAC cistern
- **AICA loop**
  - Arises from basilar artery then rises into IAC
  - Continues in IAC as **internal auditory artery** (IAA)
  - May mimic cranial nerve on high-resolution T2
  - IAA supplies 3 branches to inner ear
- **Other structures in CPA cistern**
  - **Flocculus** of cerebellum in posteromedial CPA
  - **Choroid plexus** may pass from 4th ventricle though foramen of Luschka into CPA cistern
- **Other structures in IAC cistern**
  - **Crista falciformis** (horizontal crest): Horizontal bony projection from IAC fundus
  - **Vertical crest** (Bill bar): Vertical bony ridge in superior portion of IAC fundus
  - **Cochlear nerve canal**: IAC outlet for cochlear nerve to cochlea
  - **Macula cribrosa**: Perforated bone between IAC & vestibule of inner ear

ANATOMY IMAGING ISSUES

Questions

- Can you name 3 scalar cochlear chambers?
  - Scala tympani (posteriorly), media, & vestibuli (anteriorly)
  - Scala media cannot be routinely imaged

Imaging Approaches

- Cochlear portion of CNVIII
  - Principal impetus for imaging CNVIII
  - Bone CT used in trauma, otosclerosis, & Paget disease
  - MR used to diagnose vestibular schwannoma & evaluate all other patients with sensorineural hearing loss (SNHL)
- MR imaging approach to **uncomplicated** unilateral SNHL
  - Screening MR involves high-resolution thin-section T2 imaging through CPA-IAC
- MR imaging approach to **complex** SNHL (unilateral SNHL + other symptoms)
  - Whole-brain & posterior fossa sequences
  - Begin with whole-brain axial T2 & FLAIR sequences
  - Conclude with axial & coronal T1 thin-section C+ MR of posterior fossa & CPA-IAC

Imaging Pitfalls

- Normal variants in CPA-IAC
  - Normal structures, when unusually prominent, trouble radiologist evaluating CPA-IAC
  - **AICA loop** flow void on high-resolution T2 MR
    - Will not prominently enhance on T1 C+ MR
    - Subtle enhancement in IAC on T1 C+ MR may be mistaken for small vestibular schwannoma
  - **Marrow space foci** in walls of IAC can mimic IAC tumor on T1 C+ MR images
    - Correlate location of foci with IAC cistern
    - Bone CT of temporal bone may be necessary to identify this normal variant

CLINICAL IMPLICATIONS

Function Dysfunction

- CPA-IAC lesions most commonly present with SNHL
  - **Uncomplicated unilateral SNHL**: Patient otherwise healthy & presents with unilateral SNHL
  - **Complicated SNHL**: Patient has other symptoms in addition to unilateral SNHL
    - Symptoms include other cranial neuropathy, long tract signs, & headache
- Cochlear nerve injury
  - SNHL & tinnitus are primary symptoms
- Facial nerve injury, CPA-IAC portion
  - Peripheral facial neuropathy
    - Lacrimation, stapedial reflex, anterior 2/3 tongue taste loss, & complete loss of muscles of facial expression on side of lesion
    - CNVII rarely injured by lesion in CPA-IAC
    - If lesion in CPA-IAC & CNVII is out, consider nonvestibular schwannoma causes, such as facial nerve schwannoma or metastatic disease

CPA-IAC Anatomy

GRAPHICS

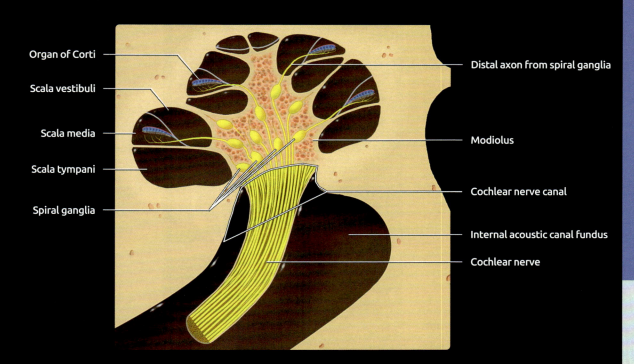

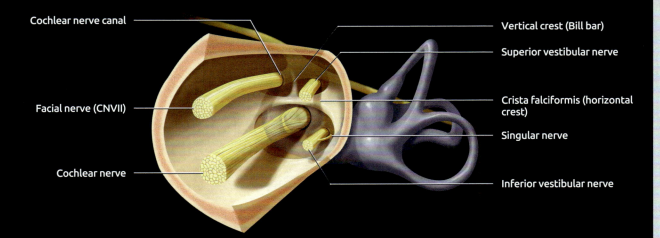

(Top) Axial graphic of a magnified cochlea shows the modiolus, cochlear nerve canal, & cochlear nerve in the internal auditory canal fundus. The spiral ganglia cells are bipolar, contributing proximal axons that constitute the cochlear nerve & distal fibers to the organ of Corti. High-resolution CT & MR imaging that is now available routinely identifies the scala tympani & vestibuli but not the scala media. (Bottom) Graphic depicts the fundus of the internal auditory canal. Notice that the crista falciformis separates the cochlear nerve & inferior vestibular nerve below from the facial nerve & superior vestibular nerve above, while the vertical crest (Bill bar) separates the facial nerve from the superior vestibular nerve. Sagittal oblique high-resolution T2 imaging has become critically important in the work-up of cochlear implant candidates because it is now possible to determine if a cochlear nerve is present with this type of imaging. No cochlear nerve significantly diminishes cochlear implant outcome.

CPA-IAC Anatomy

AXIAL BONE CT

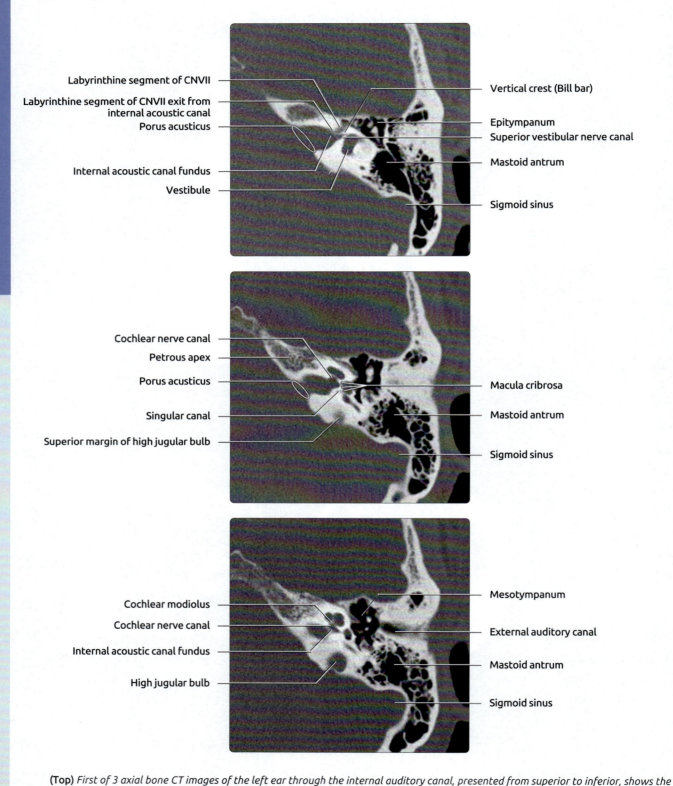

(Top) First of 3 axial bone CT images of the left ear through the internal auditory canal, presented from superior to inferior, shows the labyrinthine segment of the facial nerve exiting the anterosuperior fundus of the internal auditory canal. Note also that the vertical crest separates the anterior labyrinthine segment of CNVII from the posterior superior vestibular nerve canal. (Middle) In this image, the cochlear nerve canal is seen connecting the anteroinferior fundus of the internal auditory canal to the cochlea. The cochlear nerve accesses the modiolus of the cochlea through the cochlear nerve canal. Note the posterolateral fundal bony wall abutting the medial vestibule. Multiple branches of the vestibular nerves pass through this wall (the macula cribrosa) to the vestibule & semicircular canals. (Bottom) The cochlear modiolus is visible as a high-density structure at the cochlear base directly inside the cochlea from the cochlear nerve canal. The high jugular bulb projects cephalad behind the internal auditory canal.

SAGITTAL T2 MR

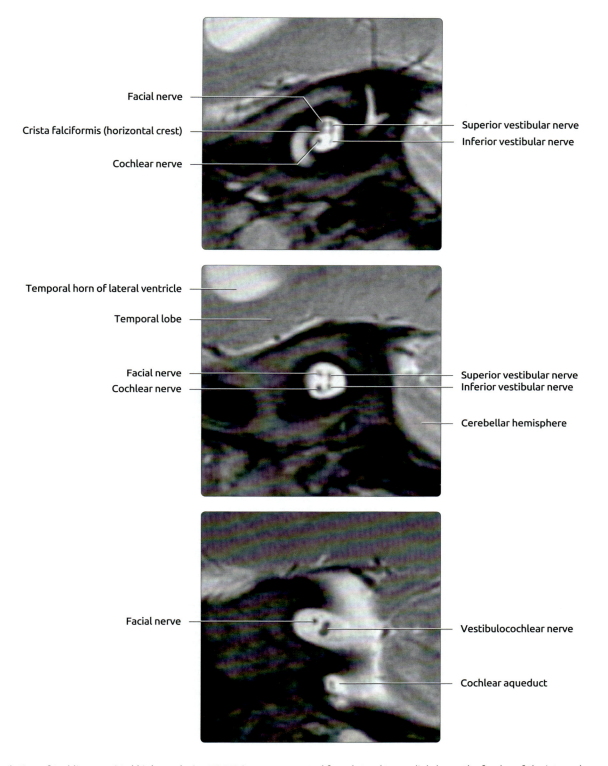

(Top) First of 3 oblique sagittal high-resolution T2 MR images presented from lateral to medial shows the fundus of the internal auditory canal filled with high-signal cerebrospinal fluid. The horizontal low-signal line in the fundus is the crista falciformis. The facial nerve is anterosuperior, whereas the cochlear nerve is anteroinferior. (Middle) In this image through the mid internal auditory canal, the 4 discrete nerves are well seen. Notice that the anteroinferior cochlear nerve is normally slightly larger than the other 3 nerves in the internal auditory canal. (Bottom) At the level of the porus acusticus, the facial nerve is visible just anterior to the vestibulocochlear nerve. The overall appearance of these 2 nerves is that of a ball (facial nerve) in a catcher's mitt (vestibulocochlear nerve). The vestibulocochlear nerve contains the cochlear, inferior, & superior vestibular nerves.

CPA-IAC Anatomy

AXIAL T2 MR

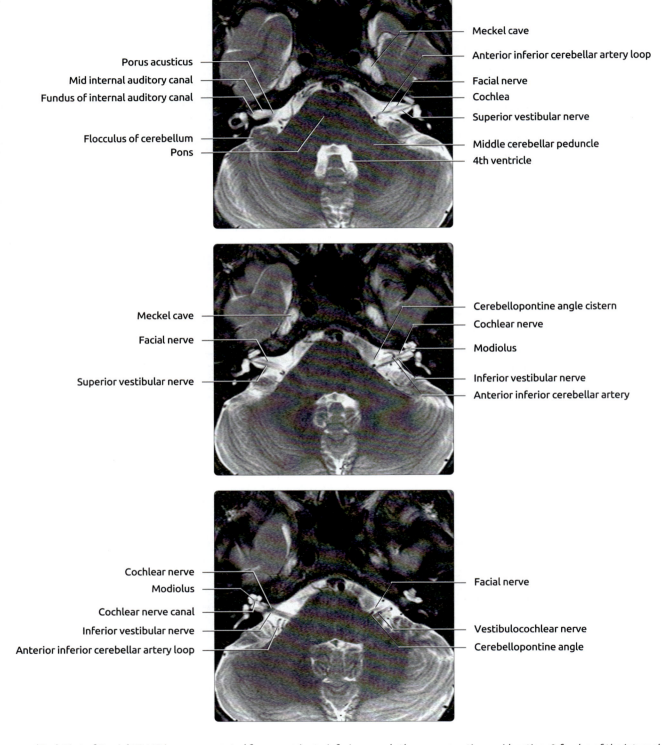

(Top) First of 3 axial T2 MR images presented from superior to inferior reveals the porus acusticus, midportion, & fundus of the internal auditory canal on the right. On the left, the anterior inferior cerebellar artery is seen looping through the cerebellopontine angle cistern. Also note the facial nerve & superior vestibular nerve on the left within the internal auditory canal. (Middle) In this image, the facial nerve & superior vestibular nerve are seen in the right internal auditory canal, & the cochlear nerve & inferior vestibular are visible on the left. (Bottom) In this image, the cochlear nerve is seen in the right internal auditory canal exiting through the cochlear nerve canal to reach the modiolus of the cochlea. On the left, the cerebellopontine angle is seen with the vestibulocochlear nerve emerging from the brainstem at this point.

CPA-IAC Anatomy

CORONAL T2 MR

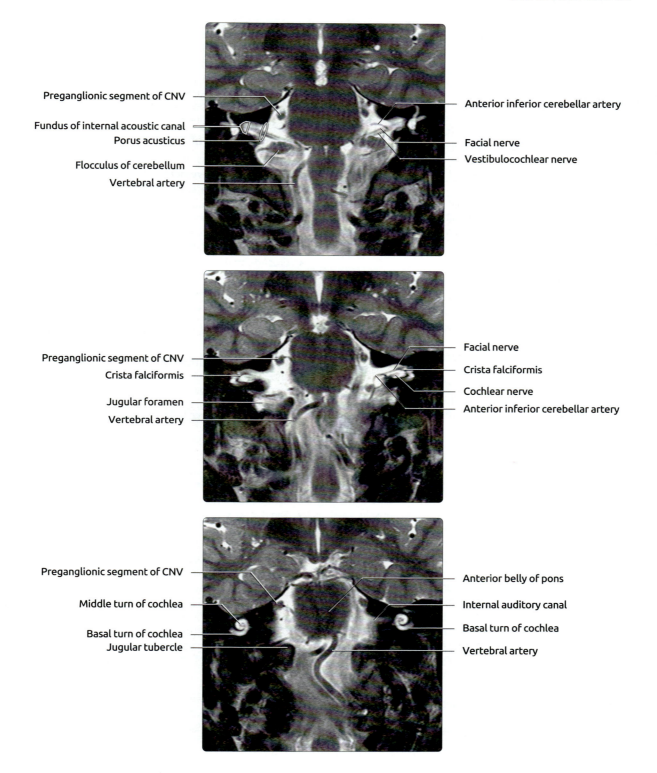

(Top) First of 3 coronal T2 MR images presented from posterior to anterior through the cerebellopontine angle & internal auditory canal cisterns shows important regional structures, including the preganglionic segment of CNV, anterior inferior cerebellar artery loop, flocculus of cerebellum, & vertebral artery. (Middle) In this image, the crista falciformis in the fundus of the internal auditory canal is seen. The facial nerve & superior vestibular nerve are above, & the cochlear nerve & inferior vestibular nerve are below the crista falciformis. (Bottom) At the level of the cochlea, the anterior belly of the pons is visible. The preganglionic segment of the trigeminal nerve is in the anterosuperior portion of the cerebellopontine angle cistern, while the jugular tubercle is in the anteroinferior portion.

Temporomandibular Joint

TERMINOLOGY

Definitions

- Temporomandibular joint (**TMJ**): Articulation between mandible & T-bone

IMAGING ANATOMY

Overview

- Complex diarthrodial joint with 2 functional movements: Rotation & translation ("ginglymoarthrodial" joint) to allow for 40-50 mm of normal mouth opening [maximum incisal opening (MIO)]
  - Initial hinge (rotatory) movement in inferior compartment between mandibular condyle & articular disc accounts for first 20 mm of MIO
  - Subsequent sliding (translational) component in superior compartment between disc & mandibular fossa accounts for remaining 20-30 mm of opening

Internal Contents

- **Articular surfaces of TMJ**
  - Undersurface of squamosal portion of T-bone contains mandibular fossa & articular eminence
    - **Mandibular fossa** (articular fossa) located anterior to external auditory meatus
    - **Articular eminence** (articular tubercle) located anterior to mandibular fossa
  - **Mandibular condyle**: Condylar H&N: Posterior protrusion from ramus of mandible
- **Articular disc**: Oval, dumbbell-shaped biconcave plate of type I collagen
  - Disc superior surface: Concavoconvex to fit articular eminence & mandibular fossa; disc inferior surface: Concave to conform to condylar head
  - **Intermediate zone** of disc found between anterior & posterior bands
  - **Anterior band**: Anteriorly attaches to joint capsule; portion is integrated into superior aspect of lateral pterygoid muscle
  - **Posterior band**: Posterior disc margin is bilaminar = **bilaminar zone**
    - **Superior portion** composed of **loose** fibroelastic tissue; attached to posterior mandibular fossa
    - **Inferior portion** composed of **taut** fibrous material; attached to posterior margin of mandibular condyle
  - Medially & laterally, disc attaches to joint capsule & medial & lateral mandibular condyle
- **TMJ compartments**: Disc creates superior & inferior compartments
  - **Superior joint compartment**: Between disc & mandibular fossa of T-bone
    - Volume: 2 mL normally but can increase up to 6 mL with pathology
  - **Inferior joint compartment**: Between disc & condyle; 2 distinct recesses
    - **Anterior recess**: Anterior to condylar head
    - **Posterior recess**: Posterior to condylar head, deep to posterior insertion of articular disc onto posterior condylar neck
    - Volume: 1 mL normally but can increase up to 2 mL with pathology

- **TMJ capsule & ligaments**
  - **Joint capsule**: Funnel-shaped; extends inferiorly from T-bone to attach to condylar neck
  - **TMJ ligaments**
    - Temporomandibular ligament: Lateral ligament attached to tubercle on zygoma root above & lateral surface of mandibular neck below
    - Sphenomandibular ligament: Medial ligament that attaches above on spine of sphenoid & below to lingula of mandibular foramen

MR Appearances of TMJ

- **Articular disc**: Low signal on T1 & T2
- **Articular disc movement**
  - Initially upon mouth opening, inferior joint rotates
  - When mouth fully opens, mandibular condyle slides forward & downward onto articular eminence
  - Articular disc slides in same direction until its posterior fibroelastic attachments are stretched to their limits
- **Closed-mouth sagittal MR**: Disc is sigmoid-shaped in anterior 1/2 of joint space on sagittal closed-mouth MR
  - Junction between low-signal posterior band of disc & intermediate-signal bilaminar zone is at "12 o'clock" position relative to mandibular condyle
  - Anterior band is located immediately inferior to articular eminence
- **Open-mouth sagittal MR**: Disc is bow tie-shaped anteroinferiorly beneath condylar eminence & above mandibular condyle

ANATOMY IMAGING ISSUES

Imaging Recommendations

- Most TMJ imaging requested for internal derangement (abnormal disc position) or TMJ degenerative disorders
- MR best imaging modality to evaluate TMJ soft tissues, especially articular disc
- Sagittal MR mainstay of TMJ imaging evaluation & largely replaced arthrography
  - Coronal closed-mouth T1, sagittal T1 & T2 with closed- & open-mouth acquisitions needed; FS T2 best for evaluation of joint effusion
- Bone CT may be needed to assess osseous structures
  - Multislice bone CT scan with 1-mm axial images; sagittal & coronal reformations helpful
  - Wilkes classification of internal derangement combines clinical & radiographic features of progressive degeneration of condyle & articular disc

Imaging Pitfalls

- When apparent limited motion between open & closed mouth series, look closely for articular disc abnormalities
- Review coronal images to evaluate lateral displacement of articular disc

CLINICAL IMPLICATIONS

Clinical Importance

- True internal derangement of TMJ represents fraction of causes of TMJ pain or hypomobility (most due to myofascial pain disorder); TMJ tumors, though rare, consist of developmental & odontogenic cysts or tumors & rarely malignancies, such as chondrosarcoma

Temporomandibular Joint

GRAPHICS

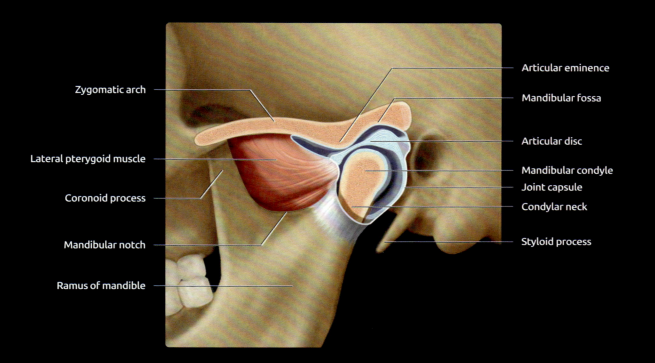

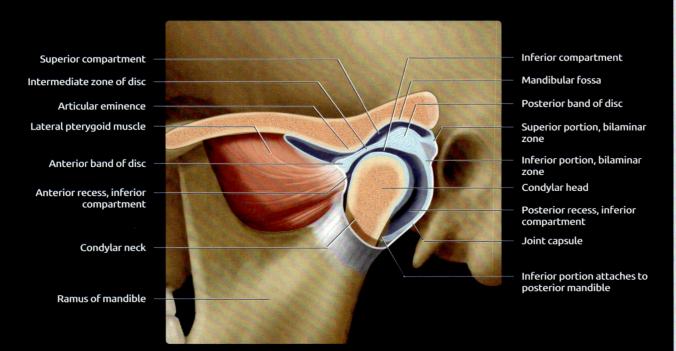

(Top) Lateral graphic shows the relationship of the condylar head to base of skull at the temporomandibular joint (TMJ). Key global features of the TMJ include the mandibular condyle, articular disc, mandibular fossa, and articular eminence. (Bottom) Magnified lateral graphic of the TMJ shows the articular disc with its anterior and posterior bands. The thinner part of the disc connecting these bands is called the intermediate zone. The disc separates the joint into a superior and inferior compartment. Note the anterior band connecting to the lateral pterygoid muscle. The posterior margin of the posterior band is referred to as the bilaminar zone with the superior strut attaching to the posterior mandibular fossa, while the inferior strut attaches to the posterior margin of the mandibular condyle.

Temporomandibular Joint

3D-VRT BONE CT

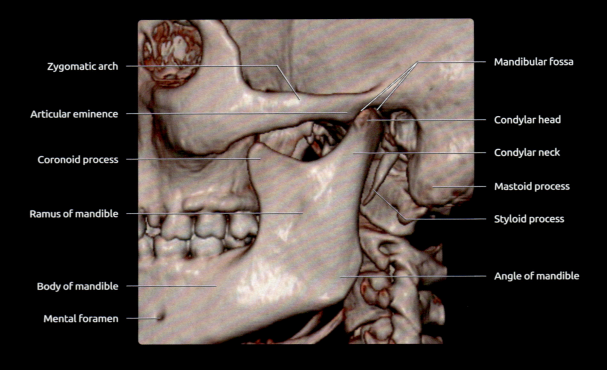

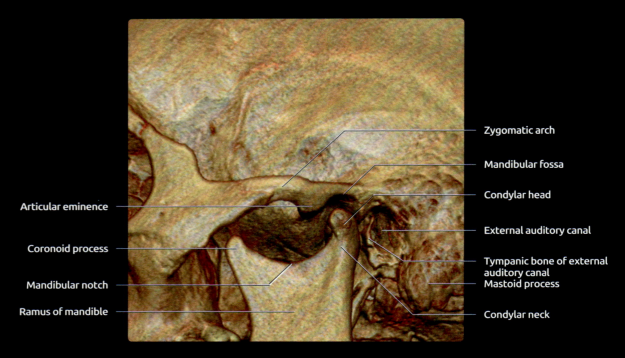

(Top) Sagittal 3D-VRT image shows the osseous anatomy of the TMJ. The condylar head is situated in the mandibular fossa deep to the posterior zygomatic arch. The zygomatic arch provides some protection laterally for the TMJ in the setting of trauma. The TMJ must be fully evaluated on all mandibular trauma cases to ensure no dislocation of the mandibular condyle has occurred. (Bottom) Sagittal 3D-VRT magnified image shows the osseous anatomy of the TMJ area. In this closed or occlusal position, the condylar head is within the mandibular fossa. In the open mouth position (not shown), the condylar head slides anteroinferiorly onto the articular eminence. Notice the close relationship between the condylar head and tympanic bone of the external auditory canal. An upward blow to the mandible can easily fracture the bony external auditory canal.

Temporomandibular Joint

BONE CT

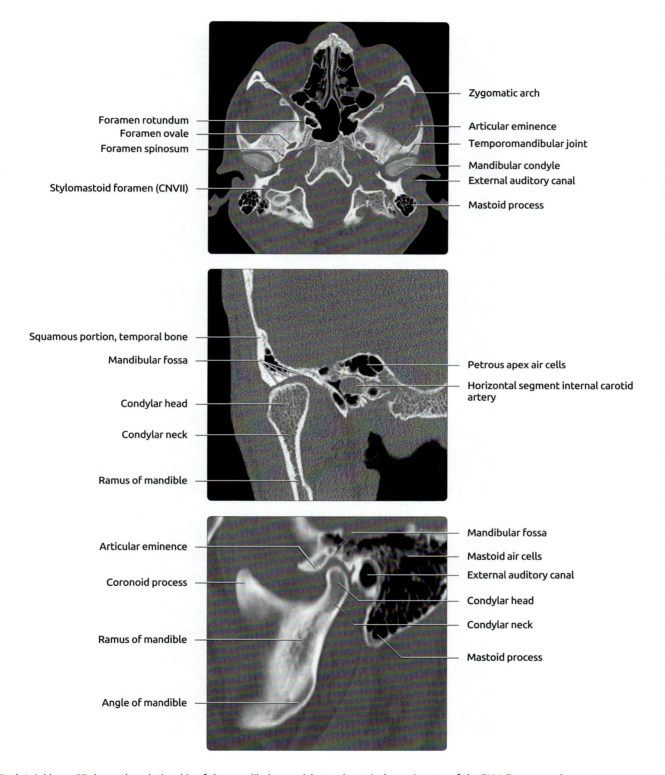

(Top) Axial bone CT shows the relationship of the mandibular condyles to the articular eminences of the TMJ. Foramen spinosum, transmitting the middle meningeal artery, is immediately anteromedial to the TMJ. In this plane, the articular eminence is seen as the posterior attachment of the zygomatic arch. (Middle) Coronal bone CT of the right TMJ shows the coronal relationship of right mandibular condyle and fossa of the TMJ. The coronal plane in the closed-mouth position shows the horizontal segment of the carotid canal medial to the TMJ and variable aeration of the temporal bone air cells superior to the TMJ. (Bottom) Sagittal bone CT reformatted image shows the sagittal relationship of osseous TMJ with the mandibular condyle normally seated within the mandibular fossa in the closed-mouth position.

Temporomandibular Joint

SAGITTAL T1 MR

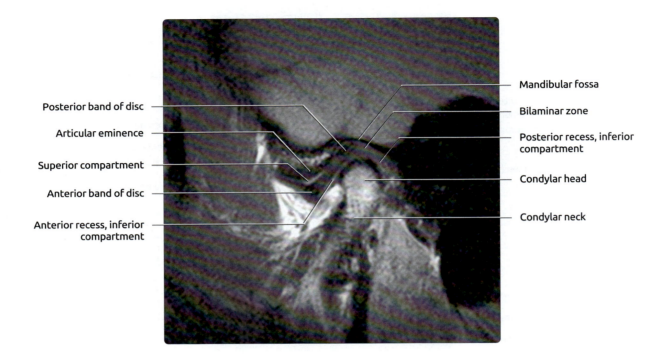

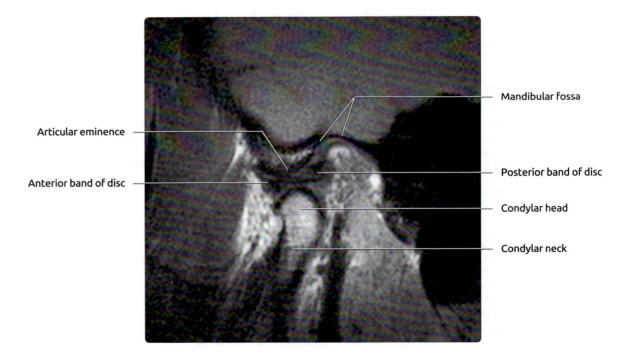

(Top) *Closed-mouth sagittal T1 MR shows the condylar head seated in the mandibular fossa. The low-signal articular disc has a sigmoid shape and is seen in the anterior 1/2 of the joint space. The junction between the low-signal posterior band of the disc and intermediate signal of the bilaminar zone is normally found at "12 o'clock" relative to the condylar head in the closed-mouth position.* **(Bottom)** *Open-mouth sagittal T1 MR is shown. The condylar head has translated anteroinferiorly onto the articular eminence. The articular disc has moved to a position between the articular eminence and mandibular condyle, taking on a bow tie appearance. Both disc and mandibular condyle must complete this anterior movement for the TMJ to function normally. When the disc fails to complete this movement, internal derangement of the TMJ results. (Courtesy J. Fuentes, MD.)*

Temporomandibular Joint

SAGITTAL T2 MR

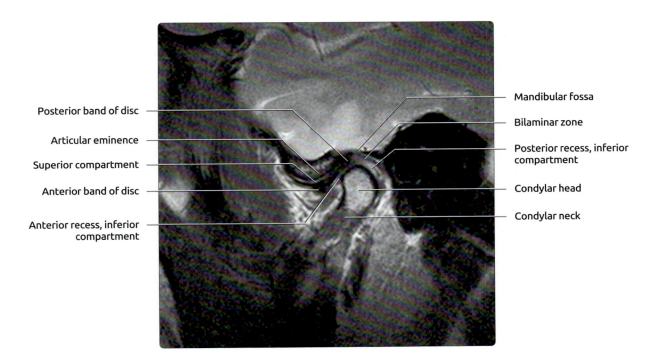

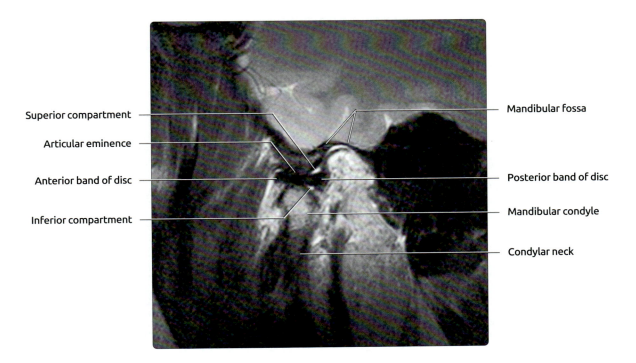

(Top) *Closed-mouth sagittal T2 MR shows the condylar head seated in mandibular fossa. The low-signal articular disc has a sigmoid shape and is seen in the anterior 1/2 of the joint space. Notice that the junction between the low-signal posterior band of the disc and the intermediate signal of the bilaminar zone is normally found at "12 o'clock" relative to the condylar head in the closed-mouth position.* (Bottom) *Open-mouth T2 MR sagittal image reveals the condylar head has translated anteroinferiorly onto the articular eminence. The disc has also moved to a position between the articular eminence and mandibular condyle, taking on a bow tie appearance in the process. Both disc and mandibular condyle must complete this anteroinferior movement for the TMJ to function normally. (Courtesy J. Fuentes, MD.)*

SECTION 2
Cranial Nerves

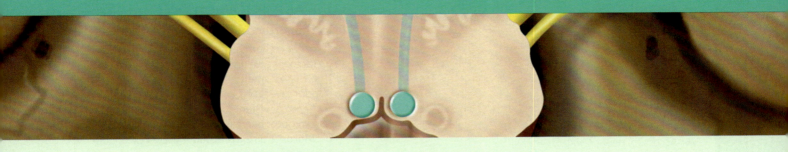

Cranial Nerves Overview	**116**
CNI (Olfactory Nerve)	**128**
CNII (Optic Nerve)	**132**
CNIII (Oculomotor Nerve)	**140**
CNIV (Trochlear Nerve)	**148**
CNV (Trigeminal Nerve)	**152**
CNVI (Abducens Nerve)	**164**
CNVII (Facial Nerve)	**168**
CNVIII (Vestibulocochlear Nerve)	**176**
CNIX (Glossopharyngeal Nerve)	**182**
CNX (Vagus Nerve)	**188**
CNXI (Accessory Nerve)	**194**
CNXII (Hypoglossal Nerve)	**198**

Cranial Nerves Overview

TERMINOLOGY

Abbreviations

- Olfactory nerve: CNI
- Optic nerve: CNII
- Oculomotor nerve: CNIII
- Trochlear nerve: CNIV
- Trigeminal nerve: CNV
- Abducens nerve: CNVI
- Facial nerve: CNVII
- Vestibulocochlear nerve: CNVIII
- Glossopharyngeal nerve: CNIX
- Vagus nerve: CNX
- Accessory nerve: CNXI
- Hypoglossal nerve: CNXII

IMAGING ANATOMY

Overview

- Cranial nerve groupings based on area of brainstem origin
  - Diencephalon: CNII
  - Mesencephalon (midbrain): CNIII and CNIV
  - Pons: CNV, CNVI, CNVII, and CNVIII
  - Medulla: CNIX, CNX, CNXI, and CNXII

ANATOMY IMAGING ISSUES

Imaging Recommendations

- Best imaging modality for any simple or complex cranial neuropathy is **MR**
  - Single exception to this directive is distal vagal neuropathy where it is necessary to image to aortopulmonic window on left
    - CECT better here as less affected by breathing, swallowing, and coughing movements
- If lesion located in bony area such as skull base, sinuses, or mandible, bone CT highly recommended to provide complementary bone anatomy and lesion-related information
  - Contrast enhancement of CT is not necessary if full T1, T2, and T1 C+ MR available

Imaging Approaches

- Remember: Cranial nerves do **not** stop at skull base
- Radiologist must image entire extent of affected cranial nerve
  - **CNI, CNII, CNIII, CNIV and VI**: Include focused **orbital sequences**
  - **CNV**: Include entire **face to inferior mandible if V3** affected
  - **CNVII**: Include **CPA, temporal bone, and parotid space**
  - **CNVIII**: Include **CPA-IAC and inner ear**
  - **CNIX-XII**: Include **basal cistern, skull base, nasopharyngeal carotid space**
    - **CNX**: To fully evaluate for recurrent laryngeal nerve lesion, follow carotid space to aortopulmonic window on left, cervicothoracic junction on right
    - **CNXII**: Remember to reach hyoid bone to include distal loop as it rises into sublingual space

Imaging Pitfalls

- Radiologist forgets to image extracranial structures associated with cranial nerve affected

CLINICAL IMPLICATIONS

Clinical Importance

- Cranial nerves and their functions
  - Olfactory nerve (CNI)
    - Sense of **smell**
  - Optic nerve (CNII)
    - Sense of **vision**
  - Oculomotor nerve (CNIII)
    - **Motor** to all **extraocular muscles** except lateral rectus and superior oblique
    - **Parasympathetic** supply to ciliary and pupillary constrictor muscles
  - Trochlear nerve (CNIV)
    - **Motor** to **superior oblique**
  - Trigeminal nerve (CNV)
    - **Motor** (V3) to **muscles of mastication**, anterior belly digastric, mylohyoid, tensor tympani and palatini
    - **Sensory** to surface of **forehead and nose** (V1), **cheek** (V2), and **jaw** (V3)
    - **Sensory** to surfaces of nose, sinuses, meninges and external surface of tympanic membrane (auriculotemporal nerve)
  - Abducens nerve (CNVI)
    - **Motor** to **lateral rectus** muscle
  - Facial nerve (CNVII)
    - **Motor** to **muscles of facial expression**
    - **Motor** to **stapedius muscle**
    - **Parasympathetic** to lacrimal, submandibular, and sublingual glands
    - Anterior 2/3 tongue taste (chorda tympanic nerve)
    - General sensation for periauricular skin, external surface of tympanic membrane
  - Vestibulocochlear nerve (CNVIII)
    - Senses of **hearing and balance**
  - Glossopharyngeal nerve (CNIX)
    - **Motor** to **stylopharyngeus** muscle
    - **Parasympathetic** to parotid gland
    - Visceral sensory to carotid body
    - Posterior 1/3 tongue **taste**
    - General sensation to posterior 1/3 of tongue and internal surface of tympanic membrane
  - Vagus nerve (CNX)
    - **Motor** to **pharynx-larynx**
    - Parasympathetic to pharynx, larynx, thoracic and abdominal viscera
    - Visceral sensory from pharynx, larynx, and viscera
    - General sensation from small area around external ear
  - Accessory nerve (CNXI)
    - **Motor** to **sternocleidomastoid and trapezius** muscles
  - Hypoglossal nerve (CNXII)
    - **Motor** to intrinsic and extrinsic **tongue muscles** except palatoglossus

Cranial Nerves Overview

GRAPHICS, GLOBAL CRANIAL NERVES

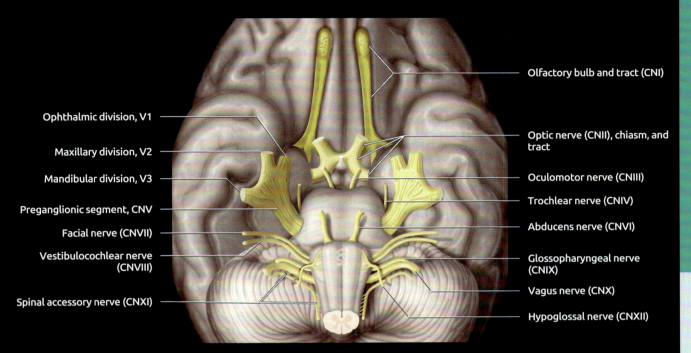

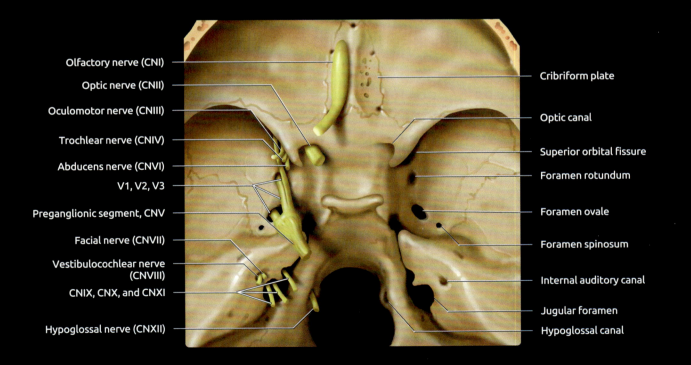

(Top) Graphic shows all cranial nerves, viewing the brainstem from below. Remember that CNs III-IV are associated with the midbrain (mesencephalon), while CNs V-VIII are affiliated with the pons. CNs IX-XII emerge from various aspects of the medulla. **(Bottom)** In this graphic of the skull base viewed from above, the foramina are illustrated on the right, and the associated cranial nerves are illustrated on the left. The terminal branches of CNI exit the skull base through many openings in the cribriform plate of the ethmoid bone. CNII exits via the optic canal, while CNs III, IV, VI, and V1 all go through the superior orbital fissure. V2 traverses foramen rotundum, and V3 is seen exiting the foramen ovale. CNVII and CNVIII are seen in internal auditory canal with CNs IX-XI found in the jugular foramen. Finally, CNXII uses its own hypoglossal canal to leave the basal cistern.

Cranial Nerves Overview

GRAPHICS, UPPER CRANIAL NERVES

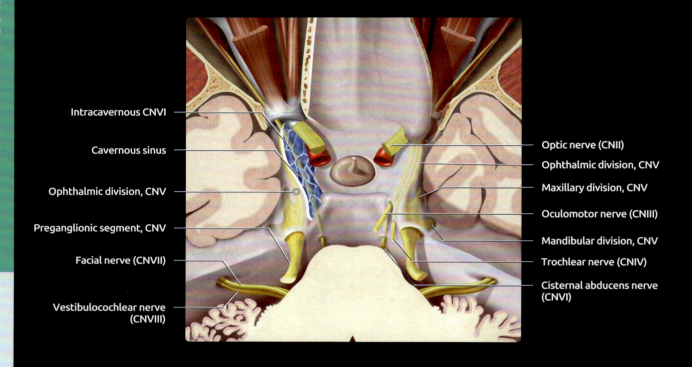

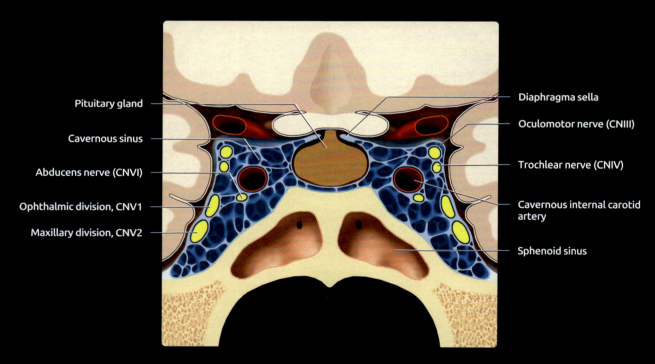

(Top) Axial graphic shows the prepontine cistern and cavernous sinus areas viewed from above. The preganglionic segment of CNV can be seen in the lateral prepontine cistern, entering the Meckel cave through the porus trigeminus. CNIII, IV, and VI are seen piercing the dura to enter the cavernous sinus. Only CNVI is within the venous sinusoids of the cavernous sinus, while CNIII and IV remain in its wall.
(Bottom) Coronal graphic shows posterior view through the cavernous sinus. The abducens nerve (CNVI) is the only cranial nerve with a purely intracavernous course. CNIII and IV enter the roof of the cavernous sinus. CNIII travels short distance in a tubular CSF-containing cistern before becoming incorporated into the lateral wall of the sinus. CNIV becomes immediately embedded in the lateral wall. V1 and V2 are in the lateral wall of the cavernous sinus, while V3 bypasses the cavernous sinus altogether. Remember sympathetic nerves travel along the intracavernous internal carotid artery as well.

Cranial Nerves Overview

GRAPHICS, LOWER CRANIAL NERVES

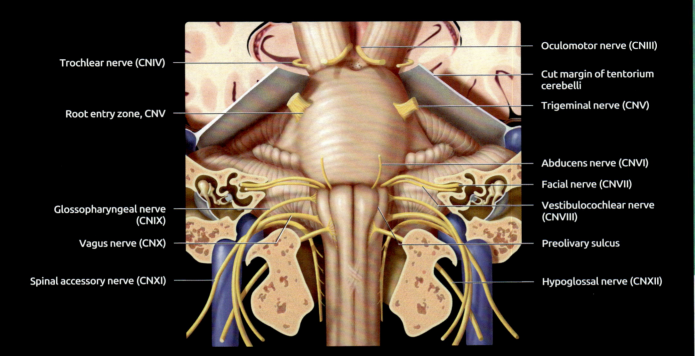

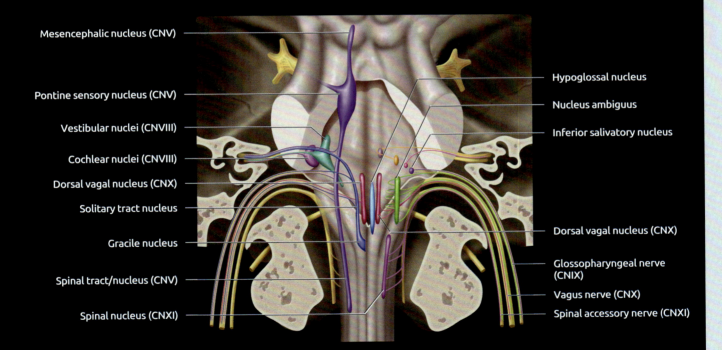

(Top) Graphic shows frontal view of brainstem and exiting cranial nerves. CNIII is seen exiting the midbrain into the interpeduncular cistern. CNIV wraps around the lateral midbrain in the tentorial margin. CNVI exits at the pontomedullary junction. CNVII and CNVIII exit the brainstem at the cerebellopontine angle. Inferiorly, CNIX-XI leave the lateral medulla in the postolivary sulcus. CNXII exits via the preolivary sulcus. (Bottom) Graphic shows brainstem from behind, emphasizing the lower cranial nerve nuclei. On the right are efferent fibers, and on left are afferent fibers connecting to brainstem nuclei. Highlights of this drawing include nucleus ambiguus providing voluntary motor fibers for CNIX and CNX. Inferior salivatory nucleus provides secretomotor fibers to the parotid via CNIX. Dorsal motor nucleus provides involuntary motor and sensory fibers to CNX. Solitary tract receives taste from CNVII and CNIX.

Cranial Nerves Overview

AXIAL BONE CT

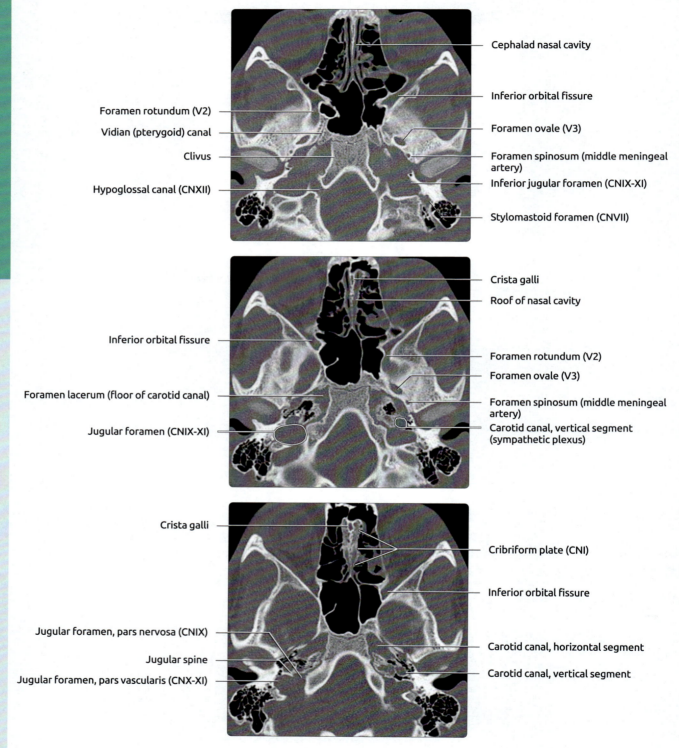

(Top) First of 6 sequential axial bone CT images through skull base, presented from inferior to superior, shows foramina of sphenoid bone including foramen rotundum (CNV2) and foramen ovale (CNV3). More posteriorly oblique, the hypoglossal canal is visible bilaterally in the occipital bone. *(Middle)* At the level of the inferior jugular foramen, the entry to the vertical segment of the carotid canal is also seen just anterior to the jugular foramen. Notice the ovoid shape of the jugular foramen at this level. The floor of the anteromedial aspect of the horizontal segment of the petrous ICA is called the foramen lacerum. *(Bottom)* At the level of the cribriform plate, the jugular foramen is now divided by the jugular spine into the more anterior pars nervosa (CNIX, Jacobsen nerve, and inferior petrosal sinus) and the more posterolateral pars vascularis (CNX, CNXI, Arnold nerve, and jugular bulb).

Cranial Nerves Overview

AXIAL BONE CT

Cranial Nerves

Superior orbital fissure (CNIII, IV, VI and V1)

Jugular foramen, pars nervosa (CNIX)

Jugular foramen, pars vascularis (CNX-XI)

Crista galli

Subfrontal cistern (olfactory bulb here)

Internal carotid artery, lacerum segment

Carotid canal, horizontal segment

Jugular spine

Facial nerve canal, mastoid segment (CNVII)

Jugular tubercle

Superior orbital fissure (CNIII, IV, VI, and V1)

Petrooccipital fissure, cephalad aspect (CNVI)

Facial nerve canal, cephalad mastoid segment

Roof of jugular bulb

Superior orbital fissure

Cavernous sinus area (CNIII, IV, VI, V1, and V2)

Inferior bony margin of porus trigeminus (CNV)

Cochlea

Roof of jugular bulb

Greater wing of sphenoid bone

Anterior clinoid process

Dorsum sellae

Internal auditory canal (CNVII and VIII)

Mastoid air cells

Optic canal (CNII)

Petrous apex

Facial nerve canal, labyrinthine segment (CNVII)

(Top) *At the level of the mid-horizontal portion of the petrous ICA, the superior orbital fissure is seen. Remember that CNs III, IV, and VI as well as the ophthalmic division of CNV and the superior ophthalmic vein all enter the orbit through this structure.* **(Middle)** *At the level of the cochlea and upper petrous apex, the petrooccipital fissure is seen. This is approximately the location of CNVI after it pierces the dura to leave the prepontine cistern on its way to the cavernous sinus. On bone CT, the area of the cavernous sinus can only be approximated. Notice also the inferior margin of the porus trigeminus.* **(Bottom)** *The internal auditory canal is visible on this most cephalad CT image. The facial (CNVII) and vestibulocochlear (CNVIII) nerves pass through the IAC. The optic nerve (CNII) enters orbit via the optic canal, which lies medial to the anterior clinoid process.*

Cranial Nerves Overview

AXIAL T2 MR

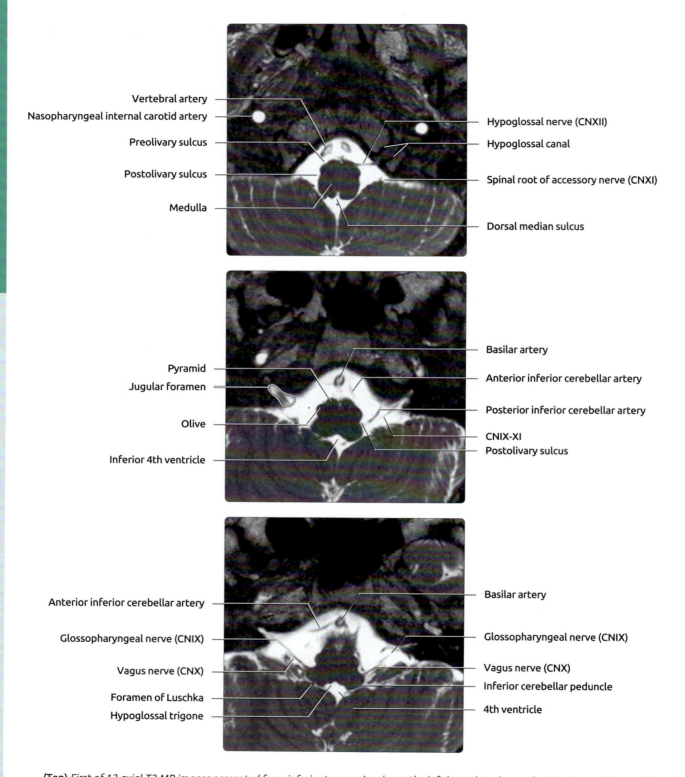

(Top) First of 12 axial T2 MR images presented from inferior to superior shows the left hypoglossal nerve leaving the preolivary sulcus of the medulla. Spinal root of accessory nerve (CNXI) ascends through the foramen magnum, lateral to the brainstem, to unite with the cranial roots of the accessory nerve before exiting via the jugular foramen. **(Middle)** Glossopharyngeal (CNIX), vagus (CNX), and cranial (bulbar) roots of spinal accessory (CNXI) nerves emerge from lateral brainstem posterior to olive in the postolivary sulcus and exit the skull base via jugular foramen. Do not confuse the posterior or anterior inferior cerebellar arteries for cranial nerves. **(Bottom)** Nucleus of hypoglossal nerve (CNXII) forms a characteristic bulge on the floor of the 4th ventricle called the hypoglossal trigone. It is often difficult to separate CNIX from CNX in the basal cistern.

Cranial Nerves Overview

AXIAL T2 MR

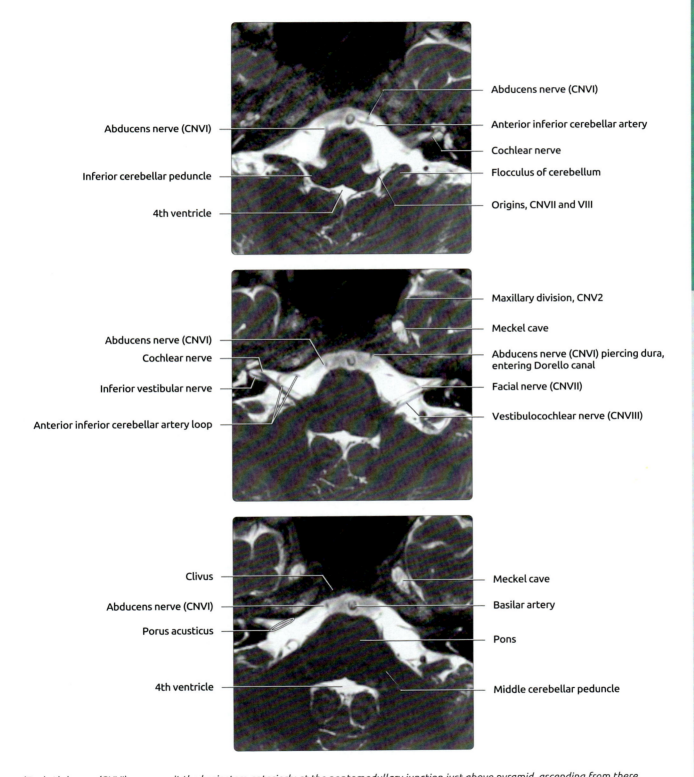

(Top) Abducens (CNVI) nerves exit the brainstem anteriorly at the pontomedullary junction just above pyramid, ascending from there through the prepontine cistern toward the clivus. Cochlear nerve nuclei are found on the lateral surface of the inferior cerebellar peduncle (restiform body). **(Middle)** CNVII and CNVIII exit the brainstem laterally at the pontomedullary junction to enter the cerebellopontine angle cistern. CNVII lies anterior to CNVIII in cerebellopontine angle cistern. Notice CNVI piercing dura on the patient's left to enter the Dorello canal, an interdural channel passing along the dorsal surface of the clivus within the basilar venous plexus toward the cavernous sinus. **(Bottom)** Meckel cave is formed by a dural reflection, lined with arachnoid and containing cerebrospinal fluid. The Gasserian ganglion (trigeminal ganglion) is semilunar in shape and lies anteroinferiorly in the Meckel cave.

Cranial Nerves Overview

AXIAL T2 MR

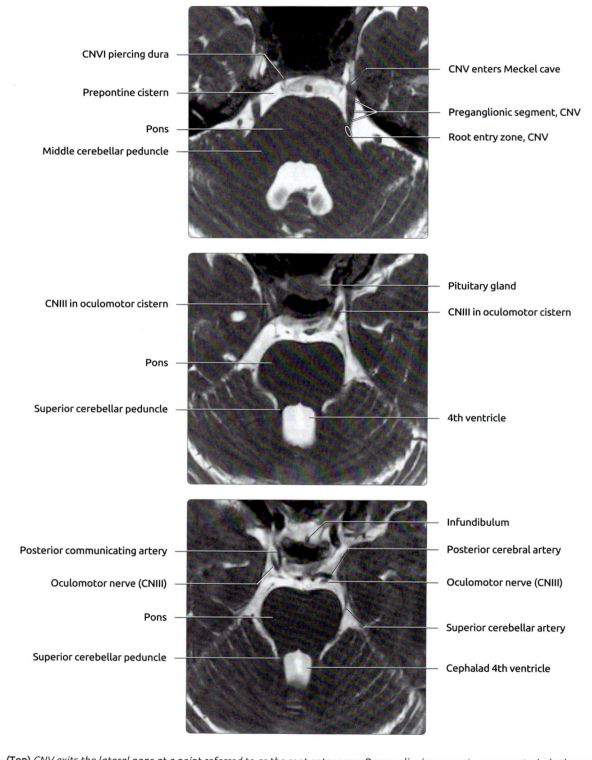

(Top) CNV exits the lateral pons at a point referred to as the root entry zone. Preganglionic segment courses anteriorly through the prepontine cistern and passes over the petrous apex to enter the Meckel cave via the porus trigeminus (entrance to Meckel cave). **(Middle)** In this image, the oculomotor nerve (CNIII) can be seen surrounded by high-signal cerebrospinal fluid as it enters the roof of the cavernous sinus. This area is referred to as the oculomotor cistern. CNIII travels anterolaterally, becoming incorporated into the lateral wall of the cavernous sinus near the anterior clinoid process. **(Bottom)** At the level of the upper pons, important vascular relationships of CNIII passing between the posterior cerebral and superior cerebellar arteries are visible. Notice CNIII coursing anteriorly within the suprasellar cistern adjacent to the posterior communicating artery. An aneurysm of the posterior communicating artery will result in compression of CNIII.

Cranial Nerves Overview

AXIAL T2 MR

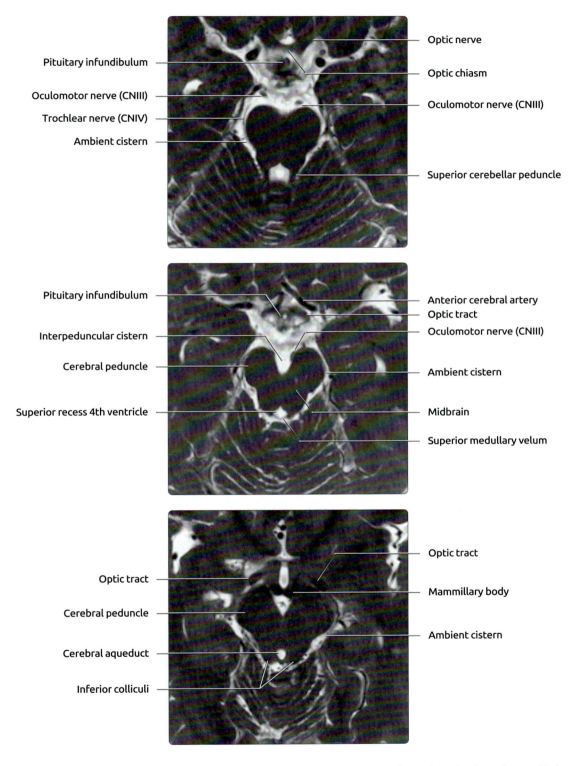

(Top) Anteriorly, note the optic nerves (CNII) form the optic chiasm in the suprasellar cistern. Fibers originating from the nasal halves of the retina cross within the optic chiasm. CNIII courses anteriorly within the suprasellar cistern toward the cavernous sinus. (Middle) CNIII is seen on the patient's left, exiting the brainstem along the medial aspect of the cerebral peduncle, where it enters the interpeduncular cistern. The trochlear nerve (CNIV) decussates in the superior medullary velum, then exits along the dorsal surface of the midbrain below the inferior colliculus to enter the quadrigeminal plate cistern. From there, CNIV courses around the brainstem below the tentorium cerebelli in ambient cistern passing between the posterior cerebral and superior cerebellar arteries. (Bottom) Optic tracts connect the lateral geniculate body to the optic chiasm. Only a portion of the optic tracts are visible here.

Cranial Nerves Overview

CORONAL T2 MR

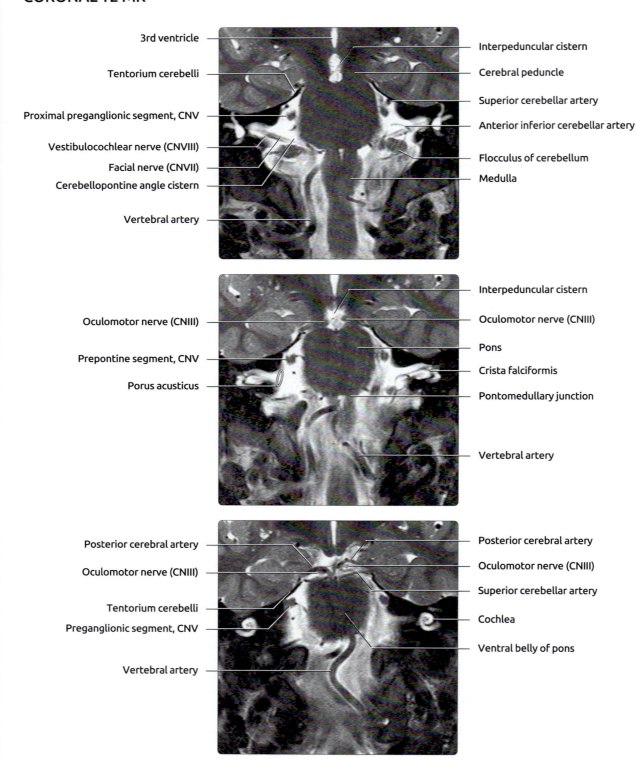

(Top) First of 6 coronal T2 MR images of the brainstem, cisterns, and cranial nerves, presented from posterior to anterior, is shown. Preganglionic segment of the trigeminal nerve is seen arising from the lateral pons. Also seen are the facial and vestibulocochlear nerves traversing the cerebellopontine angle cistern into the internal auditory canal. *(Middle)* Oculomotor nerves are seen emerging from the medial aspect of the cerebral peduncle into the interpeduncular cistern. Basal cistern cranial nerves are not visible. The abrupt transition between the pons and the medulla is termed the pontomedullary junction. *(Bottom)* In this image, notice the oculomotor nerves passing between the posterior cerebral artery above and the superior cerebellar artery below. The distal preganglionic segment of CNV is poised to enter the porus trigeminus on its way into the Meckel cave.

Cranial Nerves Overview

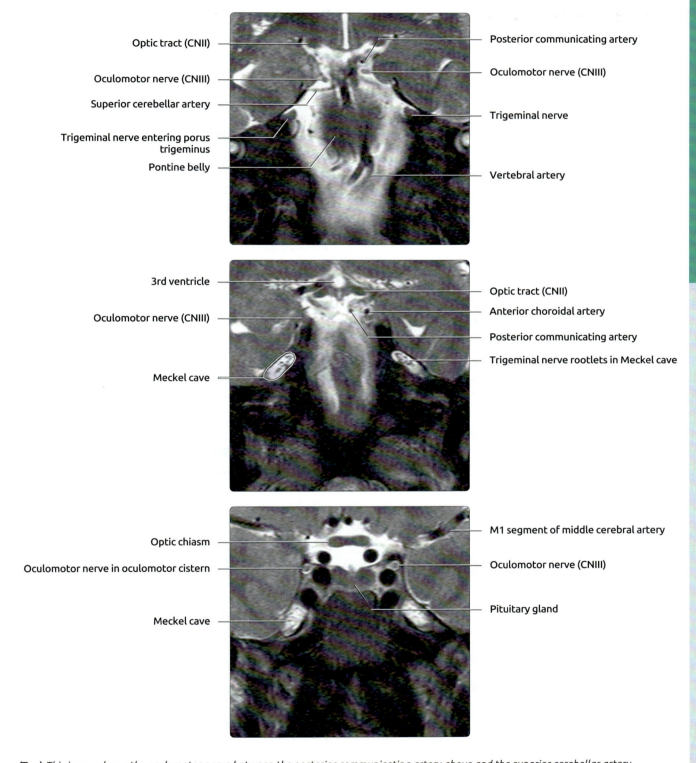

CORONAL T2 MR

(Top) This image shows the oculomotor nerve between the posterior communicating artery above and the superior cerebellar artery below. The trigeminal nerve is visible entering the porus trigeminus of the Meckel cave. **(Middle)** Here, the optic tracts are seen converging toward the optic chiasm. Note a large left anterior choroidal artery coursing posterolaterally within the suprasellar cistern. Preganglionic fibers of the trigeminal nerve are seen within the Meckel cave. The Meckel cave is formed by a reflection of dura, which is lined with arachnoid, contains cerebrospinal fluid, and communicates freely with prepontine cistern. **(Bottom)** In this most anterior coronal T2 image, the pituitary is seen below the optic chiasm. Notice the oculomotor nerve is entering the cavernous sinus in the oculomotor cistern. The high-signal ring around CNIII is cerebrospinal fluid.

CNI (Olfactory Nerve)

TERMINOLOGY

Abbreviations

- Olfactory nerve: CNI

Synonyms

- 1st cranial nerve

Definitions

- CNI: Visceral afferent cranial nerve for sense of smell

IMAGING ANATOMY

Overview

- Olfactory nerve segments
  - Receptor neurons in olfactory epithelium in nasal vault
  - Transethmoidal segment through cribriform plate
  - Intracranial olfactory bulb, tract, and cortex

Nasal Epithelium

- Pseudostratified columnar epithelium (~ 2 cm²), classically described in roof of each nasal cavity, adjacent septum, and lateral nasal cavity wall, including superior turbinates
  - Recent studies show more extensive distribution up to middle turbinate, posterior and middle septum
- This epithelium contains **bipolar olfactory receptor cells**
  - Their peripheral processes (or dendrites) act as sensory receptors for smell, each neuron expressing single type of odorant receptors out of ~ 400-500 types
- Olfactory glands (of Bowman) secrete mucous, which solubilizes inhaled scents (odorant molecules)

Transethmoidal Segment

- Hundreds of central processes (or axons) of receptor cells are bundled into unmyelinated fascicles (fila olfactoria) interleaved with specialized glial cells called olfactory ensheathing cells
  - **Fila olfactoria** are true **olfactory nerves**
  - ~ 20 fila traverse **cribriform plate** on each side of nasal cavity to synapse with olfactory bulb neurons

Intracranial Olfactory Bulb and Tract

- Olfactory bulb and tracts are extensions of brain, not nerves, but historically referred to as 1st cranial nerve
- **Olfactory bulb** (mean volume 125 ±17 mm³) is closely apposed to cribriform plate at ventral surface medial frontal lobe
  - Histologically, bulb contains 6 concentric cell layers
  - Axons within fila from receptor cells expressing same type of odorant receptor converge to spherical "glomerulus" in glomerular layer of bulb where they synapse with processes of secondary neurons (mitral and tufted cells) in deeper layers of bulb
    - Short axon and granule cells modulate secondary neurons
  - Axons of mitral and tufted cells coalesce to form lateral olfactory tract
- **Olfactory tract** (mean length 28-30 mm) trifurcates to medial, intermediate, lateral striae at **anterior perforated substance**, where intermediate striae terminate
  - This trifurcation creates **olfactory trigone**
  - Anterior olfactory nucleus formed by some neurons along olfactory tract
  - Olfactory tubercle is immediately behind division of olfactory stria, fused with anterior perforated substance

Intracranial, Central Pathways

- Complex connections, incompletely elucidated in humans
- **Olfactory cortex**
  - Cortical areas that receive input from olfactory bulb
  - Composed of anatomically distinct areas: Piriform cortex, olfactory tubercle, anterior olfactory nucleus, anterior cortical nucleus of amygdala and periamygdaloid cortex and anterior parts of entorhinal cortex
- **Lateral olfactory striae**
  - Formed by majority of fibers of olfactory tracts
  - Course over limen of insula to piriform (previously called prepiriform) cortex anterior to uncus and then to medial surface of amygdala
  - Projections from piriform cortex go to orbitofrontal cortex, thalamus (medial dorsal thalamic nucleus), hypothalamus, amygdala, and hippocampal formation
- **Medial olfactory striae**
  - Majority terminate in parolfactory area of Broca (medial surface in front of subcallosal gyrus), some in subcallosal gyrus and anterior perforated substance
  - Few fibers go contralaterally in anterior commissure
- **Medial forebrain bundle**
  - Formed by fibers from basal olfactory region, periamygdaloid area, and septal nuclei
  - Some fibers terminate in hypothalamic nuclei
  - Most fibers go to autonomic areas in brainstem (reticular formation, salivatory nuclei, dorsal vagus nucleus)
  - In human imaging studies, olfactory tubercle seen between uncus and medial forebrain bundle.

ANATOMY IMAGING ISSUES

Imaging Recommendations

- Olfactory dysfunction imaging depends on clinical context
  - Sinus CT with coronal reconstructions typically done in post-URI anosmia, head trauma, or sinus surgery
  - MR of brain and sinonasal region used with suspected neurodegenerative disease (Alzheimer, Parkinson), neurologic symptoms, olfactory hallucinations, hypogonadism, or lifelong anosmia

Imaging Pitfalls

- Coronal sinus CT includes nasal vault and cribriform plate but insensitive to intracranial pathology
- Remember to include medial temporal lobes in assessment

CLINICAL IMPLICATIONS

Clinical Importance

- CNI dysfunction produces **unilateral anosmia**
- **Esthesioneuroblastoma** arises from olfactory epithelium
- Olfactory ensheathing cells can give rise to schwannomas
- Head trauma may cause anosmia: Cribriform plate fracture or shear forces; anterior temporal lobe injury
- Seizures involving olfactory network produce "uncinate fits" with olfactory hallucinations, variable oroglossal automatisms, and impaired awareness
- Olfactory bulb volumes decreased in head trauma, chronic rhinosinusitis, Alzheimer disease, multiple sclerosis, and schizophrenia

CNI (Olfactory Nerve)

GRAPHICS

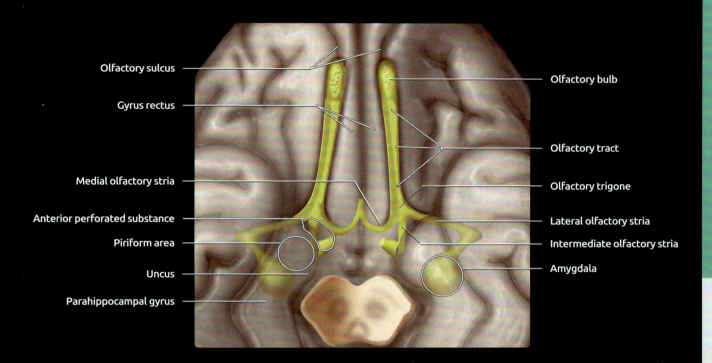

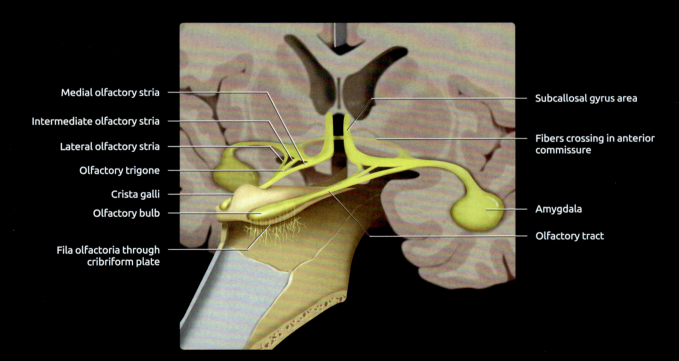

(Top) Graphic of olfactory system viewed from below shows olfactory tracts coursing from olfactory bulbs to the olfactory trigone. In the olfactory trigone, fibers split up into lateral, intermediate, and medial striae. The majority of fibers course through the lateral stria to the piriform area and amygdala. Some fibers in the medial stria course through the anterior commissure to connect to the opposite tract. The majority of intermediate stria fibers terminate in the anterior perforated substance. (Bottom) Graphic of olfactory system seen from an anterolateral oblique perspective shows central processes from bipolar olfactory cells in the olfactory epithelium crossing the cribriform plate bundled as fila olfactoria (~ 20 per side) and connecting with secondary neurons in the olfactory bulbs. The olfactory trigone is visible dividing into lateral, intermediate, and medial striae.

CNI (Olfactory Nerve)

CORONAL NECT

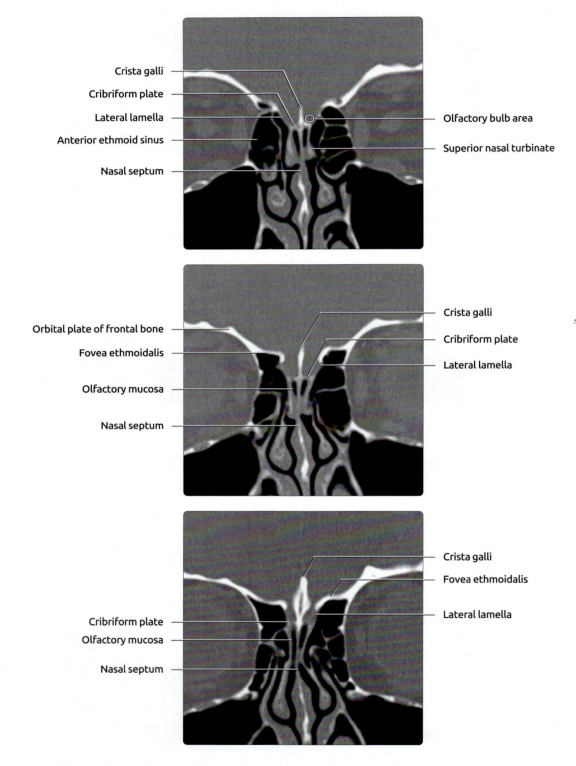

(Top) First of 3 coronal bone CTs through the anterior cranial fossa are presented from posterior to anterior. The olfactory epithelium is found on the roof of the nasal cavity, extending inferolaterally on the superior turbinate and inferomedially on the nasal septum. The olfactory nerves pass through perforations in the cribriform plate. The olfactory bulbs sit just above the cribriform plates. *(Middle)* In this CT, the ethmoid bone forms the medial floor of the anterior cranial fossa and consists of the cribriform plate and crista galli. The fenestrated cribriform plate is depressed relative to the orbital plate of the frontal bone. The fovea ethmoidalis is the most medial portion of the orbital plate of the frontal bone and separates the ethmoid labyrinth from the anterior cranial fossa. *(Bottom)* The anterior cribriform plate is seen at the base of the larger anterior crista galli.

CNI (Olfactory Nerve)

CORONAL T2 MR

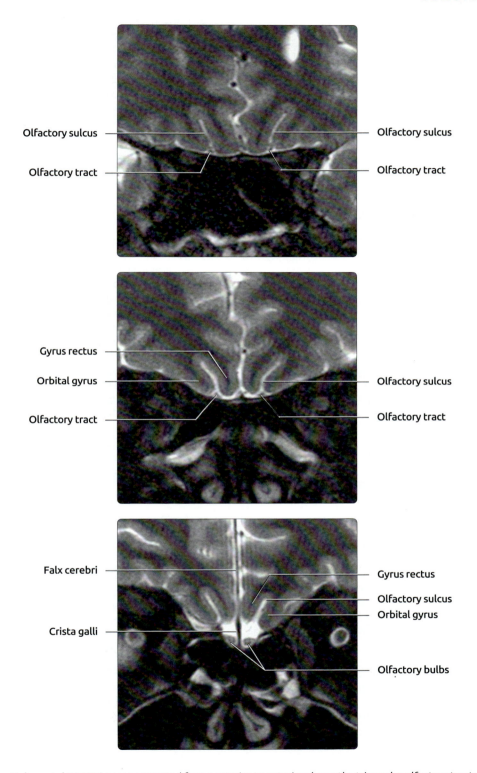

(Top) First of 3 sequential coronal T2 MR images presented from posterior to anterior shows the triangular olfactory tracts, which are composed of centrally projecting axons, embedded within the olfactory sulcus. (Middle) The olfactory sulcus is easily identified separating the gyrus rectus medially from the orbital gyrus laterally. Again note the olfactory tracts at the base of the olfactory sulcus. (Bottom) In this image through the anterior cribriform plate, note the olfactory bulbs. The olfactory bulbs are rostral enlargement of the olfactory tracts, which lie on either side of the midline on the intracranial surface of the cribriform plate. The olfactory nerves arise from the olfactory epithelium located in the roof nasal cavity and pass through the fenestrated cribriform plate to end in the olfactory bulbs.

CNII (Optic Nerve)

TERMINOLOGY

Abbreviations
- Optic nerve: CNII

Synonyms
- 2nd cranial nerve

Definitions
- CNII: Nerve of sight
- Visual pathway consists of optic nerve, optic chiasm, and retrochiasmal structures

IMAGING ANATOMY

Overview
- Optic nerve **not** true cranial nerve but rather **extension of brain**
  - Represents collection of retinal ganglion cell axons
  - Myelinated by **oligodendrocytes** not by Schwann cells as with true cranial nerves
  - Enclosed by meninges
  - Throughout its course to visual cortex, nerve fibers are arranged in **retinotopic order**
- Optic nerve has 4 segments
  - Intraocular, intraorbital, intracanalicular, and intracranial
- Partial decussation CNII fibers within optic chiasm
  - Axons from medial portion of each retina cross to join those from lateral portion of opposite retina
- Retrochiasmal structures: Optic tract, lateral geniculate body, optic radiation, and visual cortex

Optic Pathway
- **Optic nerve: Intraocular segment**
  - 1 mm in length
  - Region of sclera termed **lamina cribrosa** where ganglion cell axons exit globe
- **Optic nerve: Intraorbital segment**
  - 20-30 mm in length
  - Extends posteromedially from back of globe to orbital apex within intraconal space of orbit
  - CNII longer than actual distance from optic chiasm to globe allowing for movements of eye
  - Covered by same 3 meningeal layers as brain
    - Outer dura, middle arachnoid, and inner pia
    - Subarachnoid space (SAS) between arachnoid and pia contains cerebrospinal fluid (CSF); continuous with SAS of suprasellar cistern
    - Fluctuations in intracranial pressure transmitted via SAS of optic nerve-sheath complex
  - Central retinal artery
    - 1st branch of ophthalmic artery
    - Enters optic nerve ~ 1 cm posterior to globe with accompanying vein to run to retina
- **Optic nerve: Intracanalicular segment**
  - 4- to 9-mm segment within bony optic canal
  - Ophthalmic artery lies inferior to CNII
  - Dura of CNII fuses with orbit periosteum (periorbita)
- **Optic nerve: Intracranial segment**
  - ~ 10 mm in length from optic canal to chiasm
  - Covered by pia and surrounded by CSF within suprasellar cistern

- Ophthalmic artery runs inferolateral to nerve
- **Optic chiasm**
  - Horizontally oriented; X-shaped structure within suprasellar cistern
  - Forms part of floor of 3rd ventricle between optic recess anteriorly and infundibular recess posteriorly
  - Immediately anterior to infundibulum (pituitary stalk), superior to diaphragma sellae
  - Anteriorly chiasm divides into optic nerves
  - In chiasm nerve, fibers from medial 1/2 of retina cross to opposite side
  - Posteriorly chiasm divides into optic tracts
  - Medial fibers of optic tracts cross in chiasm to connect lateral geniculate bodies of both sides (commissure of Gudden)
- **Optic tracts**
  - Posterior extension of optic chiasm
  - Fibers pass posterolaterally, curving around cerebral peduncle and divide into medial and lateral bands
    - Lateral band (majority of fibers) ends in **lateral geniculate body** of thalamus
    - Medial band goes by medial geniculate body to pretectal nuclei deep to superior colliculi
- **Optic radiation and visual cortex**
  - Axons from lateral geniculate body form **optic radiations** (geniculocalcarine tracts)
  - Fan out from lateral geniculate body and run as broad fiber tract to calcarine fissure
    - Initially pass laterally behind posterior limb internal capsule and basal ganglia
    - Extend posteriorly around lateral ventricle passing through posterior temporal and parietal lobes
    - Terminate in calcarine cortex (primary visual cortex) on medial surface of occipital lobes

ANATOMY IMAGING ISSUES

Imaging Recommendations
- CT best for skull base and optic canal bony anatomy
- MR for CNII, optic chiasm, and retrochiasmal structures
  - Axial and coronal thin-section T2, T1, and T1 C+

Imaging Pitfalls
- Orbital CT may see subtle calcified optic sheath meningioma when MR may not

CLINICAL IMPLICATIONS

Clinical Importance
- Lesion location
  - Optic nerve pathology: **Monocular visual loss**
  - Optic chiasm pathology: **Bitemporal heteronymous hemianopsia** (loss of bilateral temporal visual fields)
  - Retrochiasmal pathology: **Homonymous hemianopsia** (vision loss in contralateral eye)
- Increased intracranial pressure transmitted along SAS of optic nerve-sheath complex
  - Manifests clinically as **papilledema**
  - Imaging shows flattening of posterior sclera, tortuosity and elongation of intraorbital optic nerves, and dilatation of perioptic SAS

CNII (Optic Nerve)

GRAPHICS

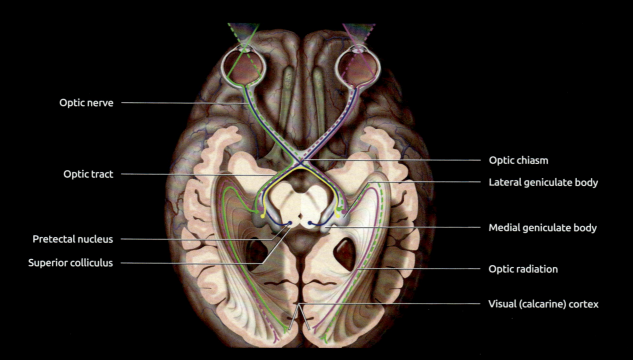

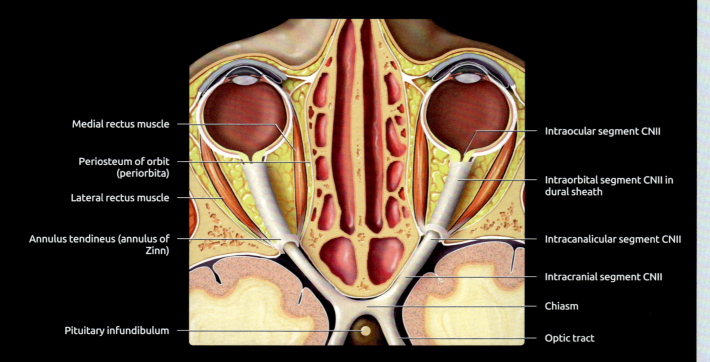

(Top) *Axial graphic through the visual pathway shows medial retinal fibers crossing in the optic chiasm so that fibers from left 1/2 of both retinas course in left optic tract, and fibers in right 1/2 of both retinas course in right optic tract (purple and green, respectively). Majority of retinal nerve fibers terminate in lateral geniculate bodies, where synaptic neuronal cell bodies give rise to optic radiations, which extend to visual cortices. A few retinal nerve fibers (blue) involved in optic reflexes bypass lateral geniculate bodies and terminate in pretectal nuclei. Medial fibers of optic tracts cross in chiasm to connect lateral geniculate bodies of both sides (yellow).*
(Bottom) *Axial graphic of the orbit shows the 4 segments of the optic nerve (intraocular, intraorbital, intracanalicular, and intracranial). At the annulus of Zinn, the dural sheath of the intraorbital segment becomes contiguous with periorbita.*

CNII (Optic Nerve)

GRAPHICS

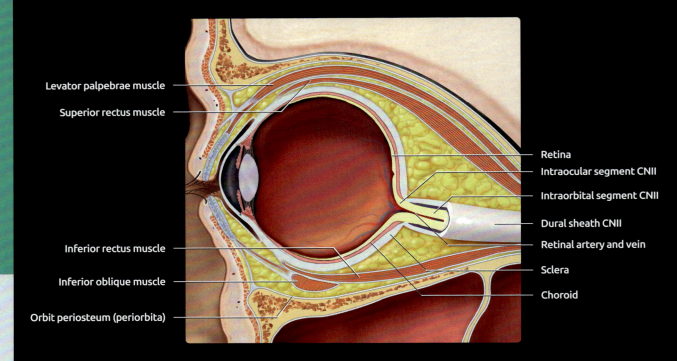

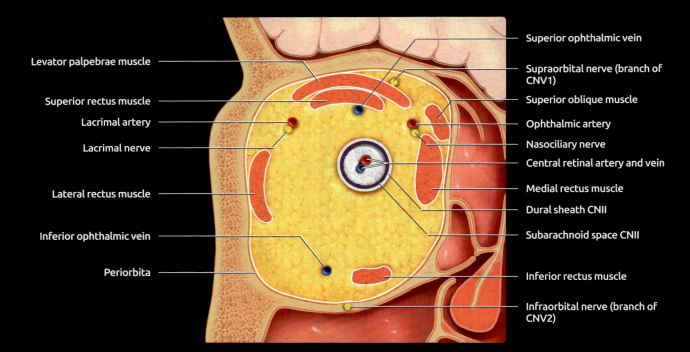

(Top) Sagittal graphic through the orbit shows continuity of the dural sheath of the intraorbital segment of CNII with the sclera. At the annulus of Zinn, the dural sheath is continuous with the periorbita (not seen in this graphic). Central retinal artery and vein enter the distal intraorbital segment of CNII to supply the retina. **(Bottom)** Coronal graphic through the distal optic nerve shows encasement of the optic nerve by the arachnoid and dura. Subarachnoid space of CNII is continuous with the cerebral subarachnoid space. Central retinal artery and vein pierce the dura of the distal intraorbital segment and continue to the retina in the center of CNII.

CNII (Optic Nerve)

AXIAL STIR MR

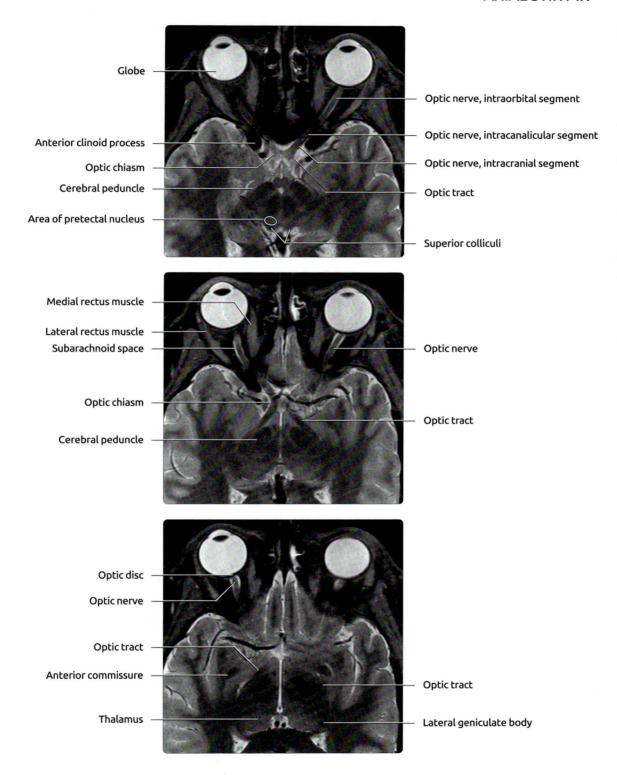

(Top) First of 3 axial STIR MR images from inferior to superior demonstrate intraorbital, intracanalicular, and intracranial segments of the optic nerve. Intraorbital segment extends from the back of the globe posteromedially to the orbital apex within the intraconal space. Intracanalicular segment passes through the bony optic canal. Intracranial segment is ~ 10 mm long from optic canal to chiasm. (Middle) Subarachnoid space with cerebrospinal fluid surrounds the optic nerve and is continuous with the subarachnoid space of the suprasellar cistern. Optic chiasm lies within the suprasellar cistern. Optic tracts extend posteriorly around the cerebral peduncles to the lateral geniculate body. (Bottom) Majority of fibers from optic tracts terminate in the lateral geniculate body located at the posteroinferior aspect of the thalamus. Efferent axons from lateral geniculate body form optic radiation extending to the calcarine cortex.

CNII (Optic Nerve)

CORONAL T1 MR

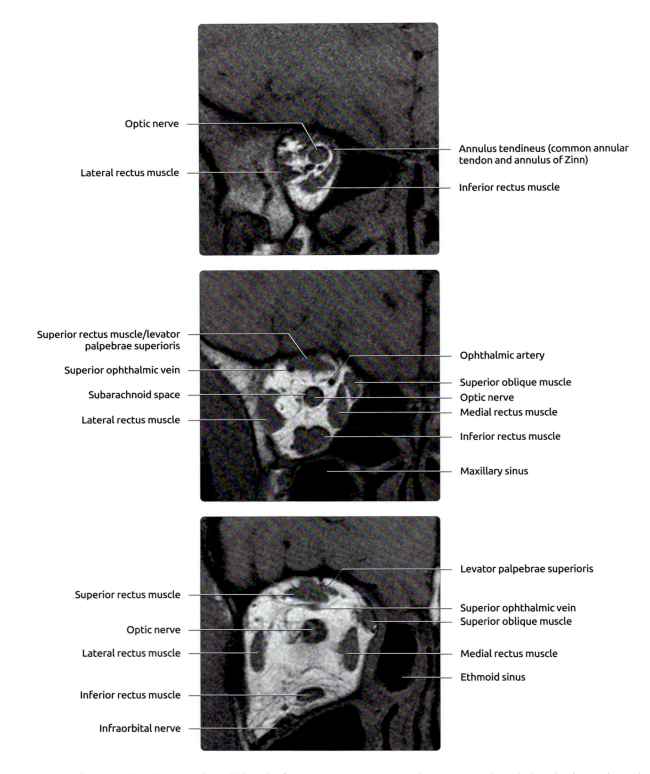

(Top) First of 3 coronal T1 MR images through the orbit from posterior to anterior is shown. Section through the orbital apex shows the optic nerve passing through the common annular tendon, which serves as the site of origin of the rectus muscles. *(Middle)* In this image, both the superolateral ophthalmic vein and the superomedial ophthalmic artery are visible. Note that the subarachnoid space is visible as a thin, black line surrounding the optic nerve, a finding often not seen on routine T1 imaging of the orbit. *(Bottom)* In this image just behind the globe, all the extraocular muscles are clearly visible. Notice the levator palpebrae superioris muscle may be difficult to distinguish from the superior rectus muscle even with high-resolution MR imaging.

CNII (Optic Nerve)

CORONAL T2 MR

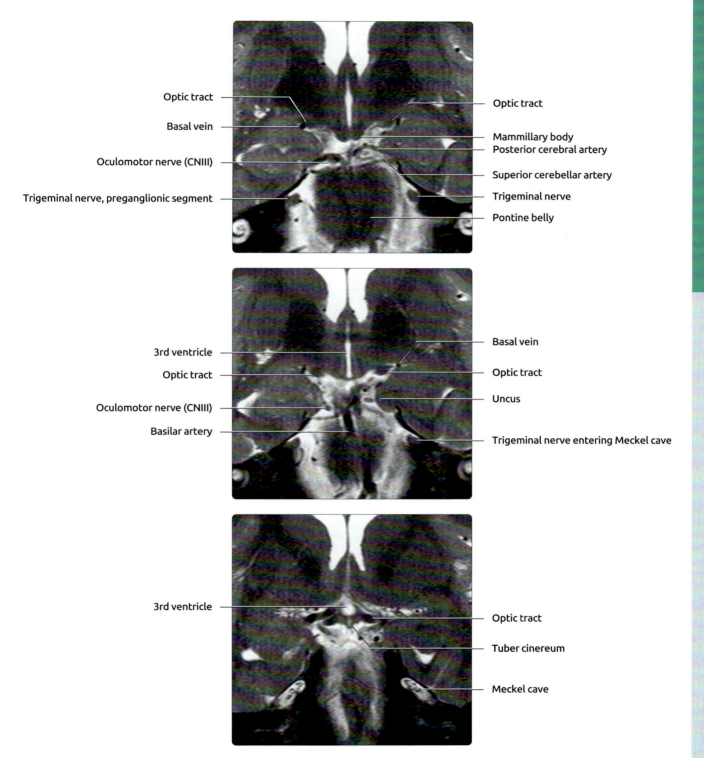

(Top) First of 6 coronal T2 MR images shows the optic tracts and chiasm from posterior to anterior. The optic tracts course posterolaterally, curving around the cerebral peduncle to eventually terminate in lateral geniculate body (lateral root) and pretectal nuclei at the superior colliculi (medial band). (Middle) Optic tracts course through the posterior suprasellar cistern toward the ambient cistern, closely related to basal vein (of Rosenthal). (Bottom) In this image through the back of the optic chiasm, the optic tracts are shown as the posterior extension of the optic chiasm carrying fibers from the ipsilateral 1/2 of both retinae. The tuber cinereum leads to the infundibulum (pituitary stalk). Notice the 3rd ventricle just above the posterior optic chiasm.

CNII (Optic Nerve)

CORONAL T2 MR

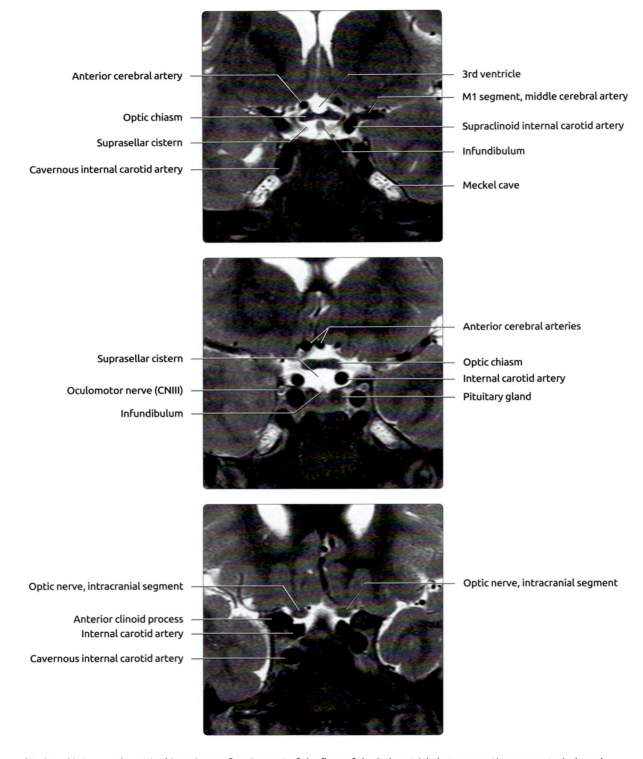

(Top) In this image, the optic chiasm is seen forming part of the floor of the 3rd ventricle between optic recess anteriorly and infundibular recess posteriorly. It is immediately anterior to the infundibulum (pituitary stalk). (Middle) Optic chiasm is a horizontally oriented, X-shaped structure within the suprasellar cistern. Nerve fibers from the medial halves of both retinae cross to continue to lateral geniculate bodies. Interruption of crossing chiasmatic fibers leads to bitemporal hemianopia. (Bottom) The intracranial segment of the optic nerves are visible in this image. This segment is ~ 10 mm in length from the optic canal anteriorly to the optic chiasm posteriorly. The nerves are covered by pia at this point. The bright CSF within the suprasellar cistern surrounds the nerves.

CNII (Optic Nerve)

AXIAL & SAGITTAL T1 MR

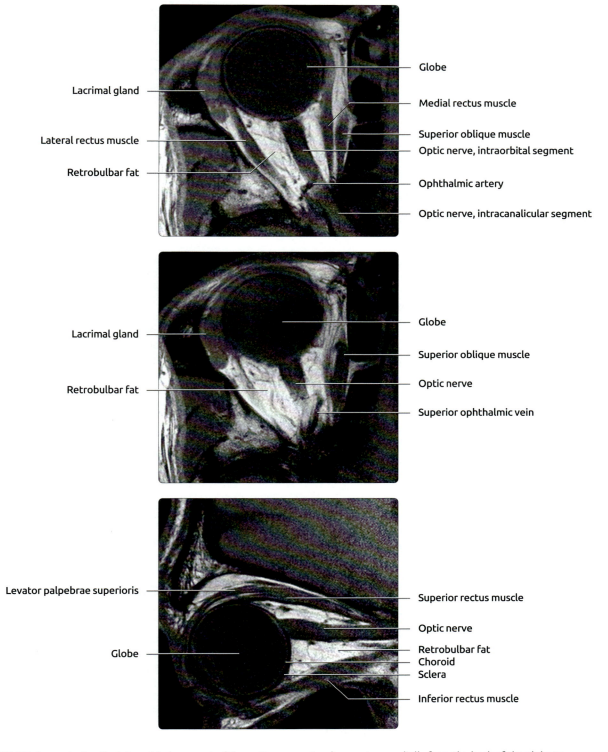

(Top) Axial T1 MR demonstrates the intraorbital segment of the optic nerve extending posteromedially from the back of the globe to the orbital apex, surrounded by fat within the intraconal space. Note the intracanalicular segment passing through the bony optic canal. (Middle) Axial T1 MR shows the origin of the optic nerve from the globe. Nerve fibers of the retina unite, forming the optic nerve before exiting the eyeball through the lamina cribrosa, a thin, perforated portion of the sclera. In the superior orbit, the lacrimal gland is seen in its superolateral fossa. (Bottom) Sagittal T1 MR through the optic nerve demonstrates the intraorbital segment of the optic nerve. Sclera of the globe is hypointense, while the pigmented choroid of the uvea is hyperintense due to T1-shortening effects of melanin.

CNIII (Oculomotor Nerve)

TERMINOLOGY

Abbreviations

- Oculomotor nerve (CNIII; CN3)
- Oculomotor nuclear complex (ONC)
- Extraocular muscle (EOM)
- Medial longitudinal fasciculus (MLF)
- Edinger-Westphal nucleus (EWn)
- Superior orbital fissure (SOF)

Synonyms

- 3rd cranial nerve

Definitions

- CNIII: Motor nerve to EOMs except lateral rectus (CNVI) and superior oblique muscles (CNIV); parasympathetic motor to pupillary sphincter and ciliary muscle

IMAGING ANATOMY

Overview

- Purely motor cranial nerve with general somatic efferent fibers as well as general visceral efferent (parasympathetic)
- Supplies all EOMs except superior oblique and lateral rectus muscles via general somatic efferent innervation
- Innervates pupillary sphincter and ciliary muscles via parasympathetic innervation
- Nerve originates from ONC in posterior midbrain
- Nerve can be divided into 7 segments: Intramesencephalic, interpeduncular cisternal, petroclinoid, trigonal, cavernous, fissural, and orbital

Oculomotor Nerve Complex

- There are paired paramedian ONCs located in posterior aspect of midbrain at level of superior colliculus
- Partially embedded in periaqueductal gray matter anterior (ventral) to cerebral aqueduct
- ONC has complex cytoarchitecture with multiple motor nuclei and parasympathetic nucleus
- Contains motor neurons of medial, inferior, and superior recti, inferior oblique, and levator palpebrae muscles
- Motor neurons are arranged into subgroups generally referred to as nuclei
- Motor nuclei are arranged in 2 paramedian clusters or stacks referred to as columns or somatic columns
- Each paramedian somatic column consists of 4 relatively distinct nuclei, providing axons to EOMs
  - **Ventral nucleus**: Ipsilateral medial rectus
  - **Central nucleus**: Contralateral superior rectus and ipsilateral inferior oblique
  - **Dorsolateral nucleus**: Ipsilateral medial rectus
  - **Dorsomedial nuclei**: Ipsilateral inferior rectus
- Just inferior to paired columns is single midline motor nucleus, **central caudal nucleus**
  - Central caudal nucleus contains motor neurons for levator palpebrae muscle, possibly provides crossed and uncrossed axons
- **EWn**
  - More complex than classically considered
    - Anatomy is confounded by differences in primates and humans

- Nomenclature confusing given inconsistent application of term EWn to 2 different groups of neurons that contain different cell types and provide different function
  - 1st group: Preganglionic parasympathetic component (EWpg)
  - 2nd group: Nonpreganglionic centrally projecting component (EWcp)
- **EWnp** (parasympathetic component)
  - Provides parasympathetic motor to pupillary sphincter and ciliary muscles of eye
  - In humans, preganglionic parasympathetic neurons are located posteromedial to somatic columns near midline but do not form compact or distinct nucleus
- **EWncp** (centrally projecting components)
  - Located posteromedial to somatic columns, in between columns and parasympathetic neurons of EWpg
  - Forms compact and distinct nucleus
  - Consists of peptidergic neurons that project to brainstem, spinal cord, and prosencephalic regions
  - Not definitely related to ocular function; may function in feeding behavior, stress responses, addiction, and pain
- **Nucleus of Perlia**
  - Small linear nucleus medial to main motor nuclei near midline of midbrain
  - Function less clear; may function in ocular convergence
  - May provide some motor fibers to superior rectus
- Arterial supply to ONC and intramesencephalic nerves is via group of small penetrating arteries that arise from terminal regions of basilar artery at near origins of superior cerebellar and posterior cerebral arteries

Intramesencephalic Segment

- Intraaxial segment resides within midbrain and extends from ONC to interpeduncular cistern
- CNIII fascicles course anteriorly at least partially through MLF, red nucleus, substantia nigra, and medial cerebral peduncle
- Oculomotor nerve fascicles converge in posterior-to-anterior direction
- Exit midbrain into interpeduncular cistern

Interpeduncular Cisternal Segment

- Each CNIII leaves midbrain medially to cerebral peduncle in lateral part of interpeduncular fossa
- Each nerve may arise as tiny rootlets that immediately unite and extend as single root
- Cisternal segment extends from exit point of nerve along medial side of cerebral peduncle through interpeduncular and prepontine cisterns to posterior petroclinoid fold, posterior margin of oculomotor triangle
- Passes between posterior cerebral artery (PCA) above and superior cerebellar artery (SCA) below
- Courses inferior to posterior communicating artery and medial to free edge of tentorium cerebelli
- Measures ~ 2.1 mm in diameter within cistern
- Topographically, pupillary fibers are superficially located in cisternal portion of CNIII

CNIII (Oculomotor Nerve)

Petroclinoid Segment

- Located between cisternal and trigonal segments
- Defined posteriorly by posterior petroclinoid fold and anteriorly by oculomotor porus (opening) of roof of cavernous sinus
- Oculomotor triangle represents floor of petroclinoid segment

Trigonal Segment

- Petroclinoid segment ends at oculomotor porus where nerve pierces roof of cavernous sinus, near center of oculomotor triangle
- Oculomotor cistern, CSF-filled arachnoid and dural cuff, begins at oculomotor porus and extends ~ 6 mm
- Trigonal segment of oculomotor nerve travels within oculomotor cistern as it enters superolateral cavernous sinus roof
- Trigonal segments terminates when nerve is incorporated into fibrous lateral wall of cavernous sinus
- Cistern and trigonal segment is recognized surgically as avascular space used to mobilize nerve during cavernous sinus surgery

Cavernous Segment

- Incorporated into lateral dural wall of cavernous sinus just under tip of anterior clinoid process
- This wall consists of 2 layers
  - Superficial dense and formed from dura
  - Deep endosteal layer that invests nerves running in lateral wall
- Cavernous segment on CNIII extends just past anterior clinoid process where SOF begins
- Carotid-oculomotor membrane: Layer of dura that lines lower margin of anterior clinoid process and extends medially to form proximal dural ring; it separates lower margin of anterior clinoid process from cavernous segment CNIII and extends medially around carotid artery
- CNIII remains most cephalad of all cranial nerves within cavernous sinus
- CNIII superolateral to cavernous internal carotid artery
- This segment is ~ 14 mm in length

Fissural Segment

- CNIII courses along lateral margin of optic strut as it passes through medial part of SOF
- Fissural segment of oculomotor nerve splits into its superior and inferior divisions
- ~ 6 mm long
- Fissural segment extends from anterior clinoid process to oculomotor foramen of SOF

Orbital Segment

- Superior and inferior branches of CNIII enter orbit through SOF and pass through annulus tendineus (annulus of Zinn)
- Annulus of Zinn partially segments SOF into lateral component and medial component; medial component is referred to as oculomotor foramen
- Superior branch supplies levator palpebrae superioris and superior rectus muscles
- Inferior branch supplies inferior rectus, medial rectus, and inferior oblique muscles

- Preganglionic parasympathetic fibers follow inferior branch to ciliary ganglion of orbit
  - Postganglionic parasympathetic fibers continue as short ciliary nerves to enter globe with optic nerve
  - In globe short ciliary nerves to ciliary body and iris
  - Control papillary sphincter function and accommodation via ciliary muscle

ANATOMY IMAGING ISSUES

Imaging Recommendations

- Bone CT best for skull base, bony foramina
- MR for intraaxial, cisternal, cavernous segments
  - Thin-section, high-resolution T2 MR sequences in axial and coronal planes
    - Depicts cisternal CNIII surrounded by CSF with high contrast and high spatial resolution

Imaging Sweet Spots

- CNIII nuclear complex and intraaxial segment not directly visualized
  - Find periaqueductal gray matter to localize
- Identification of distal basilar artery and branches can be reliable landmark for finding cisternal CNIII; it passes between posterior cerebral artery above and SCA below

Imaging Pitfalls

- Negative MR and MRA does **not** completely exclude posterior communicating artery aneurysm
  - CTA or conventional angiography recommended to exclude this diagnosis

CLINICAL IMPLICATIONS

Clinical Importance

- Uncal herniation pushes CNIII on petroclinoid ligament
- During trauma downward shift of brainstem upon impact can stretch CNIII over petroclinoid ligament
- CNIII susceptible to compression by PCA aneurysms
- CNIII neuropathy divided into **simple** if isolated and **complex** if with other CN involvement (CNIV and CNVI)
  - **Simple** CNIII with pupillary involvement
    - Must exclude **PCA aneurysm** as cause
    - Explanation: Parasympathetic fibers are peripherally distributed
  - Simple CNIII with pupillary sparing
    - Presumed microvascular infarction involves vessels supplying core of nerve with relative sparing of peripheral pupillary fibers

Cranial Nerves

CNIII (Oculomotor Nerve)

GRAPHICS

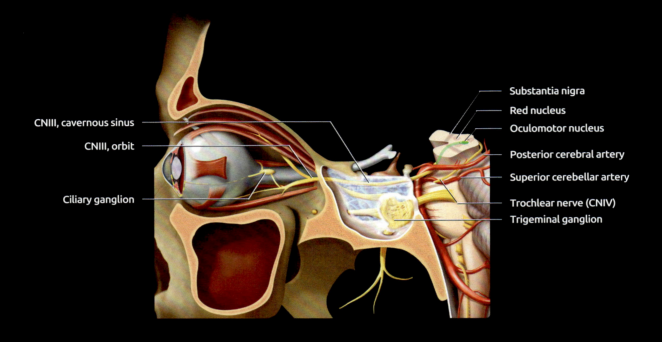

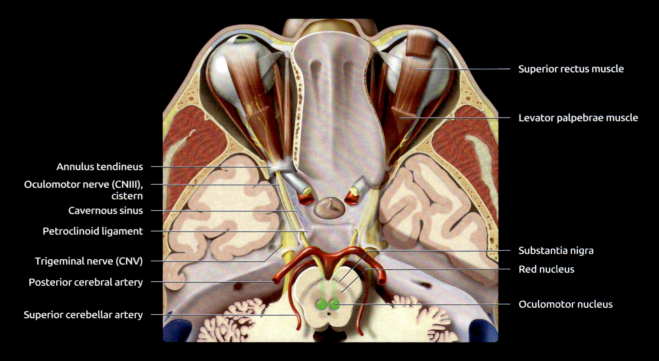

(Top) Sagittal graphic shows the oculomotor nerve exiting from the anterior brainstem. After passing medially to the trochlear nerve (CNIV) between the superior cerebellar artery and posterior cerebral artery, it enters the cavernous sinus. CNIII is the most superior nerve coursing through the cavernous sinus. Once in orbit, it divides into the superior and inferior divisions. Preganglionic parasympathetic fibers travel with the inferior division to join the ciliary ganglion. (Bottom) Axial graphic clearly depicts CNIII originating from the oculomotor nuclei complex to travel through the medial aspect of the red nucleus and substantia nigra before exiting into the prepontine cistern. After traversing the cavernous sinus, surrounded by the CSF-filled oculomotor cistern, it enters the orbit through the superior orbital fissure, dividing into superior and inferior branches and passing through the annulus tendineus (annulus of Zinn).

CNIII (Oculomotor Nerve)

AXIAL T2 MR

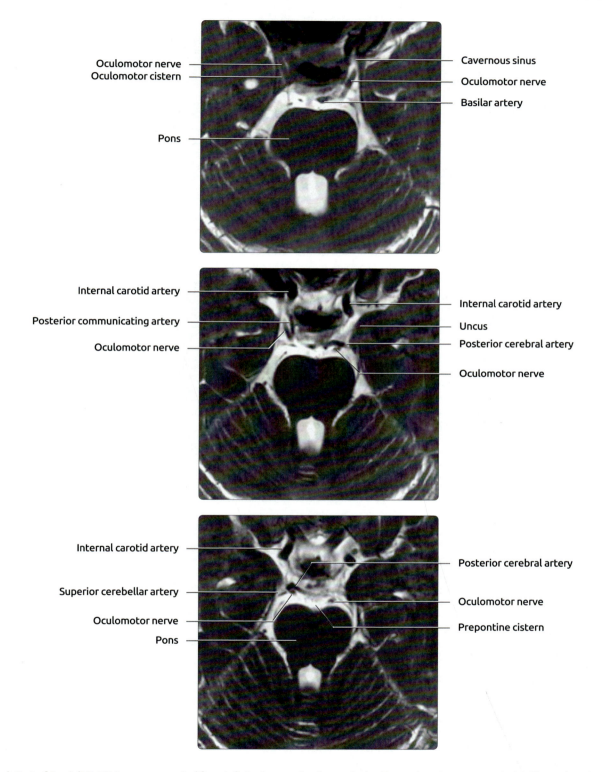

(Top) First of 6 axial T2 MR images presented from inferior to superior demonstrates the oculomotor nerves entering the oculomotor cisterns in the posterior roof of the cavernous sinus. Notice the nerves are surrounded by high-signal cerebrospinal fluid. From here the oculomotor nerves course anteriorly in the lateral wall of the cavernous sinus above the trochlear nerve and enters orbit via the superior orbital fissure. (Middle) Oculomotor nerves course anteriorly through the prepontine cistern inferolateral to the posterior communicating artery and medial to the uncus of the temporal lobe. The left oculomotor nerve is seen passing below the posterior cerebral artery. (Bottom) After exiting the brainstem, the oculomotor nerves course anteriorly through the interpeduncular and prepontine cisterns towards the cavernous sinus, passing between the posterior cerebral and superior cerebellar arteries.

CNIII (Oculomotor Nerve)

AXIAL T2 & T1 MR

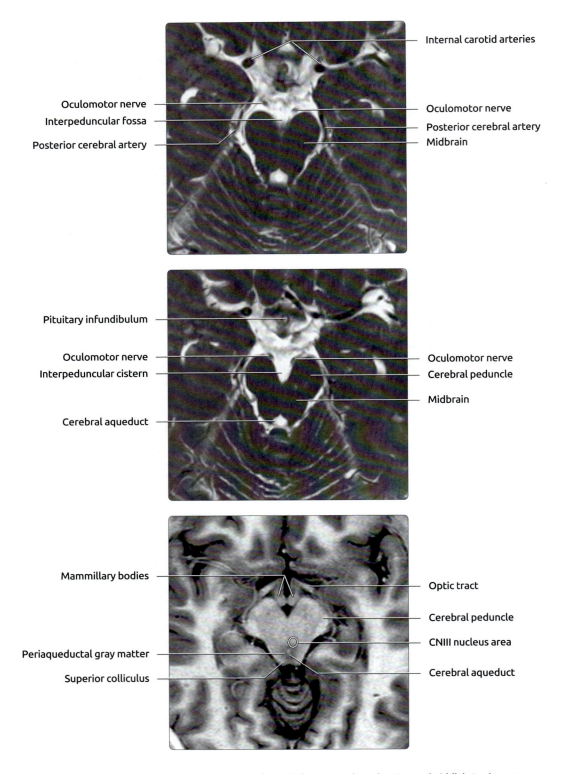

(Top) This image shows both oculomotor nerves coursing through the interpeduncular cistern. (Middle) Oculomotor nerves exit midbrain from the medial surface of the cerebral peduncle to enter the interpeduncular cistern and continue anteriorly underneath the posterior cerebral arteries. (Bottom) Axial inversion recovery prepared T1-weighted MR through the brainstem at the level of superior colliculus is shown. The paired oculomotor nuclear complex is not directly visualized. However, since it is partially embedded in periaqueductal gray matter anterior to cerebral aqueduct at the level of superior colliculus, its position can be inferred by these landmarks. The approximate location of the oculomotor nucleus in marked on the left.

CNIII (Oculomotor Nerve)

CORONAL T2 MR

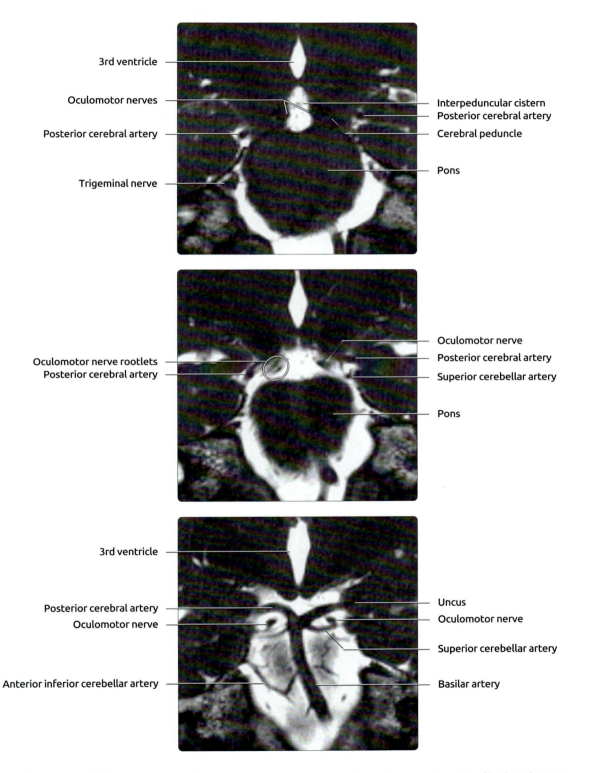

(Top) First of 6 coronal T2 MR images presented from posterior to anterior reveals the most proximal aspects of both oculomotor nerves exiting the midbrain from the medial surface of the cerebral peduncle to enter the interpeduncular cistern. (Middle) Oculomotor nerves often emerge from the midbrain by several rootlets, as seen in this T2 coronal image (circle), which subsequently fuse to form a single trunk. (Bottom) Oculomotor nerves pass between the posterior cerebral artery above and superior cerebellar artery below. The proximity of the oculomotor nerve to the uncus makes the nerve vulnerable to injury through uncal herniation. Its nearness to the posterior communicating, posterior cerebral, and superior cerebellar arteries makes it easily injured by an aneurysm.

CNIII (Oculomotor Nerve)

CORONAL T2 MR

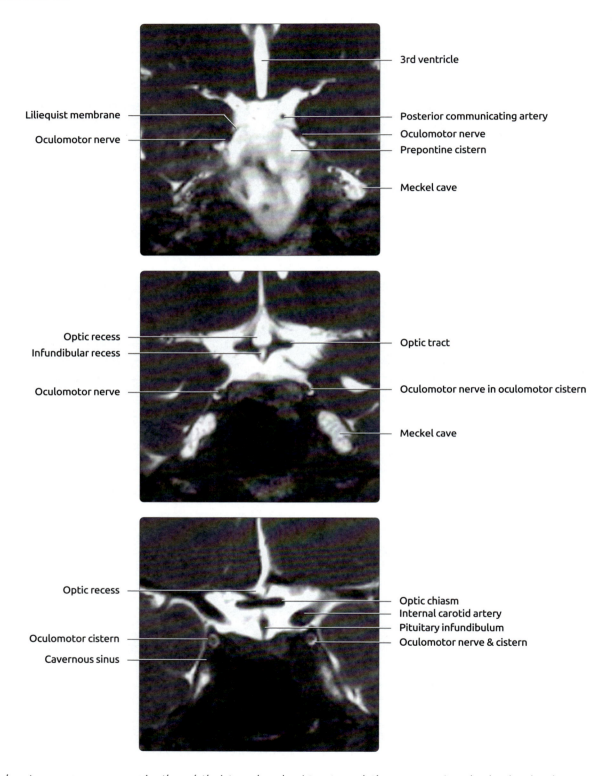

(Top) Oculomotor nerves are seen coursing through the interpeduncular cistern towards the cavernous sinus closely related to the posterior communicating artery. An aneurysm of the posterior communicating artery can result in compression of the oculomotor nerve. The lateral margin of the Liliequist membrane attaches to the arachnoidal sheath surrounding oculomotor nerves. *(Middle)* The oculomotor nerve crosses the petroclinoid ligament and is situated medial to and slightly beneath the level of free edge of the tentorium at the point of entry into the roof of the cavernous sinus. *(Bottom)* A short length of the oculomotor nerve is surrounded by a dural and arachnoid cuff to create the oculomotor cistern within the roof and lateral wall of the cavernous sinus. The oculomotor nerve courses anteriorly above the trochlear nerve within the lateral wall of the cavernous sinus and enters the orbit via the superior orbital fissure.

CNIII (Oculomotor Nerve)

CLINICAL CORRELATION

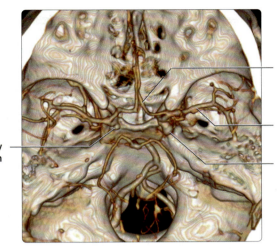

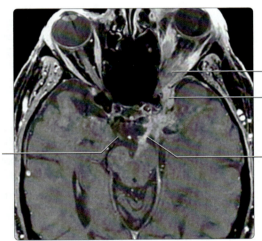

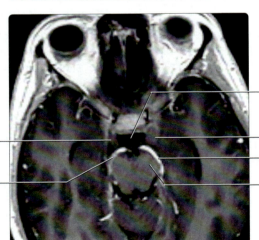

(Top) CTA with 3D reformation in a patient with new-onset right-sided 3rd nerve palsy demonstrates bilateral posterior communicating artery origin aneurysms, right greater than left. Posterior communicating artery origin aneurysms classically cause 3rd nerve palsy with associated pupillary dysfunction. *(Middle)* Middle-aged man with a history of squamous cell carcinoma of the left forehead developed progressive disease of the orbit, and perineural tumor spread to the superior orbital fissure and cavernous sinus. This axial contrast-enhanced image though the level of interpeduncular cistern demonstrates abnormal thickening and enhancement of the cisternal CNIII as tumor extends in retrograde fashion along the nerve from the cavernous sinus. *(Bottom)* Axial contrast-enhanced MR in a patient with acute lymphocytic leukemia and leukemic infiltration of several cranial nerves, including bilateral CNIII, is shown. The nerves show enlargement and abnormal enhancement of the cisternal portions, left worse than right. Notice the proximal posterior cerebral arteries pass medial to the cisternal CNIII and then pass over the nerves en route to the occipital lobes.

CNIV (Trochlear Nerve)

TERMINOLOGY

Abbreviations
- Trochlear nerve: CNIV

Synonyms
- 4th cranial nerve

Definitions
- CNIV: Motor nerve to superior oblique muscle

IMAGING ANATOMY

Overview
- CNIV is pure motor nerve (general somatic efferent) that innervates superior oblique muscle
- Segments: Intramesencephalic, cisternal, tentorial, cavernous, and extracranial

Trochlear Nuclei
- Paired nuclei located in paramedian midbrain, ventral to cerebral aqueduct, and immediately dorsal to medial longitudinal fasciculus
- Caudal to oculomotor nuclear complex at level of inferior colliculus

Intramesencephalic Segment
- Trochlear nerve fascicles course posteriorly and inferiorly around cerebral aqueduct
  - Fibers then cross (decussate) within **superior medullary velum**
  - **Key concept**: Each superior oblique muscle is innervated by ipsilateral CNIV that originates in **contralateral** trochlear nucleus
- CNIV exists dorsal midbrain just inferior to inferior colliculus **(only cranial nerve to exit dorsal brainstem)**

Cisternal Segment
- CNIV courses anterolaterally in through quadrigeminal and ambient cisterns
- Surrounded by CSF in subarachnoid space
- In ambient cistern, passes between posterior cerebral artery above and superior cerebellar artery below, just inferolateral to CNIII

Tentorial Segment
- CNIV passes anteriorly into groove along lower surface of free edge of tentorium
- From groove CNIV pierces dura near posterior margin of oculomotor triangle, along rostrolateral free edge of tentorium
- This segment extends from entrance of CNIV into tentorial groove to anterior petroclinoid fold where nerve enters cavernous sinus

Cavernous Segment
- CNIV enters roof of cavernous sinus in posterolateral apex of oculomotor triangle
- CNIV courses in lateral wall inferior to CNIII, superior to CNV1

Extracranial Segment
- CNIV enters orbit through **superior orbital fissure** together with CNIII and CNVI

- Crosses over CNIII and courses medially
- Passes **above** annulus of Zinn (CNIII and CNVI go through annulus)
- Supplies motor innervation to superior oblique muscle

ANATOMY IMAGING ISSUES

Imaging Recommendations
- CT best for skull base, bony foramina
- High-resolution MR best for brainstem, cisternal, cavernous, and intraorbital imaging
- Intraorbital segment not visualized by any imaging modality or sequence

Imaging Sweet Spots
- CNIV nucleus and intraaxial segment not directly visualized
  - Nuclei position inferred by identifying periaqueductal gray matter and cerebral aqueduct at level of inferior colliculi on high-resolution MR
- MR for intraaxial, cisternal, and cavernous segments
  - Thin-section, high-resolution T2 and T1 C+ MR in axial and coronal planes
    - Coronal imaging margins: 4th ventricle to anterior globe; axial imaging margins: Orbital roof-diencephalon to maxillary sinus roof-medulla

Imaging Pitfalls
- Difficult to visualize normal CNIV despite best MR imaging efforts
- During image interrogation by radiologist, view known landmarks along its course
  - Midbrain → tentorial margin → cavernous sinus → superior orbital fissure → extraconal orbit

Normal Measurements
- CNIV is smallest cranial nerve (.75-1.0 mm)
- CNIV has longest intracranial course (~ 7.5 cm)

CLINICAL IMPLICATIONS

Clinical Importance
- CNIV neuropathy divided into **simple and complex**
  - **Simple** CNIV neuropathy (isolated)
    - Most common form; usually secondary to trauma
    - Cisternal segment injury by free edge of tentorium cerebelli or from posterior cerebral or superior cerebellar artery aneurysm
    - Contusion of superior medullary velum
  - **Complex** CNIV neuropathy (associated with other CN injury, CNIII ± CNVI)
    - Brainstem stoke or tumor
    - Cavernous sinus thrombosis, tumor
    - Orbital tumor

Clinical Findings
- Paralysis of superior oblique muscle results in **extorsion** (outward rotation) of affected eye
- Extorsion is secondary to unopposed action of inferior oblique muscle
- Patient complaints: Diplopia, weakness of downward gaze, neck pain from head tilting
- Physical exam: Compensatory head tilt usually away from affected side

CNIV (Trochlear Nerve)

GRAPHICS

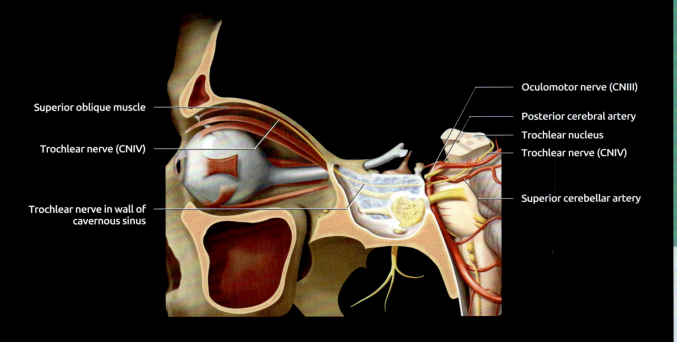

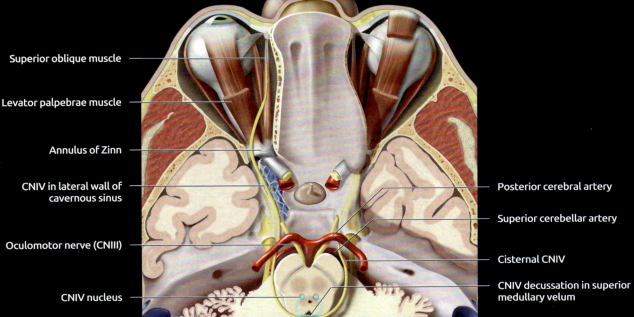

(Top) Sagittal graphic shows that the trochlear nucleus give rise to fibers that form the contralateral trochlear nerve. After exiting the dorsal brainstem, CNIV courses lateral to the oculomotor nerve between the posterior cerebral artery and superior cerebellar artery. After its long cisternal course, CNIV enters the cavernous sinus and runs inferolateral to CNIII and superior to the ophthalmic division of trigeminal nerve (CNV1). (Bottom) Axial graphic shows the trochlear nerves originating from the trochlear nuclei and decussating in the superior medullary velum. CNIV runs lateral to the oculomotor nerve between the posterior cerebral artery and superior cerebellar artery and continues inferolateral with CNIII through the cavernous sinus. It crosses over CNIII to enter orbit above the annulus of Zinn, then courses medially over the levator palpebrae muscle to innervate the superior oblique muscle.

CNIV (Trochlear Nerve)

AXIAL T2 MR

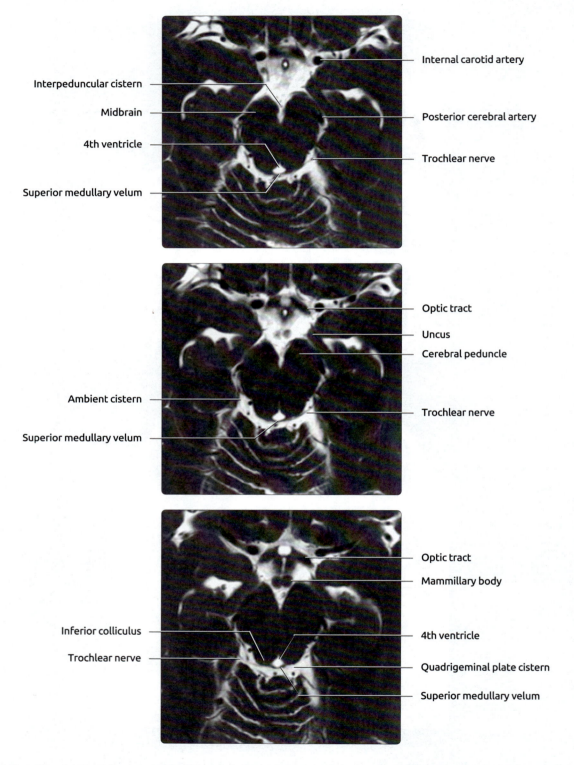

(Top) First of 3 axial T2 MR images presented from inferior to superior through the midbrain is shown. The left trochlear nerve passes around the brainstem within the ambient cistern, where it courses anteriorly below the tentorium cerebelli. The trochlear nerves decussate in the superior medullary velum with fibers from the nucleus passing to the contralateral CNIV. *(Middle)* Trochlear nerve (CNIV) is the smallest cranial nerve (0.75-1.00 mm diameter) and is not routinely visualized. In addition, the trochlear nerve may easily be confused with numerous small arteries and veins in the ambient cistern. *(Bottom)* After decussating in the superior medullary velum, the trochlear nerve exits dorsal surface of the brainstem below the inferior colliculus to enter the quadrigeminal plate cistern. The trochlear nerve is the only cranial nerve to exit the dorsal brainstem.

CNIV (Trochlear Nerve)

CORONAL T2 MR

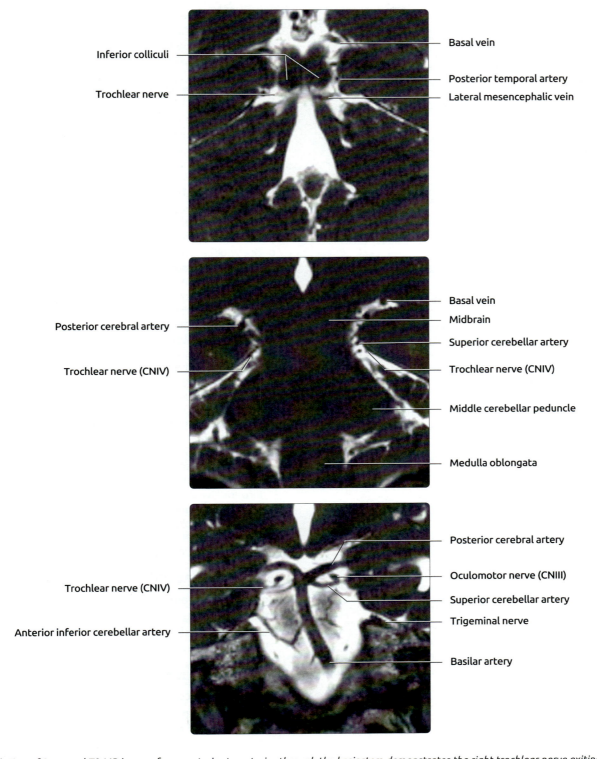

(Top) First of 3 coronal T2 MR images from posterior to anterior through the brainstem demonstrates the right trochlear nerve exiting from the dorsal brainstem below the inferior colliculus as multiple discrete rootlets enter the quadrigeminal plate cistern. The left trochlear nerve is obscured by the lateral mesencephalic vein. (Middle) Trochlear nerves can be visualized bilaterally coursing anteriorly within the ambient cistern below the free margin of the tentorium cerebelli. Only very focused thin-section high-resolution T2 MR imaging has any chance of seeing CNIV in this location. (Bottom) At the level of the basilar artery, the trochlear nerve is hidden on the left but visible on the right inferolateral to the oculomotor nerve. Both nerves pass between the posterior cerebral artery and the superior cerebellar artery.

CNV (Trigeminal Nerve)

TERMINOLOGY

Abbreviations

- Trigeminal nerve: CNV
- Ophthalmic division, trigeminal nerve: CNV1
- Maxillary division, trigeminal nerve: CNV2
- Mandibular division, trigeminal nerve: CNV3

Definitions

- CNV: Great sensory cranial nerve of head and face; motor nerve for muscles of mastication

IMAGING ANATOMY

Overview

- Mixed nerve (both sensory, motor components)
- 4 segments: Intraaxial, cisternal, interdural, and extracranial

Intraaxial Segment

- 4 nuclei (3 sensory, 1 motor) in brainstem, upper cord
  - **Mesencephalic nucleus CNV**
    - Slender column of cells projecting cephalad from pons to level of inferior colliculus
    - Found anterior to upper 4th ventricle/aqueduct near lateral margin of central gray
    - Afferent fibers for **facial proprioception** (teeth, hard palate, and temporomandibular joint)
    - Sickle-shaped mesencephalic tract descends to motor nucleus, conveys impulses that **control mastication and bite force**
  - **Main sensory nucleus CNV**
    - Nucleus lies lateral to entering trigeminal root
    - Provides **facial tactile sensation**
  - **Motor nucleus CNV**
    - Ovoid column of cells anteromedial to principal sensory nucleus
    - Supplies **muscles of mastication** (medial/lateral pterygoids, masseter, temporalis), tensor veli palatini/tensor tympani, mylohyoid and anterior belly of digastric
  - **Spinal nucleus CNV**
    - Extends from principal sensory root in pons into upper cervical cord (between C2 to C4 level)
    - Conveys **facial pain, temperature**

Cisternal (Preganglionic) Segment

- 2 roots: Smaller motor, larger sensory
- Emerges from lateral pons at **root entry zone** (REZ)
- Courses anterosuperiorly through prepontine cistern
- Enters middle cranial fossa by passing beneath tentorium at apex of petrous temporal bone
- Passes through opening in dura matter called **porus trigeminus** to enter Meckel cave

Interdural Segment

- **Meckel cave** formed by meningeal layer of dura lined by arachnoid
  - Cave filled with cerebrospinal fluid (CSF) (90%) and continuous with prepontine subarachnoid space
- Pia covers CNV in trigeminal cave
- Preganglionic CNV ends at **trigeminal ganglion** (TG)
  - TG located in inferior aspect of Meckel cave
  - TG synonyms: Gasserian or semilunar ganglion

Divisions (Postganglionic) of CNV

- **Ophthalmic nerve**
  - Courses in lateral cavernous sinus wall below CNIV
  - Exits skull through superior orbital fissure
  - Enters orbit, divides into lacrimal, frontal, and nasociliary nerves
    - Sensory innervation of **scalp, forehead, nose, globe**
- **Maxillary nerve**
  - Courses in cavernous sinus lateral wall below CNV1
  - Exits skull through **foramen rotundum**
  - Traverses roof of pterygopalatine fossa, inclines laterally on back of maxilla, and enters orbit through inferior orbital fissure
  - Continues as **infraorbital nerve** in floor of orbit
  - Exits orbit through infraorbital foramen
    - Sensory innervation of **cheek and upper teeth**
- **Mandibular nerve**
  - Does **not** pass through cavernous sinus
  - Exits directly from Meckel cave, passing inferiorly through foramen ovale into masticator space
  - Carries both motor and sensory fibers; motor root bypasses TG, joins V3 as it exits through **foramen ovale**
  - **Main trunk** of CNV3 gives off meningeal branch and nerve to medial pterygoid; latter provides nonrelaying motor root to otic ganglion (OG), which supplies tensor veli palatini and tensor tympani muscles
  - Main trunk divides into small **anterior division** (giving off masseteric, 2 deep temporal and nerve to lateral pterygoid motor branches and buccal nerve sensory branch) and large **posterior division**
  - **Auriculotemporal nerve** (secretomotor to parotid gland via otic ganglion) arises from 2 roots of proximal posterior division
  - Posterior division then divides into terminal branches: **Inferior alveolar** (posterior) and **lingual** (anterior) nerves
    - **Mylohyoid nerve** (motor to anterior belly of digastric and mylohyoid muscles) arises from inferior alveolar nerve just before it enters mandible and contains all motor fibers of posterior division of V3

ANATOMY IMAGING ISSUES

Imaging Recommendations

- CT best for skull base and bony foramina
- 3D T2 MR for intraaxial, cisternal, and intradural segments
- T1 C+ fat-saturated MR of entire extracranial course

CLINICAL IMPLICATIONS

Clinical Importance

- Sensory complaints: Pain, burning, numbness in face
- Motor (V3 only): Weakness in chewing
  - Proximal V3 injury causes motor atrophy of masticator muscles within 6 weeks to 3 months
  - Distal V3 injury (above mylohyoid nerve takeoff) affects only anterior belly of digastric and mylohyoid
- Tic douloureux (trigeminal neuralgia)
  - Sharp, excruciating pain in V2-3 distributions

CNV (Trigeminal Nerve)

GRAPHICS

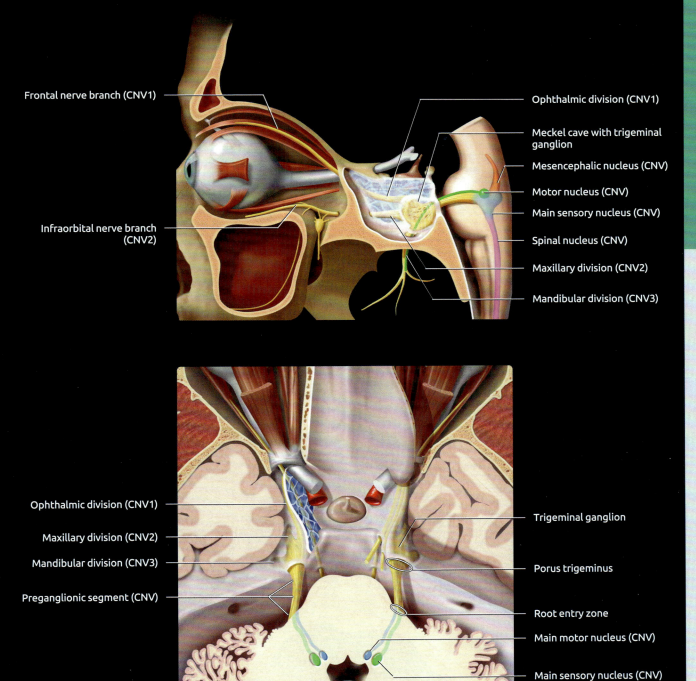

(Top) Sagittal graphic shows the 4 nuclei of the trigeminal nerve (CNV). From superior to inferior, note the mesencephalic nucleus in the midbrain, the motor nucleus and main sensory nucleus in the pons, and the spinal nucleus extending from the lower pons into the upper cervical spinal cord. The motor root of CNV sends fibers along the mandibular division only. (Bottom) Axial graphic depicts the course of CNV from its pontine nuclei (main sensory and motor nuclei) to its main 3 branches (CNV1, CNV2, CNV3). Notice the large preganglionic segment exiting the lateral pons at the root entry zone. It then enters the Meckel cave through the porus trigeminus to become the trigeminal ganglion. Vascular loop compression of the root entry zone is the most common cause of trigeminal neuralgia.

CNV (Trigeminal Nerve)

GRAPHICS

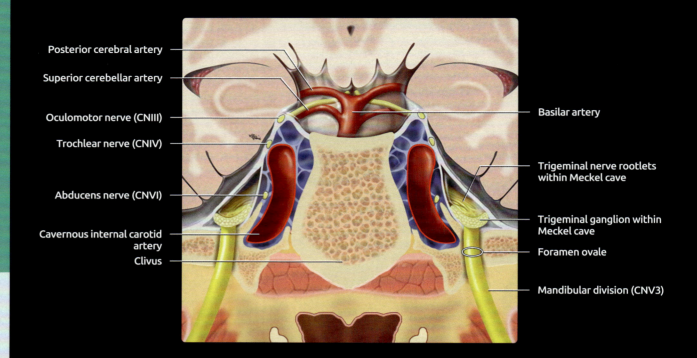

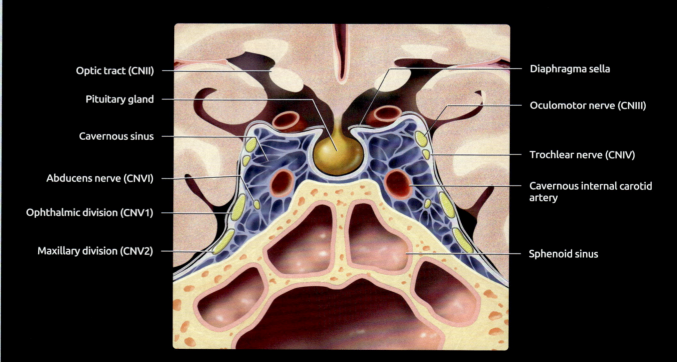

(Top) Coronal graphic shows the mandibular division of the trigeminal nerve (CNV3), which never enters the cavernous sinus. Instead, CNV3 exits directly from the Meckel cave, passing inferiorly through the foramen ovale into the nasopharyngeal masticator space. The Meckel cave is actually a small anterior extension of the lateral prepontine cistern, containing both the trigeminal nerve rootlets and the trigeminal ganglion. Remember it is CNV3 that possesses the motor fibers of the trigeminal nerve. (Bottom) Coronal graphic through the cavernous sinus shows CNV2 in the lateral wall of the cavernous sinus, just inferior to CNV1. CNV1 is embedded in the lateral wall of the cavernous sinus, as are CNIII and CNIV. The only centrally located intracavernous cranial nerve is the abducens nerve (CNVI).

CNV (Trigeminal Nerve)

GRAPHICS

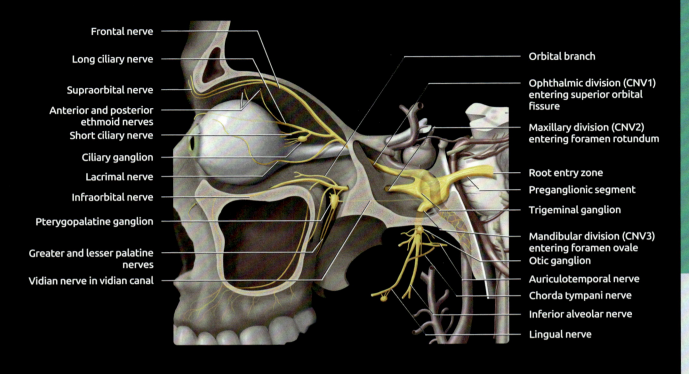

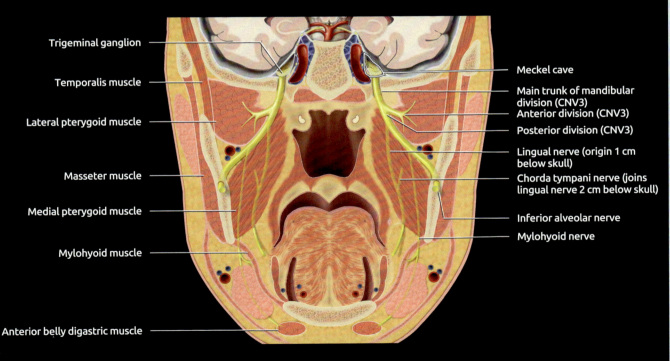

(Top) Sagittal graphic of CNV shows major branches & exiting foramina. Ophthalmic division enters into orbit via superior orbital fissure, dividing into frontal, nasociliary, & lacrimal branches. Maxillary division exits via foramen rotundum. Mandibular division exits through foramen ovale. Otic ganglion (OG) lies just below skull base between CNV3 & tensor veli palatini muscle. Lesser petrosal nerve provides preganglionic parasympathetics to OG from medullary inferior salivatory nucleus & sympathetic root is from plexus on middle meningeal artery. Postganglionic secretomotor fibers to parotid join auriculotemporal nerve (V3 branch). *(Bottom)* Coronal graphic shows CNV3 exiting skull through foramen ovale without entering cavernous sinus. Main trunk gives off a meningeal branch & nerve to medial pterygoid & soon divides into a small anterior division (giving rise to other masticator muscle branches & a buccal sensory branch) & a large posterior division, which gives rise to auriculotemporal, inferior alveolar (gives off mylohyoid nerve), & lingual nerves.

CNV (Trigeminal Nerve)

AXIAL BONE CT

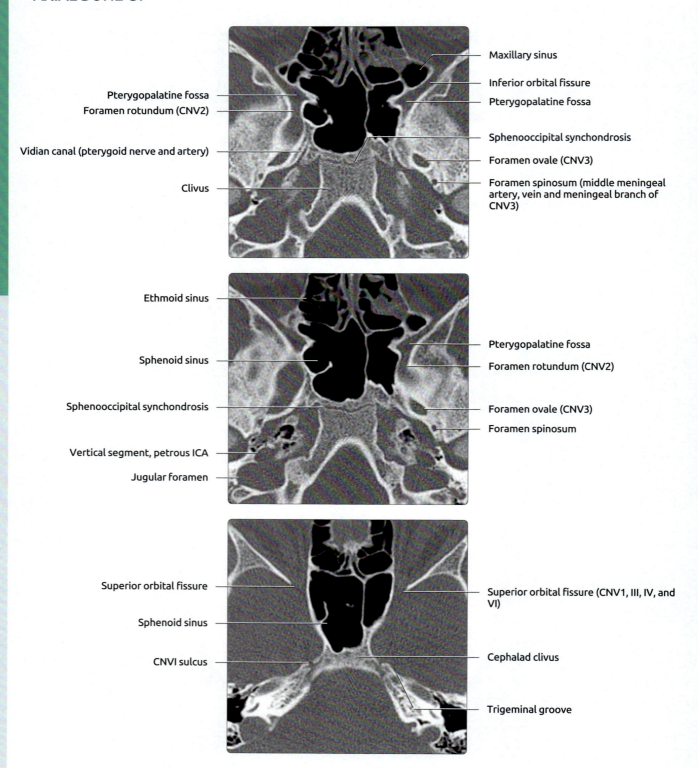

(Top) First of 3 axial bone CT images presented from inferior to superior through the central skull base is shown. CNV2 exits the skull base through the foramen rotundum to enter the superior margin of the pterygopalatine fossa. CNV3 exits via the foramen ovale to enter the masticator space where it supplies motor innervation to muscles of mastication and sensory branches inferior alveolar, lingual, and auriculotemporal nerves. *(Middle)* In this image, the foramen ovale (CNV3) and foramen rotundum (CNV2) are now best seen on the patient's left. The left foramen rotundum is seen opening into the superior pterygopalatine fossa. *(Bottom)* The superior orbital fissure transmits the ophthalmic division of CNV from cranium to orbit. Other structures passing through the superior orbital fissure include the oculomotor nerve (CNIII), trochlear nerve (CNIV), abducens Nerve (CNVI), and the superior ophthalmic vein.

CNV (Trigeminal Nerve)

AXIAL T2 MR

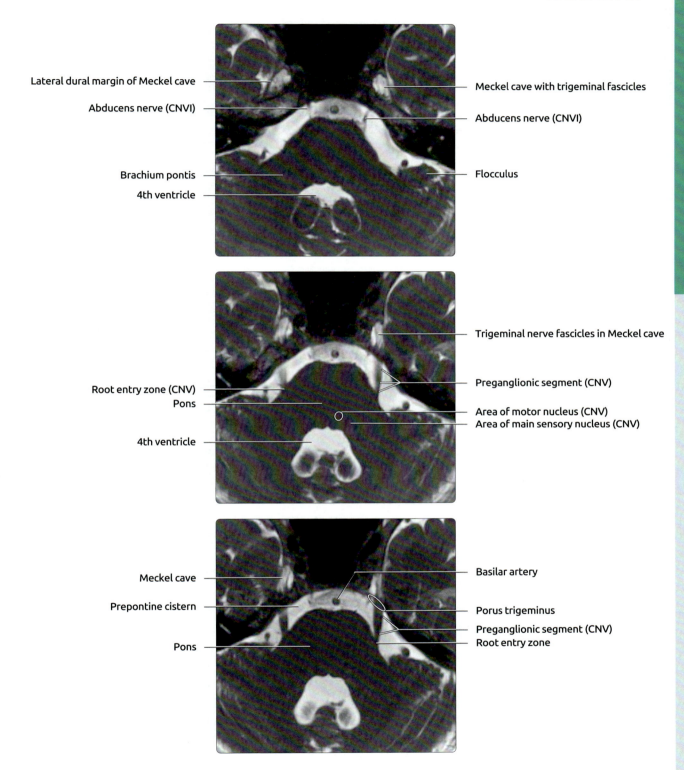

(Top) First of 3 axial T2 MR images through CNV and Meckel cave presented from inferior to superior shows a layer of hypointense dura mater forming the lateral wall and roof of Meckel cave. Right abducens nerve is seen penetrating dura to enter the Dorello canal. CNV fascicles can be seen with the cerebrospinal fluid of Meckel cave. (Middle) Preganglionic fascicles of CNV are seen within the Meckel cave, which is an arachnoid-lined, dural diverticulum protruding from the lateral aspect of the prepontine cistern. It contains cerebrospinal fluid, trigeminal fascicles, and trigeminal ganglion. Note approximate location of the main sensory and motor nuclei of CNV. (Bottom) In this image, the preganglionic segment of CNV is seen spanning the distance between the root entry zone on the lateral pons and the porus trigeminus of the Meckel cave.

CNV (Trigeminal Nerve)

AXIAL T1 C+ MR

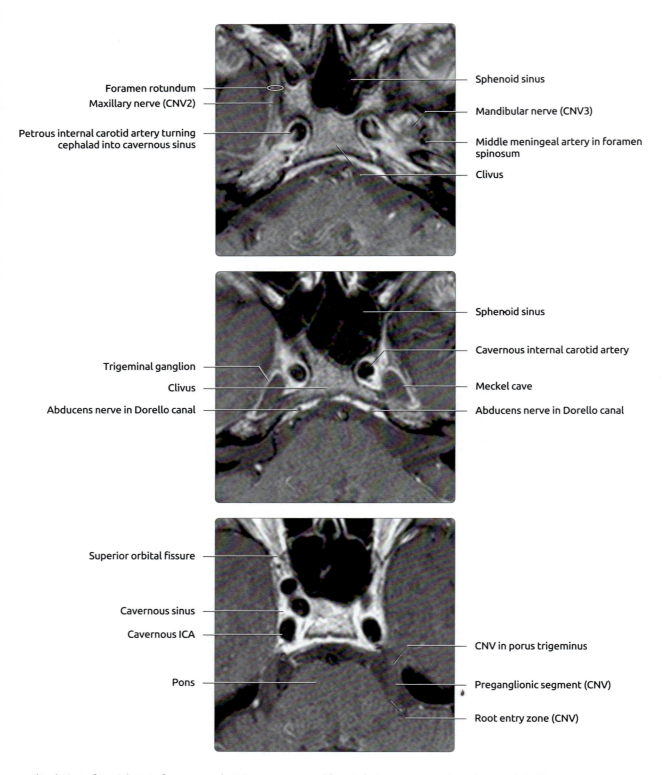

(Top) First of 3 axial T1 C+ fat-saturated MR images presented from inferior to superior through central skull base shows the right maxillary nerve (CNV2) passing anteriorly into the foramen rotundum and the left mandibular nerve (CNV3) passing inferiorly through the foramen ovale. Both nerves are surrounded by enhancing veins communicating with extracranial venous system. *(Middle)* This more superior image demonstrates the ovoid shape of the cerebrospinal fluid-filled Meckel cave. The trigeminal ganglion is the linear anteroinferior structure in the Meckel cave. It lacks a blood-nerve barrier and therefore normally enhances with contrast. *(Bottom)* Preganglionic segment of CNV arises from the lateral pons at root entry zone. Right internal carotid artery is tortuous within the cavernous sinus.

CNV (Trigeminal Nerve)

CORONAL T2 MR

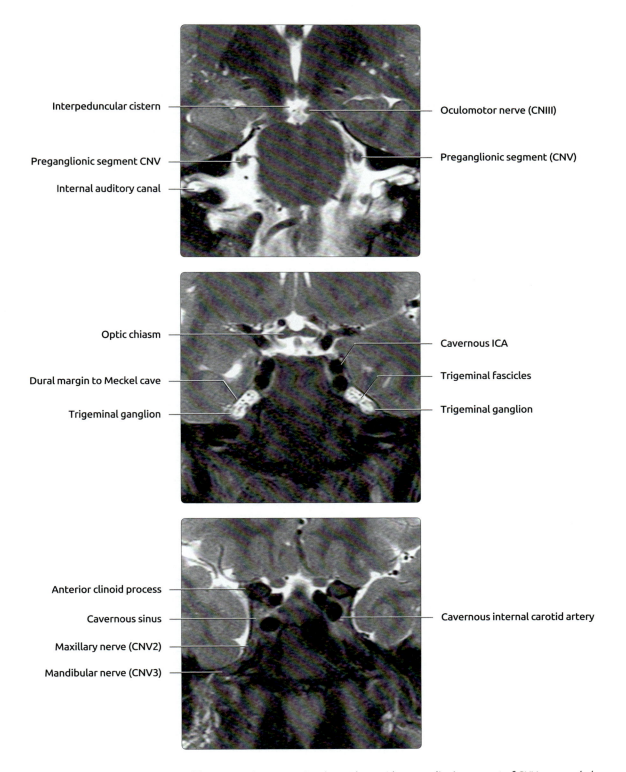

(Top) First of 3 coronal T2 MR images presented from posterior to anterior shows the ovoid preganglionic segment of CNV surrounded by high-signal cerebrospinal fluid. The preganglionic segment has just exited the lateral pons root entry zone area. (Middle) This more anterior image through the Meckel cave delineates the trigeminal fascicles of the preganglionic trigeminal nerve. The trigeminal ganglion is visible as a semilunar structure in the floor of the Meckel cave bilaterally. (Bottom) This image through the anterior cavernous sinus shows the maxillary nerve (CNV2) passing anteriorly within lateral wall of the cavernous sinus and the mandibular nerve (CNV3) passing inferiorly to its exit point in the skull base (foramen ovale).

CNV (Trigeminal Nerve)

CORONAL T1 C+ MR

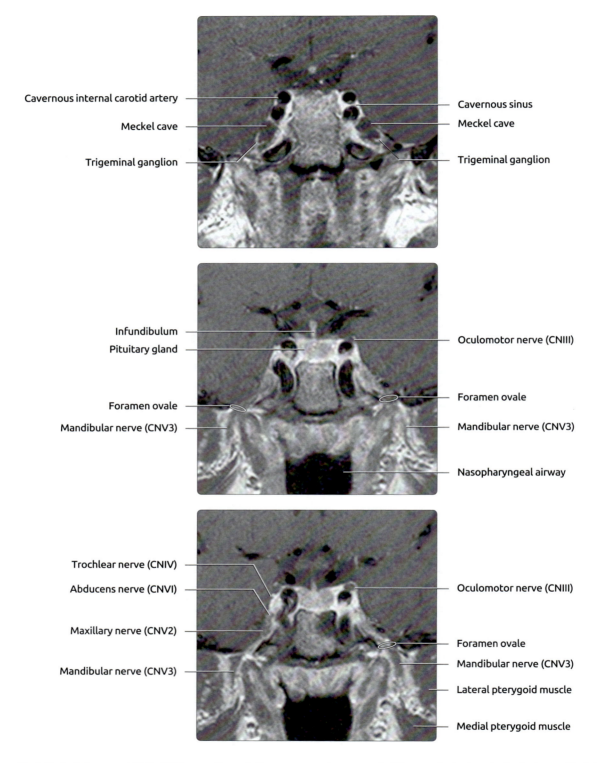

(Top) First of six coronal T1 C+ MR images through the cavernous sinus presented from posterior to anterior is shown. The trigeminal ganglion is seen as a crescentic area of enhancement in the floor of the Meckel cave. Trigeminal ganglion enhances because it lacks a blood-nerve barrier. *(Middle)* In this image through the foramen ovale, the mandibular nerve (CNV3) is visible exiting inferiorly into the masticator space. *(Bottom)* In this image, the patient's left foramen ovale and mandibular nerve are seen. The motor branches from CNV3 are to the medial pterygoid, which also supplies the tensor veli palatini and tensor tympani (from main trunk), the masseteric nerve, 2 deep temporal nerves to the temporalis and nerve to the lateral pterygoid (from anterior division), and the mylohyoid nerve, which supplies the mylohyoid and anterior belly of the digastric muscles (branch of inferior alveolar nerve; mylohyoid nerve contains all the motor fibers of posterior division). The main sensory branches are the meningeal branch (from main trunk), buccal nerve (from anterior division), auriculotemporal nerve, and the terminal lingual and inferior alveolar nerves (branches of posterior division).

CNV (Trigeminal Nerve)

CORONAL T1 C+ MR

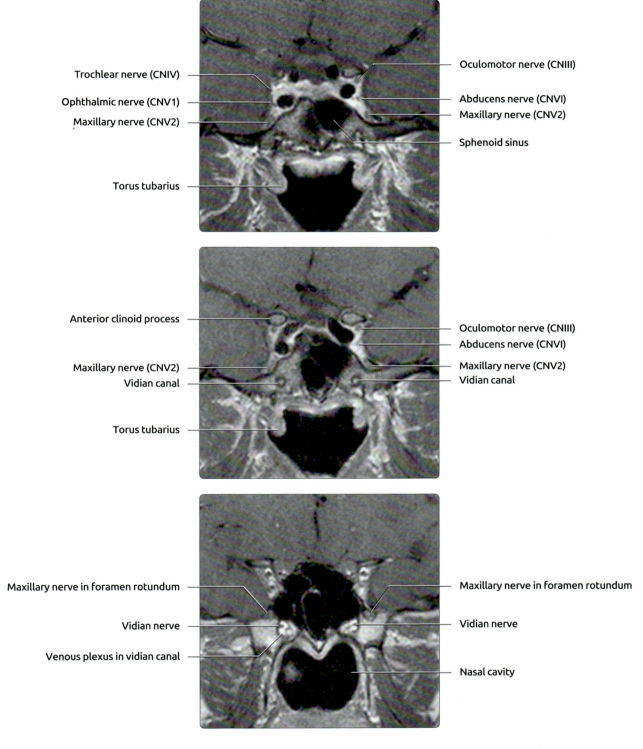

(Top) In this image through the anterior margin of the pituitary gland, the maxillary nerve (CNV2) is well seen bilaterally in the inferolateral wall of the cavernous sinus. (Middle) In this more anterior image, the maxillary nerves are seen in the inferolateral wall of the cavernous sinus just prior to its entry into the foramen rotundum. Inferomedially, note the vidian canals. (Bottom) In this image, the maxillary nerve can be seen in the foramen rotundum. Notice also the vidian canal widening on its extracranial side with the vidian nerve visible surrounded by a venous plexus. The vidian nerve carries secretomotor fibers originally in the facial nerve, which are responsible for lacrimation.

CNV (Trigeminal Nerve)

SAGITTAL T2 AND AXIAL T1 MR

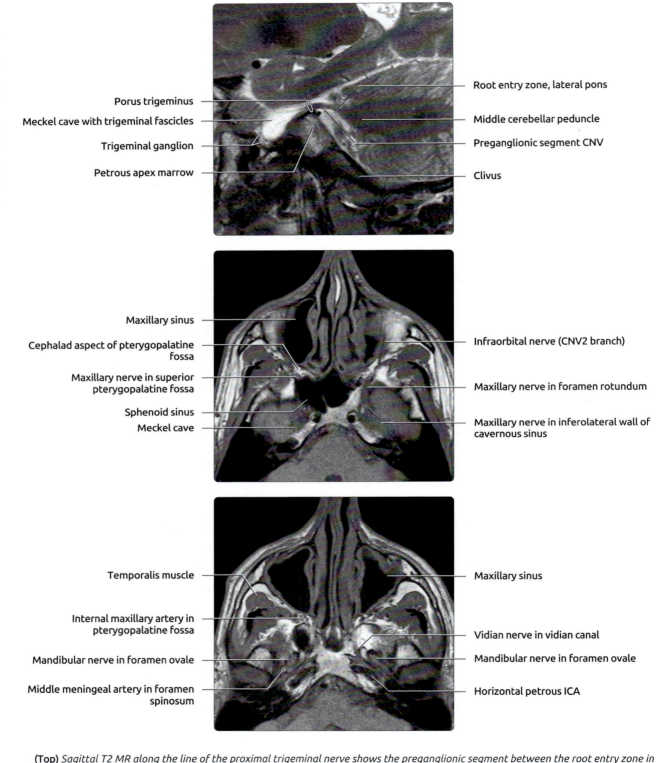

(Top) Sagittal T2 MR along the line of the proximal trigeminal nerve shows the preganglionic segment between the root entry zone in the lateral pons and the trigeminal ganglion in the anteroinferior Meckel cave. The cerebrospinal fluid within the Meckel cave communicates with the prepontine cistern through the porus trigeminus. (Middle) First of 5 axial T1 unenhanced MR images extending from the skull base to the mandibular body from superior to inferior is shown. Notice the left maxillary nerve in the foramen rotundum and then traversing the roof of pterygopalatine fossa. It then inclines laterally on the back of maxilla and enters the orbit through the inferior orbital fissure, after which it continues as the infraorbital nerve in the floor of the orbit that in turn exits the orbit through the infraorbital foramen (not shown). (Bottom) Image through the foramen ovale of the skull base is shown. Notice the mandibular nerves exiting the skull base. The vidian canal and nerve are also visible connecting the foramen lacerum to the pterygopalatine fossa. The many black dots within the pterygopalatine fossa are from the normal terminal internal maxillary artery.

CNV (Trigeminal Nerve)

AXIAL T1 MR

Cranial Nerves

Pterygopalatine fossa

Pterygoid process marrow

Mandibular nerve (CNV3)

Location of otic ganglion

Tensor veli palatini muscle

Vertical segment petrous ICA

Temporalis muscle

Lateral pterygoid muscle

Mandibular nerve (CNV3)

Mandibular condyle

Masseter muscle

Location of lingual nerve contacting mandible medial to 3rd molar tooth

Marrow space of mandibular ramus

Inferior alveolar nerve in mandibular foramen

Parotid gland

Medial pterygoid muscle

Inferior alveolar nerve in mandibular foramen

Mental foramen

Inferior alveolar nerve

Location of lingual nerve in superolateral aspect of lateral sublingual space compartment

Mylohyoid muscle

Hyoglossus muscle

Mental foramen with exiting inferior alveolar nerve

Inferior alveolar nerve

Mylohyoid muscle

Submandibular gland

(Top) *Image just under the skull base shows mandibular nerves entering medial upper masticator space. OG lies just below skull base between CNV3 and tensor veli palatini muscle. Main trunk of CNV3 gives off a meningeal branch and nerve to medial pterygoid with motor root to OG and divides soon into a small anterior division (giving off masseteric, 2 deep temporal nerves to lateral pterygoid motor branches, and a buccal nerve sensory branch) and a large posterior division. Auriculotemporal nerve arises from 2 roots of the proximal posterior division, runs backwards encircling the middle meningeal artery and forms single trunk. The posterior division then divides into terminal branches, inferior alveolar (posterior) and lingual (anterior) nerves.* **(Middle)** *Image at level of mandibular foramina shows inferior alveolar nerve runs downward lateral to medial pterygoid and enters mandibular foramen, giving off mylohyoid nerve just before entering mandible.* **(Bottom)** *Image at mandible body level shows inferior alveolar nerve course.*

CNVI (Abducens Nerve)

TERMINOLOGY

Abbreviations
- Abducens nerve: CN6, CNVI

Synonyms
- Abducens nerve: 6th cranial nerve

Definitions
- CNVI: Motor nerve to lateral rectus muscle only

IMAGING ANATOMY

Overview
- CNVI is pure motor nerve, with pontine nucleus 5 anatomic segments

Abducens Nucleus
- Paired CNVI nuclei located in pontine tegmentum near midline, just ventral to 4th ventricle
- **Facial colliculus**: Axons of facial nerve (CNVII) loop around abducens nucleus, creating bulge in floor of 4th ventricle
  - Isolated lesion to facial colliculus can cause ipsilateral CNVI and CNVII palsy

Intraaxial Segment
- Ipsilateral axons from CNVI nucleus course anteroinferiorly through pontine tegmentum

Cisternal Segment
- Emerges from anterior brainstem near midline through groove between pons and pyramid of medulla oblongata (pontomedullary sulcus)
- Usually exits as single trunk but occasionally duplicated
- CNVI ascends anterosuperiorly in prepontine cistern toward site where it penetrates dura along upper clivus laterally
- Posterior to anterior inferior cerebellar artery in 85%; anterior in 15%

Interdural Segment
- Extends from point where CNVI pierces inner layer dura posteriorly to its entrance into cavernous sinus anteriorly
- Thin sleeve of arachnoid (and occasionally dura) travels with nerve through this segment
- After penetrating dura, CNVI passes superiorly through basilar venous plexus
  - Basilar venous plexus is dorsal to upper clivus and located between inner and outer (endosteal) layers of dura; it is interdural
- Nerve remains interdural and passes superiorly over junction of petrous apex and clivus, into adjacent venous region referred to as sphenopetroclival venous confluence [or simply petroclival confluence or petroclival venous confluence (PCVC)]
  - PCVC located at junction of posterior part of cavernous sinus, lateral part of basilar plexus, and anterior part of superior and inferior petrosal sinuses
- In this location, PCVC and interdural segment of CNVI are considered to be within **classic Dorello canal**
- Classic **Dorello canal** is zone/space bounded by petrous apex (inferolateral), clivus (inferomedial), and petrosphenoidal ligament of Gruber (superiorly)

Cavernous Segment
- After exiting Dorello canal, abducens nerve enters cavernous sinus and passes laterally around proximal aspect of cavernous internal carotid artery (ICA)
- Abducens nerve is **only cranial nerve to lie within cavernous sinus**, passing lateral to cavernous ICA
- Cranial nerves III, IV, V1, and V2 are all embedded within lateral wall of cavernous sinus

Extracranial (Intraorbital) Segment
- CNVI enters orbit through **superior orbital fissure** together with CNIII and CNIV
- Passes through annulus of Zinn
- Supplies **motor innervation** to **lateral rectus muscle**

ANATOMY IMAGING ISSUES

Imaging Recommendations
- MR for intraaxial, cisternal, interdural, and cavernous segments
  - Thin-section, high-resolution T2 and contrast-enhanced T1 in axial and coronal planes
    - Depicts small structures including cranial nerves surrounded by cerebrospinal fluid with high contrast and high spatial resolution
- Bone CT best for skull base and its bony foramina

Imaging Sweet Spots
- Axial and coronal MR sequences should include brainstem, 4th ventricle, cavernous sinus, and orbit
- CNVI nucleus and intraaxial segment not directly visualized
  - Position of CNVI inferred by identifying facial colliculus in floor of 4th ventricle on high-res, thin-section T2 MR
- Cisternal segment routinely visualized on high-res T2 MR
- CNVI entrance into Dorello canal may be visualized due to invagination of cerebrospinal fluid into proximal canal
- Enhancement of basilar plexus may demonstrate CNVI as tiny, linear, nonenhancing structures

Imaging Pitfalls
- Use of fat saturation on postcontrast T1 MR sequences can amplify blooming (susceptibility) artifact around well-aerated sphenoid sinus
  - Cavernous sinus and orbital apex subtle lesions may be obscured by this artifact
  - Remove fat saturation and repeat T1 postcontrast MR if this artifact obscures key areas of interest

CLINICAL IMPLICATIONS

Clinical Importance
- In abducens neuropathy, affected eye will not **abduct** (rotate laterally)
- CNVI neuropathy divided into **simple** if isolated and **complex** if associated with other CN involvement (CNIII, CNIV, and CNVII)
  - Simple **CNVI neuropathy most common ocular motor nerve palsy**
  - Usually presents as complex cranial neuropathy
    - Pontine lesions affect CNVI with CNVII
    - Cavernous sinus, superior orbital fissure lesions affect CNVI with CNIII, CNIV, and CNV1

CNVI (Abducens Nerve)

GRAPHICS

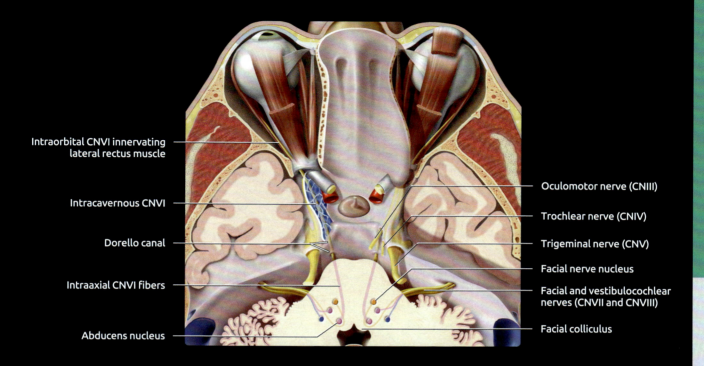

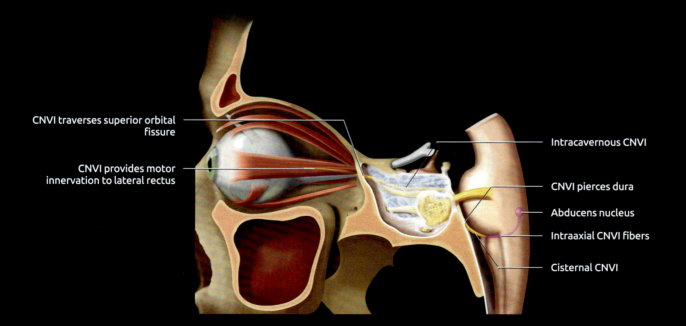

(Top) Axial graphic shows the entire length of the abducens nerve from its pontine tegmentum nuclear origin to its motor endplate in the lateral rectus muscle. Follow its progress from nucleus to its exit at the anteromedial bulbopontine sulcus. From there, note the dural penetration into the Dorello canal leading to its intracavernous portion. Finally, it passes through the superior orbital fissure and the ring of Zinn into the orbit. (Bottom) Sagittal graphic shows the abducens nerve depicted from its origin in the pontine tegmentum to its motor endplate in the lateral rectus muscle. Notice the intraaxial CNVI fibers descend before exiting the bulbopontine sulcus anteriorly. Prepontine cistern CNVI then ascends to pierce the dura into the Dorello canal. Intracavernous CNVI proceeds anteriorly to pass through the superior orbital fissure and the ring of Zinn before innervating the lateral rectus muscle in orbit.

CNVI (Abducens Nerve)

AXIAL T2 AND T1 C+ MR

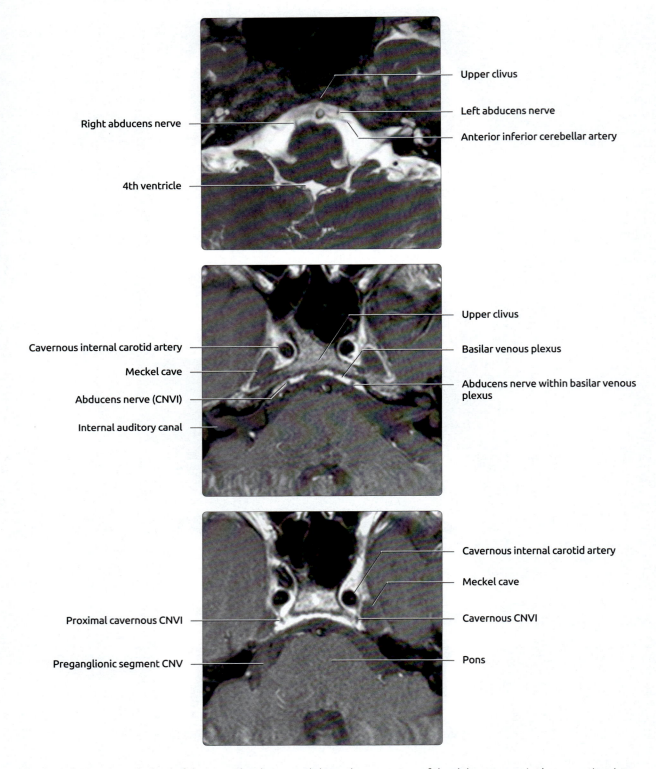

(Top) Axial T2 MR near the level of the internal auditory canal shows the appearance of the abducens nerve in the prepontine cistern. On the patient's right, CNVI is just exiting the bulbopontine sulcus while on the left, it is poised to penetrate the dura. Both nerves are rising in the prepontine cistern. (Middle) Axial T1 C+ MR demonstrates the interdural segment of the abducens nerve within the Dorello canal surrounded by brightly enhancing basilar venous plexus. (Bottom) Axial T1 C+ MR just above the internal auditory canal shows the abducens nerves passing through the superior basilar venous plexus to enter the posterior margin of the cavernous sinus. At this point, CNVI is arching over the petrous apex below the petrosphenoidal ligament into the upper posterior region of the cavernous sinus.

CNVI (Abducens Nerve)

SAGITTAL T2 MR

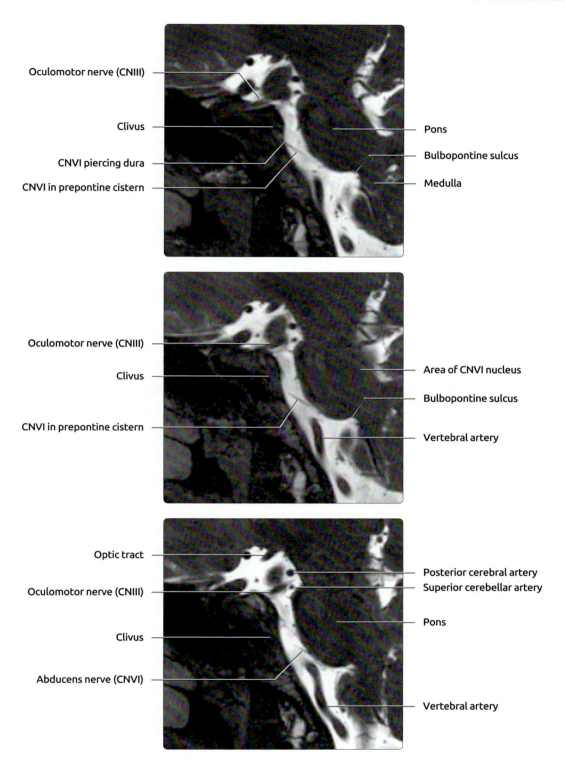

(Top) First of 3 sagittal T2 MR images presented from lateral to medial reveals the abducens nerve traversing the prepontine cistern toward the clivus. In this image, the abducens nerve is visible penetrating the dura to enter the Dorello canal, which lies between the cranial dura and periosteum surrounded by basilar venous plexus. **(Middle)** Image of the brainstem area shows the abducens nerve coursing anterosuperiorly from its exit point from the brainstem (bulbopontine sulcus) toward its point of dural penetration into the Dorello canal. Notice the approximate location of the CNVI nucleus and the steep course that the intraaxial fibers take to reach the bulbopontine sulcus. **(Bottom)** Image of the brainstem and prepontine cisterns shows the proximal cisternal CNVI closely associated with the belly of the pons. CNIII is seen passing between the posterior cerebral and superior cerebellar arteries.

CNVII (Facial Nerve)

TERMINOLOGY

Abbreviations

- Facial nerve (CN7, CNVII)

Definitions

- CNVII: Cranial nerve that carries motor nerves to muscles of facial expression; parasympathetics to lacrimal, submandibular, and sublingual glands; and taste from anterior 2/3 of tongue

IMAGING ANATOMY

Overview

- Mixed nerve: Motor, parasympathetic, and special sensory (taste)
- 2 roots: Motor and sensory (nervus intermedius) roots
  - Nervus intermedius exits lateral brainstem between motor root of facial and vestibulocochlear nerves, hence its name
- 3 nuclei and 4 segments: Intraaxial, cisternal, intratemporal, and extracranial (parotid)

Nuclei and Intraaxial Segment

- 3 nuclei (1 motor, 2 sensory)
- **Motor nucleus of facial nerve**
  - Located in ventrolateral pontine tegmentum
  - Efferent fibers loop dorsally around CNVI nucleus in floor of 4th ventricle, forming facial colliculus
  - Fibers then course anterolaterally to exit lateral brainstem at pontomedullary junction
- **Superior salivatory nucleus**
  - Located lateral to CNVII motor nucleus in pons
  - Efferent **parasympathetic fibers** exit brainstem posterior to CNVII as nervus intermedius
    - To submandibular, sublingual, and lacrimal glands
- **Solitarius tract nucleus**
  - Termination of taste sensation fibers from anterior 2/3 of tongue
  - **Cell bodies** of these fibers in **geniculate ganglion**
  - Fibers travel within nervus intermedius

Cisternal Segment

- 2 roots in cisternal CNVII
  - Larger motor root anteriorly
  - Smaller sensory nervus intermedius posteriorly
- Emerge from lateral brainstem at **root exit zone** in pontomedullary junction to enter cerebellopontine angle (CPA) cistern
  - CNVIII exits brainstem posterior to CNVII
- 2 roots join together and pass anterolaterally through CPA cistern with CNVIII to internal auditory canal (IAC)

Intratemporal Segment

- CNVII further divided in T-bone into 4 segments: IAC, labyrinthine, tympanic, and mastoid
- **IAC segment**: Porus acusticus to IAC fundus; anterosuperior position above crista falciformis
- **Labyrinthine segment**: Connects fundal CNVII to geniculate ganglion (anterior genu)
- **Tympanic segment**: Connects anterior to posterior genu, passing under lateral semicircular canal
- **Mastoid segment**: Inferiorly directed from posterior genu to stylomastoid foramen

Extracranial Segment

- Main CNVII exits skull base through **stylomastoid foramen** to enter parotid space
- Parotid CNVII passes lateral to retromandibular vein
- Ramifies within parotid, passes anteriorly to innervate muscles of facial expression

CNVII Branches

- **Greater superficial petrosal nerve**
  - Arises at geniculate ganglion, passes anteromedially, exits temporal bone via facial hiatus
  - Carries **parasympathetic** fibers to **lacrimal gland**
- **Stapedius nerve**
  - Arises from high mastoid segment of CNVII
  - Provides **motor** innervation to **stapedius muscle**
- **Chorda tympani nerve**
  - Arises from lower mastoid segment
  - Courses across middle ear to exit anterior T-bone
  - Carries **taste** fibers from **anterior 2/3 of tongue**
    - These fibers travel with lingual branch of mandibular division of trigeminal nerve
- **Terminal motor branches** to muscles of facial expression
  - Superior to inferior: Temporal, zygomatic, buccal, mandibular, cervical

ANATOMY IMAGING ISSUES

Imaging Recommendations

- Bone CT best for intratemporal segment of CNVII
- MR for intraaxial, cisternal, IAC, and extracranial segments
- Do not image routine Bell palsy!

Imaging Sweet Spots

- Include brainstem, CPA cistern, IAC, T-bone, and **parotid** when MR completed for CNVII palsy

Imaging Pitfalls

- Mild enhancement of labyrinthine segment, geniculate ganglion, and proximal tympanic segments of CNVII can be normal on postcontrast T1 MR
  - Secondary to circumneural arteriovenous plexus
- Always check parotid in peripheral CNVII paralysis

Clinical Issues

- Facial nerve paralysis can be central or peripheral
  - **Central**: Supranuclear injury resulting in paralysis of contralateral muscles of facial expression with forehead sparing
  - **Peripheral**: Injury to CNVII from brainstem nucleus peripherally, resulting in paralysis of all ipsilateral muscles of facial expression
    - If lesion proximal to geniculate ganglion, lacrimation, sound dampening and taste are affected
    - If CNVI involved, check pons for lesion
    - If CNVIII involved, check CPA-IAC for lesion
    - If lacrimation, sound dampening and taste are variably affected, T-bone lesion possible
    - If lacrimation, sound dampening and taste are spared, extracranial CNVII implicated

CNVII (Facial Nerve)

GRAPHICS

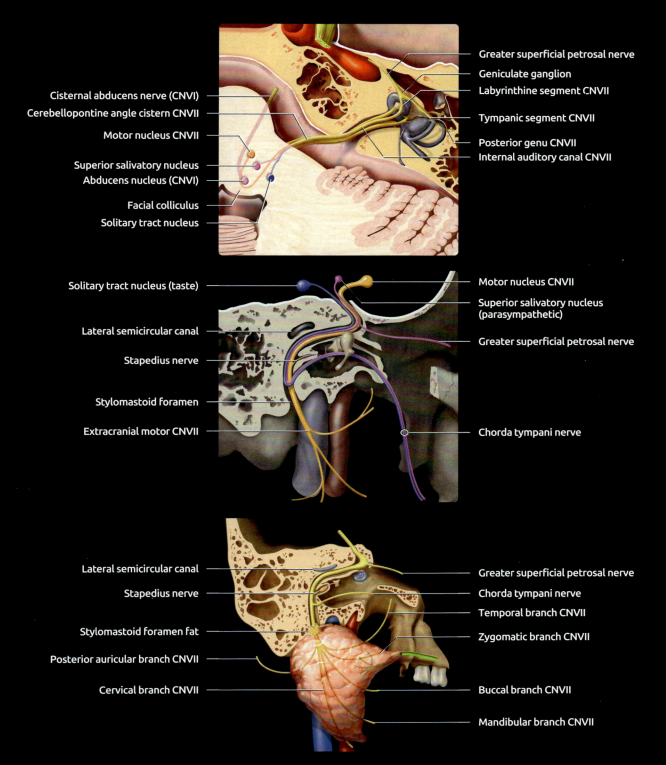

(Top) Axial graphic shows CNVII nuclei. Motor nucleus sends out its fibers to circle CNVI nucleus before reaching root exit zone at pontomedullary junction. Superior salivatory nucleus sends parasympathetic secretomotor fibers to lacrimal, submandibular, and sublingual glands. Solitary tract nucleus receives taste information from anterior 2/3 of tongue. (Middle) Sagittal graphic depicts CNVII within temporal bone. Motor fibers pass through T-bone, dropping stapedius nerve to stapedius muscle, then exits via stylomastoid foramen to extracranial CNVII (entirely motor). Parasympathetic fibers from superior salivatory nucleus reach lacrimal gland via greater superficial petrosal nerve and submandibular-sublingual glands via chorda tympanic nerve. Anterior 2/3 tongue taste fibers come via chorda tympani nerve. (Bottom) Sagittal graphic depicts extracranial motor branches of the facial nerve.

CNVII (Facial Nerve)

AXIAL BONE CT

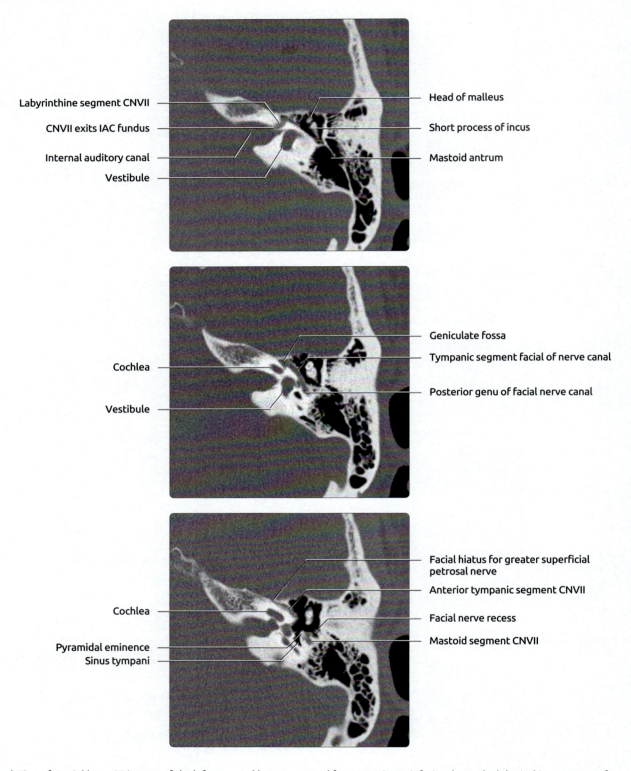

(Top) First of 6 axial bone CT images of the left temporal bone presented from superior to inferior shows the labyrinthine segment of the facial nerve canal as a C-shaped structure arching anterolaterally over the top of the cochlea. *(Middle)* In this image, the labyrinthine segment CNVII canal terminates in the geniculate fossa. The facial nerve canal turns abruptly at the geniculate fossa (anterior genu). The tympanic segment arises from the geniculate fossa, coursing posterolaterally in axial plane, running under the lateral semicircular canal before turning 90 degrees inferiorly at the posterior genu to become the mastoid segment. *(Bottom)* At the level of the oval window, the mastoid segment is visible deep to the facial nerve recess. Notice the more medial pyramidal eminence and sinus tympani.

CNVII (Facial Nerve)

AXIAL BONE CT

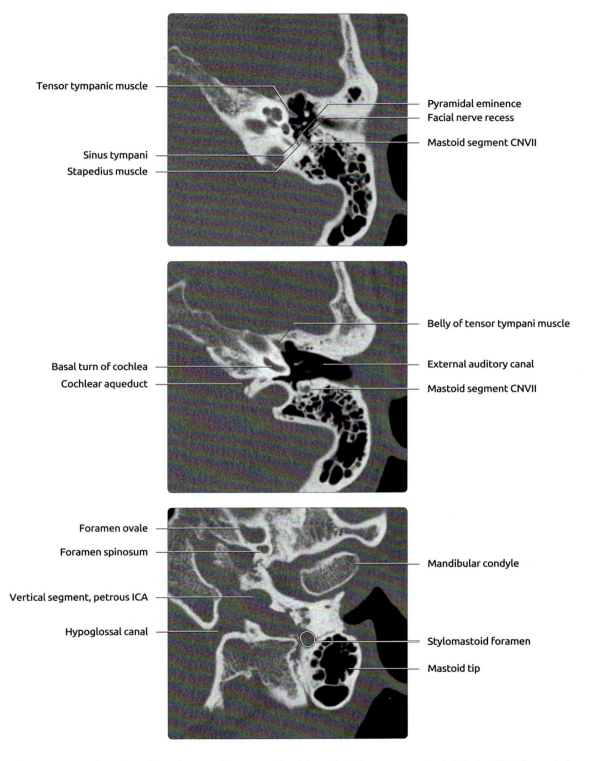

(Top) *Mastoid segment extends ~ 13 mm from the posterior genu to the stylomastoid foramen, coursing inferiorly within the posterior wall of the middle ear cavity. Mastoid segment is related anteriorly to the facial nerve recess and medially to the stapedius muscle within the pyramidal eminence on the posterior wall of the middle ear cavity.* (Middle) *At the level of the basal turn of the cochlea, the mastoid segment of the facial nerve is still visible. Both the nerve to stapedius muscle proximally and chorda tympani distally branch off the mastoid segment CNVII.* (Bottom) *Image at the level of the stylomastoid foramen is shown. Notice the "bell" of the stylomastoid foramen is just anteromedial to the mastoid tip. The mastoid tip protects the facial nerve from traumatic injury as it exits the skull base.*

CNVII (Facial Nerve)

CORONAL BONE CT

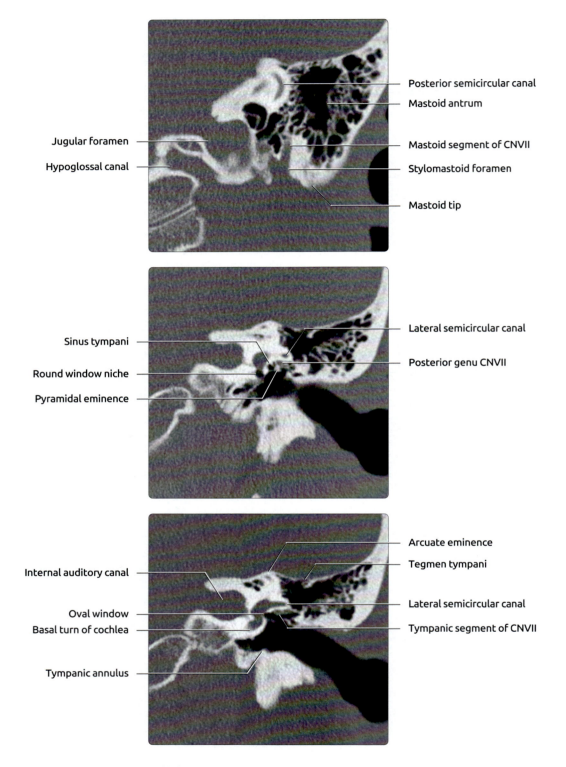

(Top) First of 6 coronal bone CT images of left temporal bone presented from posterior to anterior shows lower mastoid segment of the facial nerve (CNVII) and stylomastoid foramen. *(Middle)* At the level of the round window, the posterior genu of the facial nerve can be seen just lateral to the pyramidal eminence. Notice the sinus tympani is medial to the pyramidal eminence. *(Bottom)* At the level of the oval window, the tympanic segment of the facial nerve can be seen coursing under the lateral semicircular canal. Notice the fine bony covering (thin white line) surrounding the facial nerve. Also note the location relative to the upper margin of the oval window. In patients with oval window atresia, the facial nerve is found near or within the oval window niche.

CNVII (Facial Nerve)

CORONAL BONE CT

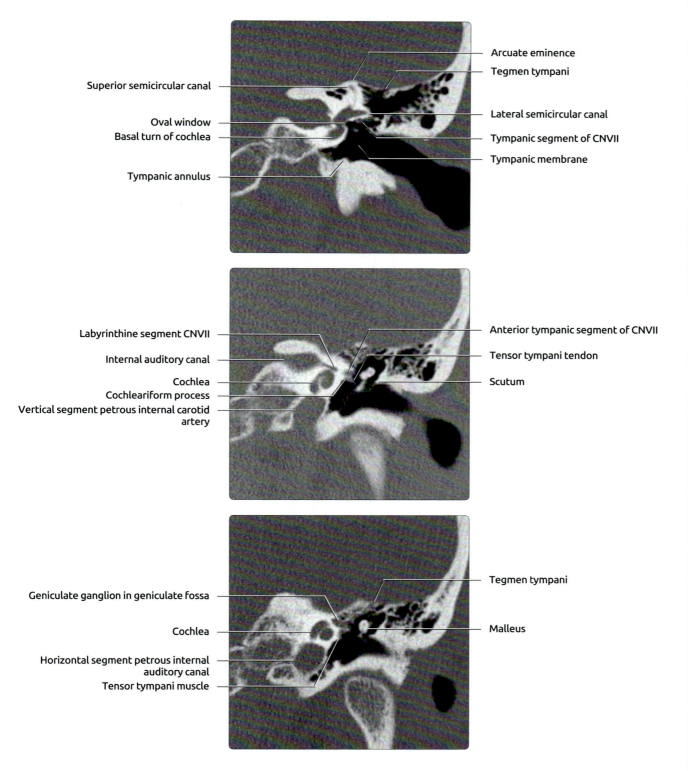

(Top) At the level of the anterior margin of the oval window, the tympanic segment of the facial nerve can be seen under the lateral semicircular canal. Notice the fine bony covering (thin white line) surrounding the facial nerve is now not seen. The facial nerve canal bony covering in this area is normally incomplete. (Middle) In the anterior middle ear cavity, the labyrinthine segment of the facial nerve can be seen exiting the internal auditory canal over the top of the cochlea. The anterior tympanic segment of the facial nerve is also visible. Do not confuse the muscle-tendon of the tensor tympani in the cochleariform process with the facial nerve. (Bottom) In the most anterior portion of middle ear cavity (where both the carotid and the cochlea are visible), the geniculate ganglion is seen within the geniculate fossa as an ovoid structure just above the cochlea.

CNVII (Facial Nerve)

AXIAL T2 & T1 MR

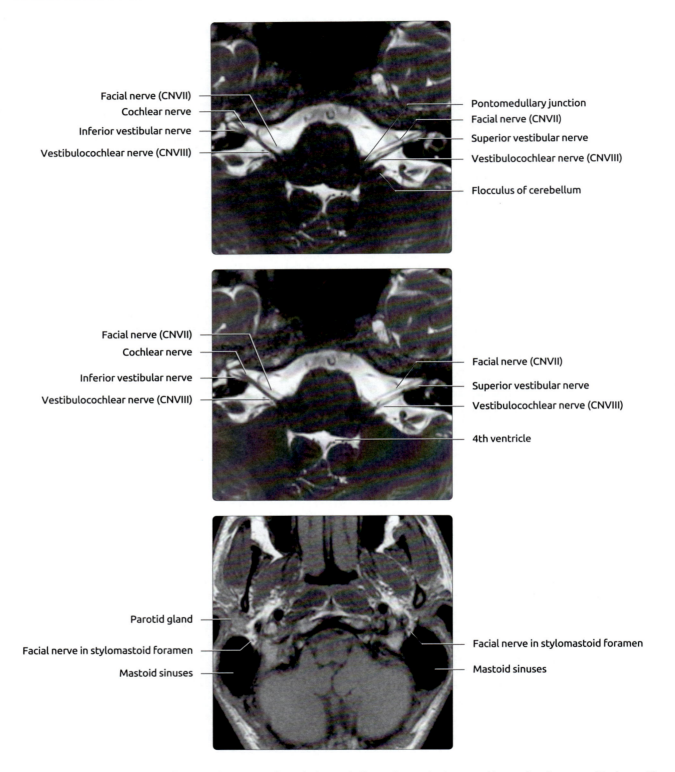

(Top) First of 2 axial high-resolution T2 MR images through the cerebellopontine angle cistern and internal auditory canal is shown. The facial nerve root exit zone is seen anterior to the vestibulocochlear nerve in the pontomedullary junction bilaterally. Notice the facial nerve maintains an anterior relationship with the vestibulocochlear nerve as it crosses through the cerebellopontine angle cistern. (Middle) Image through cephalad internal auditory canal on the patient's left shows the facial nerve anterior to the superior vestibular nerve throughout its internal auditory canal course. (Bottom) Axial T1 MR at the level of the stylomastoid foramen shows the exiting low-signal facial nerve surrounded by high-signal fat in the "bell" of the stylomastoid foramen. If perineural parotid malignancy is present, the fat in this area is obscured.

CNVII (Facial Nerve)

OBLIQUE SAGITTAL T2 MR

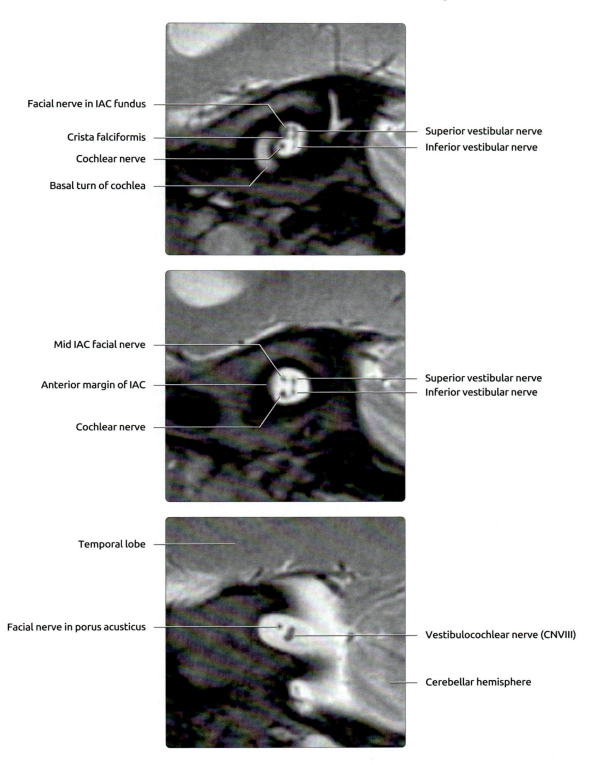

(Top) First of 3 oblique sagittal T2 MR images presented from lateral to medial shows normal fundal anatomy. The horizontal crista falciformis separates the fundus into upper and lower portions. Facial nerve is anterosuperior, separated from superior vestibular nerve by a vertical bony septum called "Bill bar," which is not resolved. Below the falciform crest are the larger anterior cochlear nerve and posterior inferior vestibular nerve. (Middle) In the mid internal auditory canal, 4 nerves are clearly identified. The facial nerve is anterosuperior. (Bottom) This image through the porus acusticus reveals the characteristic ball in catcher's mitt appearance of the facial and vestibulocochlear nerves. The facial nerve is the "ball" and the vestibulocochlear nerve is the "catcher's mitt."

CNVIII (Vestibulocochlear Nerve)

TERMINOLOGY

Abbreviations
- Vestibulocochlear nerve: CN8, CNVIII

Synonyms
- Eighth cranial nerve

Definitions
- CNVIII: Afferent sensory nerve of hearing & balance

IMAGING ANATOMY

Overview
- Sensory (special sensory afferent) nerve consisting of 2 parts
  - Vestibular part: Balance
  - Cochlear part: Hearing
- CNVIII best described from peripheral to central

Cochlear Nerve
- Arises from bipolar neurons located in **spiral ganglion** within modiolus of cochlea
  - Peripheral fibers pass to organ of Corti in cochlear duct (scala media) within cochlea
  - Central fibers coalesce & pass as auditory component of CNVIII (cochlear nerve) to brainstem
- Central fibers pass from modiolus through cochlear aperture into internal auditory canal (IAC)
  - **Cochlear aperture** defined as bony opening into anteroinferior quadrant of fundus of IAC
  - Maximum diameter of cochlear aperture: ~ 2 mm
- **Cochlear nerve** passes from IAC fundus to porus acusticus within **anteroinferior quadrant of IAC**
- Near porus acusticus, cochlear nerve joins together with superior & inferior vestibular nerves to form vestibulocochlear nerve (CNVIII)
- CNVIII crosses cerebellopontine angle (CPA) cistern posterior to facial nerve
- CNVIII enters lateral brainstem at pontomedullary junction posterior to facial nerve
- Cochlear nerve fibers bifurcate, ending in dorsal & ventral cochlear nuclei
- **Dorsal & ventral cochlear nuclei**
  - Cochlear nuclei found on lateral surface of inferior cerebellar peduncle (restiform body)

Vestibular Nerve
- Arises from bipolar neurons located in vestibular (Scarpa) ganglion located within vestibular nerve in fundal portion of IAC
  - Vestibular ganglion not visible on imaging
  - Peripheral fibers pass to sensory epithelium of utricle, saccule, & semicircular canals
    - Traverse multiple foramina in cribriform plate in lateral wall of IAC fundus
  - Central fibers coalesce to form superior & inferior vestibular nerves that pass medially to brainstem
- Fundus of IAC
  - Superior & inferior vestibular nerves are separated by **falciform crest** (transverse crest)
  - Superior vestibular nerve separated from facial nerve anteriorly by vertical bony structure called **Bill bar**
    - Bill bar not visible on imaging (CT or MR)
- Superior & inferior vestibular nerves pass medially from IAC fundus to porus acusticus within posterosuperior & posteroinferior quadrants of IAC
- Near porus acusticus, superior & inferior vestibular nerves join together with cochlear nerve to form vestibulocochlear nerve (CNVIII)
- Vestibulocochlear nerve crosses CPA cistern posterior to facial nerve
- Enters lateral brainstem at junction pons & medulla posterior to facial nerve
- Vestibular nerve fibers divide into ascending & descending branches, which mainly terminate in vestibular nuclear complex
- **Vestibular nuclear complex**
  - 4 nuclei (lateral, superior, medial, & inferior)
  - Located beneath lateral recess along floor of 4th ventricle (rhomboid fossa) in lower pons
  - Complex connections exist between vestibular nuclei, cerebellum, spinal cord (vestibulospinal tract), & nuclei controlling eye movement

ANATOMY IMAGING ISSUES

Imaging Recommendations
- Sensorineural hearing loss (SNHL)
  - **Intracochlear lesion suspected**
    - CT & MR both useful for imaging
    - Congenital lesions of membranous labyrinth seen as abnormalities of fluid spaces on MR or in bony labyrinth shape on T-bone CT
    - T-bone CT better for otosclerosis, Paget disease, labyrinthine ossificans, or if trauma suspected
    - Only MR will demonstrate labyrinthitis or intralabyrinthine tumor
  - **CNVIII lesion suspected (CPA-IAC)**
    - MR imaging method of choice
    - Thin-section, high-resolution T2 sequence in axial & coronal planes may be used to screen patients with unilateral SNHL
    - T1 C+ MR remains gold standard

Imaging Sweet Spots
- Unilateral SNHL
  - Focus on brainstem (inferior cerebellar peduncle)-CPA-IAC-cochlea
  - Central acoustic pathway (intraaxial pathways above cochlear nuclei) rarely site of offending lesion
- Cisternal & IAC segments of CNVIII routinely visualized on high-resolution T2 MR

Imaging Pitfalls
- Beware small lesions of IAC (≤ 2 mm)
  - Follow-up imaging recommended as may be transient finding where surgery not needed

CLINICAL IMPLICATIONS

Clinical Importance
- Vestibular nerve dysfunction (dizziness, vertigo, imbalance) alone usually has negative MR
- 95% of lesions causing unilateral SNHL found by MR are **vestibulocochlear schwannoma**

CNVIII (Vestibulocochlear Nerve)

GRAPHICS

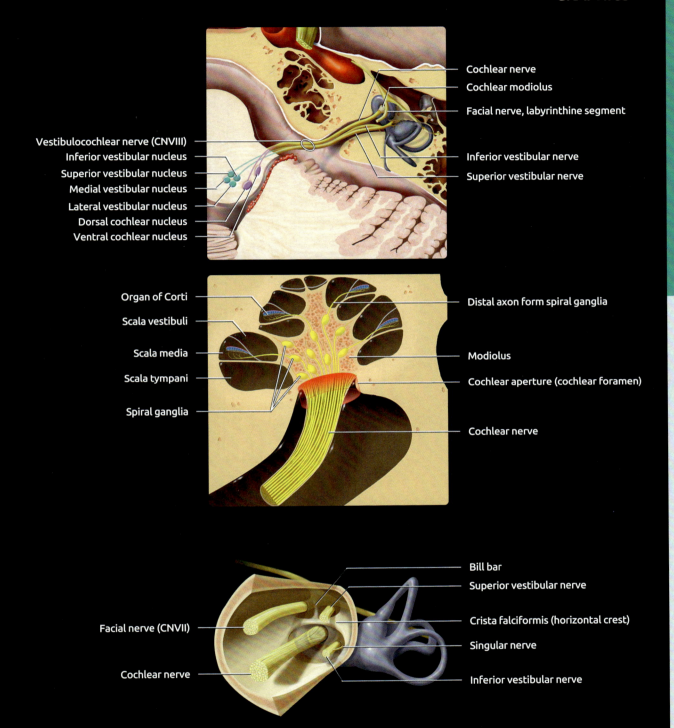

(Top) Axial graphic of the cerebellopontine angle (CPA), internal auditory canal (IAC), & inner ear is shown. Cochlear component of CNVIII begins in bipolar cell bodies in spiral ganglion of cochlear modiolus. Central fibers run in the cochlear nerve to dorsal & ventral cochlear nuclei in the inferior cerebellar peduncle. The inferior & superior vestibular nerves begin in cell bodies in the vestibular ganglion, from there coursing centrally to 4 vestibular nuclei. **(Middle)** Axial graphic of magnified cochlea, modiolus, & cochlear nerve is shown. Notice the bipolar spiral ganglion cells within modiolus contribute distal fibers to the organ of Corti as well as proximal axons that constitute the cochlear nerve. **(Bottom)** Graphic depicting fundus of the IAC is shown. Notice the crista falciformis separates the cochlear nerve & inferior vestibular nerve below from CNVII & superior vestibular nerve above. Also note Bill bar separating CNVII from the superior vestibular nerve.

CNVIII (Vestibulocochlear Nerve)

AXIAL & CORONAL BONE CT

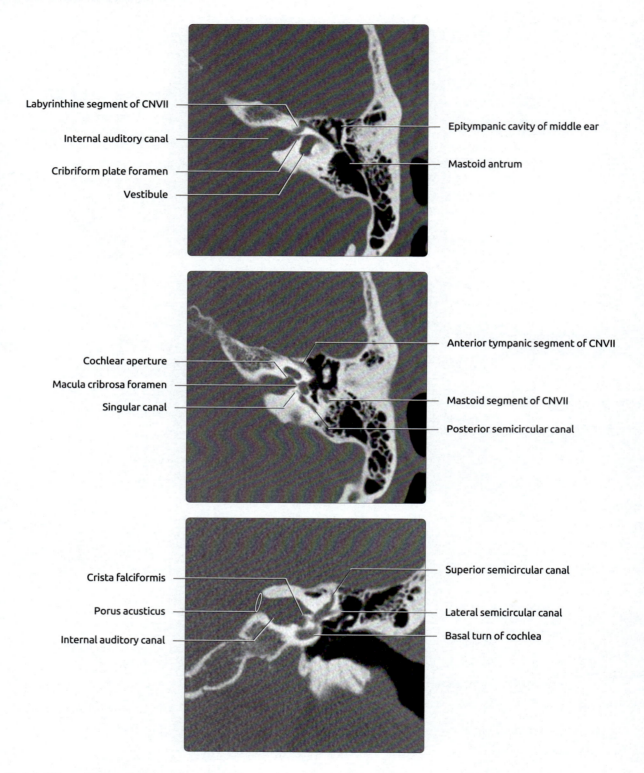

(Top) Axial bone CT through the upper portion of the IAC shows the C-shaped labyrinthine segment of the facial nerve & a main canal of the superior vestibular nerve crossing the cribriform plate toward the vestibule. (Middle) Axial bone CT through the lower IAC shows anterolateral cochlear aperture through which the cochlear nerve passes on its way from the cochlear modiolus into the IAC. Also notice the cribriform plate foramen through which the inferior vestibular nerve reaches the vestibule & the smaller singular canal. (Bottom) Coronal bone CT through the IAC demonstrates the horizontal falciform crest, which divides the fundus of the IAC into upper & lower portions. Facial & superior vestibular nerves pass above, & cochlear & inferior vestibular nerves pass below the falciform crest. Porus acusticus is a bony aperture of the IAC.

CNVIII (Vestibulocochlear Nerve)

AXIAL T2 MR

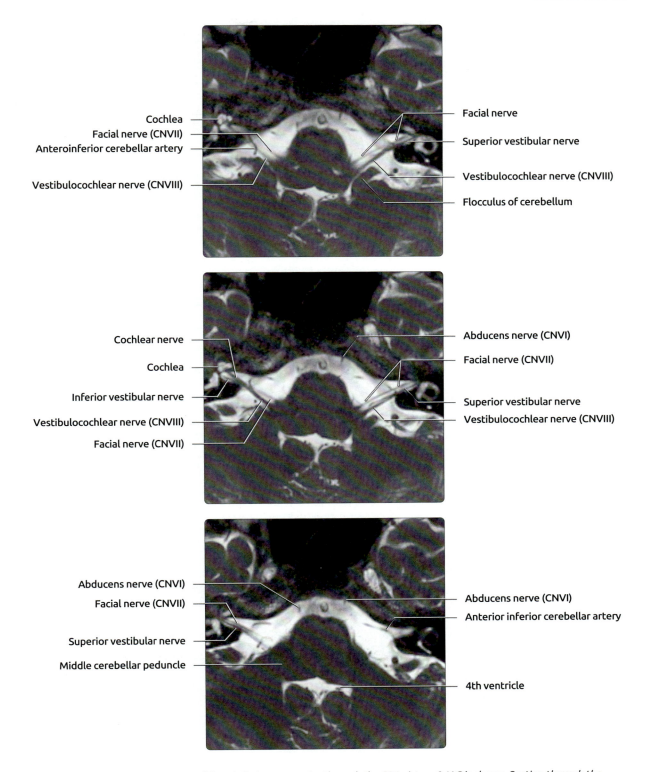

(Top) First of 3 axial T2 MR images presented from inferior to superior through the CPA cistern & IAC is shown. Section through the superior left IAC demonstrates the cochlear nerve anteriorly & inferior vestibular nerve posteriorly at the fundus. (Middle) Vestibulocochlear nerve arises posterior to the facial nerve from the brainstem at the pontomedullary junction & maintains a posterior position throughout its course through the CPA/IAC. On the patient's right, the cochlear nerve is anterior to inferior vestibular nerve within the fundus of the IAC. On the left, the superior fundus of the IAC is seen with the anterior facial nerve & posterior superior vestibular nerve. (Bottom) MR slice through the superior IAC area demonstrates the superior vestibular nerve posterior to facial nerve on the patient's right.

CNVIII (Vestibulocochlear Nerve)

CORONAL T2 MR

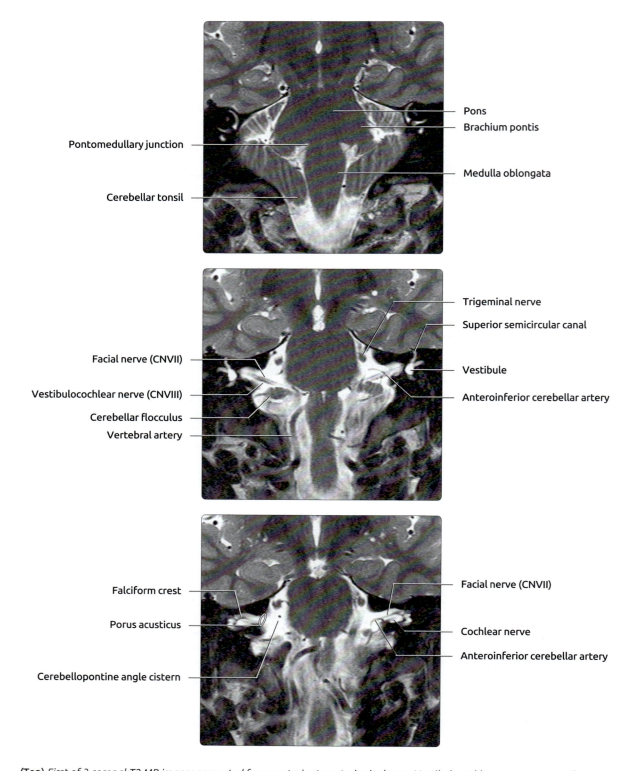

(Top) First of 3 coronal T2 MR images presented from posterior to anterior is shown. Vestibulocochlear nerve emerges from the brainstem posterior to the facial nerve at the pontomedullary junction. *(Middle)* Facial & vestibulocochlear nerves course through the CPA into the IAC. Facial nerve is anterior & superior to the vestibulocochlear nerve within the CPA & IAC. Notice the somewhat cephalad course of CNVIII as it rises into the IAC from its origin at the pontomedullary junction. *(Bottom)* Section through the fundus of the IAC demonstrates the horizontal falciform crest separating the fundus into upper & lower portions. At this level, the facial nerve is above & the cochlear nerve is below the falciform crest. The anteroinferior cerebellar artery loop is a constant fixture in the normal anatomy of the CPA & IAC area.

CNVIII (Vestibulocochlear Nerve)

OBLIQUE SAGITTAL T2 MR

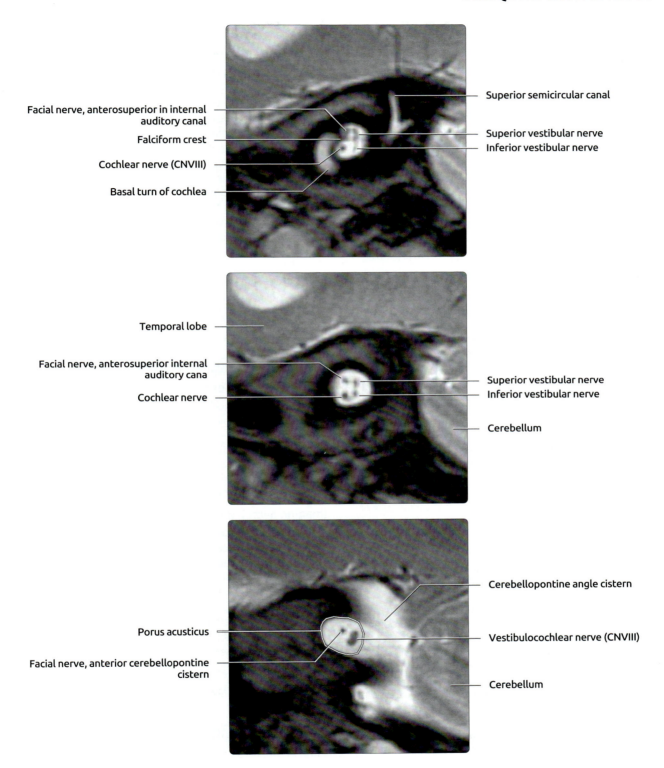

(Top) First of 3 sequential oblique sagittal T2 MR images through the IAC presented from lateral to medial is shown. Slice is through the fundus of the IAC showing the horizontal falciform crest separating the fundus into upper & lower portions. Facial nerve is anterosuperior, separated from the superior vestibular nerve by a vertical bony septum called "Bill bar," which is not resolved with even focused imaging. Below the falciform crest are the cochlear nerve anteriorly & inferior vestibular nerve posteriorly. (Middle) In the mid IAC, this image shows 4 discrete nerves. (Bottom) At the level of porus acusticus, both the superior & inferior vestibular nerves join together with the cochlear nerve to form a C-shaped vestibulocochlear nerve. The facial nerve remains discrete as it travels across the CPA cistern.

CNIX (Glossopharyngeal Nerve)

TERMINOLOGY

Abbreviations
- Glossopharyngeal nerve (CN9, CNIX)

Synonyms
- 9th cranial nerve

Definitions
- Mixed nerve with complex functions
  - Taste & sensation to posterior 1/3 of tongue
  - Sensory nerve to middle ear & pharynx
  - Parasympathetic to parotid gland
  - Motor to stylopharyngeus muscle
  - Viscerosensory to carotid body & sinus

IMAGING ANATOMY

Overview
- 4 segments: Intraaxial, cisternal, skull base, & extracranial

Intraaxial Segment
- Glossopharyngeal nuclei are in upper & middle medulla
  - **Motor fibers** to stylopharyngeus muscle originate in **nucleus ambiguus**
  - **Sensory fibers** from tympanic membrane, soft palate, tongue base, & pharynx terminate in **spinal nucleus CNV**
  - **Taste fibers** from posterior 1/3 of tongue terminate in **solitary tract nucleus**
  - **Parasympathetic fibers** to parotid gland originate in **inferior salivatory nucleus**

Cisternal Segment
- Exits lateral medulla in **postolivary sulcus** as 3-5 rootlets uniting to form cisternal segment just above vagus nerve
- Mean nerve length from medulla to jugular foramen is ~ 14-18 mm
- Transition zone (TZ) located ~ 1.1-1.8 mm from medulla or root entry/exit zone (REZ)
  - TZ is area between central & peripheral myelin with increased vulnerability to mechanical irritation & relevant in neurovascular compression
  - REZ is portion of nerve including TZ, central myelin root portion, & adjacent brainstem surface
  - Glossopharyngeal neuralgia caused by neurovascular compression occurs 95% in proximal REZ, overlapping proximal location of TZ
- Nerve travels anterolaterally through basal cistern with vagus nerve & bulbar portion of accessory nerve
- Passes through glossopharyngeal meatus into **pars nervosa** portion of **jugular foramen**

Skull Base Segment
- Passes through anterior **pars nervosa**
  - Accompanied by inferior petrosal sinus
  - CNX & CNXI are posterior within pars vascularis portion of jugular foramen
  - Superior & inferior sensory ganglia of CNIX are found within jugular foramen

Extracranial Segment
- Exits into anterior **nasopharyngeal carotid space**
- Passes lateral to internal carotid artery, innervates stylopharyngeus, & contributes to carotid sinus nerve
- Gives branches to pharyngeal plexus & terminates as tonsillar and lingual branches

Extracranial Branches
- **Tympanic branch (Jacobson nerve)**
  - Sensation from middle ear & parasympathetic to parotid gland via lesser petrosal nerve & otic ganglion
  - Arises from inferior sensory ganglion in jugular foramen
  - Via **inferior tympanic canaliculus** to hypotympanum
    - Aberrant internal carotid artery enters via this canal
  - Forms tympanic plexus on cochlear promontory
    - Glomus bodies associated with this nerve form glomus tympanicum paraganglioma
- **Stylopharyngeus branch**
- **Carotid sinus nerve**
  - Supplies viscerosensory fibers to carotid sinus & body
  - Conducts impulses from mechanoreceptors of sinus & chemoreceptors of carotid body to medulla
- **Pharyngeal branches**
  - Sensory to posterior oropharynx & soft palate (pharyngeal plexus)
- **Lingual branch**
  - Sensory & taste to posterior 1/3 of tongue

ANATOMY IMAGING ISSUES

Imaging Recommendations
- MR imaging method of choice
  - Superior sensitivity to skull base, meningeal, cisternal, & brainstem pathology
  - Sequences should include combination of T2, T1 without fat-saturation, & contrast-enhanced T1 with fat-saturation in axial & coronal planes
- Supplemental bone CT for complex skull base pathology

Imaging Sweet Spots
- Image from pontomedullary junction to hyoid bone
- CNIX nuclei & intraaxial segment not directly visualized
  - Position inferred by identifying upper medulla, posterior to postolivary sulcus
  - Cisternal segment not always visualized on routine MR
    - High-resolution, thin-section T2 sequences often identify cisternal segments of CNIX-XI nerve complex
    - Bone algorithm CT for bony anatomy of pars nervosa
- Extracranial segment not visualized

Imaging Pitfalls
- Remember to image entire extracranial course of CNIX beyond skull base

CLINICAL IMPLICATIONS

Clinical Importance
- Complex CNIX-XI neuropathies (Vernet syndrome) caused by disease in medulla, basal cistern, jugular foramen, or nasopharyngeal carotid space
  - Isolated CNIX neuropathy exceedingly rare
- Glossopharyngeal neuralgia mostly caused by compression by PICA > AICA; minority from trauma, neoplasm, infection, multiple sclerosis, or elongated styloid process (Eagle syndrome)

CNIX (Glossopharyngeal Nerve)

GRAPHICS

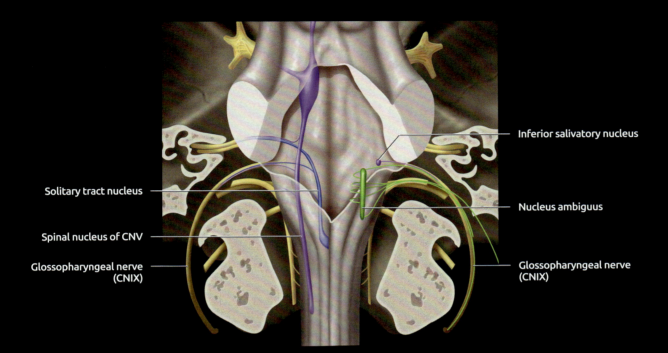

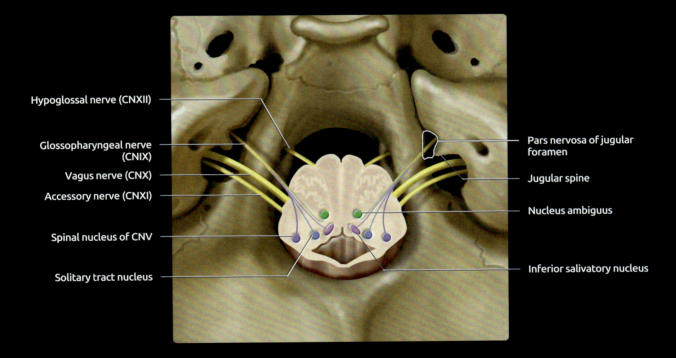

(**Top**) *Posterior view of the brainstem emphasizes the 4 nuclei participating in the functions of the glossopharyngeal nerve. Notice the 2 efferent nuclei, the nucleus ambiguus and inferior salivatory nucleus labeled on the right. The nucleus ambiguus supplies motor fibers to the stylopharyngeus muscle, while the inferior salivatory nucleus supplies parasympathetic fibers to the parotid gland. On the left, the afferent nuclei are the solitary tract nucleus and the spinal nucleus of CNV. The solitary tract nucleus receives taste fibers from the tongue base, while the spinal nucleus of CNV receives sensation from the middle ear, soft palate, tongue base, and pharynx.* (**Bottom**) *Axial graphic through medullary brainstem from above shows the 4 nuclei of the glossopharyngeal nerve.*

CNIX (Glossopharyngeal Nerve)

GRAPHIC, EXTRACRANIAL

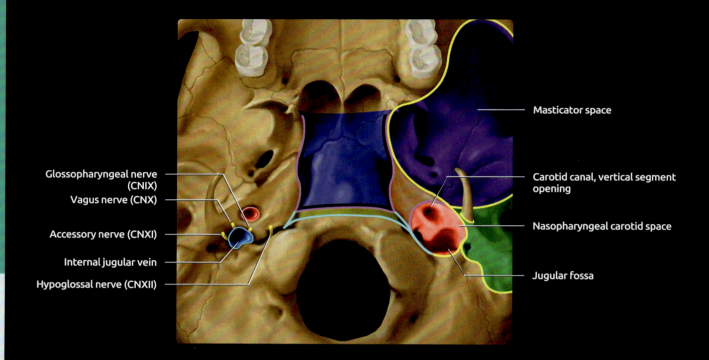

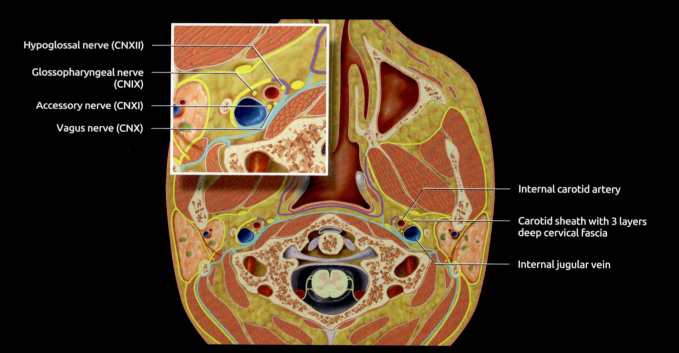

(Top) Graphic of skull base viewed from below depicts the 4 cranial nerves emerging into the nasopharyngeal carotid space. The glossopharyngeal nerve is just anteromedial to the internal jugular vein as it exits the pars nervosa of the jugular foramen. (Bottom) Axial graphic of nasopharyngeal carotid spaces shows the extracranial glossopharyngeal nerve situated anteriorly in the gap between the internal carotid artery and the internal jugular vein. Notice that at this level, CNX, CNXI, and CNXII are all still within the carotid space. The glossopharyngeal nerve exits the carotid space at the level of the high oropharynx.

CNIX (Glossopharyngeal Nerve)

GRAPHIC, EXTRACRANIAL

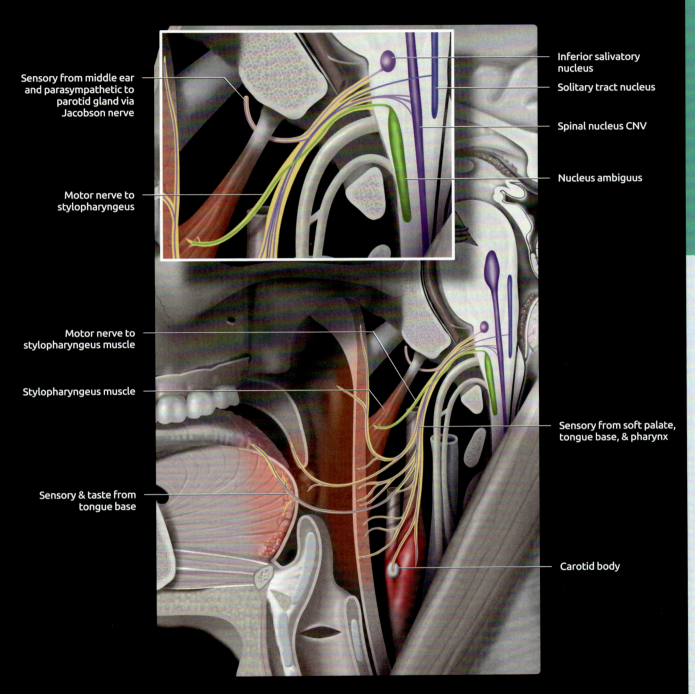

Sagittal graphic emphasizing the extracranial component of the glossopharyngeal nerve is shown. Only 1 muscle is innervated by the fibers in CNIX from the nucleus ambiguus, the stylopharyngeus. Sensory information from the middle ear, tongue base, soft palate, and oropharyngeal surface are transmitted via CNIX to the spinal nucleus of the trigeminal nerve. Taste sensation from the tongue base travels via CNIX to the solitary tract nucleus. Parasympathetic secretomotor fibers from the inferior salivatory nucleus bound for the parotid gland also travel in CNIX.

CNIX (Glossopharyngeal Nerve)

AXIAL BONE CT

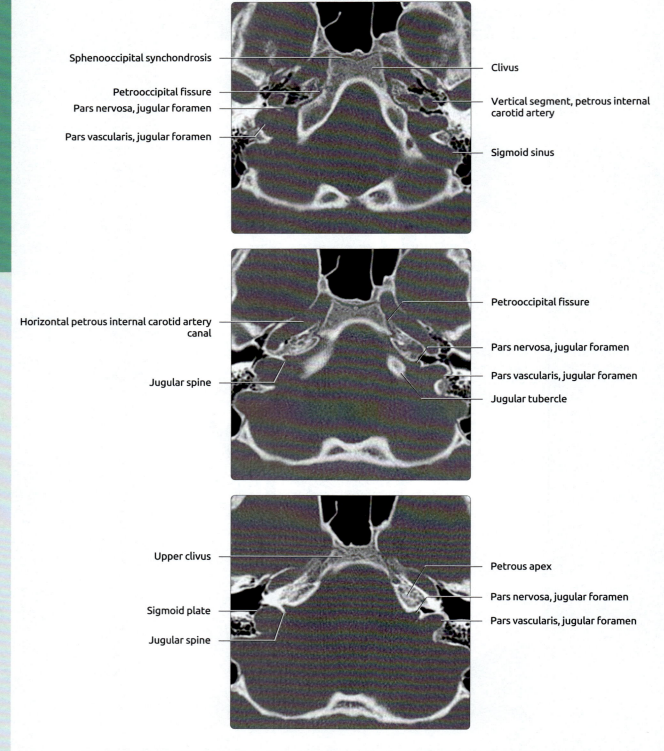

(Top) First of 3 axial bone CT images presented from inferior to superior through posterior skull base emphasizes the bony anatomy of the jugular foramen. The jugular foramen is located on the floor of the posterior cranial fossa between the petrous temporal bone anterolaterally and occipital bone posteromedially. It is therefore a venous channel between these bones. (Middle) The jugular foramen is seen here as 2 discrete pieces, the smaller anteromedial pars nervosa and larger posterolateral pars vascularis, separated by jugular spine of petrous bone. (Bottom) The 2 parts of the jugular foramen are visibile. The pars nervosa transmits the glossopharyngeal nerve (CNIX), Jacobsen nerve, and inferior petrosal sinus. The pars vascularis transmits the vagus (CNX) and accessory (CNXI) cranial nerves, Arnold nerve, and sigmoid sinus, which becomes the internal jugular vein.

CNIX (Glossopharyngeal Nerve)

AXIAL T2 MR

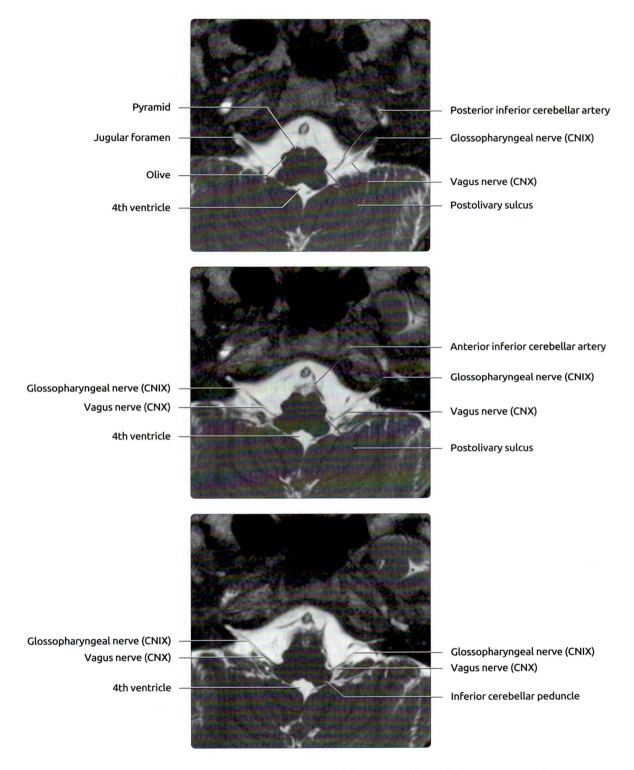

(Top) First of 3 axial high-resolution T2 MR images through the brainstem medulla presented from inferior to superior is shown. Glossopharyngeal nerve is seen passing laterally into the pars nervosa of the jugular foramen. (Middle) The glossopharyngeal nerve (CNIX), vagus nerve (CNX), and bulbar accessory nerve (CNXI) all exit the medulla laterally in the postolivary sulcus. CNIX is the most cephalad of these. With routine MR imaging it is not possible to see these 3 cranial nerves individually. (Bottom) In the upper medulla, the vagus nerve is well seen leaving the brainstem via the postolivary sulcus. The glossopharyngeal nerve is seen more laterally, as it has already exited the brainstem above the vagus nerve.

CNX (Vagus Nerve)

TERMINOLOGY

Abbreviations
- Vagus nerve: CNX

Definitions
- CNX: Longest and one of most complex cranial nerves (CN) with diverse functions including parasympathetic (PS) innervation of neck, thoracic and abdominal viscera
- Involved in autonomic regulation of cardiovascular, respiratory, and gastrointestinal systems
- Additional innervation
  - Motor to majority of soft palate, pharynx, larynx, and palatoglossus tongue muscle
  - Visceral sensation from larynx, esophagus, trachea, thoracic and abdominal viscera
  - Sensory nerve to external tympanic membrane (TM), external auditory canal (EAC), and external ear
  - Taste from epiglottis

IMAGING ANATOMY

Overview
- Longest of CN, extending from medulla to colon
- Segments: Intraaxial, cisternal, skull base, and extracranial

Intraaxial Segment
- Vagal nuclei are in upper and middle medulla
  - **Motor fibers** originate in **nucleus ambiguus**
  - **Taste** from epiglottis goes to **solitary tract nucleus**
  - **Sensory fibers** from viscera go to **dorsal vagal nucleus** (afferent component)
  - **PS fibers** project from **dorsal vagal nucleus** (efferent component)
  - Sensations from meninges and ear to spinal nucleus CNV

Cisternal Segment
- Nerve fibers exit lateral medulla in **postolivary sulcus** inferior to CNIX and superior to bulbar portion of CNXI

Skull Base Segment
- Enters **pars vascularis** portion of jugular foramen (JF)
  - With CNXI (shared fibrous sheath) and jugular bulb
  - **Superior vagal (jugular) ganglion** is found within JF

Extracranial Segment
- Exits JF into nasopharyngeal **carotid space**
- Inferior vagal (nodose) ganglion lies just below skull base
- Travels posterolateral to carotid artery into thorax
  - Passes anterior to aortic arch on left and subclavian artery (SCA) on right
- Forms plexus around esophagus and major blood vessels to heart and lungs
- Esophageal plexus nerves provide PS supply to stomach
- Innervation to intestines and visceral organs follows arterial blood supply

Extracranial Branches in Head and Neck
- **Auricular branch (Arnold nerve)**
  - Sensation from external surface of TM, EAC, external ear
  - Arises from superior vagal ganglion within JF, also has CNIX branches
  - Passes through **mastoid canaliculus** extending from posterolateral JF to mastoid segment CNVII canal
  - Enters EAC via tympanomastoid fissure
- **Pharyngeal branches**
  - **Pharyngeal plexus** exits just below skull base
  - Sensory to epiglottis, trachea, and esophagus
  - Motor to soft palate [except tensor veli palatini muscle (CNV3)] and pharyngeal constrictor muscles
  - **Carotid sinus branch (Hering nerve)**
    - Formed by small CNIX branch and branch from CNX
    - Supplies carotid sinus wall baroreceptors and carotid body chemoreceptors
- **Superior laryngeal nerve**
  - Motor to **cricothyroid** muscle (external branch)
  - Sensory internal branch to hypopharynx and supraglottis
- **Recurrent laryngeal nerve (RLN)**
  - On right, recurs at cervicothoracic junction, passes posteriorly around SCA
  - On left, recurs in mediastinum, passes posteriorly under aorta at aortopulmonary window (APW)
  - Travels in **tracheoesophageal groove** (TEG) posteromedial to thyroid lobe and enters larynx at cricothyroid joint level
  - Motor to all laryngeal muscles except cricothyroids
  - Sensory to mucosa of infraglottis

ANATOMY IMAGING ISSUES

Imaging Recommendations
- **Proximal vagal neuropathy**
  - Image from medulla to hyoid bone
  - MR imaging method of choice: Superior sensitivity for skull base, meningeal, cisternal, and brainstem pathology
    - Should include axial and coronal T2, T1 (without fat saturation and contrast enhanced with fat saturation)
    - Include heavily T2-weighted steady state (FIESTA or CISS) sequence
    - Bone CT complementary in complex skull base pathology
- **Distal vagal neuropathy**
  - Image skull base to mediastinum; **to carina for left side**
  - Key areas to evaluate are carotid space, TEG, APW
  - CECT imaging method of choice

CLINICAL IMPLICATIONS

Clinical Importance
- **Vagal nerve dysfunction: Proximal symptom complex**
  - Injury site: Between medulla and hyoid bone
  - Multiple CN involved (CNIX-XII, Vernet syndrome) with oropharyngeal and laryngeal dysfunction
- **Vagal nerve dysfunction: Distal symptom complex**
  - Injury site: Below hyoid bone
  - Isolated larynx dysfunction with vocal cord (VC) paralysis (RLN involvement > > infrahyoid CNX)
  - Imaging features of VC paralysis: Medialization of ipsilateral true VC, anteromedial arytenoid cartilage rotation, enlarged laryngeal ventricle = sail sign, medialized, thickened aryepiglottic fold, enlarged pyriform sinus

CNX (Vagus Nerve)

GRAPHICS, PROXIMAL CNX

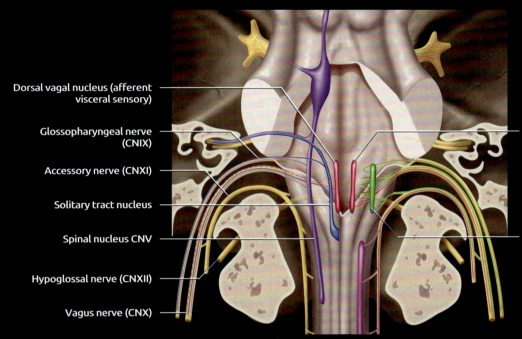

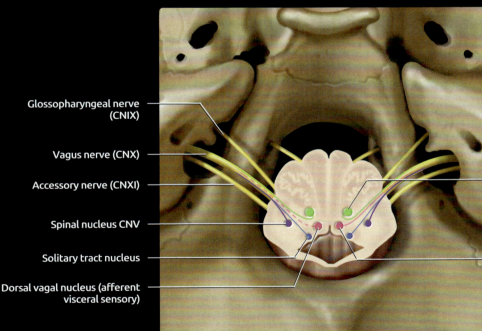

(Top) *Graphic of brainstem viewed from behind shows critical nuclear columns of CNX. Note the nucleus ambiguus supplies motor fibers to CNX. Dorsal vagal nucleus is a mixed nucleus, sending efferent parasympathetic fibers to the viscera while receiving afferent sensory fibers from these same viscera. The solitary tract nucleus receives taste information from the epiglottis and vallecula via CNX.* **(Bottom)** *Axial graphic through the medulla shows principal nuclei associated with vagus nerve function. Skeletal motor fibers to pharynx and larynx come from the nucleus ambiguus. Parasympathetic fibers to the viscera are associated with the dorsal nucleus of the vagus nerve (solid pink line). Sensory information transmitted from the viscera is also transmitted to the dorsal nucleus of the vagus nerve (dashed pink line). The solitary tract nucleus receives taste information for the epiglottis.*

CNX (Vagus Nerve)

GRAPHIC, EXTRACRANIAL VAGUS NERVE

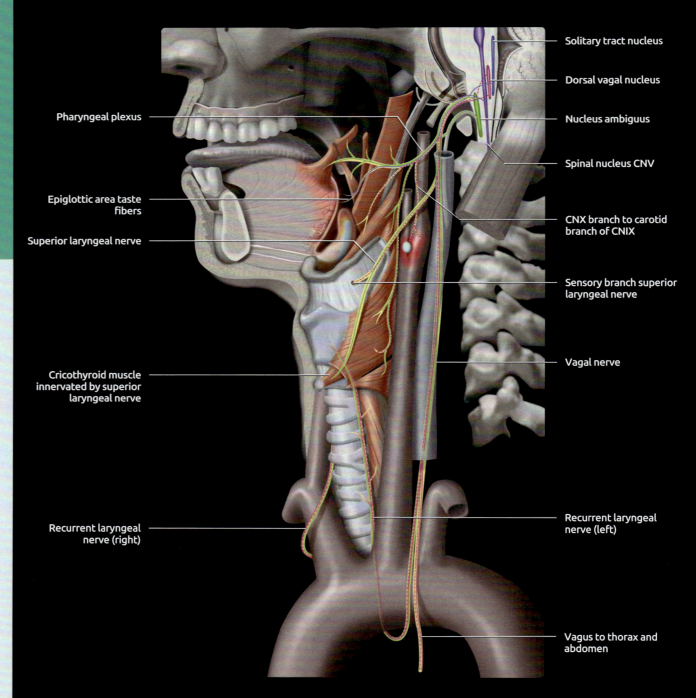

Lateral graphic shows the neck and upper mediastinal portions of CNX, including the 4 brainstem nuclei. The nucleus ambiguus supplies efferent motor innervation (green lines) via the pharyngeal plexus to the soft palate and pharynx (superior, middle, and inferior constrictor muscles) and via the recurrent laryngeal nerves to all laryngeal muscles except the cricothyroids. The dual-functioning dorsal vagal nucleus both sends out efferent fibers for involuntary motor activity in the viscera (solid pink line) as well as receives sensations from these same viscera (dashed pink line). The solitary tract nucleus receives taste information from the region of the epiglottis and vallecula. The spinal nucleus of CNV receives external ear and skull base-meninges sensory information. Only the visceral motor and sensory fibers from dorsal vagal nucleus continue on CNX to the rest of the body.

CNX (Vagus Nerve)

GRAPHICS, EXTRACRANIAL CNX

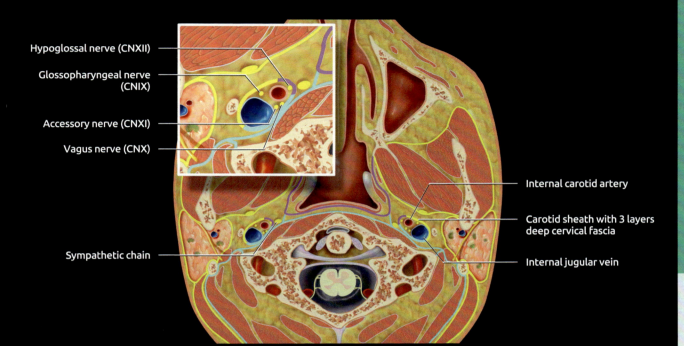

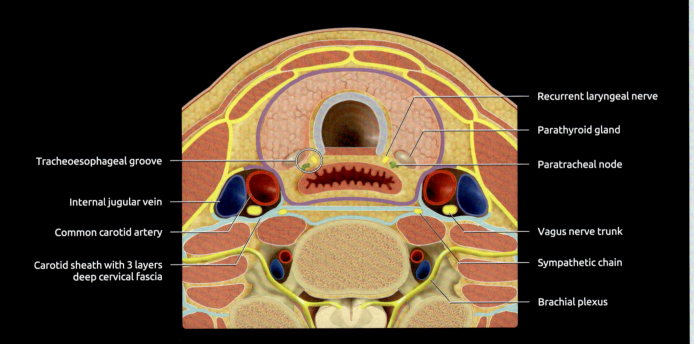

(Top) Axial graphic of nasopharyngeal carotid spaces shows the extracranial vagus nerve situated posteriorly in the gap between the internal carotid artery and the internal jugular vein. Notice that at this level, CNIX, CNXI, and CNXII are all still within the carotid space. (Bottom) Axial graphic through the infrahyoid carotid spaces at the level of the thyroid gland demonstrates the vagus trunk is the only remaining cranial nerve within the carotid space. It remains in the posterior gap between the common carotid artery and the internal jugular vein. Note the recurrent laryngeal nerve in the tracheoesophageal groove with the visceral space. Remember the left recurrent laryngeal nerve turns cephalad in the aortopulmonic window in the mediastinum, whereas the right recurrent nerve turns at the cervicothoracic junction around the subclavian artery.

CNX (Vagus Nerve)

AXIAL BONE CT

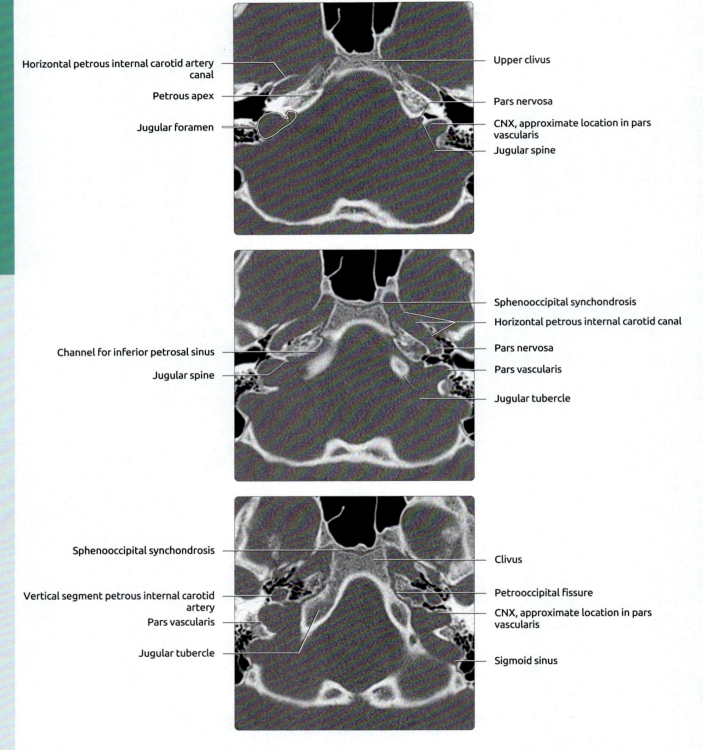

(Top) First of 3 axial bone CT images of the skull base presented from superior to inferior is shown. The jugular foramen is divided by the jugular spine into the anteromedial, smaller pars nervosa, and posterolateral pars vascularis. The pars vascularis transmits the vagus and accessory cranial nerves, Arnold nerve, and jugular bulb, which becomes the internal jugular vein. *(Middle)* In this image, the pars nervosa is seen to connect anteromedially to the inferior petrosal sinus. CNIX, Jacobsen nerve, and the inferior petrosal sinus are all found within the pars nervosa. *(Bottom)* Image through the lower jugular foramen shows the sigmoid sinuses emptying into the pars vascularis of the jugular foramen. Notice the jugular foramen is located on the floor of the posterior cranial fossa in the seam between the petrous temporal bone anterolaterally and occipital bone posteromedially.

CNX (Vagus Nerve)

AXIAL T2 MR

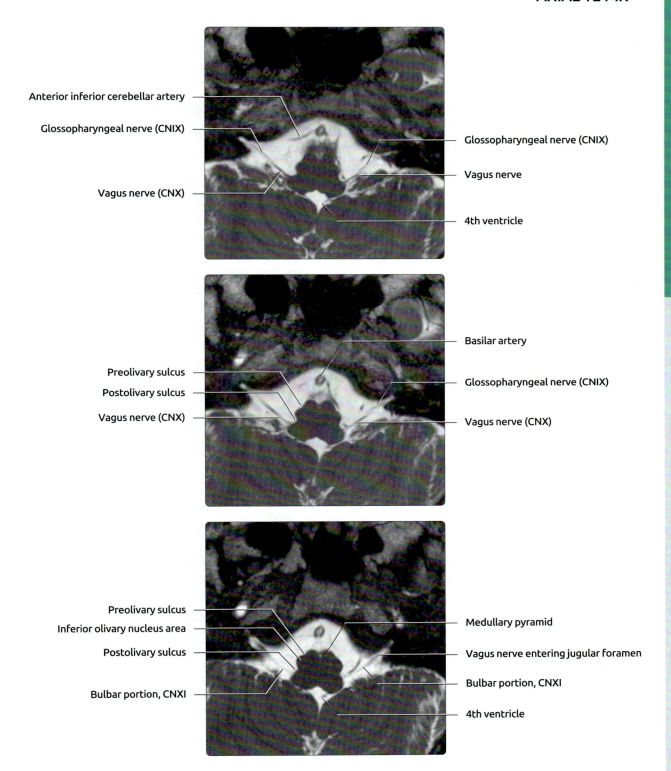

(Top) First of 3 axial T2 MR images of the low brainstem presented from superior to inferior is shown. The vagus nerve is seen exiting the lateral medulla in the postolivary sulcus inferior to the glossopharyngeal nerve. (Middle) In this image, the vagus nerve is clearly seen exiting the postolivary sulcus into the lateral basal cistern bilaterally. CNIX exits this sulcus just above the vagus nerve, while the bulbar CNXI exits it just inferiorly. (Bottom) At the level of the cephalad margin of the jugular foramen, the bulbar root of the accessory nerve is seen exiting the postolivary sulcus. The vagus nerve is entering the jugular foramen laterally. Without thin-section-focused T2 imaging, it is often difficult to separate the glossopharyngeal nerve, vagus nerve, and bulbar root of the accessory nerve in the basal cisterns.

CNXI (Accessory Nerve)

TERMINOLOGY

Abbreviations
- Accessory nerve: CN 11, CNXI

Synonyms
- 11th CN

Definitions
- CNXI: Pure motor CN, supplying sternocleidomastoid, trapezius muscles (through spinal component) and palatal, pharyngeal, laryngeal muscles (through cranial component)

IMAGING ANATOMY

Overview
- Motor CN only
- 4 CNXI segments are defined
  - Intraaxial, cisternal, skull base, and extracranial

Intraaxial Segment
- 2 distinct nuclear origins
  - **Bulbar** (cranial) motor fibers originate in lower **nucleus ambiguus**
    - Fibers course anterolaterally to exit lateral medulla in postolivary sulcus inferior to CNIX and CNX (vagus nerve)
  - **Spinal** motor fibers originate from **spinal nucleus** of accessory nerve
    - Narrow column of cells along lateral aspect of anterior horn from CI to CV
    - Nerve fibers emerge from lateral aspect of cervical spinal cord between anterior and posterior roots
    - Fibers combine forming bundle that ascends entering skull base via **foramen magnum**

Cisternal Segment
- Bulbar portion travels anterolaterally through basal cistern along similar course as CNIX and CNX
- Spinal portion enters lower lateral basal cistern, exits thorough jugular foramen
- Bulbar root joins spinal component of accessory nerve either in lower cistern or within jugular foramen

Skull Base Segment
- Passes through posterior **pars vascularis portion of jugular foramen**
  - CNX and jugular bulb are also in pars vascularis
- Bulbar and spinal portions remain together in jugular foramen

Extracranial Segment
- Fibers from bulbar portion, which arise within nucleus ambiguus separate from main nerve and merge with vagus nerve
  - Travel via CNX to supply muscles of palate, pharynx, and larynx
    - Palate: Levator veli palatini, palatoglossus, palatopharyngeus, and musculus uvulae
    - Pharynx: Superior constrictor and soft palate via pharyngeal plexus
    - Larynx: Except cricothyroid muscle via recurrent laryngeal nerve
- Fibers from spinal portion remain in extracranial CNXI
  - Diverges posterolaterally from carotid space
  - Descend along medial aspect of sternocleidomastoid muscle
  - **Innervates sternomastoid muscle**
  - Continues across floor of posterior cervical space in neck
  - Terminate in and **innervate trapezius muscle**

ANATOMY IMAGING ISSUES

Imaging Recommendations
- MR imaging method of choice
  - Superior sensitivity to skull base, meningeal, cisternal, and brainstem pathology
  - Sequences should include combination of T2, T1 without fat saturation, and contrast-enhanced T1 with fat saturation in axial and coronal planes
- Bone CT used to supplement MR when complex skull base pathology is present

Imaging Sweet Spots
- CNXI nuclei and intraaxial segment not directly visualized
- Cisternal segment is often not visualized on routine MR imaging
  - High-resolution thin-section T2 MR sequence usually demonstrates CNIX-XI nerve complex passing through basal cisterns from postolivary sulcus to pars vascularis of jugular foramen
- Bone CT clearly demonstrates bony anatomy of pars vascularis of jugular foramen
- Extracranial CNXI segment not directly visualized
  - Location inferred from its constant position deep to sternocleidomastoid muscle in floor of posterior cervical space

Imaging Pitfalls
- Hypertrophic levator scapulae muscle following serious CNXI injury may mimic tumor
- **Do not mistake this enlarged muscle for mass**

CLINICAL IMPLICATIONS

Clinical Importance
- CNXI innervates sternocleidomastoid and trapezius muscles

Function Dysfunction
- CNXI dysfunction: Isolated CNXI injury
  - Most common cause is radical neck dissection because jugular nodal chain intimately associated with CNXI
  - Initial symptoms of spinal accessory neuropathy
    - Downward and lateral rotation of scapula
    - Shoulder droop resulting from loss of trapezius tone
  - Long-term findings in spinal accessory neuropathy
    - Within 6 months results in **atrophy** of ipsilateral sternocleidomastoid and trapezius muscles
    - **Compensatory hypertrophy** of ipsilateral **levator scapulae muscle** occurs over months

CNXI (Accessory Nerve)

GRAPHICS

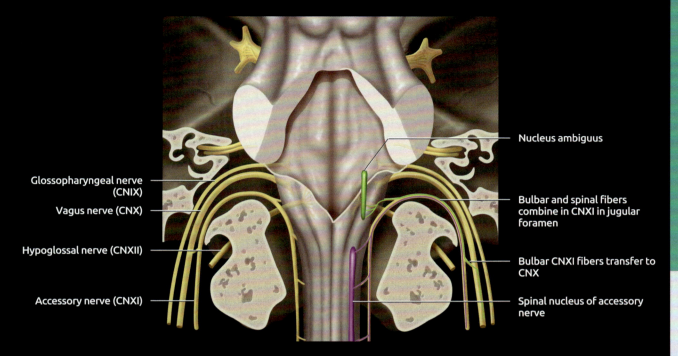

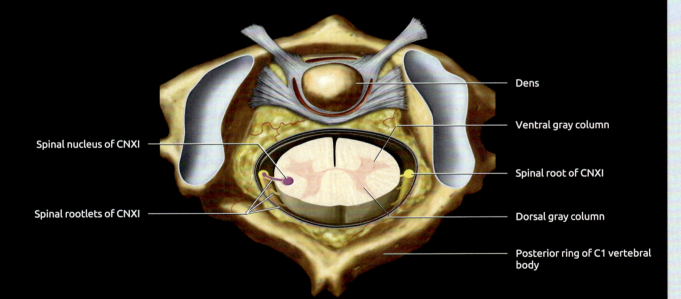

(Top) Graphic of the posterior brainstem reveals both the spinal and the bulbar roots of the accessory nerve (CNXI). Note the lower nucleus ambiguus gives rise to multiple rootlets of the bulbar root of CNXI. Both the spinal and the bulbar roots combine in the lateral basal cistern and jugular foramen. The spinal root continues as extracranial CNXI to innervate the sternocleidomastoid and trapezius muscles. The bulbar root fibers cross to the vagus nerve extracranially or within the jugular foramen to supply motor innervation to the pharynx (superior constrictor and soft palate) and the larynx (except the cricothyroid muscle). (Bottom) Axial graphic shows the upper cervical spinal cord cut to reveal the spinal nucleus of the accessory nerve giving rise to multiple rootlets that unite to form the spinal root of the accessory nerve. The rootlets exit the posterolateral sulcus just anterior to the posterior cervical roots.

CNXI (Accessory Nerve)

GRAPHIC, INTRACRANIAL & EXTRACRANIAL

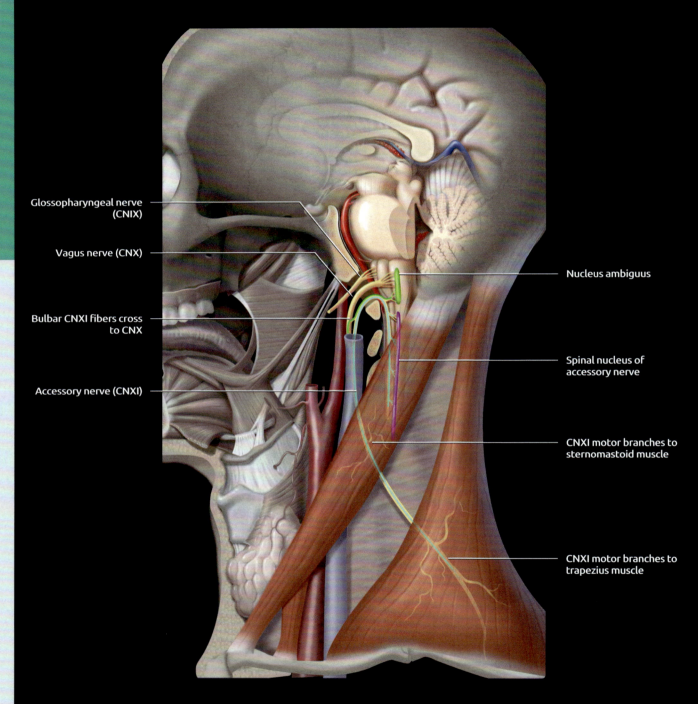

Overview graphic of the intracranial and extracranial accessory nerve (CNXI) shows the lower nucleus ambiguus at the origin of the bulbar root of CNXI while the spinal nucleus gives rise to the spinal root. Both roots combine in the jugular foramen. Extracranially, the bulbar fibers cross to the vagus nerve to eventually provide motor innervation via the pharyngeal plexus to the soft palate and superior constrictor muscles and via the recurrent laryngeal nerve to the majority of the endolaryngeal muscles. The spinal fibers that remain in the accessory nerve provide motor innervation to the sternocleidomastoid and trapezius muscles. Notice extracranial CNXI runs in the floor of the posterior cervical space.

CNXI (Accessory Nerve)

AXIAL BONE CT & T2 MR

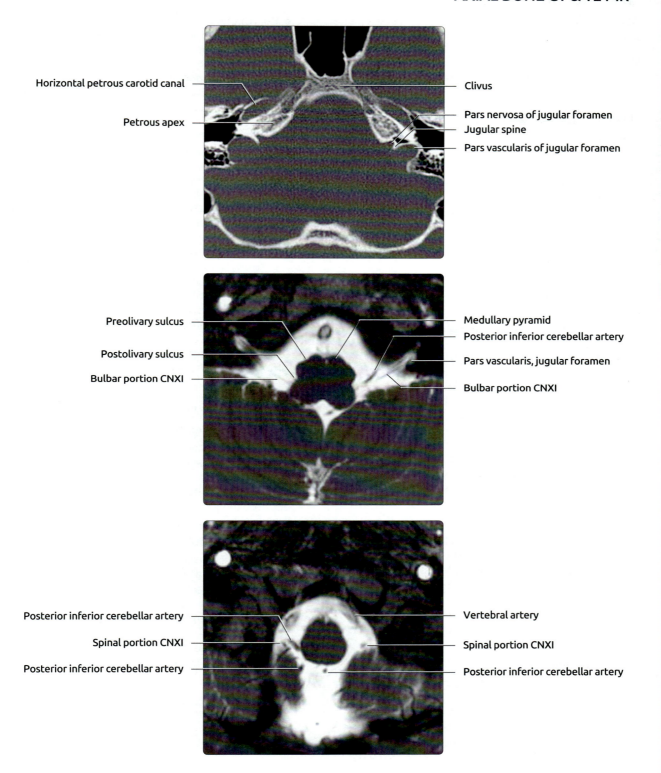

(Top) Axial bone CT through the jugular foramen shows the anteromedial pars nervosa, the jugular spine, and the posterolateral pars vascularis. The pars nervosa transmits CNIX, the Jacobsen nerve, and the inferior petrosal sinus. The pars vascularis transmits CNX, CNXI, the Arnold nerve, and the sigmoid sinus, which becomes the internal jugular vein. (Middle) Axial T2 MR at the level of the medulla shows the bulbar portion of CNXI emerging from the postolivary sulcus just inferior to CNX. The bulbar portion travels anterolaterally through the basal cistern together with CNX and CNIX. (Bottom) Axial T2 MR through the lower medulla reveals the spinal root of CNXI climbing cephalad through the foramen magnum to join the bulbar root of the CNXI before they enter the pars nervosa of the jugular foramen. It is the spinal root that eventually becomes the extracranial CNXI with motor fibers to the sternocleidomastoid and trapezius muscles.

CNXII (Hypoglossal Nerve)

TERMINOLOGY

Abbreviations

- Hypoglossal nerve: CNXII

Definitions

- Motor nerve supplying intrinsic and extrinsic tongue muscles

IMAGING ANATOMY

Overview

- Motor cranial nerve to intrinsic and extrinsic tongue muscles
  - Only extrinsic muscle **not** innervated by CNXII is **palatoglossus muscle** (by CNX)
- Hypoglossal nerve anatomic segments
  - Intraaxial segment
  - Cisternal segment
  - Skull base segment
  - Extracranial

Intraaxial Segment

- **Hypoglossal nucleus**
  - In dorsal medulla between dorsal vagal nucleus and midline
  - Long, thin nucleus that is ~ same length as ventrolateral olive (15- to 18-mm craniocaudal dimension)
  - Extends from level of hypoglossal eminence (trigone) in floor of 4th ventricle just inferior to medullary striae of 4th ventricle to proximal medulla
- Hypoglossal intraaxial axonal course
  - Efferent fibers from hypoglossal nucleus extend ventrally through medulla, lateral to medial lemniscus
  - Efferent fibers exit between olivary nucleus and pyramid (root exit zone) at **ventrolateral sulcus** (also called **preolivary sulcus)**

Cisternal Segment

- Efferent fibers coalesce to form multiple (6-14) **rootlets**
  - In premedullary cistern, course between posterior inferior cerebellar artery and vertebral artery
- Rootlets fuse into hypoglossal nerve (2-4 trunks) just as it exits skull base through hypoglossal canal
- Hypoglossal filaments may merge with vagal fibers
- Total length of cisternal segment ranges from 8-15 mm, mean width from 0.3-0.6 mm

Skull Base Segment

- Hypoglossal nerve exits occipital bone via **hypoglossal canal**, surrounded by venous plexus
  - Canal is in occipital bone caudal to jugular foramen
    - "Empties" into medial nasopharyngeal carotid space
    - Osseous septa may bisect hypoglossal canal
  - Mean length of hypoglossal canal reported to range from 9.5-16.0 mm, mean width from 1.3-3.0 mm

Extracranial Segment

- **Carotid space component of CNXII**
  - Hypoglossal canal "empties" into medial nasopharyngeal carotid space
  - Hypoglossal nerve immediately gives off **dural branches** after exiting hypoglossal canal
  - Descends in posterior carotid space, closely apposed with CNX
  - Exits carotid space anteriorly between jugular vein and internal carotid artery, crosses lateral surface of external carotid artery at inferior margin of posterior belly of digastric muscle
- **Transspatial component of CNXII**
  - From carotid space, nerve runs anteroinferiorly toward hyoid bone, lateral to carotid bifurcation
  - At level of occipital artery base, nerve turns anterior, continuing as muscular branch below posterior belly of digastric muscle, medial to submandibular gland
  - Gives off superior root of ansa cervicalis from horizontal segment of nerve to anastomose with lower root
- Distal branches of imaging importance
  - **Muscular branch** travels on lateral margin of hyoglossus muscle in posterior sublingual space close to lingual artery, medial to mylohyoid muscle
    - Innervates extrinsic (styloglossus, hyoglossus, and genioglossus) and intrinsic tongue muscles
    - **Geniohyoid** innervated by **C1** spinal nerve
  - **Ansa cervicalis**: Formed from superior and inferior (C1-C3 spinal nerves) roots
    - Innervates infrahyoid strap muscles (sternothyroid, sternohyoid, omohyoid)
- Direct CT or MR identification of CNXII in these spaces is difficult, position is inferred by adjacent anatomical structures

ANATOMY IMAGING ISSUES

Imaging Recommendations

- MR is preferred imaging study
  - Best for brainstem, cisterns, skull base, and suprahyoid neck
  - Should include heavily T2-weighted sequence
- CECT with bone algorithm of skull base for skull base and suprahyoid neck (cover from orbital roof to below hyoid)

Imaging Sweet Spots

- CT or MR evaluation requires entire coverage of nerve from brainstem to hyoid bone
- Asymmetric appearance of tongue is clue to denervation
  - Acute/subacute: Denervated hemitongue may show T1 hypointensity and T2 hyperintensity and contrast enhancement
  - Chronic: Tongue atrophy (fatty infiltration and volume loss) on CT or MR; infrahyoid strap muscle atrophy

Imaging Pitfalls

- Denervated hemitongue may appear enlarged due to edema (acute) or flaccidity (chronic); may mimic infiltrative tongue mass
- Not imaging hyoid bone will result in missed diagnoses

CLINICAL IMPLICATIONS

Clinical Importance

- Unilateral lesion causes tongue protrusion to "side of lesion"
- Nearly 50% of CNXII neuropathies are from neoplastic processes, mostly malignant

CNXII (Hypoglossal Nerve)

GRAPHICS, INTRACRANIAL

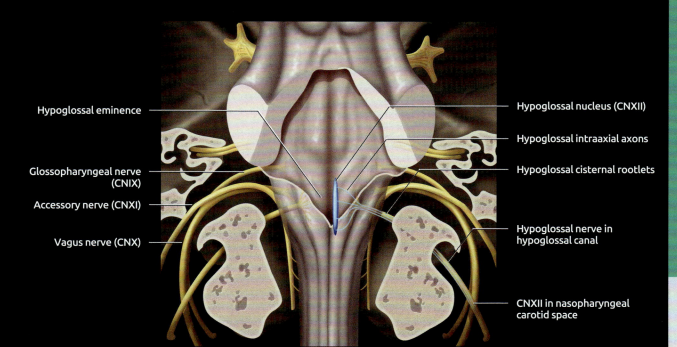

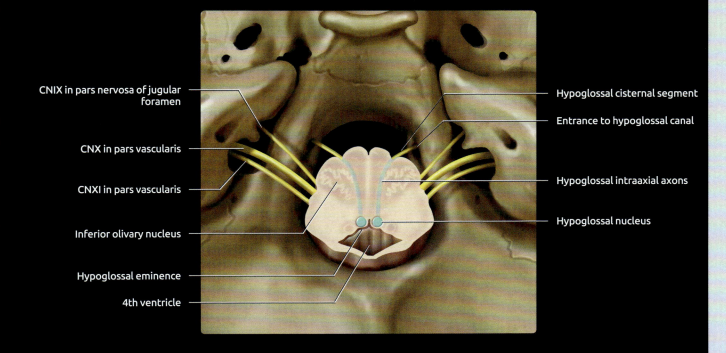

(Top) Graphic of lower brainstem seen from behind illustrates key features of the proximal hypoglossal nerve. Notice the hypoglossal nucleus in the dorsal paramedian medulla feeding intraaxial axons that exit the preolivary sulcus into the anterolateral basal cistern. Cisternal rootlets fuse into the hypoglossal nerve that traverses the skull base through the hypoglossal canal. Exiting the hypoglossal canal, CNXII immediately enters the nasopharyngeal carotid space. **(Bottom)** Axial graphic through lower medulla shows the hypoglossal nucleus feeding intraaxial axons that dive ventrally to curve around the inferior olivary nucleus to exit the medulla ventrolaterally via the preolivary sulcus. Note that the hypoglossal nucleus gives the floor of the 4th ventricle an arch (hypoglossal eminence/trigone). The cisternal rootlets combine in the hypoglossal canal to become the hypoglossal nerve (CNXII). Note the hypoglossal canal is anterior and inferior to the jugular foramen.

CNXII (Hypoglossal Nerve)

GRAPHIC, EXTRACRANIAL

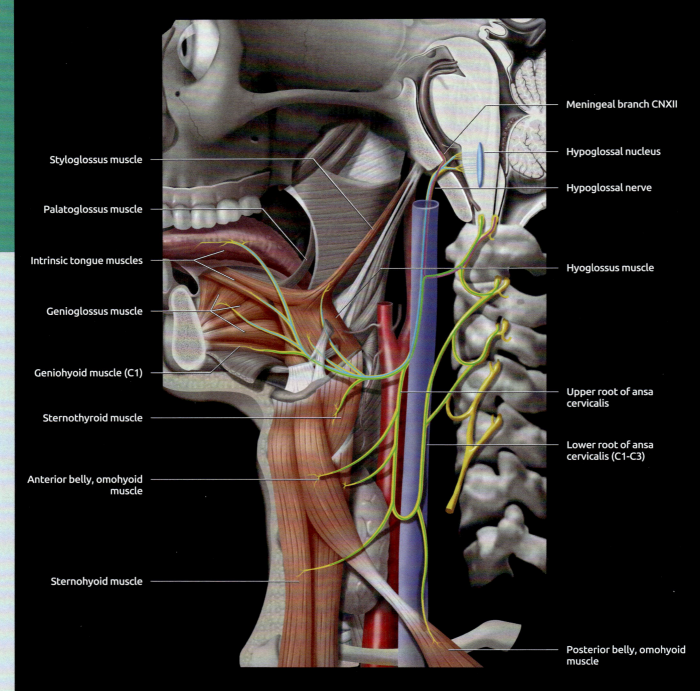

Lateral graphic depicts the entire course of the hypoglossal nerve. The nerve originates in the hypoglossal nucleus in the floor of the 4th ventricle. As CNXII exits the skull base, it immediately enters the nasopharyngeal carotid space just medial to the internal carotid artery. It travels inferiorly in the carotid space to exit anteriorly between the carotid artery and the internal jugular vein. CNXII supplies motor innervation to intrinsic and extrinsic (styloglossus, hyoglossus, genioglossus) tongue muscles. C1 spinal nerve supplies motor to the geniohyoid muscle. Ansa cervicalis (C1-C3 spinal nerves) supplies motor innervation to the infrahyoid strap muscles, including sternothyroid, sternohyoid, and omohyoid muscles. Also note the meningeal sensory branch from C1 following CNXII retrograde to supply clival meninges.

CNXII (Hypoglossal Nerve)

AXIAL BONE CT AND T2 MR

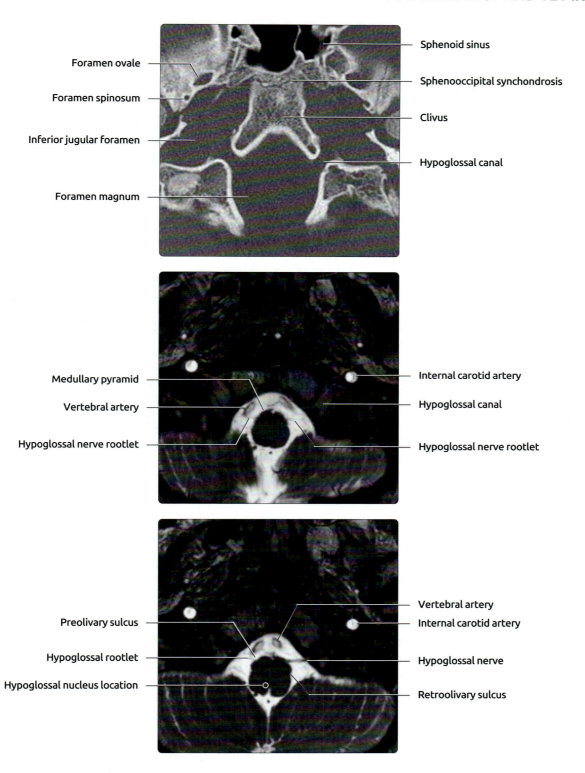

(Top) Axial bone CT at the level of the hypoglossal canal is shown. Notice the margins of the hypoglossal canals are well corticated. (Middle) First of 2 axial T2 MR images through the lower medulla demonstrates cisternal segment of hypoglossal nerves. Anatomy of cisternal segment is variable, but usually, multiple rootlets emerge from the preolivary sulcus and merge into 2 trunks, which penetrate the dura to enter the hypoglossal canal. The trunks abut or pass near the vertebral arteries in the basal cisterns. (Bottom) Hypoglossal nerves emerge from the medulla in the preolivary sulcus between the olive and pyramid. Cisternal segment of the patient's left hypoglossal nerve is seen as a thick, discrete trunk entering the hypoglossal canal. The right hypoglossal nerve consists of multiple small rootlets.

CNXII (Hypoglossal Nerve)

CORONAL BONE CT

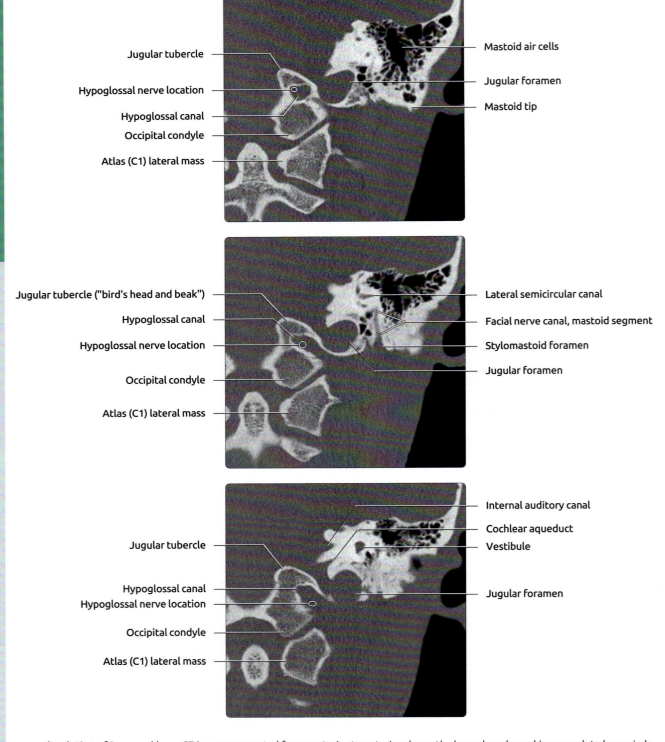

(Top) First of 3 coronal bone CT images presented from posterior to anterior shows the hypoglossal canal is a complete bony circle, indicating that the image is at the level of the entry into the canal. The location of CNXII is in the upper medial quadrant within the hypoglossal canal. *(Middle)* In this image of the mid hypoglossal canal, the surrounding bone appears as a "bird's head and beak" with the head and beak made up of the jugular tubercle. The jugular foramen is directly lateral to the hypoglossal canal. *(Bottom)* At the level of the distal hypoglossal canal, the hypoglossal nerve leaves the skull base to emerge inferiorly into the nasopharyngeal carotid space. Notice the lateral jugular foramen also empties its contents into the carotid space, including the jugular vein and cranial nerves IX, X, and XI.

CNXII (Hypoglossal Nerve)

CORONAL T1 C+ MR

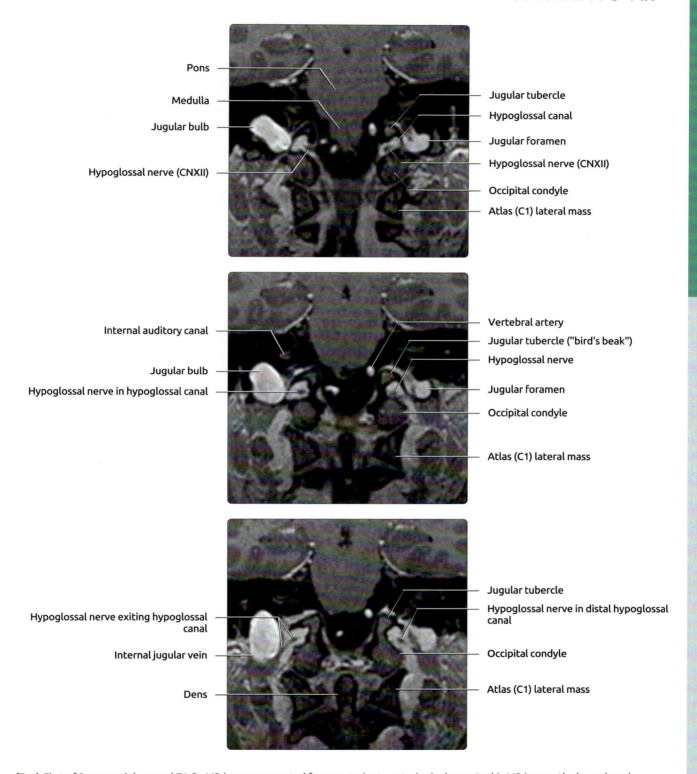

(Top) First of 3 sequential coronal T1 C+ MR images presented from posterior to anterior is shown. In this MR image, the hypoglossal nerve is seen entering the proximal hypoglossal canal. The hypointense hypoglossal nerve is surrounded by the strongly enhancing venous plexus and is therefore easily seen on thin-section enhanced MR. The hypoglossal canal also carries a branch of the ascending pharyngeal artery. *(Middle)* In this coronal MR of the mid hypoglossal canal, the low-signal hypoglossal nerve is visible surrounded by the enhancing venous plexus just beneath the "bird's beak" of the jugular tubercle. *(Bottom)* In this coronal image through the distal hypoglossal canal, the hypoglossal nerves can be seen exiting inferolaterally into the nasopharyngeal carotid space. Notice also the internal jugular vein exiting inferiorly on the patient's right into this same nasopharyngeal carotid space.

SECTION 3
Orbit

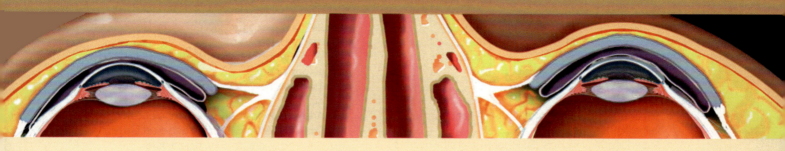

Orbit Overview	**206**
Bony Orbit and Foramina	**216**
Optic Nerve/Sheath Complex	**220**
Globe	**224**
Cavernous Sinus	**226**

Orbit Overview

TERMINOLOGY

Abbreviations

- Cranial nerves
  - Optic nerve (CNII)
  - Oculomotor nerve (CNIII)
  - Trochlear nerve (CNIV)
  - Trigeminal nerve (CNV)
    - Branches (V1, V2, and V3)
  - Abducens nerve (CNVI)
- Orbital structures
  - Superior ophthalmic veins (SOV), inferior ophthalmic veins (IOV)
  - Superior orbital fissures (SOF), inferior orbital fissures (IOF)
  - Extraocular muscles (EOM)
  - Ophthalmic artery (OphA)

IMAGING ANATOMY

Overview

- Each orbit consists of conical-shaped bony cavity or socket (bony orbit) and its internal contents that extend from eyelids anteriorly to orbital apex posteriorly
- Orbit contains globe and intraorbital optic nerve
- Also contains lacrimal gland, EOM, various nerves (motor, autonomic, and sensory), fat, arteries, and veins

Extent

- Margins of orbit are largely determined by bony orbital walls arranged in cone or pyramid shape
- Ventral aspect of orbit (or base) is formed by orbital rim peripherally and soft tissues centrally; anterior soft tissue margin is defined by orbital septum
- 7 different bones that contribute to bony orbit
  - Roof of orbit: Sphenoid and frontal bones
  - Medial wall: Formed from lesser wing of sphenoid bone, ethmoid bone, lacrimal bone, and frontal process of maxilla
  - Orbital floor: Formed from sphenoid bone, orbital process of palatine bone, and orbital process of maxillary bone
  - Lateral wall: Greater wing of sphenoid bone near apex and frontal and zygomatic bones anteriorly toward face
- Size and extent of orbit is influenced by age, race, and sex of individual
  - Height of orbit measured anteriorly at rim is ~ 3.5 cm
  - Width of orbit is ~ 4.0 cm
  - Medial orbital wall measures ~ 4.5 cm from rim to apex
  - Lateral wall is shorter than medial wall, measuring ~ 3.5 cm
  - Volume of each orbit is variable but ranges from 16-30 cubic centimeters

Anatomy Relationships

- Orbit is superior to maxillary sinus and lateral to ethmoid sinus
- Roof of orbit forms floor of anterior cranial fossa
- Apex of orbit is at transition zone between anterior skull base and central skull base

Internal Contents

- **Globe**
  - Occupies 1/3 of volume of orbit
  - Spherical organ of vision, functions in refraction of light so that photons are focused on retina
  - Retina is specialized layer of globe that contains neurons that are sensitive to light
  - Globe is mobile and is maneuvered by EOMs
- **CNII (optic nerve)**
  - Transmits nerve impulses from retina to visual center of brain
  - Arises from posterior margin of globe at optic disc
  - Contains nerve fibers from nerve cells in retina
  - Covered by pia, arachnoid, and dura
- **EOMs**
  - Responsible for movement of eye
    - Lateral and medial rectus are pure abductor and pure adductor, respectively
    - Other EOMs have component of torsion that must be coordinated with other EOM
  - Most EOMs arise from annulus of Zinn and insert upon globe
  - Inferior rectus originates from anterior floor of orbit, not annulus
  - Levator palpebrae superioris originates from annulus but inserts on upper eye lid, not globe
  - Have similar density on CT and similar signal on MR as other skeletal muscle
  - EOMs demonstrate prominent gadolinium enhancement on MR
  - **Superior rectus**
    - Located upper aspect of orbit, inferior to levator palpebrae muscle
    - Originates from superior rim of annulus
    - Primary function is upward gaze, rotation of superior margin globe posteriorly
    - Innervated by CNIII (oculomotor)
  - **Medial rectus**
    - Located along medial orbital wall, just lateral to lamina papyracea
    - Originates along medial aspect of annulus and attaches to medial margin of globe
    - Medial rectus rotates medial margin of globe posteriorly allowing for medial gaze
    - Innervated by CNIII (oculomotor)
  - **Lateral rectus**
    - Located along lateral orbital wall
    - Originates along lateral margin of of annulus and attaches to lateral margin of globe
    - Contraction results in posterior rotation of lateral margin of globe for lateral gaze
    - Innervated by abducens CNVI (abducens)
  - **Inferior rectus**
    - Located along floor of orbit
    - Originates along inferior margin of annulus and attaches to inferior margin of globe
    - Rotates inferior margin of globe posteriorly for downward gaze
    - Innervated by CNIII (oculomotor)
  - **Superior oblique**

Orbit Overview

- Origin at medial margin of annulus of Zinn
- Passes through trochlea at superomedial rim of bony orbit
- Inserts posterolaterally on sclera superiorly
- Rotates the globe inferiorly
- Innervated by CNIV (trochlear nerve)
  - ○ **Inferior oblique**
    - Origin at anteroinferior orbital rim
    - Insertion posterolaterally on sclera inferiorly
    - Rotates eye superiorly
    - Innervated by CNIII (oculomotor)
  - ○ **Levator palpebrae superioris**
    - Unlike other EOMs, does not attach to or move globe
    - Origin at annulus of Zinn
    - Courses above superior rectus, divides in 2
    - Superior aponeurosis insertion at upper eyelid
    - Inferior Müller insertion at tarsal plate
    - Elevates upper eye lid
    - Innervated by CNIII (oculomotor)
- **Orbital fat**
  - ○ Occupies ~ 50% of orbital volume
  - ○ Functions to stabilize globe, cushion globe, and facilitates movement of intraorbital structures
  - ○ Fat can be divided into intraconal (behind globe and within conical boundaries of rectus muscles) and extraconal components
  - ○ Normal orbital fat density on CT and fat signal on MR scans allow for delineation of most important intraorbital structures
- **Intraorbital nerves**
  - ○ CNII: Optic nerve represents collection of axons derived from retinal ganglion cells that transmit visual information from retina to brain
  - ○ CNIII: Motor to medial, superior and inferior recti, and levator palpebrae; parasympathetic motor to iris
  - ○ CNIV: Motor to superior oblique
  - ○ CNVI: Motor to lateral rectus
  - ○ CNV: Sensory from orbit and eyelids (V1)
- **OphA**
  - ○ Major arterial supply of orbit
  - ○ 1st intradural branch of internal carotid artery (ICA); measures 0.7- to 1.5-mm diameter at origin
  - ○ Typical origin is just above distal dural ring
  - ○ **Variant origin**: 1-2% originate from middle meningeal artery; < 1% originate from cavernous ICA
  - ○ OphA courses along inferolateral optic canal, piercing proximal dural sleeve of CNII laterally
  - ○ Intraorbital course
    - At apex (1st segment), passes along inferolateral aspect on CNII
      - □ Then passes medially (becoming 2nd segment), most often **over** CNII
      - □ Finally extends forward (3rd segment) in medial aspect of orbit, medial to CNII
  - ○ OphA branches can be classified into ocular, orbital, extraorbital, and dural branches
  - ○ **Ocular** branches include **central retinal artery**, lateral posterior ciliary artery, and medial posterior ciliary artery
    - These arteries arise near junction of 1st and 2nd segments of intraorbital OphA

- ○ **Orbital** branches include muscular and lacrimal
- ○ **Extraorbital**: Supraorbital, anterior and posterior ethmoidal, palpebral, dorsal nasal, and supratrochlear branches
- ○ **Dural**: Recurrent branches of OphA, 1 superficial and other deep, course back through SOF and supply dura of cavernous sinus
- **Ophthalmic veins**
  - ○ **SOV**
    - Formed by confluence of angular vein and supraorbital vein at medial margin of supraorbital rim
    - Passes by trochlea and medial to superior oblique muscle, crosses anterior portion of CNII, and passes posteriorly along superolateral border of CNII
    - Extends through SOF before draining into cavernous sinus
  - ○ **IOV**
    - Smaller and more variable than SOV Located adjacent to inferior rectus
    - Located just superior to inferior rectus
    - Usually anastomoses with SOV but may drain into cavernous sinus directly or drain through IOF into pterygoid venous plexus
- **Connective Tissue and Supporting Structures**
  - ○ **Periorbita**
    - a.k.a .orbital periosteum or orbital fascia
    - Dense connective tissue membrane that covers inner margins of bones of orbit, serves as attachment for muscles, tendons, and ligaments
    - Continuous anteriorly with periosteal covering of facial bones
    - Continuous posteriorly through orbital foramina and fissures with periosteal layer of dura mater
    - Posteriorly, periorbita thickens to form fibrous ring that encircles optic nerve canal and portions of SOF, annulus of Zinn
    - Attached loosely to underlying bone except at orbital margins, along sutures, and at edges of fissures and foramina
  - ○ **Annulus of Zinn**
    - Annulus is tendinous ring formed by thickened periorbita at apex of orbit
    - Ring passes over optic nerve canal and partially encircles medial aspect of SOF
    - 4 rectus and superior oblique muscles and levator palpebrae superioris arise from annulus
    - CNIII (upper and lower divisions of oculomotor), CNVI (abducens), and nasociliary branch of ophthalmic division of CNV (trigeminal) all enter apex of orbit through annulus of Zinn
    - CNII (optic nerve) also passes through annulus as nerve passes through optic canal
  - ○ **Tenon capsule**
    - Dense elastic and vascular fibrous connective tissue that surrounds globe and separates globe from retrobulbar fat
    - Extends from insertion site of optic nerve to margins of cornea
    - Capsule separated from episclera by loose potential space providing smooth inner surface; allows for ocular motility

Orbit Overview

- – EOMs must penetrate capsule before inserting on globe
- o **Orbital septum**
  - – Thin anterior band of connective tissue arising from orbital periosteum of orbital rim
  - – Inserts into levator palpebrae aponeurosis and superior tarsal plate (upper lid) and inferior tarsal plate (lower lid)
  - – Essentially separates orbital contents from lid structures
  - – Location is inferred on routine CT and MR scans
  - – High-resolution MR scans can occasionally demonstrate septum
- o **Tarsal plates**
  - – Dense connective tissue that adds rigidity to upper and lower eyelids
  - – Contain large sebaceous glands (meibomian glands)
- o **Lateral canthal ligament**
  - – Anchors tarsal plates of both lids to zygomatic bone laterally at Whitnall tubercle
- o **Medial canthal ligament**
  - – Medial tendinous attachment of orbicularis oculi and upper and lower tarsal plates
  - – Anchor is primarily at anterior lacrimal crest, located on frontal process of maxilla
- o **Whitnall ligament (superior transverse ligament)**
  - – Primary suspensory support for upper lid found at intersection of muscular and aponeurotic portions of levator palpebrae
  - – Extends from trochlea medially to lateral orbit wall
  - – Attaches to levator aponeurosis and superior rectus muscle as well as conjunctiva and Tenon capsule
  - – May function as fulcrum for levator palpebrae superioris
  - – Passes between orbital and palpebral lobes of lacrimal gland
- o **Intermuscular transverse ligament (ITL)**
  - – Also originates from trochlea and inserts into lateral orbital wall on deeper part of Whitnall ligament
  - – ITL passes only behind palpebral lobe
- o **Lockwood ligament**
  - – Thickened lower part of Tenon capsule
  - – Serves as suspensory ligament for globe
  - – Blends with lateral canthus and lateral check ligament laterally and attaches to lacrimal crest medially
- **Müller muscle**
  - o Sympathetically innervated smooth muscle that functions as upper eyelid retractor
  - o Extends from inferior aspect of levator palpebra muscle to superior edge of tarsal plate, posterior to levator aponeurosis
- **Nasolacrimal apparatus**
  - o **Lacrimal gland**
    - – Orbital lobe: Larger, lies in bony fossa at anterior aspect of superotemporal orbit
    - – Palpebral lobe: Smaller, lies inferiorly, separated by levator aponeurosis
  - o Drainage via puncta at medial lower lids → canaliculi → lacrimal sac → nasolacrimal duct

ANATOMY IMAGING ISSUES

Questions

- Approach to orbital lesions
  - o Localize to region and involved structures
    - – Globe: Intraocular vs. transscleral
    - – Optic nerve vs. nerve-sheath complex
    - – Intraconal vs. conal vs. extraconal orbit
    - – Lacrimal gland: Unilateral vs. bilateral (systemic)
    - – Isolated vs. multifocal vs. transspatial process
    - – Intracranial: Direct extension vs. secondary
  - o Assess CT, MR, &/or ultrasound characteristics
    - – Solid or cystic; heterogeneity
    - – Fluid, fat, blood, or soft tissue
    - – Bony remodeling vs. destruction
    - – Well defined vs. infiltrative
    - – Degree and homogeneity of enhancement

Imaging Recommendations

- CT
  - o Axial + coronal planes; thin sections (≤ 2 mm)
  - o Multislice isovoxel acquisition with MPR
  - o Soft tissue algorithm; bone in at least 1 plane
  - o Excellent evaluation of orbit aided by natural contrast between fat, bone, air, and soft tissues
  - o Easily detects calcifications
  - o Noncontrast CT alone for thyroid orbitopathy
  - o Bone windows for evaluation of fracture, hyperostosis, or permeative changes
- MR
  - o Optimal soft tissue contrast for globe, optic nerve, orbital structures, and intracranial findings
  - o Stronger gradients, faster sequences, surface coils, fat suppression + gadolinium improve image quality
  - o Axial: Above orbital roof to orbital floor
  - o Coronal: Back of pons through globe
  - o Thin section (3-4 mm); small FOV (12-16 cm)
  - o T1 precontrast (axial + coronal)
  - o STIR or T2 FSE fat saturation (axial + coronal)
  - o T1 C+ with fat saturation (axial + coronal)
- Ultrasound
  - o 1st-line modality for intraocular lesions
  - o Noninvasive, readily available
- CT and MR are complementary, especially with complex lesions

Orbit Overview

BONY ORBIT

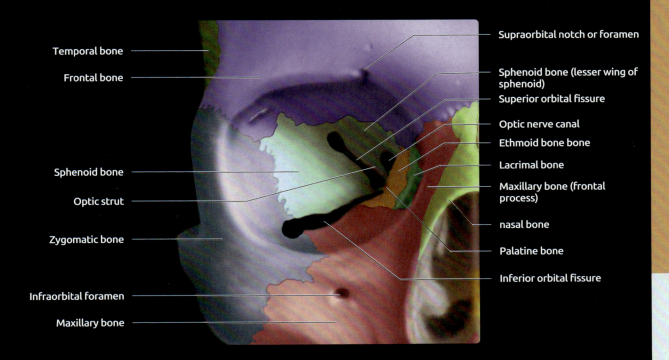

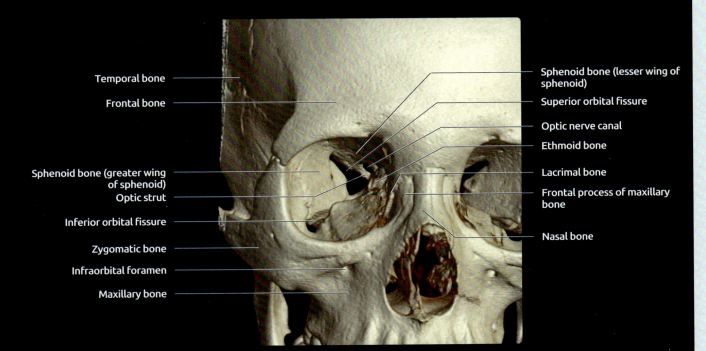

(Top) Frontal graphic shows the bones of the right orbit. A total of 7 embryologically distinct bones contribute to the bony orbit (lacrimal, ethmoid, palatine, maxillary, zygomatic, sphenoid, and frontal bones). The sphenoid bone has greater and lesser sphenoid wings. The complex orbital fissures and optic canal at the apex are formed largely by the wings of the sphenoid bone and associated relationships. Notice that the optic canal has the lesser wing of sphenoid and ethmoid bone components. **(Bottom)** Oblique frontal projection through the right orbit demonstrates the 3D characteristics of the cone-shaped bony confines of the orbit and illustrates several of the important foramina and fissures. Notice that the optic canal is separated from the superior orbital fissure by the optic strut.

Orbit Overview

GRAPHIC AND AXIAL STIR MR

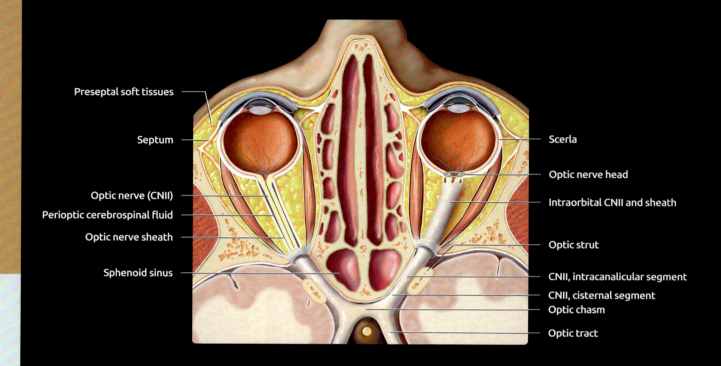

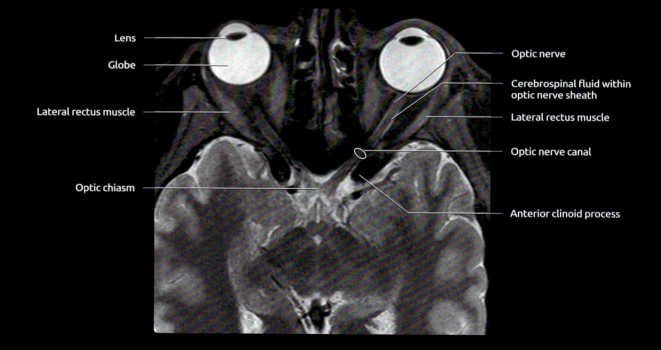

(Top) Axial graphic shows intraorbital and intracranial segments of CNII. The extraaxial optic pathways can be segmented (posterior to anterior) into the optic tract, optic chiasm, cisternal nerve, intracanalicular nerve, and intraorbital nerve. The optic sheath is a dural reflection that is contiguous with intracranial dura mater. Optic glioma, optic melanoma, and retinoblastoma may all follow the orbital segment of the optic nerve to reach intracranial structures. (Bottom) Axial STIR MR is shown through the level of the optic nerves. In this sequence, the fat is suppressed so that all fat is hypointense. Fluid signal is hyperintense. Muscle is intermediate in signal.

Orbit Overview

GRAPHICS AND OBLIQUE SAGITTAL T1 MR

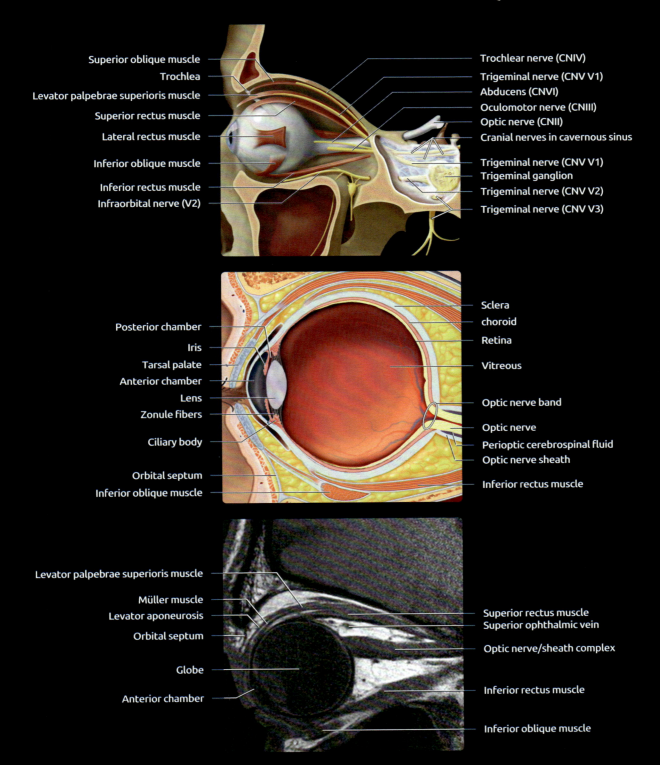

(Top) Lateral graphic of the left orbit is shown. Intricate mechanics and innervation of the extraocular muscles provide for complementary and complex control of eye motion. CNII-VI enter the orbit via the complex foramina. (Middle) Sagittal graphic reveals an anterior segment composed of anterior and posterior chambers, which are contiguous through the pupil. The choroid and iris are anterior extensions of the uveal tract. The posterior segment is filled by the vitreous chamber. The retina and sclera are contiguous with the optic nerve and sheath, respectively, at the nerve head. (Bottom) Oblique sagittal T1 MR at the mid orbit shows the intimate relationship between the superior oblique and levator palpebrae superioris muscles. The distinct division of the Müller muscle and levator aponeurosis anteriorly is evident. Inferiorly, the inferior oblique muscle is seen in oblique cross section, distinct from the inferior rectus muscle.

Orbit Overview

EXTRAOCULAR MUSCLES

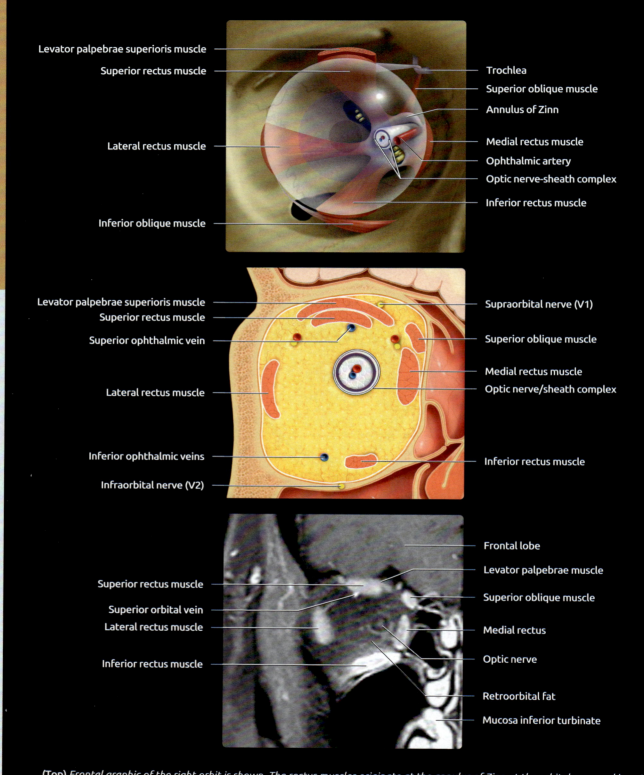

(Top) Frontal graphic of the right orbit is shown. The rectus muscles originate at the annulus of Zinn at the orbital apex and insert at the corneoscleral junction of the eye, forming a muscle cone. The superior oblique muscle courses through the trochlea, providing for the angled pulley motion of this muscle. The inferior oblique inserts at the inferolateral aspect of the eye. (Middle) Coronal graphic of the right orbit is shown. The optic nerve-sheath complex courses in the intraconal space behind the eye. Branches of CNIII-VI, branches of the ophthalmic artery, and ophthalmic veins are located in the intraconal and extraconal spaces. (Bottom) T1 C+ FS MR demonstrates normal enhancement of the extraocular muscles. The optic nerve itself should not demonstrate intrinsic enhancement. Normally, the optic nerve sheath dura can demonstrate subtle enhancement. Beware of fat saturation artifacts in the orbit related to air in the maxillary and ethmoid sinus. In this case, there is subtle increased signal (incomplete fat saturation) in the fat inferiorly and medially.

Orbit Overview

CORONAL T1 MR

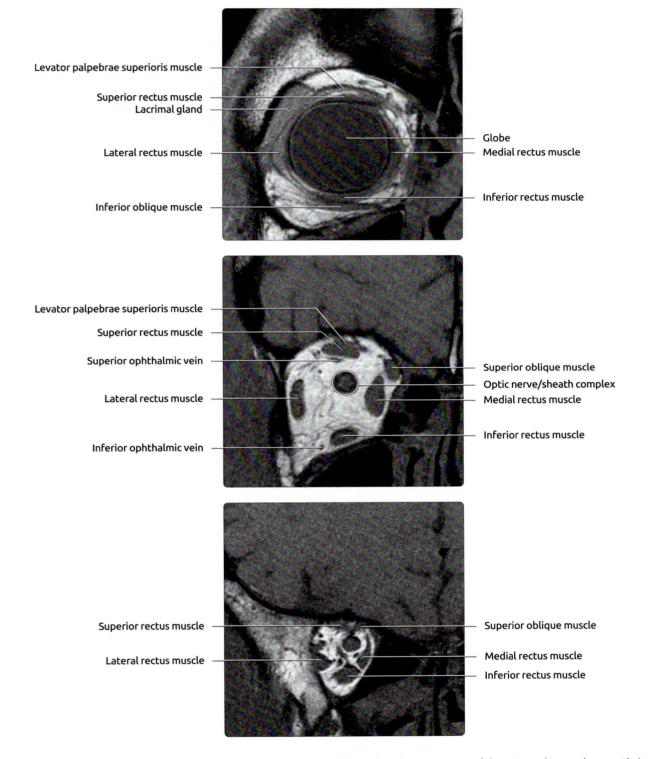

(Top) Coronal T1 MR at the level of the globe shows the flattened and thinned tendinous contours of the extraocular muscles near their insertions. The inferior oblique muscle is evident at this level. The lacrimal gland is isointense and located in the anterior aspect of the superotemporal extraconal space. (Middle) Coronal T1 MR in the mid orbit shows the muscle cone formed by the extraocular muscles with the nerve-sheath complex centrally in the intraconal space. Complex and variable branches of the ophthalmic artery are seen as small flow voids within the intraconal and extraconal fat. (Bottom) Coronal T1 MR at the orbital apex shows the close proximity of the extraocular muscles, nerve-sheath complex, and ophthalmic vessels.

Orbit Overview

AXIAL ANATOMY CECT

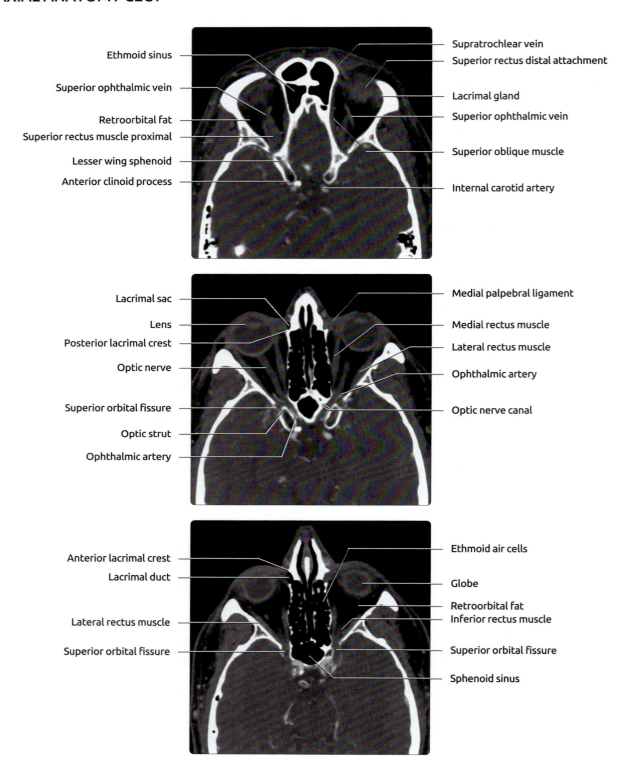

(Top) Axial CECT through the superior aspect of the orbit demonstrates partial inclusion of the superior rectus muscle (and levator palpebrae muscle) in the plane as well as the superior ophthalmic vein that is quite variable in size and can be asymmetric normally. Anterior tributaries to the superior ophthalmic vein include the supraorbital and supratrochlear veins. The superior oblique is seen medially within the superior orbit, en route to the trochlea. Notice extensive retroorbital fat. (Middle) Axial CECT through the mid orbit includes most of the intraorbital optic nerve on the left side of the image. The proximal ophthalmic arteries are seen within the optic nerve canals bilaterally, traveling just below the optic nerves. The optic strut is part of the lesser wing of the sphenoid that separates the optic nerve canal from the superior orbital fissure. (Bottom) Axial CECT is shown through the inferior aspect of the orbit. The proximal inferior rectus muscles are seen partially. The inferior ophthalmic veins are less consistent and often consist of groups of small veins. The superior orbital fissure is more conspicuous at this level.

Orbit Overview

ANATOMIC-PATHOLOGIC CORRELATION

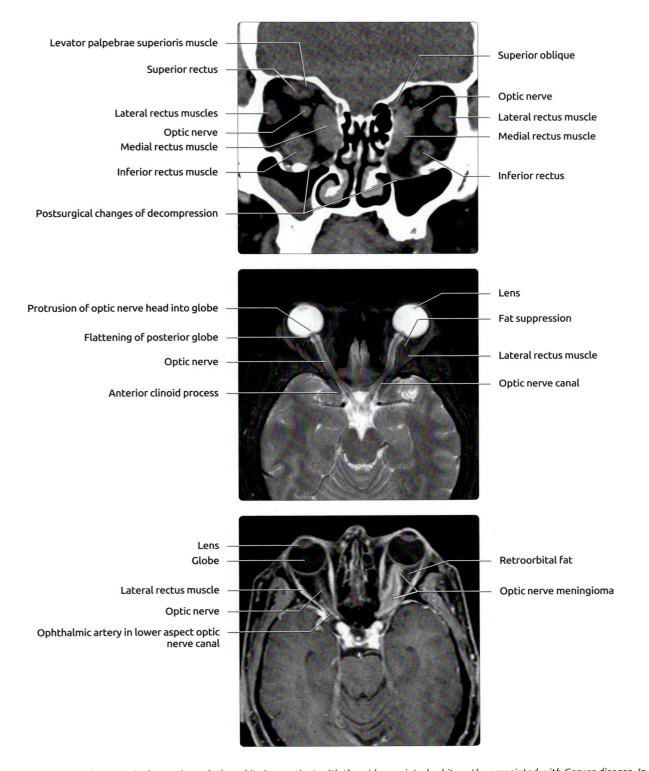

(Top) Coronal CT scan is shown through the orbits in a patient with thyroid-associated orbitopathy associated with Graves disease. In this disease, autoimmune response leads to inflammation and enlargement of the extraocular muscles. The muscles are involved bilaterally but asymmetrically. The mass effect from extraocular muscle enlargement can create considerable proptosis and lead to optic nerve compression. This patient has undergone decompression surgery that essentially expands the bony volume of the orbits inferomedially. (Middle) Axial STIR MR of papilledema in the setting of idiopathic intracranial hypertension shows excellent fat suppression and nice delineation of the optic nerves. There is mild prominence of the optic nerve sheaths bilaterally and prominent swelling of the optic nerve head, which protrudes into the posterior globe. (Bottom) Axial fat-suppressed MR through the orbit demonstrates a typical optic nerve meningioma of the left optic nerve. The meningioma arises from the dura along the optic nerve. In this case, the enhancing meningioma extends the entire length of the intraorbital optic nerve.

Bony Orbit and Foramina

TERMINOLOGY

Abbreviations

- **Bones, foramina, and fissures**
  - Greater wing of sphenoid (GWS)
  - Lesser wing of sphenoid (LWS)
  - Optic canal (OpC)
  - Superior orbital fissure (SOF)
  - Inferior orbital fissure (IOF)
  - Foramen rotundum (FR)
  - Foramen ovale (FO)
  - Vidian canal (VC)
  - Pterygopalatine fossa (PPF)
- **Cranial nerves**
  - Optic nerve (CNII)
  - Oculomotor nerve (CNIII)
  - Trochlear nerve (CNIV)
  - Trigeminal nerve (CNV)
    - Ophthalmic branch (V1)
    - Maxillary branch (V2)
    - Mandibular branch (V3)
  - Abducens nerve (CNVI)
- **Vessels**
  - Ophthalmic artery (OA)
  - Superior ophthalmic vein (SOV)
  - Inferior ophthalmic vein (IOV)

Definitions

- MPR: 2D multiplanar reformations

GROSS ANATOMY

Bones of Orbit

- **Frontal bone**
  - Forms superior rim and anterior roof (orbital process)
- **Zygomatic bone**
  - Forms inferolateral rim, anterior portion of lateral wall (orbital process), anterolateral floor (maxillary process)
- **Maxillary bone**
  - Forms inferomedial rim (frontal process) and anterior portion of inferomedial wall (orbital surface)
- **Nasal bone**
  - Forms bridge of nose
  - Anteromedial to frontal process of maxillary bone
- **Ethmoid bone**
  - Forms midportion of medial wall
  - Very thin bone (lamina papyracea)
- **Lacrimal bone**
  - Forms anterior portion of medial wall, just posterior to frontal process of maxillary bone
  - Fossa for lacrimal sac
- **Sphenoid bone**
  - Forms posterior portion of lateral wall (GWS) and posterior portion of medial roof (LWS)
  - Complex contours between GWS and LWS create elaborate apical fissures
- **Palatine bone**
  - Forms small portion of inferomedial wall posteriorly
  - Located between orbital portions of ethmoid and maxillary bones

IMAGING ANATOMY

Anatomy Relationships

- **Major foramina**
  - **OpC**
    - Formed completely by LWS
    - Separated from SOF by optic strut
  - **SOF**
    - Formed by LWS medially, GWS laterally
    - Primary connection between orbit and intracranial compartment
  - **IOF**
    - Formed by GWS and zygomatic bone laterally, maxillary and ethmoid bones medially
    - Mostly contiguous with SOF, separated only at posterior aspect by short bony roof of FR
    - Anterior continuation of FR

Internal Contents

- **Contents of foramina**
  - **OpC**: CNII and OA
  - **SOF**: CNIII, IV, V (V1), and VI, SOV
  - **IOF**: CNV (V2), IOV
  - **FR**: CNV (V2)-proximal segment
  - **FO**: CNV (V3)
  - **Supraorbital foramen**: Supraorbital nerve (V1)
  - **Infraorbital foramen and canal**: Infraorbital nerve (V2)

ANATOMY IMAGING ISSUES

Questions

- **Pathways of orbit-sinus disease spread**
  - Orbit → intracranial
    - SOF and IOF: Common pathway; extends into cavernous sinus and Meckel cave, involves CNIII-VI
    - OpC: Involves CNII, dura
  - Orbit → deep face
    - SOF and IOF: Communicate with PPF
    - Infraorbital canal to PPF
    - Supraorbital canal to SOF (rare)
  - Sinus → orbit
    - Ethmoid: Common pathway via lamina papyracea
    - Frontal: Especially postobstructive process

Imaging Recommendations

- CT
  - Preferred for assessing bony structures and foramina
- MR
  - Preferred for evaluation of tumor and inflammation

Imaging Pitfalls

- Assessing foramina
  - OpC oriented obliquely
    - MPR orthogonal to long axis may be required to demonstrate intact canal
  - FR and VC often mistaken
    - FR superolateral to VC on coronals, shorter than VC
- Artifacts
  - Dental artifact troublesome on direct coronal images
    - Axial multislice source with coronal MPR preferred if dental amalgam present

Bony Orbit and Foramina

GRAPHICS

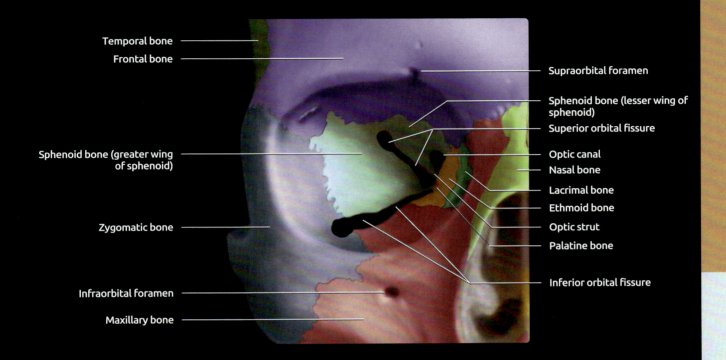

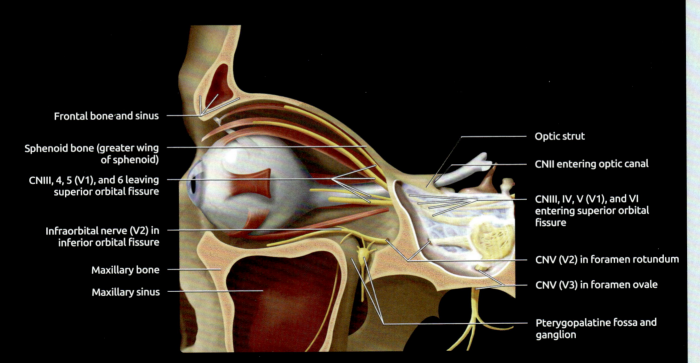

(Top) Frontal graphic of the bones of the right orbit is shown. A total of 7 embryologically distinct bones contribute to the bony orbit (lacrimal, ethmoid, palatine, maxillary, zygomatic, sphenoid, and frontal bones). The sphenoid bone has greater and lesser sphenoid wings. The complex orbital fissures and optic canal at the apex are formed largely by the wings of the sphenoid bone and associated relationships. Notice that the optic canal has lesser wing of sphenoid and ethmoid bone components. (Bottom) Lateral graphic of the left orbit is shown. The optic nerve (CNII) is relatively isolated in the optic canal, whereas the superior orbital fissure transmits CNIII, IV, V (V1), and VI as they course forward from the cavernous sinus and Meckel cave. The other branches of CNV also contribute to the complexity of the central skull base as they pass through their respective foramina.

Bony Orbit and Foramina

AXIAL BONE CT

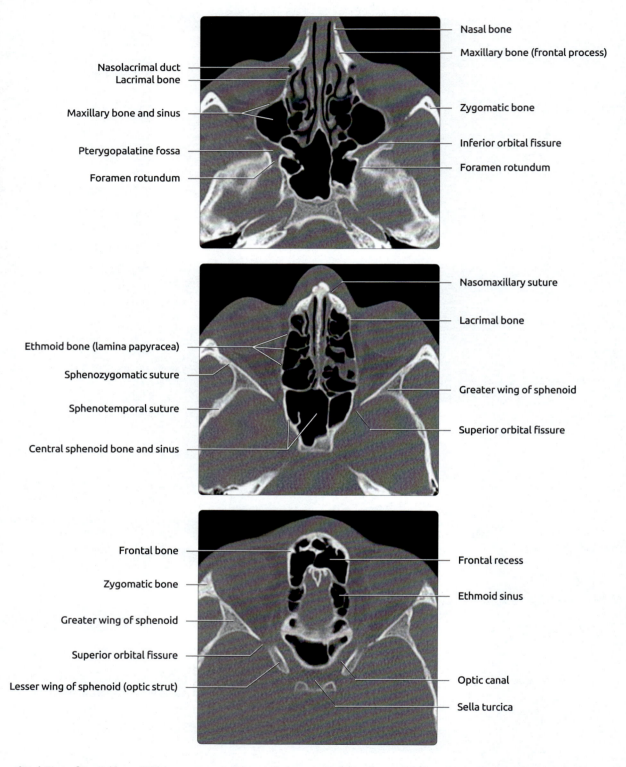

(Top) First of 3 axial bone CT images presented from inferior to superior is shown. The short, horizontally oriented foramen rotundum is seen at the posterior margin of the pterygopalatine fossa with the inferior orbital fissure extending anterolaterally in roughly the same plane. Anteriorly, relationships between the medial bony orbit and nasolacrimal structures are evident. (Middle) Image at the level of the midorbit is shown. The superior orbital fissure is seen as a gap at the orbital apex. The thin ethmoid bone forms the bulk of the medial orbital wall. (Bottom) Image at the level of the upper orbit is shown. The optic canals show characteristic angles as the nerves approach the chiasm, which is located above the sella. The superior orbital fissure is inferior and lateral to the optic canal, from which it is separated by the bony optic strut of the lesser wing of sphenoid. Sinus air space within the paramedian portions of the frontal bones is seen anteriorly.

Bony Orbit and Foramina

CORONAL BONE CT

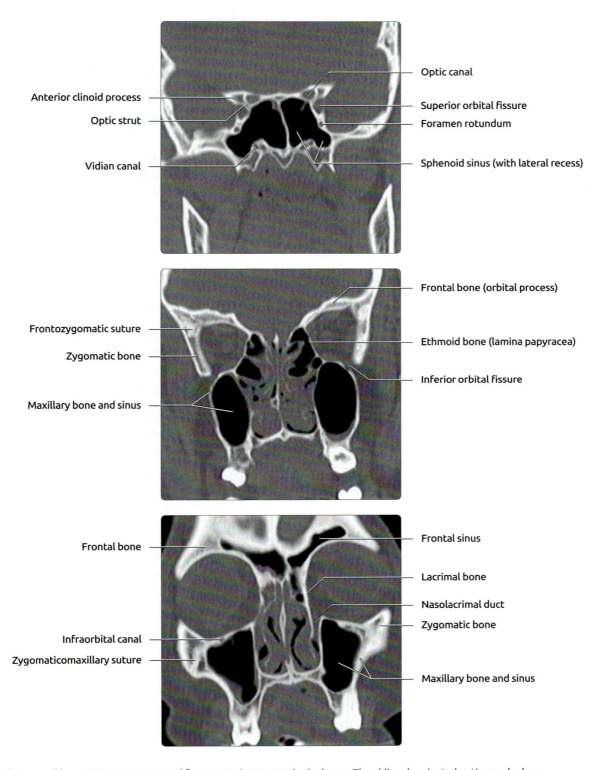

(Top) First of 3 coronal bone CT images presented from posterior to anterior is shown. The obliquely oriented optic canals show characteristic ovoid shape. The superior orbital fissure is located inferolaterally relative to the optic canal with the optic strut and attached clinoid process of the lesser wing of sphenoid separating the 2. Further inferolaterally is the foramen rotundum. The vidian canal is inferior and medial to rotundum, noting a prominent lateral recess of the sphenoid sinus separating the 2 foramina. (Middle) Image at the level of the midorbit is shown. Contours of the bony orbit, including integrity of the thin lamina papyracea of the medial wall, are best seen in this plane. (Bottom) Image at the level of the anterior orbit is shown. Contours of the bony orbital rim are best evaluated in the coronal plane. The nasolacrimal structures, as well as anterior sinonasal spaces, are well demonstrated.

Optic Nerve/Sheath Complex

TERMINOLOGY

Abbreviations

- Optic nerve-sheath complex (ONSC); optic nerve (CNII); ophthalmic artery (OA)

Definitions

- Optic nerve, chiasm, and tract: Afferent visual CNS pathways that extend from retina to visual nuclei of midbrain
- Optic sheath: Dural encasement of intraorbital CNII

GROSS ANATOMY

Optic Nerve

- Each optic nerve contains ~ 1 million axons that originate in ganglion cell layer of retina
- Nonmyelinated axons converge at optic nerve head, organize into fascicles, and then cross lamina cribrosa
- Axons then enter intraorbital segment and become myelinated from oligodendrocytes, **not** Schwann cells
- Anatomically CNS tract; differs from other cranial nerves

Optic Sheath

- All 3 membrane layers of meninges present, including pia, arachnoid, and dura mater
- Layers are separated by subarachnoid and subdural spaces
- Layers and spaces are contiguous with intracranial counterparts
  - Subarachnoid space contiguous with suprasellar cistern, transmits intracranial pressure

IMAGING ANATOMY

Extent

- **Optic nerve**
  - From optic nerve head to chiasm
  - Optic nerve segments
    - **Intraocular**: Within nerve head (1 mm)
    - **Orbital**: Nerve head to optic canal (30 mm)
    - **Canalicular**: Within optic canal (10 mm)
    - **Cisternal**: Optic canal to optic chiasm (10 mm)
- **Optic chiasm**
  - Within suprasellar cistern
    - Just anterior to pituitary stalk
  - Decussation of 1/2 of axons
    - Represents nasal portion of retina
    - Each 1/2 of visual field from each eye is afferent to contralateral visual cortex
- **Optic tract**
  - From optic chiasm to visual nuclei of midbrain

Anatomy Relationships

- Optic canal
  - Transmits ONSC and OA
  - Separated from superior orbital fissure by optic strut

Internal Contents

- **Vascular supply**
  - **OA**
    - 1st intradural branch of internal carotid artery
    - Major arterial supply to orbit

- Passes through optic canal in dural sheath
- Exits sheath laterally at orbital apex
  - **Central retinal artery**
    - Major branch of OA, supplies retina
    - Enters CNII ~ 1 cm posterior to nerve head
  - **Central retinal vein**
    - Accompanies central retinal artery
    - Drains directly into cavernous sinus

ANATOMY IMAGING ISSUES

Questions

- Orientation of optic nerve
  - **Intraorbital segment**
    - Posteromedial oblique sagittal long axis
    - Roughly horizontal plane
    - Position varies with eye movement
    - Nerve longer than distance from apex to globe, tends to form S-shaped contour
  - **Canalicular segment**
    - Oblique axis results in nonorthogonal "ovoid" cross-sectional appearance on coronal images
  - **Cisternal segment**
    - Angle changes relative to intraorbital segment as it courses posteriorly
    - Oblique sagittal long axis ~ 30° medially and superiorly

Imaging Recommendations

- Routine orbital approach appropriate for most nerve/sheath lesions
- Special circumstances
  - **Sheath mass** (possible meningioma)
    - May benefit from noncontrast CT to detect calcification
    - Additional brain imaging may be necessary to define extent of intraaxial tumor
  - **Inflammatory nerve work-up** (optic neuritis)
    - Requires concomitant brain imaging
    - High incidence of demyelinating disease

Imaging Approaches

- Dedicated optic nerve MR imaging
  - Axial sequences
    - 3.0 mm, anterior fossa floor through floor of orbit
  - Coronal sequences
    - 3.5-4.0 mm, back of pons through globe
  - T1WI, STIR, and T1 C+ with fat suppression
    - Both axial and coronal
    - May substitute axial T2WI FSE + fat suppression for STIR

Imaging Pitfalls

- Motion artifacts on MR
  - Common due to irrepressible eye motion
- Surface coils
  - Generally not adequate to visualize entire ONSC

CLINICAL IMPLICATIONS

Nerve vs. Sheath Lesions

- Important distinction, different DDx and prognoses
- Best with coronal STIR and T1 C+ with fat suppression

Optic Nerve/Sheath Complex

GRAPHICS

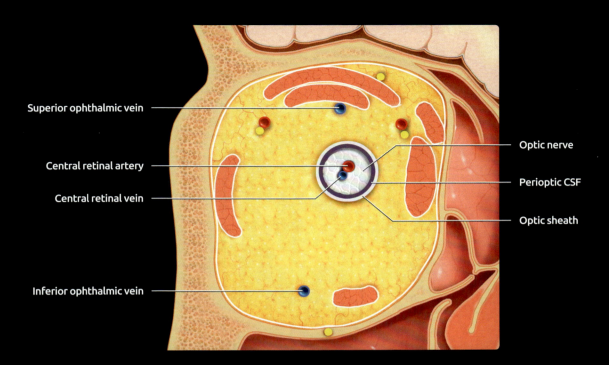

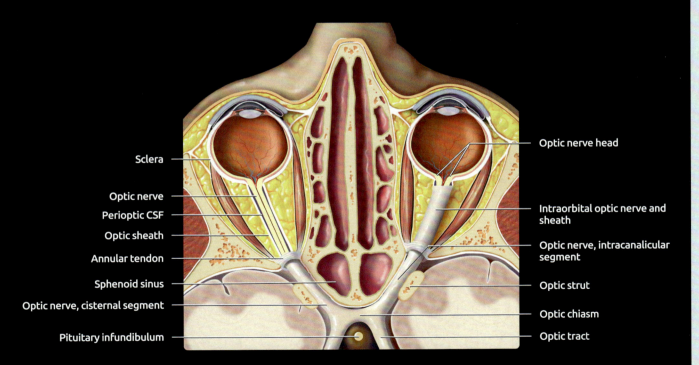

(Top) Coronal graphic of the midorbit depicting the optic nerve-sheath complex is shown. The nerve is bathed by a thin layer of CSF, which is contained by the dural optic sheath. The central retinal vessels are external to the optic sheath posteriorly in the orbit and pierce the dura in the midportion of the nerve to travel within the substance of the nerve anteriorly. (Bottom) Axial graphic of the intraorbital and intracranial segments of CNII is shown. The extraaxial optic pathways can be segmented (posterior to anterior) into optic tract, optic chiasm, cisternal nerve, intracanalicular nerve, and intraorbital nerve. The optic sheath is a dural reflection that is contiguous with intracranial dura mater. Note the relationship of the pituitary infundibulum to the optic chiasm.

Optic Nerve/Sheath Complex

CORONAL AND AXIAL T1 MR

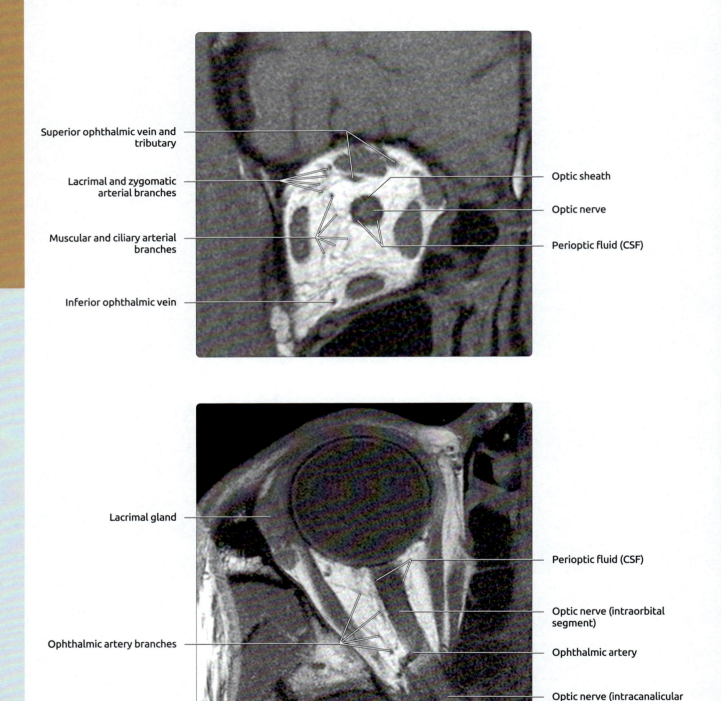

(Top) Coronal high-resolution T1 MR of the intraconal orbit is shown. The optic nerve/sheath complex is centered within the extraocular muscle cone. Perioptic fluid is contiguous with intracranial CSF and is seen as hypointense signal between the nerve centrally and the dural sheath peripherally. Intraconal branches of the ophthalmic artery are in proximity with the nerve/sheath complex; considerable variation exists in the order and anastomotic connections of these branches. (Bottom) Axial high-resolution T1 MR of the midorbit is shown. The optic nerve/sheath complex angles medially within the muscle cone as it courses toward the optic canal. The ophthalmic artery is visible near the apex as it exits laterally from within the dural sheath just beyond the optic canal.

Optic Nerve/Sheath Complex

CORONAL AND AXIAL STIR MR

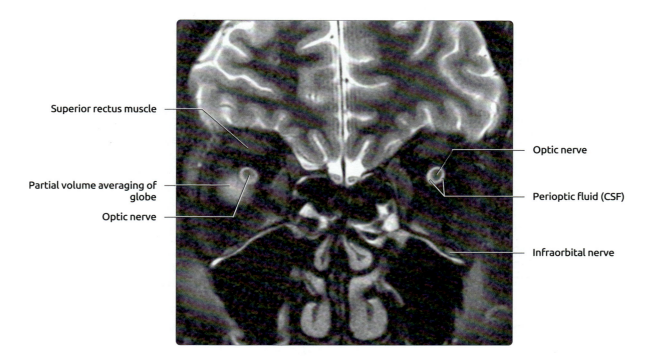

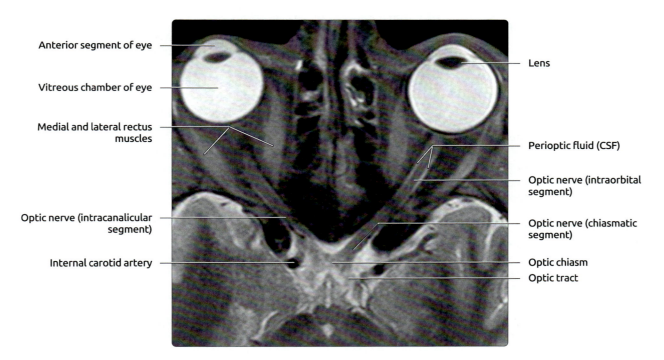

(Top) Coronal T2 STIR MR of the orbits is shown. STIR technique provides reliable and effective suppression of intraorbital fat, making the fluid signal of the perioptic cerebrospinal fluid appear conspicuous. Extraocular muscles appear relatively hypointense on STIR. Remember the arachnoid space surrounding the optic nerve is contiguous with the suprasellar cistern. Its size will therefore vary with intracranial pressure. **(Bottom)** Axial T2 STIR MR of the orbits is shown. A slightly oblique plane allows for demonstration of both intraorbital and cisternal segments of CNII. Because of the normal angulation of the nerves proximally, the chiasm and tracts are usually demonstrated on images superior to those depicting the intraorbital nerves. The anterior segment of the eye includes both the anterior and posterior chambers in front of the lens.

Globe

GROSS ANATOMY

Segments

- **Anterior segment of globe**
  - Portion of eye in front of anterior margin of vitreous (hyaloid face)
    - Ciliary body, suspensory ligaments, and lens
    - Anterior and posterior chambers
    - Iris
    - Cornea
- **Posterior segment of globe**
  - Vitreoretinal portion of eye and its layers
    - Vitreous chamber
    - Retina
    - Choroid
    - Sclera

Chambers

- **Anterior chamber**
  - Major chamber of anterior segment
  - Between cornea and iris
  - Filled with aqueous humor, which provides nutrition and structure
- **Posterior chamber**
  - Small potential space posterior to iris and anterior to lens/ligament complex
  - Contiguous with anterior chamber through pupil
- **Vitreous chamber**
  - Large chamber that fills posterior segment
  - Filled with viscoelastic transparent gel

Tunicae

- **Tunica interna (retina)**
  - Multilayered sensorineural organ
    - Photoreceptor cells (rods and cones) overlie pigment epithelium at outermost layer
    - Bipolar and ganglion cells form inner layer (next to vitreous) and assemble and convey sensory signals
  - Regions and extent
    - **Macula**: Central portion, daylight and color vision
    - **Fovea**: Macular center, highest spatial resolution
    - **Peripheral**: Outer portion, night vision and motion
    - **Ora serrata**: Anterior margin of retina
- **Tunica vasculosa (uvea)**
  - Pigmented, vascular loose connective tissue
  - **Choroid**
    - Layer between retina and sclera
    - Vascular supply to photoreceptor layer
  - **Ciliary body**
    - Uveal structure anterior to ora serrata
    - Attached to lens via zonule fibers
    - Contractile function provides for lens accommodation
    - Source of aqueous production
  - **Iris**
    - Thin elastic tissue overlying lens
    - Sphincter muscle provides pupillary response
- **Tunica fibrosa (sclera)**
  - Outer fibrous layer
  - Attachment site for extraocular muscles
    - Contiguous with dura of optic sheath as well as fibrous diaphragm (lamina cribrosa) at nerve head
    - Contiguous with cornea anteriorly

IMAGING ANATOMY

Overview

- Primary imaging approaches
  - Direct funduscopy is 1st-line technique
  - Sonography readily available at most eye clinics
- Cross-sectional modalities (MR and CT)
  - Particularly useful in eyes with opaque media (i.e., obscured by vitreous or aqueous opacity)
  - Routine imaging as part of orbital evaluation
    - Extraocular extension of ocular disease
    - Ocular involvement of orbital process

Internal Contents

- **Anterior segment**
  - Aqueous chambers exhibit fluid signal
  - Lens moderately hyperdense on CT, isointense on T1WI, hypointense relative to fluid on T2WI
  - Ciliary body and iris variably distinguishable but not diagnostic detail
- **Posterior segment**
  - Vitreous chamber exhibits fluid signal

ANATOMY IMAGING ISSUES

Imaging Recommendations

- CT
  - Evaluation of calcification (e.g., retinoblastoma)
  - Evaluation in child without sedation
- MR
  - Preferred for evaluation of extraocular extent of disease
  - T2WI useful for evaluating vitreous and aqueous chambers; otherwise limited utility in eye
  - T1WI pre- and postcontrast better for assessing uveoretinal structures
  - Surface coils improve signal and resolution in globe but may be limited in assessment of posterior orbit

Imaging Pitfalls

- MR
  - Irrepressible globe movement results in ubiquitous motion artifact

EMBRYOLOGY

Embryologic Events

- **Optic fissure**
  - Extends along inferonasal aspect of optic disc and stalk
  - Fissure fusion (~ 5th week) required for normal globe and nerve formation
  - Failure of fusion results in coloboma
- **Primary vitreous**
  - Embryonic fibrovascular hyaloid with hyaloid artery in Cloquet canal
  - Normally regresses ~ 7 months gestation
    - Visible in premature infant
  - Failure of regression results in persistent hyperplastic primary vitreous

Globe

GRAPHIC AND SAGITTAL T1 MR

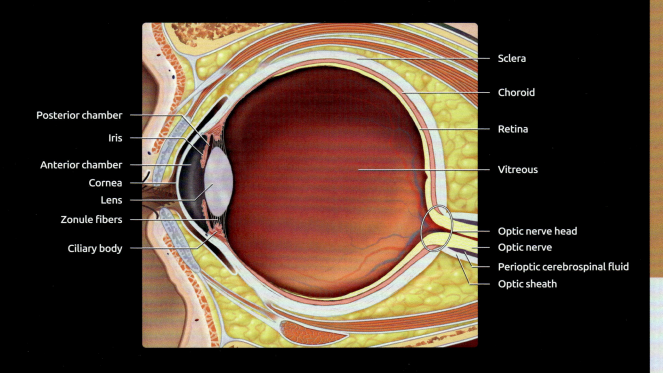

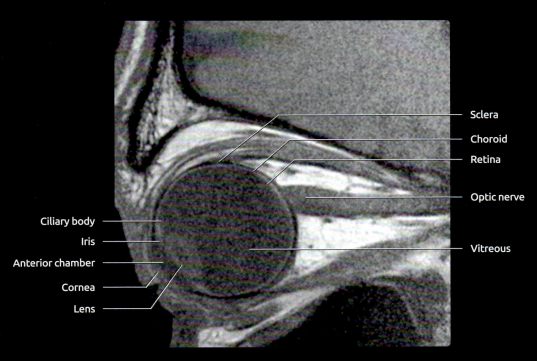

(Top) Sagittal graphic shows that the anterior and posterior chambers of the anterior segment are contiguous through the pupil. The choroid and iris are anterior extensions of the uveal tract. The posterior segment is filled by the vitreous chamber. The retina and sclera are contiguous with the optic nerve and sheath, respectively, at the nerve head. (Bottom) Sagittal T1 MR shows that the aqueous-filled anterior chamber and vitreous-filled posterior chamber exhibit essentially pure fluid signal. The lens is distinguishable; the iris and ciliary body are identifiable but not reliably diagnostic on routine MR imaging. The pigmented choroid may be seen as a thin hyperintense layer on high-resolution T1.

Cavernous Sinus

TERMINOLOGY

Abbreviations

- Cavernous sinus (CS)

Definitions

- CSs are paired parasellar dural venous sinuses of central skull base region at confluence of multiple veins draining orbit, sylvian fissure, and middle and anterior fossa; ultimately provide venous drainage posteriorly and inferiorly via inferior petrosal, superior petrosal, and basilar venous sinuses
- CSs contain several cranial nerves and internal carotid artery (ICA)

IMAGING ANATOMY

Overview

- CSs are valveless, septated dural venous sinuses of central skull base, present on either side of sella
- CSs are surrounded by dural walls, interposed between sella and pituitary gland medially and temporal lobe laterally
- CSs are important given location, relationship to sella and pituitary gland, and internal contents, including multiple cranial nerves and cavernous ICA

Anatomy Relationships

- **Osseous relationships**
  - CS rests on intracranial surface of sphenoid bone and petrous apex (PA)
  - Anteriorly, CS extends to anterior clinoid process and superior orbital fissure (SOF) below it
  - Posteriorly, CS extends to posterior clinoid process, lateral margin of upper clivus, and petroclival junction, extending laterally to point just medial to trigeminal impression
  - Superiorly, CS extends from base of anterior clinoid process to posterior clinoid process
  - Medially, CS bordered by lateral margin of sella and carotid sulcus of sphenoid bone
- **Venous communications**
  - Venous tributaries
    - Superior, inferior ophthalmic veins
    - Sphenoparietal sinus
  - Communicate with each other via intercavernous plexus (across sella) and basilar venous plexus (across clivus)
  - Communicates posteriorly with inferior petrosal sinus, superior petrosal sinus, and basilar venous sinus
  - Additional communications with veins of skull base foramina: Foramen ovale, rotundum, and spinosum, carotid canal, and sphenoidal emissary foramen
- **Roof**
  - Dural roof of CS extends from optic strut and SOF anteriorly to PA and tentorial free edge (incisura) posteriorly
  - Medial margin of CS roof is contiguous with diaphragma sella
  - **Oculomotor triangle** is triangular-shaped portion of CS roof created by 3 dural folds

- Lateral margin of roof is separated from lateral wall of CS by cord-like thickening of dura called **anterior petroclinoid fold** that extends from tentorial edge at PA to anterior clinoid process
  - Separate fold extends from tentorial edge at PA to posterior clinoid process, **posterior petroclinoid fold**
  - Thin band of dura, **interclinoid fold**, extends from anterior clinoid process to posterior clinoid process
  - CNIII, along with its sleeve of arachnoid (oculomotor cistern), pierces roof at oculomotor triangle
  - CNIV enters posterolateral aspect of oculomotor triangle just posterior to CNIII
  - Small portion of roof passes inferomedial to anterior clinoid process where dural roof merges with dura, forming proximal and distal dural rings
- **Lateral wall**
  - Sail-shaped dural sheet that extends from SOF and anterior clinoid process anteriorly to PA posteriorly; faces medial temporal lobe
  - Consists of thick dural membrane that is typically easily dissected into 2 distinct layers
    - Thin outer (meningeal) layer and thicker inner (endosteal) layer
    - Thicker inner (endosteal)
  - Inner layer envelops oculomotor nerve (CNIII), trochlear nerve (CNIV), and ophthalmic (V1) and maxillary (V2) segments of trigeminal nerve
  - Lateral and medial walls of CS merge inferiorly along lateral margin of sphenoid, just above maxillary nerve, 2nd division of trigeminal nerve (V2)
  - While V3 is invested by contiguous dura, it is not considered component of CS wall
  - Lateral wall merges inferiorly and posteriorly with dura covering Meckel cave
- **Medial wall**
  - Medial wall of CS consists of upper sellar component and lower sphenoid component
  - Upper sellar component of medial wall is thin dural membrane, typically single cell layer in thickness that separates venous compartment from lateral margin of pituitary gland
  - More inferiorly, medial wall is thicker and adherent to carotid sulcus of sphenoid bone
- **Anterior wall**
  - Anterior wall essentially rectangular in shape and extends from optic strut, beneath anterior clinoid process laterally to include SOF
  - Inferior margin is foramen rotundum
  - Anterior CS merges with venous plexus within SOF
- **Posterior wall**
  - Extends from lateral margin of dorsum sella to medial aspect of trigeminal impression of PA and superiomedial aspect of Meckel cave
  - Posterior wall is limited inferiorly by junction of PA and body of sphenoid bone at superiomedial aspect of petroclival fissure
  - **Dorello canal and CNVI**
    - Near medial and superior tip of PA, there is small gap that separates PA from clivus

Cavernous Sinus

- Small ligament, petrosphenoid ligament of Gruber, crosses from PA tip to base of posterior clinoid process
- This gap or space, called Dorello canal, contains venous tissue at confluence of posterior CS and petrosal sinuses
- CNVI passes from prepontine cistern through Dorello canal to enter CS
  - o **Petrolingual ligament (PLL)**
    - Extends from PA to lingula of sphenoid bone
    - Invariably surrounds dorsal and lateral walls of lacerum segment of ICA
    - Important surgical landmark that marks point at which ICA lacerum segment transitions to cavernous segment
    - Also marks inferior and posterior margin of CS
- **Meckel cave**
  - o Dural outpouching that begins in posterior fossa (porus trigeminus) and extends over petrosphenoid junction into medial and posterior aspect of middle cranial fossa
  - o Contains part of trigeminal nerve, including trigeminal ganglion
  - o Superior, anterior, and medial portions of Meckel cave are immediately adjacent to posterior and lateral aspects of CS
  - o Medial and inferior aspect of Meckel cave is just lateral to ICA as it arises from medial opening of carotid canal and begins to turn vertically and anteriorly into CS
  - o Trigeminal ganglion is positioned within anterior and inferior aspect of Meckel cave and divides into 3 divisions: Ophthalmic (V1), maxillary (V2), and mandibular (V3)
  - o Ophthalmic division (V1) extends medially and anteriorly and enters lateral wall of CS
  - o Maxillary division (V2) extends anteriorly, along inferior margin of CS to enter foramen rotundum
  - o Mandibular division (V3) extends inferiorly and laterally through foramen ovale

Internal Contents

- **CNIII**
  - o Pierces roof of CS in oculomotor cistern and is quickly embedded in lateral wall
  - o Surrounded by thin sleeve of arachnoid and CSF (oculomotor cistern) that travels with nerve for several millimeters to approximate anterior clinoid process
- **CNIV**
  - o Also pierces roof of CS, and nerve is positioned in lateral wall below CNIII
- **V1** (ophthalmic division of CNV) in lateral wall below CNIV
- **V2** (maxillary division of CNV) is most inferior cranial nerve in lateral CS wall
- **V3** (mandibular division of CNV) does **not** enter CS proper (passes from Meckel cave inferiorly into foramen ovale)
- **CNVI** lies within CS proper, next to ICA
- Sympathetic fibers travel along ICA within CS
- **Cavernous ICA**
  - o In 1996, Bouthillier et al described 7-segment classification system for ICA
    - Cervical
    - Petrous

- Lacerum
- Cavernous
- Clinoid
- Opthalmic
- Communicating segments
- o Cavernous segment begins as lacerum segment of ICA passes beneath PLL (fibrous band from PA to sphenoid lingula)
- o Initially ascends and then turns (posterior bend) anteriorly to assume horizontal course through CS
- o Posterior bend is usual site of origin for meningohypophyseal trunk
- o Horizontal portion of cavernous ICA lies within shallow groove along lateral margin of sphenoid bone, carotid sulcus
- o Carotid sulcus occasionally dehiscent, allowing ICA to protrude into sphenoid sinus
- o Horizontal segment gives rise to inferolateral trunk, which supplies tiny branches to intracavernous cranial nerves and tentorium
- o Near anterior margin of CS, ICA turns cephalad (anterior bend) and continues medial to anterior clinoid process
- o Along this anterior vertical course, ICA passes through 2 anatomically distinct dural rings: Proximal dural ring, which forms true roof of CS anteriorly, and distal dural ring
- o Clinoid segment is short vertical segment medial to anterior clinoid process and corresponds to interdural segment of artery between proximal and distal dural rings

ANATOMY IMAGING ISSUES

Imaging Recommendations

- High-resolution MR with T1, T2, and T1 C+ with fat saturation in 2 planes through central skull base is best overall examination
- CT angiogram is best for identifying pathology of cavernous ICA and for carotid cavernous fistula
- CT venogram can produce adequate venous-phase contrast enhancement to evaluate for CS thrombosis or thrombophlebitis

Cavernous Sinus

GRAPHICS

Top graphic labels (left): CNVI exiting cavernous sinus through superior orbital fissure; Cavernous sinus, lateral dural wall; 1st (ophthalmic or V1) division of CNV; 2nd (maxillary or V2) division of CNV; 3rd (mandibular or V3) division of CNV; Trigeminal ganglion within Meckel cave; CNVI in Dorello canal. Top graphic labels (right): Diaphragma sellae; Hypophysis; Internal carotid artery; Oculomotor nerve (CNIII), cistern; Cisternal portion of CNIV; Cisternal portion of CNV.

Middle graphic labels (left): Tuber cinereum of hypothalamus with infundibulum; Hypophysis; Internal carotid artery; Abducens nerve (CNVI); Sphenoid sinus. Middle graphic labels (right): Optic tract; Arachnoid; Oculomotor nerve (CNIII), cistern; Trochlear nerve (CNIV); Lateral dural wall of cavernous sinus; CNV1; CNV2; Nasopharynx.

Bottom graphic labels (left): Optic nerve (CNII) entering optic canal; Ophthalmic (V1) division of CNV (trigeminal); Maxillary nerve (CNV2) entering foramen rotundum; Mandibular nerve (CNV3) entering foramen ovale. Bottom graphic labels (right): Trochlear nerve (CNIV); Oculomotor nerve (CNIII); Meckel cave; Trigeminal ganglion; Abducens nerve (CNVI).

(Top) *Axial graphic of sella turcica, as viewed from above, depicts normal sellar & parasellar anatomy. Dura covering right cavernous sinus (CS) is removed to show CNV & CNVI. All cranial nerves are shown in left CS. Mandibular division of CNV does not run through CS but exits from Meckel cave inferiorly to enter foramen ovale. Note CS is not a single venous channel but is extensively septated.* **(Middle)** *Coronal graphic depicts contents of CSs. The following cranial nerves traverse CS within lateral wall of CS, from superior to inferior: Oculomotor (CNIII), trochlear (CNIV), 1st (ophthalmic or V1) & 2nd (maxillary or V2) divisions of trigeminal (CNV) nerves. The only cranial nerve actually within venous sinusoids of CS is abducens nerve (CNVI).* **(Bottom)** *Lateral graphic demonstrates cranial nerve detail in sellar region. CNIII, CNIV, CNV1, & CNV2 are in lateral dural wall of CS. CNVI courses within venous sinusoids of CS, adjacent to internal carotid artery (not shown). Meckel cave is CSF-filled, dural & arachnoid-lined invagination that communicates freely with prepontine cistern. It contains fascicles of trigeminal nerve (CNV) & trigeminal (gasserian) ganglion.*

Cavernous Sinus

AXIAL T1 C+ MR

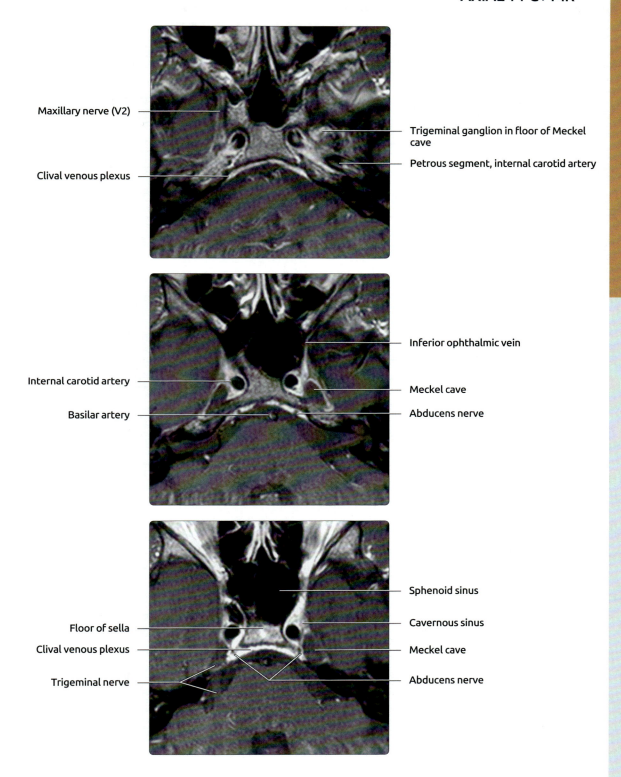

(Top) Series of 6 axial contrast-enhanced T1 MR images, presented from inferior to superior through the skull base and CS, demonstrates the right maxillary nerve (V2) passing anteriorly into the foramen rotundum and the left trigeminal ganglion. The mandibular nerve (V3) will exit inferiorly through the foramen ovale (not shown). (Middle) The Meckel cave is located posterior, inferior, and lateral relative to the CS. Dura forming the posterior part of the lateral wall of the CS also forms the upper medial 1/3 of the Meckel cave, separating the 2 structures. Note the abducens nerve (CNVI) seen here as a filling defect within the clival venous plexus, just before entering the Dorello canal. (Bottom) Both abducens nerves are seen coursing through the Dorello canal to enter the posterior CS. The right trigeminal nerve is seen entering the Meckel cave.

Cavernous Sinus

AXIAL T1 C+ MR

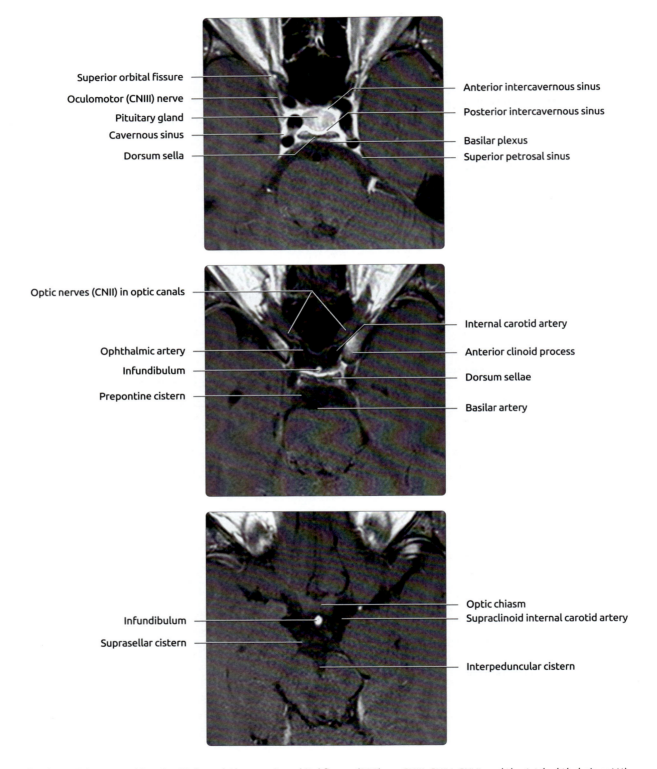

(Top) Cranial nerves exiting the CS through the superior orbital fissure (SOF) are CNIII, CNIV, CNVI, and the 1st (ophthalmic or V1) division of CNV. (Middle) The optic nerve in the optic canal is located anteromedial to the anterior clinoid and superomedial to the SOF. It is separated from the SOF by a thin, bony strut, the "optic strut." The cavernous carotid is posteromedial to the anterior clinoid. Note the origin of the ophthalmic artery from the internal carotid artery, just above the transition from the intracavernous carotid (below) to the intradural carotid (above) segments. (Bottom) Pituitary infundibulum is seen within the suprasellar cistern posterior to the optic chiasm; avid enhancement seen here is typical. The supraclinoid internal carotid artery (or terminal segment) is seen laterally.

Cavernous Sinus

CORONAL T2 MR

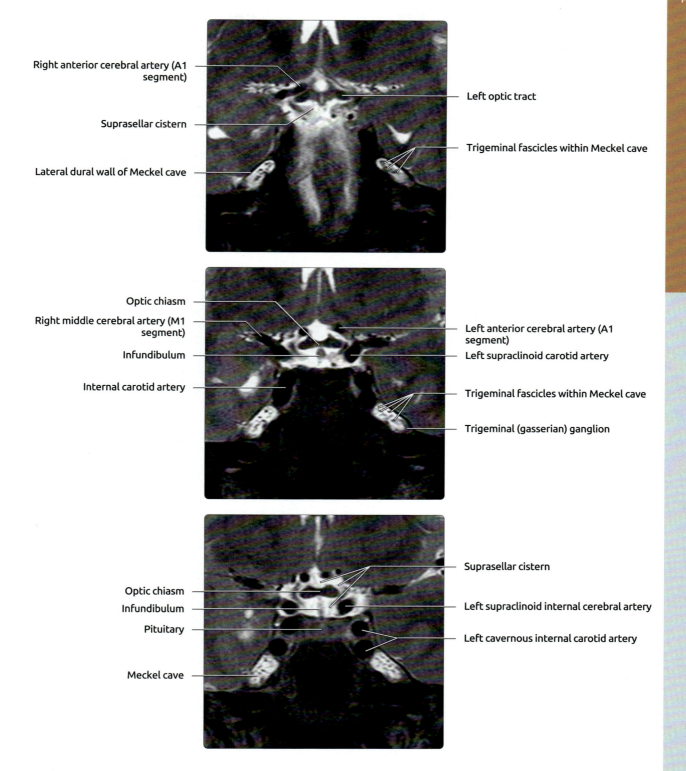

(Top) First of 6 sequential coronal T2 MR images, presented from posterior to anterior, demonstrates the optic tracts within the posterior aspect of the suprasellar cistern and the anterior cerebral and supraclinoid internal carotid arteries. (Middle) The posterior optic chiasm and part of the pituitary infundibulum are seen here. Note the internal carotid, middle cerebral, and anterior cerebral arteries. Individual trigeminal nerve rootlets are well demonstrated within the Meckel cave on thin-section imaging. (Bottom) Image at the level of the optic chiasm within the suprasellar cistern demonstrates normal pituitary gland and regional vascular anatomy. Note the normal location and appearance of the Meckel cave, seen inferior and lateral. The pituitary gland and venous blood within the CS are nearly isointense with each other on T2.

CORONAL T2 MR

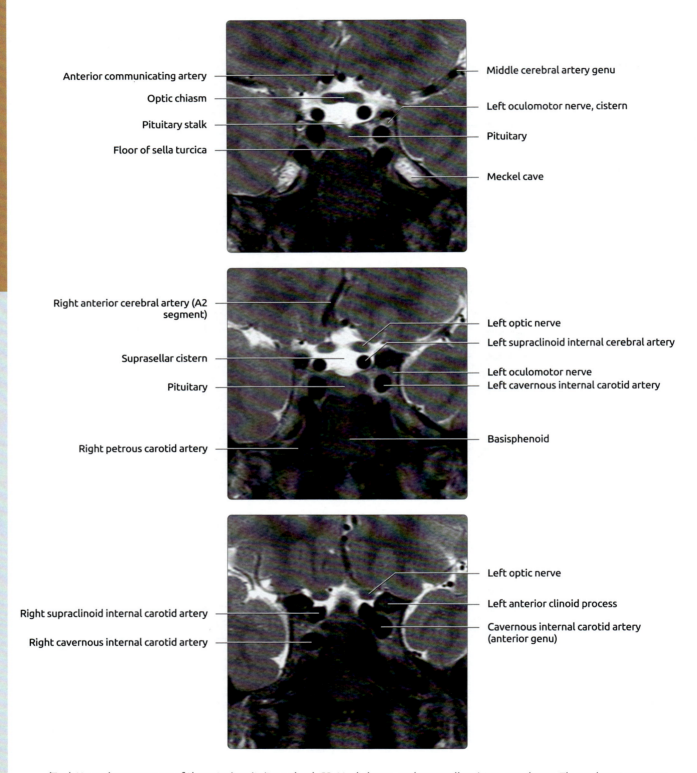

(Top) Normal appearances of the anterior pituitary gland, CS, Meckel cave, and suprasellar cistern are shown. The oculomotor nerves (CNIII) and optic nerves (CNII) are well seen. The anterior communicating artery, which connects the 2 anterior cerebral arteries and the left middle cerebral artery genu, are visible. (Middle) The most anterior aspect of the suprasellar cistern demonstrates normal optic nerves (CNII), oculomotor nerves (CNIII), cavernous internal carotid arteries, and the anterior cerebral artery within the anterior interhemispheric fissure. (Bottom) The anterior clinoid processes seen here form the anterolateral boundaries of the sella turcica. Note the normal optic nerves, located medial to the anterior clinoids, and the anterior genu of the cavernous internal carotid artery on the left.

Cavernous Sinus

CORONAL T1 C+ MR

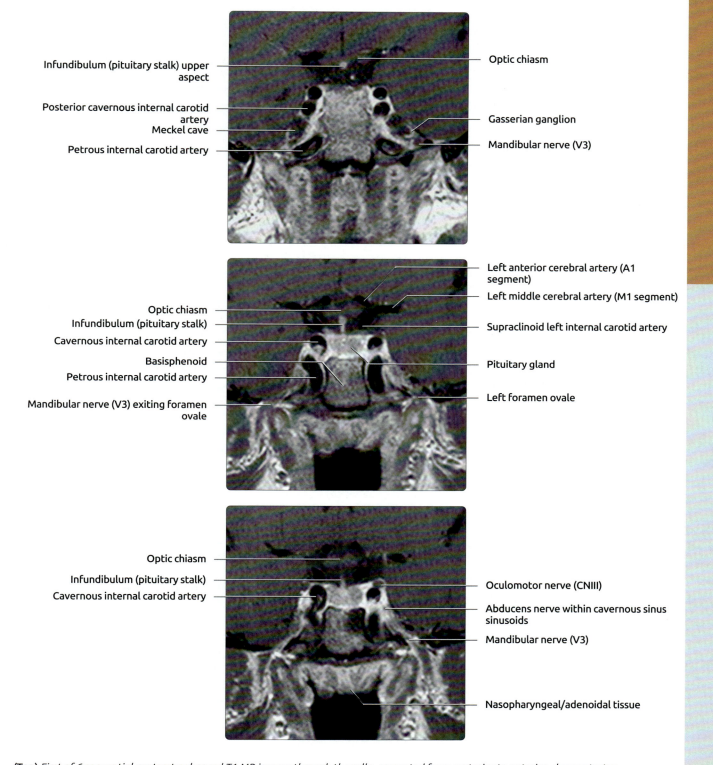

(Top) First of 6 sequential contrast-enhanced T1 MR images through the sella, presented from posterior to anterior, demonstrates details of the Meckel cave. The mandibular (V3) division of the trigeminal nerve is seen inferior to the normally enhancing gasserian ganglion. (Middle) The pituitary infundibulum insertion into the gland is well seen. Note the mandibular nerve (3rd division of trigeminal nerve, or V3), best seen on the right, as it exits through foramen ovale, entering the high masticator space. It is easy to see how extracranial tumors may gain access to the intracranial compartment without destroying the skull base, either through direct extension or via perineural spread. (Bottom) The left foramen ovale is well seen. Note the 3rd and 6th cranial nerves within the CS. All of the cranial nerves are not well seen on this image.

Cavernous Sinus

CORONAL T1 C+ MR

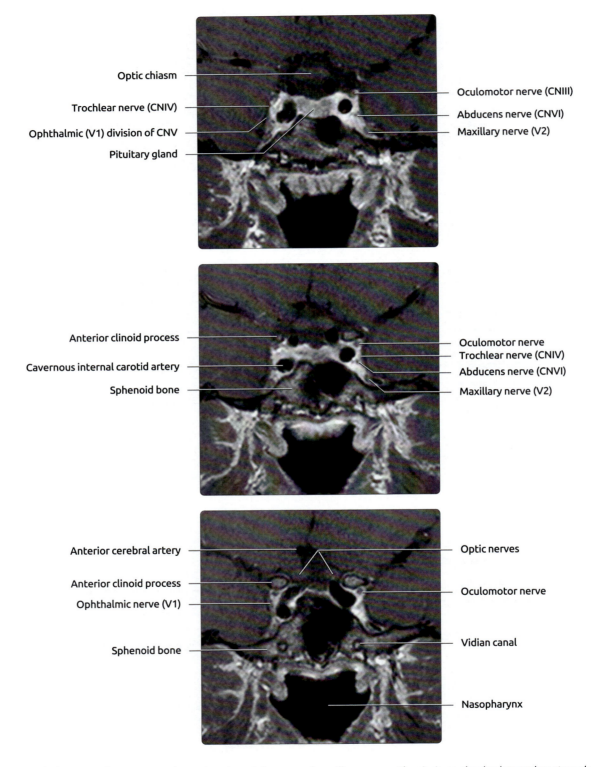

(Top) This image demonstrates the oculomotor, abducens, and maxillary nerves. The pituitary gland enhances less strongly than venous blood in the CS. (Middle) Normal cranial nerves traversing the CS from superior to inferior include the oculomotor nerve, trochlear nerve, abducens nerve, ophthalmic nerve (V1), and maxillary nerve (V2). The 4th cranial nerve (trochlear) is small and difficult to visualize but is normally located in the lateral CS between the oculomotor and trigeminal nerves, lateral to the abducens. (Bottom) The oculomotor nerve is again well seen in the anterior CS before it traverses the SOF. The vidian canal, which contains the vidian artery and nerve, is seen in the sphenoid bone. Note the optic nerves medial to the anterior clinoids before entering the optic canals.

Cavernous Sinus

ANATOMIC-PATHOLOGIC CORRELATION CAVERNOUS SINUS THROMBOSIS

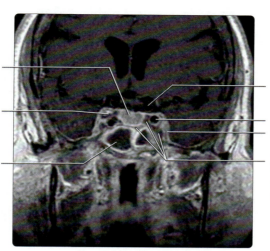

Normal pituitary
Lack of enhancement in superomedial component of right cavernous sinus
Opacified sphenoid sinus
Ophthalmic segment internal carotid artery
Cavernous internal carotid artery
Normal dural enhancement
Lack of normal enhancement in inferior intercavernous sinus and medial and inferior compartments of left cavernous sinus

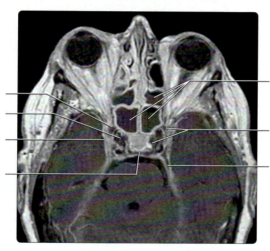

Thrombosis of anterior compartment
Internal carotid artery
Normal enhancement of lateral wall
Thrombosis of basilar venous sinus
Sinusitis with air-fluid levels
Thrombosis of medial and lateral compartments of cavernous sinus
Thrombosis of superior petrosal sinus

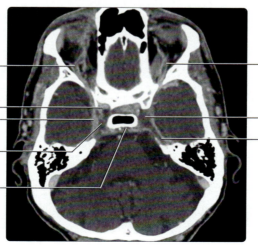

Thrombosis of superior ophthalmic vein
Internal carotid artery clinoid segment
Normal enhancement lateral wall
Thrombosis of right cavernous sinus
Thrombosis basilar venous sinus
Thrombosis of superior ophthalmic vein
Thrombosis of left internal carotid artery
Thrombosis of left superior petrosal sinus

(**Top**) *Bacterial sinusitis complicated by bilateral CS thrombosis is shown. Coronal MR through the CSs demonstrates complete opacification of the sphenoid sinus secondary to bacterial sinusitis. The lateral walls and roofs of the CSs enhance normally. However, there is conspicuous lack of enhancement in the central areas of CSs bilaterally. Normal flow voids (dark areas) are identified in the internal carotid arteries bilaterally.* (**Middle**) *Axial MR performed in the same patient with bacterial sinusitis and bilateral CS thrombosis is shown. The flow voids in the internal carotid arteries are less distinct but present. The CS walls enhance normally, but the internal venous compartments of the CSs fail to enhance bilaterally due to venous sinus thrombosis.* (**Bottom**) *Axial CECT in a patient with bacterial facial cellulitis and bilateral CS thrombosis is shown. The superior ophthalmic veins show filling defects bilaterally, consistent with thrombosis. The lateral walls of the CSs enhance normally. However, on this delayed venous-phase image, the CSs demonstrate lack of significant internal enhancement consistent with bilateral thrombosis.*

SECTION 4
Nose and Sinuses

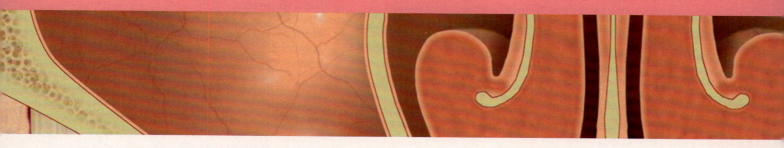

Sinonasal Overview	**238**
Ostiomeatal Unit	**248**
Pterygopalatine Fossa	**252**
Frontal Recess and Related Air Cells	**260**

Sinonasal Overview

IMAGING ANATOMY

Overview

- All paranasal sinuses lined by respiratory pseudostratified epithelium attached directly to bone (mucoperiosteum)
- **Nasal cavity**: Triangle divided in midline by septum
  - Roof formed by horizontal **cribriform plate (CP) of ethmoid**, floor by hard & soft palate, laterally by lateral nasal wall with attached turbinates
  - Nasal mucosa & sensory nerves traverse CP into anterior cranial fossa & synapse intracranially with secondary neurons in olfactory bulb & tract
  - Anteriorly **nasal pyriform aperture**; posteriorly **posterior choana** connecting to nasopharynx
- Ethmoid roof is formed by horizontal **fovea ethmoidalis** of orbital plate of frontal bone superolaterally & vertical **lateral lamella** of CP medially (just lateral to horizontal CP of nasal roof); lateral lamella 10x thinner than fovea
- **Keros classification** of ethmoid roof/olfactory fossa into 3 types according to increasing vertical height of lateral lamella & resultant depth of olfactory fossa (1-3 mm in Keros type I, 4-7 mm in type II & 8-16 mm in type III); Keros type III has max risk for iatrogenic injury to lateral lamella & CSF leak during endoscopic surgery
- **Nasal septum**: Anterior septum formed from cartilage
  - Bony septum: Perpendicular plate of ethmoid posterosuperiorly & vomer posteroinferiorly
- **Nasal turbinates (conchae)**
  - Concha bullosa: Pneumatization and expansion of middle turbinate
  - Bony superior & middle (part of ethmoidal complex), & inferior (separate bone) turbinates project inferomedially into nasal cavity
  - Define region below & lateral as superior, middle, & inferior meati, respectively
  - Tail of superior turbinate points medially toward natural ostium of sphenoid sinus in sphenoethmoid recess & is very important surgical landmark here
  - Vertical portion of basal lamella of middle turbinate attaches to CP (coronal CT), middle & posterior portions laterally to lamina papyracea (sagittal CT)
- **Nasal meati**
  - **Superior meatus**: Receives drainage from posterior ethmoid & sphenoid sinus at sphenoethmoidal recess (known as posterior ostiomeatal complex)
    - Sphenopalatine foramen (site of origin of juvenile nasopharyngeal angiofibroma) connects superior meatus with pterygopalatine fossa lateral to it
  - **Middle meatus: Ethmoid bulla**: Large ethmoid air cell at superior aspect of ostiomeatal complex
    - **Hiatus semilunaris (HS)**: Semilunar region between uncinate process & ethmoid bulla, receives drainage from anterior ethmoid air cells & maxillary sinus via infundibulum
  - **Inferior meatus**: Receives drainage from nasolacrimal duct anteriorly, covered by mucosal (Hasner) valve

Anatomy Relationships

- **Maxillary sinus**: Paired air cells within maxillary bone
  - Drain via maxillary ostium at its superomedial aspect, into infundibulum, then into HS at middle meatus

- **Ethmoid sinus**: Paired groups of 3 to 18 air cells within ethmoid labyrinths
  - Separated into anterior & posterior groups separated by basal lamella (lateral attachment of middle turbinate to lamina papyracea)
  - Ethmoid bulla: Dominant anterior ethmoid air cell that protrudes inferomedially into infundibulum or HS
  - Anterior drainage: Anterior recess of HS & middle meatus around ethmoid bulla & some into ethmoid infundibulum
  - Posterior drainage: Superior meatus & sphenoethmoidal recess
- **Frontal sinus**: Paired air cells within frontal bone; drainage through frontal recess (funnel-shaped) into middle meatus
- **Sphenoid sinus**: Paired air cells within sphenoid bone; drainage into sphenoethmoidal recess
- **Extramural paranasal air cells**
  - **Infraorbital ethmoid cells (Haller)**: Ethmoid cells that extend into inferomedial orbital floor
  - **Agger nasi cell**: Most anterior air cell that involve lacrimal bone or frontal process of maxilla
  - **Frontal recess Kuhn cells (4 types)**: Frontal recess bordered **anteriorly** by agger nasi below, Kuhn cells above
  - **Bulla ethmoidalis & frontal bullar, suprabullar (intramural) & supraorbital ethmoid (extramural) cells**: Frontal recess bordered **posteriorly** by these cells
  - **Sphenoethmoidal cells (Onodi)**: Posterior ethmoid air cells with prominent superolateral pneumatization; close relationship to optic nerve; look for horizontal septum in upper sphenoid sinus in coronal CT & trace its continuity with posterior ethmoid air cell in sagittal or axial images

ANATOMY IMAGING ISSUES

Imaging Recommendations

- CT scan ideally delayed in URIs & done after 4-6 weeks of starting sinusitis medications as mucosal thickening is nonspecific & changes due to simple sinusitis may be seen
- Unenhanced thin 0.625-mm volumetric images with sagittal & coronal reconstructions at 1- to 2-mm intervals
- Both high-resolution bone & soft tissue algorithm reconstructions in all 3 planes
- No gantry tilt; include ears, entire maxilla, tip of nose, chin, & frontal sinuses to ensure compatibility with functional endoscopic sinus surgery image navigation guidance systems
- Sinusitis complications can be imaged with CECT, but CE MR better for adjacent orbits, dura, brain, & cavernous sinuses
- MR best to differentiate solid internal enhancement of tumor from peripheral mucosal enhancement of polyp, retention cyst, or retained secretions filling sinus
- Fat saturation should be utilized on at least 1 postcontrast sequence

Sinonasal Overview

GRAPHICS

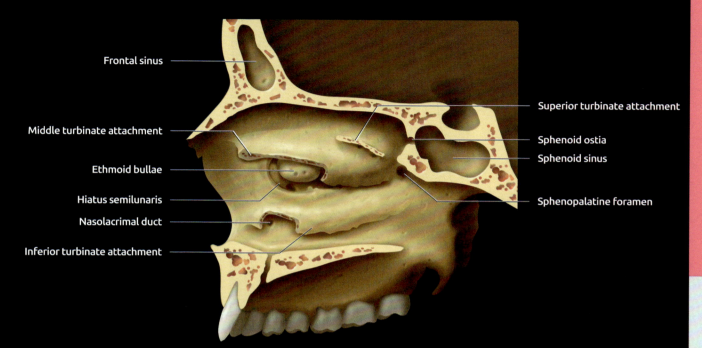

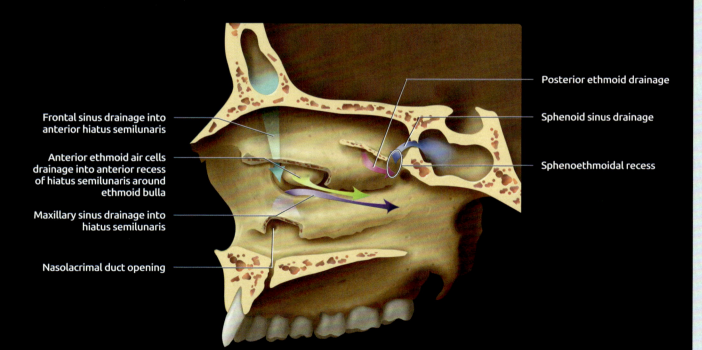

(Top) Sagittal graphic shows osseous anatomy of the lateral wall of the nose. The superior & middle turbinate have been resected. The ethmoid bullae & hiatus semilunaris are below the middle turbinate attachment. The nasolacrimal duct empties into the anterior aspect of the inferior meatus. (Bottom) Sagittal graphic shows drainage pathways of the sinuses, ultimately directed toward the nasopharynx. The sphenoid & posterior ethmoid sinuses drain into the sphenoethmoidal recess in the posterior nasal cavity; maxillary sinus drains via the ethmoid infundibulum while the anterior ethmoids mostly drain into the anterior recess of hiatus semilunaris & middle meatus around the ethmoid bulla (some into the ethmoid infundibulum). Frontal sinus drains into the anterior middle meatus through the frontal recess.

Sinonasal Overview

AXIAL BONE CT

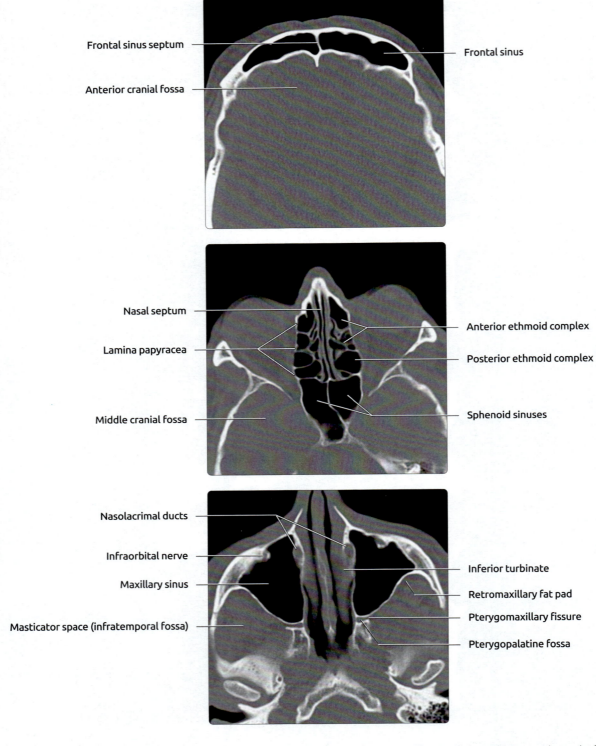

(Top) The 1st of 3 axial bone CT images of the sinuses presented from superior to inferior is shown. This image shows the frontal sinuses with their midline septum and thin posterior wall separating the sinuses from the anterior cranial fossa. Frontal sinus disease can extend posteriorly into the cranial vault. (Middle) This image shows the ethmoid air cells and sphenoid sinuses. The thin lamina papyracea is the lateral wall of the ethmoid sinuses. Ethmoid air cell disease can extend through the lamina papyracea to create a postseptal subperiosteal orbital abscess. (Bottom) This image through the maxillary sinuses shows their intimate relationship to the nasolacrimal ducts, pterygopalatine fossa, and retromaxillary fat pad. Notice the infraorbital nerve anteriorly just before it exits through the infraorbital foramen.

Sinonasal Overview

CORONAL BONE CT

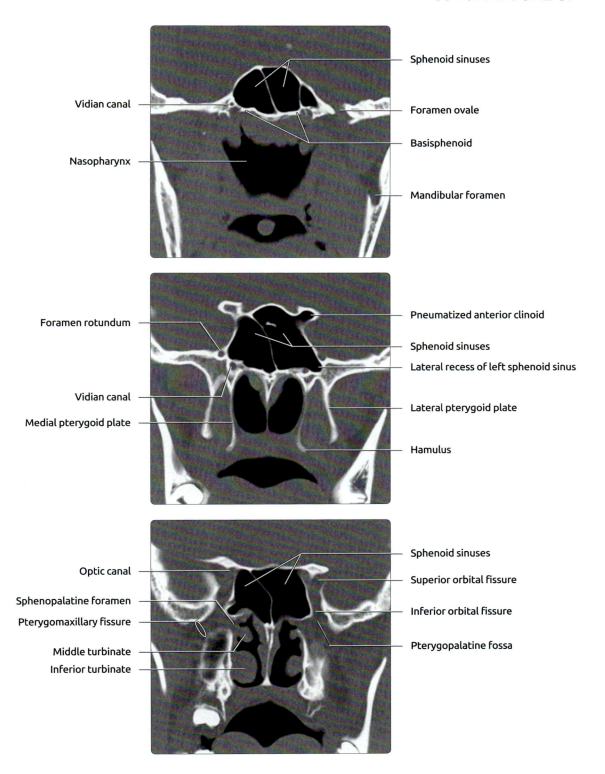

(Top) First of 9 coronal bone NECTs through paranasal sinuses presented from posterior to anterior shows sphenoid sinuses superior to nasopharynx. (Middle) Image shows pterygoid plates posterior to maxillary sinuses. Inferolateral to sphenoid sinus, note foramen rotundum & vidian canal. Note lateral (pterygoid) recess of sphenoid sinus on left side separating vidian canal in body of sphenoid bone inferomedially from foramen rotundum superolaterally. Best practical method to identify skull base foramina on coronal images is by identifying them in relation to lateral recess of sphenoid sinus. Lateral recess may hinder endoscopic repair of sphenoid sinus CSF leak, as pterygoid process acts like a pillar blocking access to recess & will need a transpterygoid approach with partial pterygoid process excision to facilitate sinus obliteration by complete removal of sinus mucosa. (Bottom) Image shows complex anatomic landscape surrounding pterygopalatine fossa (PPF). Lateral exit of PPF is pterygomaxillary fissure through which it exits into masticator space. Superiorly, PPF exits into inferior orbital fissure. Medial exit from PPF is through sphenopalatine foramen into posterolateral nose.

Sinonasal Overview

CORONAL BONE CT

(Top) In this image, the sphenoethmoidal recess is visible as vertical air-filled slits in the posterosuperior nose into which both the posterior ethmoid sinus and the sphenoid sinus empty. Note the greater palatine canal exiting the lateral hard-soft palate junction. Perineural malignancy may travel from the palate to the pterygopalatine fossa via the greater palatine nerve. **(Middle)** In this image through the anterior ethmoid air cells, the ethmoid bulla is seen projecting inferiorly into the middle meatus. The shared wall between the anterior ethmoid air cells and the orbit is paper thin, hence the term lamina papyracea. **(Bottom)** Image through the ostiomeatal complex shows the maxillary infundibulum draining the maxillary sinuses into the middle meatus. The uncinate process, middle meatus, maxillary infundibulum, and ethmoid bulla are the components of the ostiomeatal complex. The olfactory fossa depth corresponds to Keros type II (4-7 mm), which is the most common. Note that there is a lateral to medial slope of the anterior skull base, which is extremely important during transethmoidal surgical approach to anterior skull base lesions. The same axial plane of dissection that was safe along the more lateral ethmoid roof could injure the skull base, dura, and brain if extended medially to the cribriform plate region.

Sinonasal Overview

CORONAL BONE CT

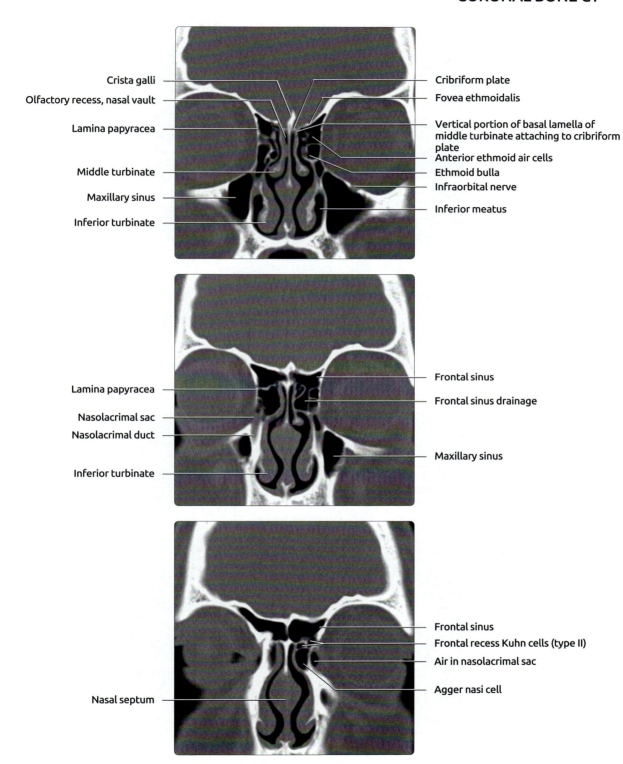

(Top) Image through anterior aspect of anterior ethmoid complex, fovea ethmoidalis (roof of ethmoid), cribriform plate, & crista galli along roof of sinuses & nose from lateral to medial is shown. Olfactory recess of nasal vault contains nasal mucosa. From nasal mucosa arises esthesioneuroblastoma. Foveal plane is horizontal plane passing through junction of fovea ethmoidalis with medial orbital wall. Foveal angle is between fovea & amina papyracea. A low-sloping fovea predisposes anterior skull base injury & intracranial penetration during FESS. The safest anatomy is when the horizontal line from ethmoid roof crosses upper 1/3 of orbit, & precautions to avoid skull base injury should be taken when horizontal plane of ethmoid roof crosses below vertical midpoint of orbit. (Middle) Image shows close relationship of nasolacrimal ducts to maxillary sinuses. Remember, nasolacrimal duct drains into anterior recess of inferior turbinate. (Bottom) In this image through the frontal sinuses, the anteroinferior extramural ethmoid air cell called agger nasi is shown. Note a normal air-filled nasolacrimal sac just lateral to agger nasi cell. Kuhn cells are frontal recess air cells seen above agger nasi (type I single, type II multiple in recess, & type III single, reaching sinus), & type IV is a single isolated cell within frontal sinus.

Sinonasal Overview

SAGITTAL BONE CT

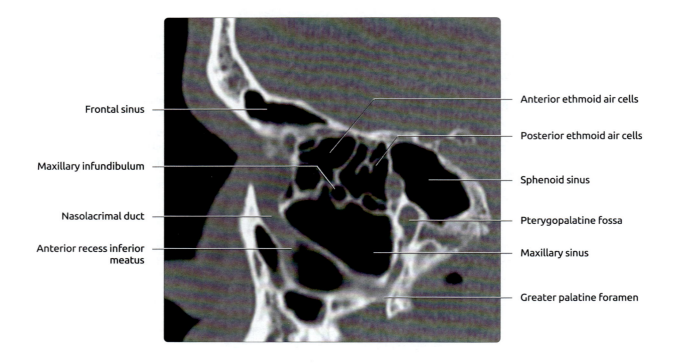

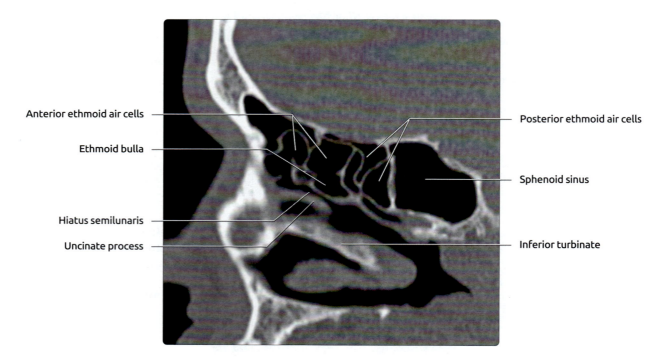

(Top) The 1st of 4 sagittal bone NECT images through the paranasal sinuses presented from lateral to medial is shown. This image shows the nasolacrimal duct draining into the inferior meatus. Also note the pterygopalatine fossa posterior to the maxillary sinus. **(Bottom)** In this image, the uncinate process can be seen just inferior to the ethmoid bulla. The gap between these 2 structures is the hiatus semilunaris. Note that there is a concept of a series of 5 obliquely oriented parallel lamellae (derived from the ridges in the lateral nasal wall of the fetus called ethmoturbinals), which are easy to recognize at surgery. The 1rst lamella is the uncinate process, the 2nd is ethmoid bulla, the 3rd is ground or basal lamella of the middle turbinate, the 4th is basal lamella of the superior turbinate, and the 5th lamella is the basal lamella of the supreme turbinate. Most important is the 3rd lamella (ground or basal lamella of the middle turbinate), which is a bony septation that separates the anterior and posterior ethmoid air cells with separate drainage pathways.

Sinonasal Overview

SAGITTAL BONE CT

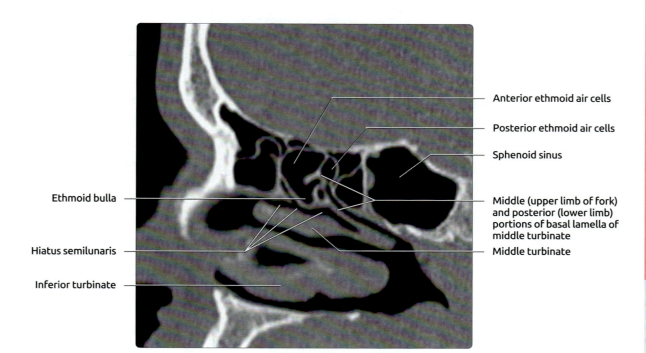

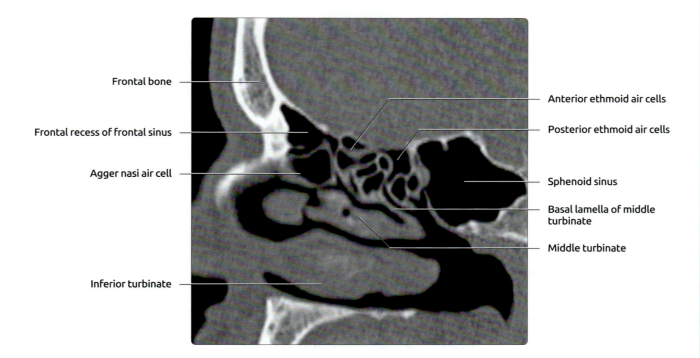

(Top) Image shows middle & inferior turbinates & basal lamella of middle turbinate. Vertical portion of basal lamella attaches to cribriform plate & is best seen in coronal CTs; it's very delicate & its detachment at surgery in this region could damage dura with resultant CSF leak. Middle & posterior portions of basal lamella extend laterally to join lamina papyracea & divides anterior from posterior ethmoid air cells. Posterior margin of basal lamella attaches to perpendicular plate of palatine bone. (Bottom) Image shows anteroinferior ethmoid air cell (agger nasi cell) extending anteroinferiorly to frontal recess of frontal sinus. If this cell is infected, frontal sinus recess & frontal sinus will also become infected secondarily. Sphenoid sinus is well pneumatized, which is most common pattern (sellar type). Sphenoid sinus can be classified into 3 types based on extent of pneumatization: "Conchal" (rudimentary or absent sphenoid sinus where area below sella is a solid block of bone), "presellar" (sphenoid is pneumatized to level of anterior plane of sella & not beyond where posterior sphenoid sinus wall is separated from sella by thick bone), & "sellar" (pneumatization extends into body of sphenoid where posterior sphenoid sinus wall is adjacent to sellar floor or beyond & may even reach clivus).

Sinonasal Overview

AXIAL T1 MR

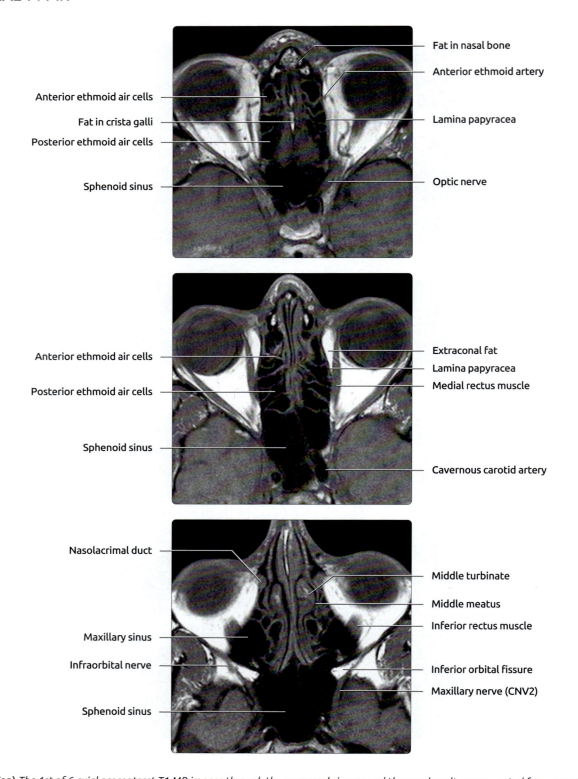

(Top) The 1st of 6 axial precontrast T1 MR images through the paranasal sinuses and the nasal vault are presented from superior to inferior. In this image, the anterior ethmoid artery is visible piercing the lamina papyracea into the anterior ethmoid air cells. The anterior ethmoidal artery (along with the vein and nerve) travels from the orbit through a canal piercing the lamina papyracea into the anterior ethmoid sinus immediately posterior to the frontal recess, crosses the sinus, and enters the anterior cranial fossa. The posterior ethmoidal foramen containing the posterior ethmoidal artery, vein, and nerve lies between the ethmoid and sphenoid bones, just posterolateral to cribriform plate of ethmoid. (Middle) In this image through the mid globes, the close relationship of the ethmoid air cells to extraconal fat and medial rectus muscle is seen. The thin lateral wall of the ethmoid sinus (lamina papyracea) is all that separates the orbit from the sinus. If the ethmoid sinuses become infected, inadequate treatment can lead to orbital infection. (Bottom) In this image through the superior portion of the maxillary sinus, the middle meatus and middle turbinate are seen in the axial plane. Note the fluid-filled normal nasolacrimal duct in the anterior aspect of the lateral nasal wall.

Sinonasal Overview

AXIAL T1 MR

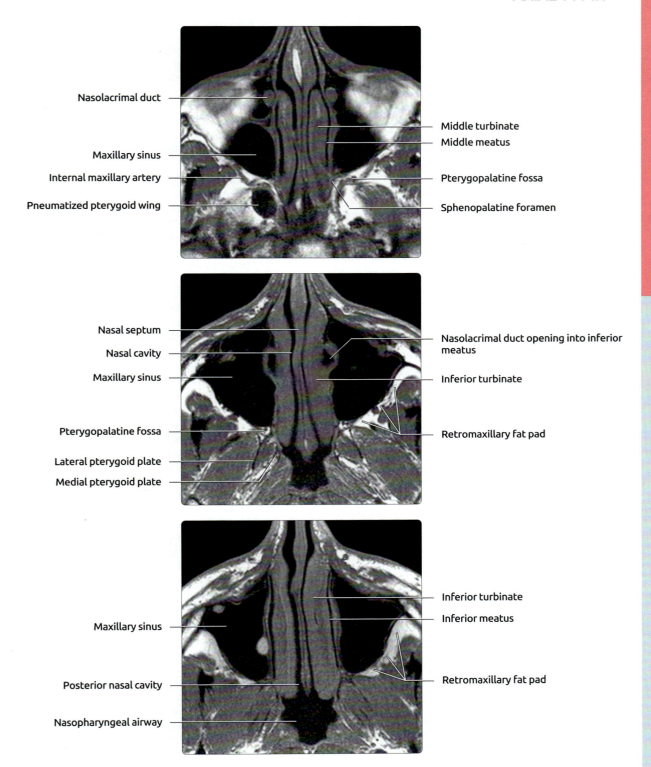

(Top) At the level of the pterygopalatine fossa, the internal maxillary artery can be seen as its principal occupant. The medial exit from the pterygopalatine fossa is the sphenopalatine foramen. Juvenile angiofibroma originates along the nasal margin of the sphenopalatine foramen. Often the 1st route of spread for this tumor is through this foramen into the pterygopalatine fossa. (Middle) In this image, the nasolacrimal duct is visible emptying inferiorly into the anterior recess of the inferior meatus. The inferior turbinate is the largest of the turbinates and can be mistaken for a mass when large and asymmetric. (Bottom) At the level of the midmaxillary sinus, the posterior nasal cavity can be seen in direct continuity with the nasopharyngeal airway. The retromaxillary fat pad sits behind the maxillary sinus. It is the superior extension of the buccal space.

Ostiomeatal Unit

TERMINOLOGY

Abbreviations

- Ostiomeatal unit (OMU), uncinate process (UP)

IMAGING ANATOMY

Overview

- OMU includes superomedial maxillary sinus, maxillary infundibulum, UP, ethmoid bulla (bulla ethmoidalis), hiatus semilunaris/middle meatus

Anatomy Relationships

- **Middle meatus** receives anterior ethmoid, maxillary, & frontal sinus drainage into crescent-shaped groove called **hiatus semilunaris** between tip of UP & ethmoid bulla
  - **Hiatus semilunaris** best seen from endoscopic vantage point; difficult to see on coronal sinus CT, but sagittal CT reconstruction somewhat demonstrates it
  - **Anterior ethmoid air cells** drain mostly into middle meatus around ethmoid bulla & some into ethmoid infundibulum
  - **Maxillary sinus** drains through maxillary ostium into ethmoid infundibulum & then into middle meatus
  - **Frontal sinus** drains through frontal recess into anterior middle meatus
    - If **UP** inserts on middle turbinate or skull base, frontal recess drains into ethmoid infundibulum & then middle meatus; hence, obstruction in infundibulum may cause combined frontal, anterior ethmoid, & maxillary sinusitis
    - If UP inserts on lamina papyracea, frontal recess drains into middle meatus directly, & ethmoid infundibulum is closed superiorly by blind-ending pouch called **recessus terminalis**; hence, infection or obstruction in infundibulum results in anterior ethmoid & maxillary sinusitis without frontal sinusitis
    - Paradoxically, presence of recessus terminalis increases incidence of frontal sinusitis, presumably due to lack of anatomic barrier between frontal recess & middle meatus against ascent of predisposing factors like allergens, irritants, & infections from nasal cavity
    - Disease in recessus terminalis can displace UP medially against middle turbinate obstructing frontal recess drainage
    - **Frontal recess**: Frontal sinus drainage funnel bordered anteriorly by agger nasi & frontal recess Kuhn cells, & posteriorly by bulla ethmoidalis & frontal bullar, suprabullar, & supraorbital ethmoid cells

Internal Contents

- **UP**: Upper medial maxillary sinus wall, projects anterosuperiorly from palate & inferior turbinate
  - Defines medial wall of maxillary (ethmoid) infundibulum & endoscopically hides hiatus semilunaris
  - UP removal (uncinectomy) is 1st step of most functional endoscopic sinus surgeries (FESS); its anterior insertion to lamina papyracea should be kept in mind to avoid medial orbital wall injury
  - Displaced laterally against orbit in maxillary sinus hypoplasia

- Nasal mass such as inverted papilloma displaces UP laterally toward orbit, while maxillary sinus mass like antrochoanal polyp displaces it medially toward nasal cavity
- **Ethmoid bulla**: Dominant anterior ethmoid air cell protruding inferomedially into ethmoid infundibulum & upper middle meatus, defining infundibular lateral wall
  - When nonpneumatized, rarely results in bony projection from lamina papyracea called **torus lateralis**
- **Middle meatus**: Space between middle turbinate & medial wall of maxillary sinus
- **Maxillary (ethmoid) infundibulum**: Drainage channel of maxillary sinus
  - Defined laterally by bulla ethmoidalis/orbit & UP medially
  - Drains into middle meatus via natural **maxillary sinus ostium**, superior border of ostium identifies orbital floor level after uncinectomy
  - **Accessory ostium** of maxillary sinus lies behind hiatus semilunaris & under ethmoid bulla in area called "posterior fontanelle" between tails of middle & inferior turbinates; can be mistaken for natural ostium during FESS if uncinectomy is incomplete
- **Potentially obstructing aeration & variants near OMU**
  - **Concha bullosa**: Aeration of nasal turbinate, most commonly **conchal cells** by ethmoid air cells invading anterior aspect of **middle turbinate**
    - When inflamed, may compress UP & obstruct OMU
    - **Complete** obstructive **OMU pattern** with frontal, maxillary, & anterior ethmoid opacification
    - **Interlamellar cells** arise from superior meatus pneumatizing vertical lamella of middle turbinate
  - **Paradoxical middle turbinate**: Middle turbinate oriented convex toward lateral nasal wall (instead of usual concave orientation) & may compress UP & obstruct OMU
  - **Turbinate sinus**: Exaggerated normal lateral concave curve of middle turbinate may envelope middle meatus; space under its concavity frequently filled by large ethmoid bulla is called turbinate sinus
  - **Haller cell** (infraorbital ethmoid air cell): Air cell located inferomedial to orbit & lateral to infundibulum
    - When inflamed, may obstruct posteroinferior infundibulum, creating **infundibular pattern** of **isolated maxillary** sinusitis
  - **Agger nasi** air cell: Most anterior ethmoid air cells
    - Found medial to lamina papyracea, adjacent to frontal recess
    - When inflamed, agger nasi air cell may obstruct frontal recess, causing **isolated** opacification of **frontal** sinus without involving anterior ethmoid or maxillary sinuses
  - **Deviated nasal septum with spurring**: May displace middle turbinate laterally, narrowing middle meatus

IMAGING RECOMMENDATIONS

CT Technique

- Unenhanced, thin 0.625-mm volumetric images with sagittal & coronal reconstructions
- No gantry tilt, & include ears, entire maxilla, tip of nose, chin, & frontal sinuses to ensure compatibility with FESS image navigation guidance systems

Ostiomeatal Unit

GRAPHICS

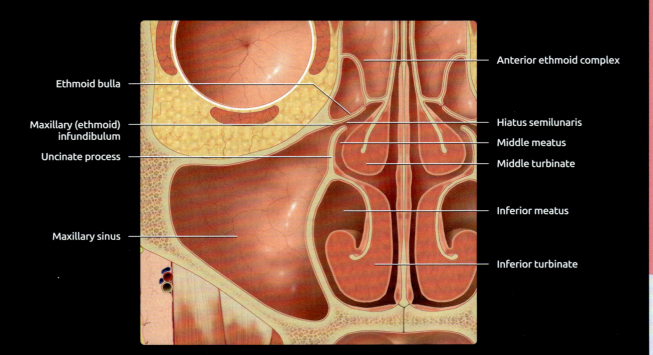

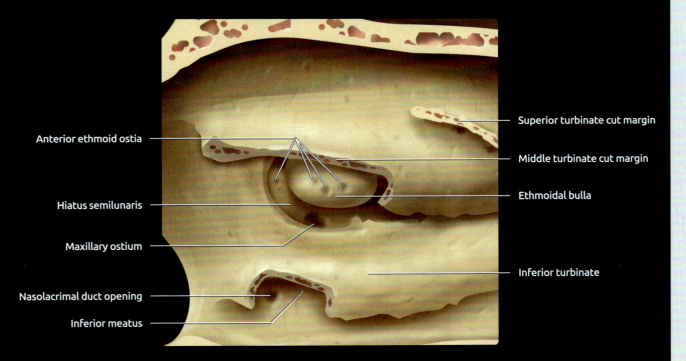

(Top) Coronal graphic of magnified right sinonasal area illustrates the important structures of the ostiomeatal unit (OMU). Note the maxillary (ethmoid) infundibulum provides drainage for the maxillary sinus, while the ethmoid bulla (dominant ethmoid air cell of the anterior ethmoid complex) protrudes inferomedially into the upper middle meatus. The middle meatus is the key area of drainage of normal secretions of the anterior ethmoid sinuses and the maxillary sinus. (Bottom) Graphic of the lateral wall of the nose focused on the region of the middle meatus with the superior turbinate removed, as well as part of the middle turbinate, is shown. Note anterior ethmoid ostia drain into the middle meatus as does the maxillary sinus via maxillary infundibulum. The nasolacrimal duct drains into the inferior meatus.

Ostiomeatal Unit

CORONAL BONE CT

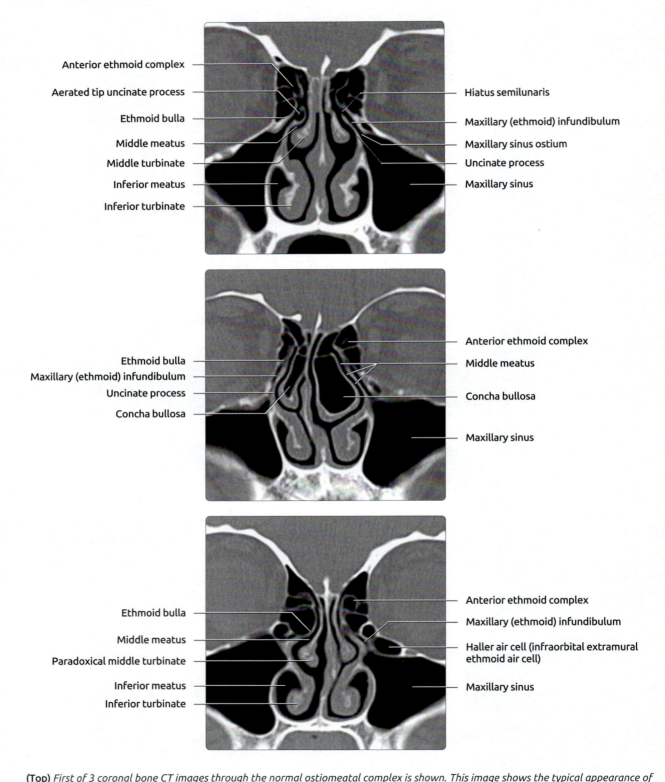

(Top) *First of 3 coronal bone CT images through the normal ostiomeatal complex is shown. This image shows the typical appearance of the maxillary (ethmoid) infundibulum and ethmoid bulla. Note the right superior tip of the uncinate process is pneumatized.* (Middle) *In this image, bilateral aerated uncomplicated concha bullosa are visible. Notice the attenuated maxillary (ethmoid) infundibulum. If the concha bullosa becomes infected (complicated), early obstruction of the middle meatus causes opacification of the ipsilateral maxillary, anterior ethmoid, and frontal sinuses (complete OMU pattern).* (Bottom) *Image through a normal OMU with Haller air cell (infraorbital air cell) seen protruding into maxillary infundibulum is shown. If the Haller cell becomes infected, it can cause an infundibular pattern of sinus disease where there is isolated maxillary sinus opacification without ethmoid or frontal sinus involvement. This happens when only the posteroinferior aspect of infundibulum is occluded, as the anterior ethmoid and frontal sinuses may also drain via the infundibulum more anterosuperiorly. Also note the bilateral paradoxical middle turbinates convex toward the lateral nasal walls (instead of usual concave orientation); this may compress the uncinate process and obstruct OMU.*

Ostiomeatal Unit

SAGITTAL BONE CT

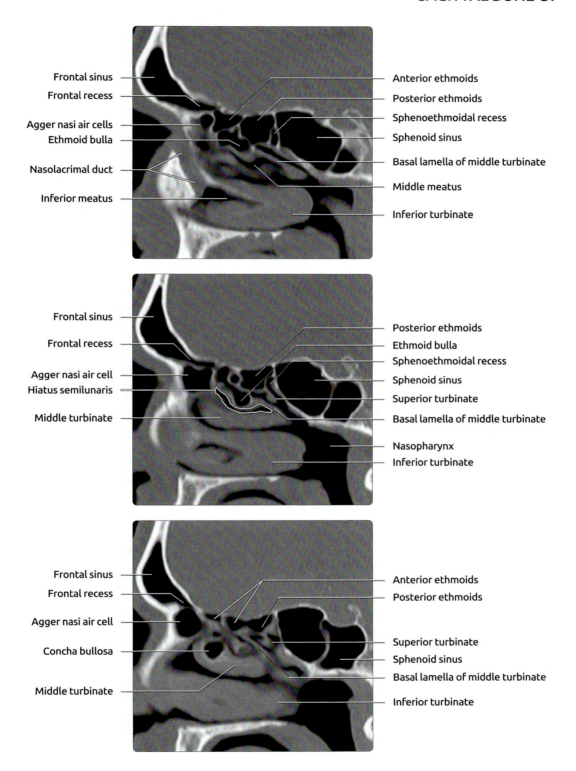

(Top) First of 3 sagittal bone CT reformations of the sinonasal region presented from lateral to medial demonstrating the structures of the OMU and its vicinity is shown. In this image, the middle meatus can be seen just inferior to the ethmoid bulla. The nasolacrimal duct is visible emptying inferiorly into the anterior aspect of the inferior meatus. (Middle) In this image, middle and inferior turbinates, as well as the basal lamella of the middle turbinate, are seen. Also note the curvilinear hiatus semilunaris. The frontal recess is visible extending around the agger nasi air cell. The sphenoethmoidal recess receives the secretions of the posterior ethmoid and sphenoid sinuses. (Bottom) Notice the air cell in the anterior middle turbinate (concha bullosa) in this image. The basal lamella of the middle turbinate is also visible.

Pterygopalatine Fossa

TERMINOLOGY

Abbreviations

- Pterygopalatine fossa (PPF)

Definitions

- PPF is small, predominantly fat-filled space located in deep face; serves as anatomic junction and neurovascular intersection between oral cavity, nasal cavity, orbit, masticator space, nasopharynx, and middle cranial fossa

IMAGING ANATOMY

Overview

- Although relatively small, PPF is clinically inaccessible and is critical landmark in head and neck imaging
- Given its anatomic relationships and multiple connections to adjacent spaces, it is important potential site of disease spread in deep face and skull base
- PPF is narrow space (fossa), roughly shaped like inverted pyramid, interposed between sinuses, oral cavity and orbit anteriorly, and central skull base posteriorly
- PPF is predominantly fat-filled but contains pterygopalatine ganglion (PPG) as well as several small nerves that communicate between sinuses, oral cavity, soft tissues of face, orbit, and central skull base foramina

Extent

- Exact margins of PPF are not defined or agreed upon in anatomic literature
- Some margins of PPF are formed by adjacent osseous structures and boundaries are relatively discrete
- However, PPF communicates with or merges with contiguous fissures and foramina; boundaries are less defined in these locations
- Anterior border: Formed from curved posterior wall of maxillary sinus
- Posterior border: Formed by base of pterygoid process superiorly and more inferiorly by ventral aspect of pterygoid process (essentially fused medial and lateral pterygoid plates)
  - Base of pterygoid process is essentially junction between inferior body of sphenoid, greater wing of sphenoid medially, and pterygoid process
- Superior recess of PPF merges with inferior orbital fissure and is ultimately contiguous with inferolateral aspect of orbital apex
- Inferior recess is funnel-shaped and tapers into vertical canal (a.k.a. pterygopalatine canal) formed at junction of palatine and maxillary bones
  - Pterygopalatine canal used synonymously with greater palatine canal since it essentially tapers to greater palatine foramen
- Medial border: Formed by perpendicular (vertical) plate of palatine bone and includes small gap in plate called sphenopalatine foramen
- Lateral boundary is formed by medial (deep) aspect of pterygomaxillary fissure

Contents, Communications, and Nerve Connections

- **Fat** is predominant tissue within PPF

- Fat is also most characteristic imaging feature that helps identify normal PPF; responsible for hypodensity on CT and hyperintensity on T1-weighted MR sequences
  - Displacement or replacement of fat by soft tissue abnormality is indication of pathology in PPF
- **Maxillary nerve (CNV2)**
  - Largest nerve directly related to PPF
  - Exits middle cranial fossa through **foramen rotundum**
  - CNV2 passes anteriorly and laterally through upper recess of PPF and enters **inferior orbital fissure**
  - After entering inferior orbital fissure, CNV2 becomes **inferior orbital nerve**
  - Provides sensory innervation to cheek, maxillary sinus, nasal cavity, and maxillary alveolar ridge
  - Number of sensory branches arise from CNV2 within PPF
    - Zygomatic nerve and posterior superior alveolar nerve
    - Includes inferior branches that pass through PPG without synapsing: Nasopalatine nerve, posterior superior nasal nerve, greater palatine nerve, lesser palatine nerve
- **PPG** is small parasympathetic ganglion within upper aspect of PPF
  - PPG receives **parasympathetic** innervation (that originates in facial nerve) via vidian nerve
  - Additional tiny nerves traverse ganglion without synapsing, including sensory innervation from CNV2 and sympathetic innervation from vidian nerve
- **Vidian nerve** is small but important mixed nerve formed in vidian canal by confluence of parasympathetic fibers from greater superficial petrosal nerve and sympathetic fibers from deep petrosal nerve
  - **Parasympathetic fibers** from superior salivatory/lacrimatory nuclei in pons pass through nervus intermedius, facial nerve, geniculate ganglion, greater superficial petrosal nerve, and **vidian** nerve to reach ganglion
    - Postganglionic fibers supply secretomotor nerves to lacrimal gland and to mucous glands of nose, paranasal sinuses, palate, and nasopharynx
  - **Sympathetic from postganglionic** fibers of superior cervical sympathetic ganglion pass through internal carotid plexus, deep petrosal nerve, and vidian nerve to reach ganglion
    - Supply vasomotor nerves to mucous membrane of nose, paranasal sinuses, palate, and nasopharynx
  - **Vidian canal**
    - Transmits vidian nerve though skull base
    - Thin, narrow canal that passes through body of sphenoid bone from proximal opening near foramen lacerum to posterior wall of PPF
    - Vidian canal is longer and narrower than foramen rotundum; positioned inferomedial to foramen rotundum
    - Vidian artery accompanies vidian nerve within canal
- **Greater palatine nerve**
  - Greater and lesser palatine nerves travel inferiorly from PPG into inferior recess of PPF and into greater palatine canal
  - Greater palatine nerve passes through greater palatine canal and exits posterolateral hard palate at greater palatine foramen

Pterygopalatine Fossa

- Provides sensory and parasympathetic fibers to ipsilateral hard palate and gingiva posterior to canine tooth
- **Greater palatine canal (pterygopalatine canal)**: Inferior canal that transmits descending palatine artery, vein, and greater and lesser palatine nerves between PPF and oral cavity
  - Formed by vertical groove on posterior part of maxillary surface of palatine bone; converted into canal by articulation with maxilla
  - Passes through maxillary and palatine bones to reach palate, ending in greater palatine foramen
  - Accessory canals branch off from this canal; known as lesser palatine canals ending in lesser palatine foramen
- **Lesser palatine nerve**
  - Like greater palatine, this nerve provides sensory and parasympathetic innervation
  - Passes inferiorly through tiny lesser palatine foramen at posterior hard palate and supplies soft palate and tonsil
- **Vascular structures**
  - **Distal internal maxillary artery** passes through masticator space, then through pterygomaxillary fissure, and into PPF
  - **Veins** accompany neurovascular bundles in PPF
  - Vascular structures can be seen normally on CT and MR as variable linear and curvilinear structures within predominantly fat-filled PPF
- **Inferior orbital fissure**
  - Superior recess of PPF merges with inferior orbital fissure
  - CNV2 passes through upper PPF and inferior orbital fissure
  - Inferior orbital fissure communicates with inferolateral aspect of orbital apex
- **Sphenopalatine foramen**
  - Perpendicular plate of palatine bone forms medial wall of PPF
  - Sphenopalatine foramen is small gap in palatine bone perpendicular plate that leads to submucosa of posterior nasal cavity
  - Represents potential communication between PPF and lateral wall of posterior nasal cavity at superior meatus
- **Pterygomaxillary fissure**: Lateral opening into nasopharyngeal masticator space, between maxilla and lateral pterygoid plate
  - Represents vertically oriented gap between posterior curved margin of maxilla and anterior curved margin of sphenoid bone
  - Fat in lateral PPF is contiguous with retromaxillary fat and fat within masticator space
  - Represents potential communication between disease in masticator space and PPF
- **Palatovaginal (palatinovaginal) canal**
  - Inconsistent short bony canal formed by articulation of sphenoidal process of palatine bone anteriorly to vaginal process of sphenoid bone posteriorly
  - Vaginal process is medial extension from upper end of medial pterygoid plate inferior to body of sphenoid to articulate with ala of vomer

- Posterior opening to roof of nasopharynx near orifice of auditory tube (transmits pterygovaginal arterial pharyngeal branches of internal maxillary artery and pharyngeal nerve from PPG); located immediately inferomedial to vidian canal

ANATOMY IMAGING ISSUES

Imaging Recommendations
- Like many lesions near skull base, CT and MR are often complimentary for comprehensive evaluation
- **CT**
  - Thin-slice bone CT with coronal and sagittal reformations best for demonstrating bony erosion or destruction involving adjacent regions of hard palate, pterygoid process, sinuses, or sphenoid bone
  - CECT can demonstrate replacement of normal fat in PPF and presence of enhancing inflammatory or neoplastic process
- **MR**
  - T1 precontrast images in axial and coronal planes best for demonstrating normal PPF fat
  - Fat-suppressed T1-weighted images with contrast best demonstrates abnormal enhancing tissue in PPF
  - Complete evaluation for perineural tumor spread (PNTS) requires imaging from distal nerve back to brainstem

Imaging Pitfalls
- Beware of fat-saturation artifact on MR; blooming at air-tissue interface may obscure PPF (or result in incomplete fat saturation) as result of maxillary sinus air
- Dental amalgam artifact may obscure subtle lesions of PPF
- There can be normal asymmetry in neurovascular structures (particularly veins) within PPF

CLINICAL IMPLICATIONS

Clinical Importance
- Primary tumors of PPF are rare (like schwannoma)
- Neoplasms involve PPF by direct invasion from adjacent space or by PNTS
- Tumors involving PPF are more difficult to treat surgically and carry worse prognosis
- Tumors in PPF can readily access central skull base and cavernous sinus by direct invasion or PNTS
- **PNTS most commonly involves CNV2**
  - **Infraorbital nerve** from cheek skin, maxillary sinus, or orbit
  - **Palatine nerves** from hard-soft palate
  - **Pharyngeal branches** from nasopharyngeal cancer along palatovaginal canal
- Intractable **epistaxis** is usually from sphenopalatine artery, but other branches of pterygopalatine internal maxillary artery may also be responsible, including enlarged **pterygovaginal artery** in palatovaginal canal seen to have descending posterior course from PPF on lateral projections of selective internal maxillary angiograms
- Pterygovaginal artery anastomoses with ascending pharyngeal and ascending palatine arteries; and may carry blood retrogradely raising probability of internal maxillary/branch arterial surgical ligation failures

Nose and Sinuses

Pterygopalatine Fossa

GRAPHICS

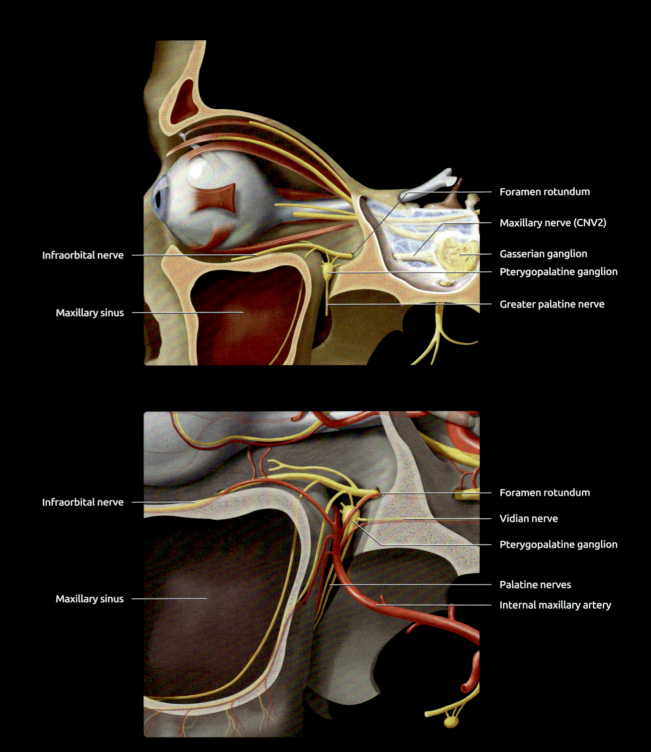

(Top) Sagittal graphic demonstrates the anatomic landscape surrounding the pterygopalatine fossa (PPF). This image shows the close relationship of the PPF to the inferior orbital foramen and its important transiting structures superiorly, as well as the vital intracranial structures posteriorly, the cavernous sinus, and Meckel cave, with the Gasserian ganglion. (Bottom) Magnified sagittal graphic demonstrates the structures traversing the PPF. This important crossroads of the deep face allows a potential pathway for disease between the orbit, sinonasal cavity, masticator space, and the intracranial cavity. The internal maxillary artery supplies the foramina surrounding the fossa, and the nervous structures are shown along their pathway from the face to the intracranial cavity through this central deep face location.

Pterygopalatine Fossa

AXIAL BONE CT

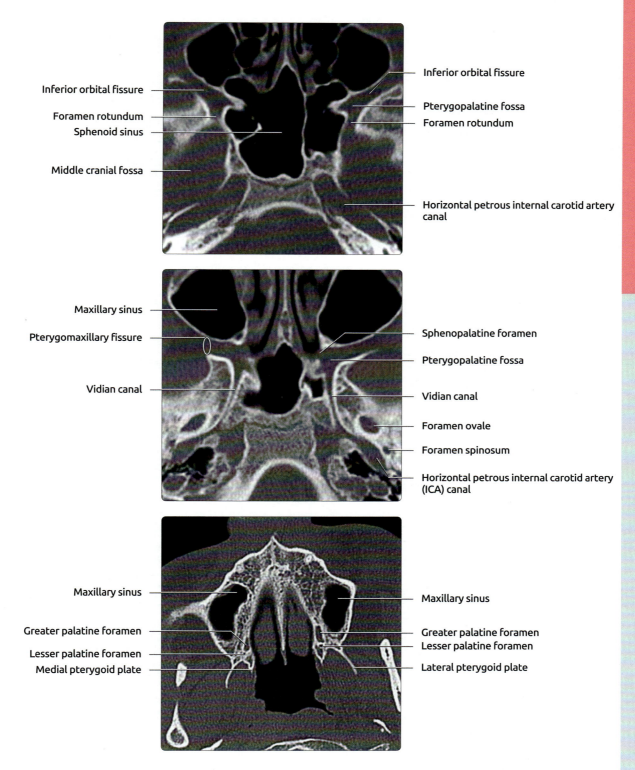

(Top) First of 3 axial bone CT images from superior to inferior shows the foramen rotundum through which the maxillary nerve traverses. (Middle) Image through PPF shows the vidian canal passing through body of sphenoid bone, connecting PPF to foramen lacerum. Foramen lacerum is the anteroinferomedial cartilaginous floor of horizontal petrous internal carotid artery (ICA) canal, between sphenoid and temporal bones. Note that the horizontal petrous ICA canal serves as a very important landmark simplifying the identification of foramen ovale and foramen spinosum lateral to the canal (likened to a high-heeled lady's shoe with the larger foramen ovale anteriorly forming the sole of the shoe, and the tiny foramen spinosum posteriorly forming its heel) and the foramen lacerum seen at its anteroinferomedial floor. Do not mistake the vidian canal for the superolateral foramen rotundum. (Bottom) This inferior image shows the greater and lesser palatine foramen, which transmit greater and lesser palatine nerves, respectively, from PPF inferiorly to palate.

Pterygopalatine Fossa

CORONAL BONE CT

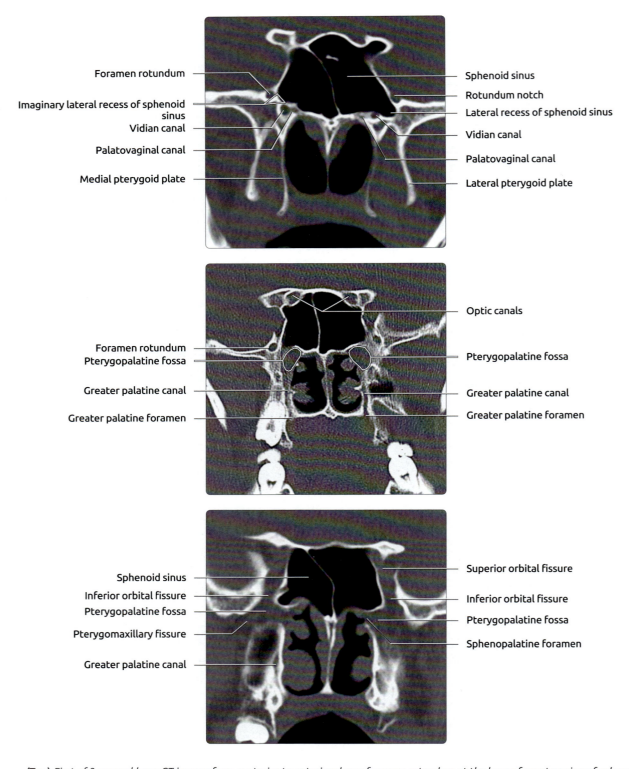

(Top) First of 3 coronal bone CT images from posterior to anterior shows foramen rotundum at the base of greater wing of sphenoid, superiorolateral to vidian canal in body of sphenoid. Practically, identify these foramina on coronal images by their relation to lateral (pterygoid) recess of sphenoid sinus, and when no lateral recess is present, draw an imaginary recess at inferolateral aspect of the sinus. Posteriorly, the inferior PPF divides into vidian canal and tiny palatovaginal canal (when present) inferomedial to it. Above mentioned, 3 foramina at posterior wall of PPF have a somewhat oblique alignment. (Middle) Image through the posterior PPF and through the vertical aspect of the greater palatine canal shows this canal connecting PPF above with greater palatine foramen below. The greater palatine nerve, which provides sensory innervation to the posterior 2/3 of the soft palate, uses greater palatine to canal to access the palate. (Bottom) Image through anterior PPF shows the communication routes to nasal vault and infratemporal fossa. Sphenopalatine foramen is covered by mucosa (site of origin of nasopharyngeal angiofibroma) but is a potential route of disease spread.

Pterygopalatine Fossa

SAGITTAL BONE CT

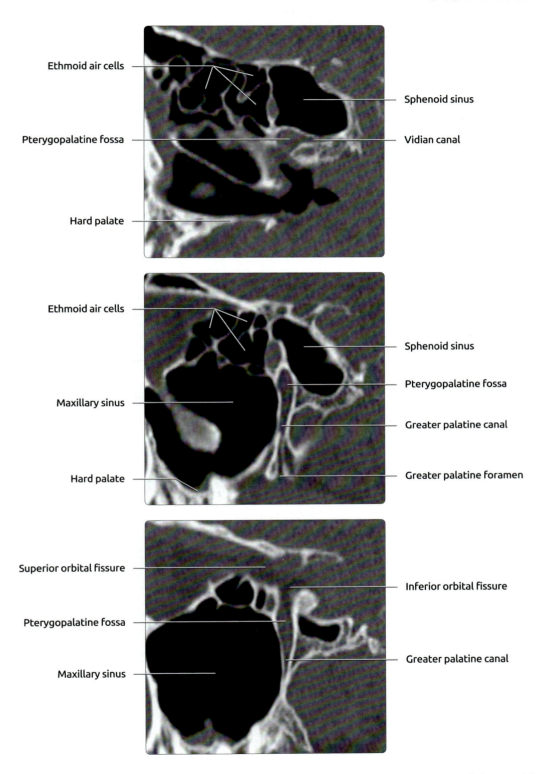

(Top) First of 3 sagittal bone CT images through the PPF from medial to lateral is shown. This image shows the medial PPF and the anterior vidian canal extending posteriorly toward the foramen lacerum. Notice the well-aerated sphenoid sinus seen immediately superior to the PPF. (Middle) This image nicely demonstrates the greater palatine canal, extending inferiorly from the PPF to the palate. This again demonstrates the importance of the PPF with potential routes of spread of disease from the oral cavity, sinonasal region, orbit, infratemporal fossa, and intracranial cavity. (Bottom) This image demonstrates the greater palatine canal, extending inferiorly from the PPF to the palate. The inferior orbital fissure is an important connection between the PPF and the orbit.

Pterygopalatine Fossa

AXIAL T1 MR

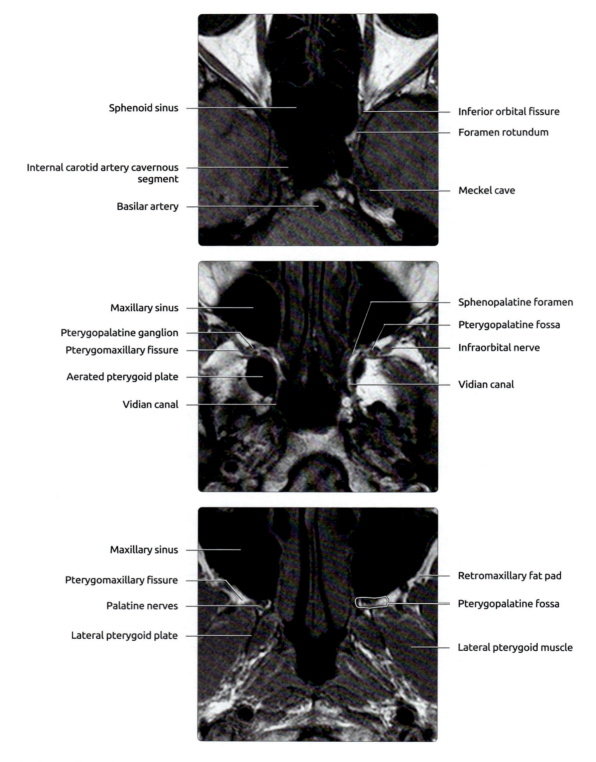

(Top) First of 3 axial T1 MR images presented from superior to inferior shows the foramen rotundum, transmitting CNV2 from cavernous sinus to PPF. The borders of the cavernous sinus are shown to be concave in this normal case, anterior to Meckel cave, containing cavernous segments of the internal carotid arteries. *(Middle)* This image shows PPF and its connections. Medially, it communicates with the nose via sphenopalatine foramen. Laterally, it communicates with the masticator space via pterygomaxillary fissure. Vidian canal connects the foramen lacerum to PPF. *(Bottom)* In this image, inferior PPF is visible with nerves and arteries seen as low-signal structures within hyperintense fat. Epistaxis is usually from sphenopalatine artery, but other internal maxillary branches may contribute, including enlarged pterygovaginal artery in palatovaginal canal.

Pterygopalatine Fossa

ANATOMIC-RADIOLOGIC CORRELATION

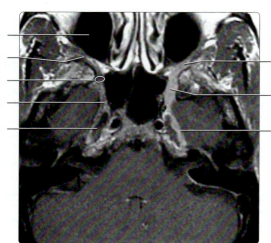

Maxillary sinus
Infraorbital nerve entering inferior orbital fissure
Foramen rotundum
Cavernous sinus
Meckel cave

Enlarged enhancing infraorbital nerve entering inferior orbital fissure
Schwannoma: Expanded CNV2 within enlarged foramen rotundum
Enhancing tissue along lateral margin of Meckel cave

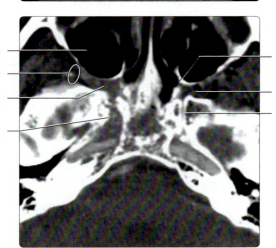

Maxillary sinus
Pterygomaxillary fissure
Enhancing tumor within pterygopalatine fossa
Expanded vidian canal secondary to perineural tumor spread

Sphenopalatine foramen
Normal fat density pterygopalatine fossa
Vidian canal

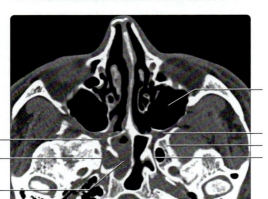

Abnormal pterygopalatine fossa
Vidian canal
Sinusitis of right sphenoid sinus

Maxillary sinus
Pterygopalatine fossa
Body of sphenoid
Vidian canal

(Top) Schwannoma of CNV2 is shown. Axial T1 C+ MR through the upper PPF demonstrates enhancing lesion along the left CNV2. Abnormal enhancement extends from the Meckel cave posterior, through the expanded foramen rotundum, and into the proximal inferior orbital fissure. (Middle) Axial CECT through the central skull base in a patient with known nasopharyngeal carcinoma and new right-sided facial pain demonstrates enhancing soft tissue within the right PPF, extending posteriorly along the vidian nerve to the foramen lacerum. CT demonstrates replacement of normal fat density in the PPF and bony erosion and widening of the right vidian canal. (Bottom) Invasive fungal sinusitis in a chemotherapy patient is shown. Axial CT through level of the mid-PPF demonstrates opacification of the sphenoid sinus indicative of sinusitis. The medial wall of the vidian canal is eroded, and there is abnormal soft tissue density infiltrating the PPF, consistent with invasion by fungal sinusitis.

Frontal Recess and Related Air Cells

TERMINOLOGY

Abbreviations

- Frontal recess (FR), agger nasi cell (AN), ethmoid bulla (EB), suprabullar cell (SBC), frontal bullar cell (FBC), supraorbital ethmoid cell (SOEC)

Definitions

- **FR**: Frontal sinus drainage pathway (inverted funnel shape) bordered anteriorly by agger nasi and FR Kuhn cells, posteriorly by bulla ethmoidalis, frontal bullar, and SBCs, and posterolaterally by SOECs

IMAGING ANATOMY

Overview

- **Frontal sinus** lies within frontal bone (right and left sinuses develop independently) with thick anterior table and thinner posterior table; medial wall is intersinus septum; thin floor corresponds to anterior aspect of orbital roof
  - Thin posterior wall and floor can be eroded by mucocele
- Funnel-shaped posteroinferomedial aspect of frontal sinus (often called **frontal infundibulum**) superiorly and inverted funnel-shaped FR inferiorly likened to "hourglass" with its waist in between at frontal sinus ostium
- **Frontal beak (nasofrontal process)** forms floor of inferior frontal sinus and is identifier for anterior landmark of **frontal sinus ostium**
- FR is formed by opposition of adjacent air cells at anteroinferior aspect of frontal bone superiorly and anterosuperior aspect of ethmoid bone inferiorly
- Upper border of FR is frontal sinus ostium; inferior drainage from FR can be either to **middle meatus** directly or via **ethmoid infundibulum**

Extent

- If uncinate process turns laterally to insert on **lamina papyracea**, FR drains into middle meatus directly, and ethmoid infundibulum is closed superiorly by blind-ending pouch called **recessus terminalis**
- If uncinate process turns medially to insert on **middle turbinate** or runs superiorly to insert on **skull base**, FR drains into ethmoid infundibulum and then middle meatus

Anatomy Relationships

- Anteriorly: AN below and Kuhn cells above
- Laterally: Lamina papyracea (or intervening AN and Kuhn cells when present)
- Posterolaterally: SOEC when present
- Medially: Middle turbinate vertical portion
- Posteriorly: EB and SBC and FBC when present

Internal Contents

- **Middle and posterior portions of basal lamella of middle turbinate**: Extend laterally to join lamina papyracea and divides anterior from posterior ethmoid air cells
  - EB, SBC, and FBC are intramural anterior ethmoid air cells anterior to basal lamella of middle turbinate and form posterior boundary of FR
  - Posterior margin of basal lamella attaches to perpendicular plate of palatine bone

- Vertical portion of basal lamella attaches to cribriform plate of ethmoid and is best seen in coronal CT; it is very delicate and its detachment at surgery in this region could damage dura with resultant CSF leak
- **EB (bulla ethmoidalis)**: Dominant anterior ethmoid air cell formed by pneumatization of bulla lamella (seen anterior to basal lamella of middle turbinate)
  - Forms lateral margin of ethmoid infundibulum and posterior margin of FR
- **SBCs**: Anterior ethmoid cells seen above EB; extends behind FR but lies entirely below level of frontal sinus ostium (no extension into frontal sinus); superior wall is skull base
  - CT correlate of suprabullar recess, which is seen as cleft above EB when viewed endoscopically
- **Suprabullar and retrobullar recesses**: Previously less correctly called sinus lateralis or lateral sinus of Grunwald; located between ethmoid roof superiorly, EB anteriorly and inferiorly, lamina papyracea laterally, and basal lamella of middle turbinate posteriorly
  - These recesses are typically separated by bony crest or mucosal projection from basal lamella of middle turbinate to EB
  - Recesses communicate medially with middle meatus through hiatus semilunaris superior
  - Suprabullar recess separated from FR by bulla lamella/EB reaching and attaching to skull base; 2 recesses do not typically communicate with FR
  - FR may rarely drain directly into suprabullar recess when bulla lamella/EB does not extend to skull base
  - Anterior ethmoidal artery (AEA) is located at roof of suprabullar recess in majority (85%)
- **FBCs**: Anterior ethmoid cells above EB; extends behind FR and **also into frontal sinus** above frontal sinus ostium; posterosuperior wall is skull base
- Both SBC and FBC may be mistaken for skull base during endoscopic surgery resulting in incomplete surgical dissection; their presence should be determined before surgery by assessing preoperative scans
- **SOECs**: Anterior ethmoid air cells that extend superolaterally over orbit from FR and are seen posterolateral to FR; its posterior wall is skull base
  - Pneumatization of orbital plate of frontal bone posterior to frontal sinus and posterolateral to FR; its ostium can be mistaken for frontal sinus ostium during FESS
  - Transillumination of SOEC with telescope during FESS shows transmitted light in inner canthal area, while that of frontal sinus shows light in supraorbital area
  - Drain into lateral aspect of FR; SOEC ostium seen just anterior to AEA canal in sequential coronal CT scan images
  - SOEC can be mistaken for septated frontal sinus in coronal images, but can be differentiated by its location posterior to frontal sinus separated by horizontally oriented septum in axial images
  - **AEA** runs in **anterior ethmoidal notch (foramen)** along medial orbital wall (lamina papyracea); crosses anterior ethmoid air cells in bony canal called **anterior ethmoidal canal**; AEA enters anterior cranial fossa at a point in lateral lamella of cribriform plate called **ethmoidal sulcus**

Frontal Recess and Related Air Cells

- AEA found endoscopically by tracing anterior wall of EB towards ethmoid roof and is 11 mm (range 6-15 mm) behind posterior wall of FR (in suprabullar recess in 85%); usually in contact with skull base, but not infrequently 1-3 mm below skull base within bony mesentery
- **Anterior ethmoidal canal** is ~ 8 mm in length with 40% showing partial or total bony dehiscence especially inferiorly; posterior ethmoidal artery is located ~ 10 mm behind AEA
- **AEA** runs obliquely in skull base behind anterior wall of EB, where skull base turns from vertical (posterior frontal sinus wall) to horizontal (cribriform plate of ethmoid); **intact bulla technique** for FR surgery can protect AEA
- If anterior wall of EB does not reach skull base and there is suprabullar recess, then AEA may be damaged even with intact bulla technique
- SOEC immediately above anterior ethmoidal notch predisposes anterior ethmoid artery at risk during FESS, since artery travels freely within ethmoid sinus/suprabullar recess
- If no SOEC, then anterior ethmoidal notch abuts fovea ethmoidalis/lateral lamella of cribriform plate, and artery is considered relatively protected during FESS
- AEA injury can lead to rapidly enlarging retroorbital hematoma due to retraction of transected artery into orbit
- Cut AEA should be prophylactically cauterized to avoid enlarging orbital hematoma
- **Interfrontal sinus septal cell**: Pneumatized interfrontal sinus septum; can extend into crista galli when extensive
  - Drain into medial aspect of FR and can obstruct frontal sinus ostium
- **AN** Latin for "nasal mound"; most anterior ethmoid air cell that involve lacrimal bone or frontal process of maxilla; forms anterior and lateral boundary of FR inferiorly
  - Key to surgical access to FR; open AN and palpate with probe to identify posterior wall of frontal sinus away from and in front of AEA for good safe visualization of frontal sinus
- **FR Kuhn cells**: Forms anterior and lateral boundary of FR superiorly
  - **Types 1 to 3** Kuhn cells are FR air cells seen **above AN** (type 1 single and type 2 multiple in FR, and type 3 single reaching sinus); but **type 4** is single isolated cell within frontal sinus **not abutting AN**
  - Type 1: Single cell above AN; posterior wall is free partition in FR
  - Type 2: Tier of 2 or more cells above AN; posterior wall is free partition in FR
  - Type 3: Single large cell above AN; extends superiorly into frontal infundibulum/sinus proper, posterior wall is free partition in FR and frontal sinus
  - FBC also extends from FR into frontal sinus and cannot be differentiated in coronal CT from type 3 Kuhn cell
  - In sagittal images, posterosuperior wall of FBC (posterior to FR) is skull base, whereas that of type 3 Kuhn cell (anterior to FR) is free partition in FR and frontal sinus, with air gap of frontal sinus between it and skull base
  - Type 4: Rare isolated cell in frontal sinus; anterior or inferior margin is anterior table or floor of frontal sinus; posterior wall is free partition in frontal sinus

- Called "cell within cell"; sometimes isolated aerated type 4 cell may be seen with opacification of surrounding diseased frontal sinus
- **Modified Kuhn classification** defines type 3 cell as extending up from FR above frontal beak but < 50% of vertical height of frontal sinus, whereas type 4 cell extends from FR into frontal sinus > 50% of its height

ANATOMY IMAGING ISSUES

Imaging Pitfalls

- Sagittal images to be reviewed in addition to coronal and axial images for FR anatomy and presence/disease of AN and Kuhn cells anteriorly; intersinus septal cell medially; EB, SBC, FBC posteriorly and SOEC posterolaterally
- Failure to identify may lead to incomplete failed FESS in FR

CLINICAL IMPLICATIONS

Clinical Importance

- Primary surgery of FR is usually avoided initially and primary surgery of anterior ethmoid/ostiomeatal unit (OMU) done 1st to reduce risk of injury to critical structures adjacent to FR like orbit, anterior ethmoid artery, and floor of anterior cranial fossa; and susceptibility of FR region to postsurgical scar formation
- Frontal sinus surgeries are mostly revision procedures after failed OMU surgeries like uncinectomy, anterior ethmoidectomy, middle meatal antrostomy and septoplasty
- Anterior ethmoid/OMU surgeries usually enough to clear FR and frontal sinus disease
- Small **size of FR** limits enlargement of frontal sinus drainage pathway during frontal sinus FESS and more extensive frontal sinusotomy will have to be done; size of FR should be evaluated in preoperative scans
- Frontal beak (nasofrontal process) anterior to frontal sinus ostium has no important structure in it and hence drilling anterior to frontal ostium with angled burr is relatively safe, whereas posterior margin of frontal sinus ostium should be never breached as it is closely related to cribriform plate and anterior cranial fossa
- **Inadequate removal** of AN or other anterior (Kuhn), medial (intersinus cell), posterior (EB, SBC, FBC) or posterolateral (SOEC) air cells in relation to FR is most common cause of failed FESS in this location
  - Residual air cells obstruct FR and also serve as scaffold for scar tissue formation
- Disease in recessus terminalis in cases where inferior FR drains into middle meatus directly (when uncinate process turns laterally to insert on lamina papyracea) can displace uncinate process medially towards FR
  - **Retained medialized uncinate process** predispose to FR restenosis after FESS
- **Lateralized middle turbinate** amputated anterior stump may obstruct FR after FESS
- **Bolgerization**: Process of medialization of middle turbinate by surgically creating small abrasions on its medial aspect and adjacent nasal septum, to correct floppy lateralized middle turbinate rather than resecting it
  - Medialized middle turbinate is normal expected postsurgical finding in this scenario

Nose and Sinuses

Frontal Recess and Related Air Cells

CORONAL AND SAGITTAL GRAPHICS OF TYPE 1 AND 2 KUHN CELLS

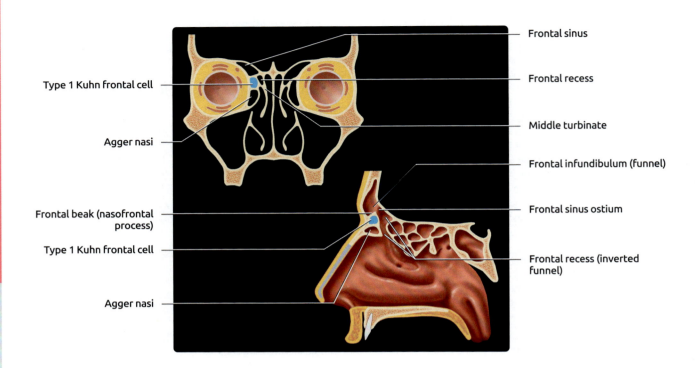

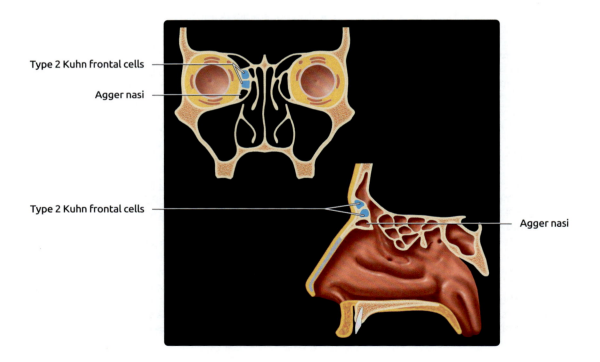

(Top) *Graphics show frontal sinus drainage pathway anatomy and a right type 1 Kuhn frontal cell. The frontal sinus drainage is through the funnel-shaped posteroinferomedial frontal sinus (often called frontal infundibulum) superiorly and the inverted funnel-shaped frontal recess (FR) inferiorly; together they resemble an hourglass with the waist in between at the frontal sinus ostium. The frontal beak (nasofrontal process) forms the floor of the inferior frontal sinus and serves as the anterior landmark of the frontal sinus ostium. The FR is bordered anterolaterally by agger nasi and FR Kuhn cells, posteriorly by the bulla ethmoidalis and frontal bullar and suprabullar cells, and posterolaterally by the supraorbital ethmoid cells (SOEC). The upper border of the FR is the frontal sinus ostium and its inferior drainage can be either to the middle meatus directly or via the ethmoid infundibulum according to attachment pattern of the uncinate process. Type 1 Kuhn cell is a single cell above agger nasi.* (Bottom) *Graphics show type 2 Kuhn cells, a tier of 2 or more cells above agger nasi. The posterior walls of both type 1 and II Kuhn cells are free partitions in the FR.*

Frontal Recess and Related Air Cells

CORONAL AND SAGITTAL GRAPHICS OF TYPE 3 AND 4 KUHN CELLS

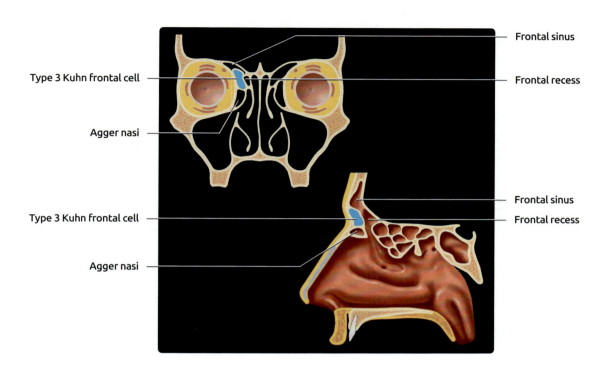

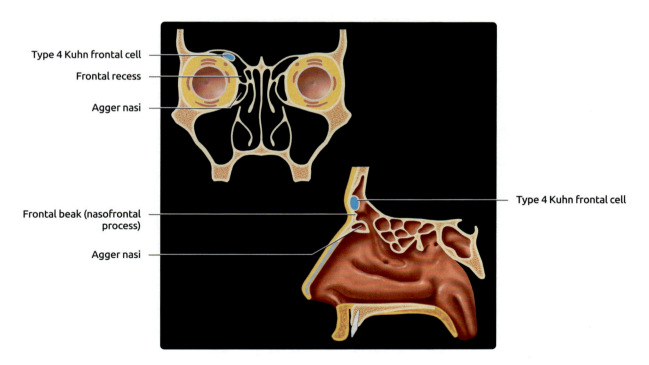

(Top) Graphics show a type 3 Kuhn frontal cell, a single large cell above agger nasi. It extends superiorly beyond the FR into the frontal infundibulum/sinus proper. The posterior wall of a type 3 cell is a free partition in the FR and frontal sinus. (Bottom) Graphics show a type 4 Kuhn frontal cell, a rare isolated cell in the frontal sinus. Its anterior or inferior margin is formed by the anterior table or floor of the frontal sinus and the posterior wall is a free partition in the frontal sinus. Note that types 1-3 Kuhn cells are FR air cells seen above agger nasi (type 1 single and type 2 multiple in FR, and type 3 single reaching sinus) and form the anterior and lateral boundary of the FR superiorly, whereas type 4 is a single isolated cell within the frontal sinus not abutting agger nasi air cell.

Frontal Recess and Related Air Cells

CORONAL AND SAGITTAL GRAPHICS OF SUPRABELLAR CELLS AND BULLAR CELLS

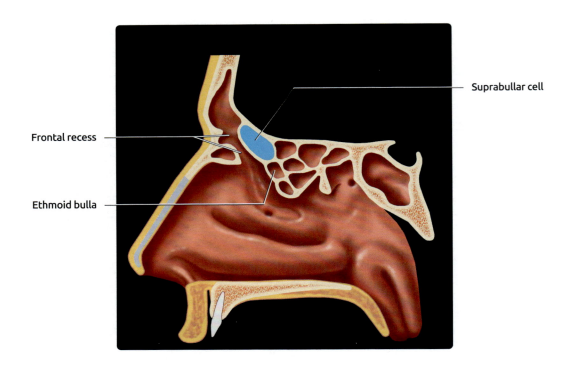

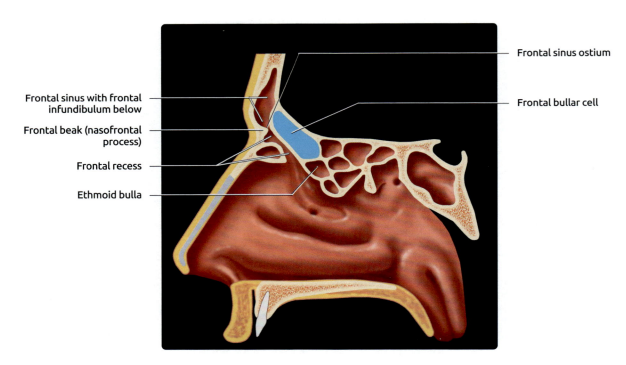

(Top) Sagittal graphic shows a suprabullar air cell. Suprabullar cells are anterior ethmoid air cells seen above the bulla ethmoidalis extending behind the FR and lying entirely below the level of frontal sinus ostium (with no extension into the frontal sinus); its superior wall is the skull base. A suprabullar cell is the CT scan correlate of a suprabullar recess, which is seen as a cleft above the ethmoid bulla when viewed endoscopically. (Bottom) Sagittal graphic shows a frontal bullar cell. Frontal bullar cells are also anterior ethmoid air cells above the bulla ethmoidalis extending behind the FR, but unlike suprabullar cells, extend into the frontal sinus above the frontal sinus ostium; its posterosuperior wall is also the skull base. Both suprabullar and frontal bullar cells may be mistaken for the skull base during endoscopic surgery, resulting in incomplete surgical dissection. Their presence should be determined before surgery by assessing preoperative scans.

Frontal Recess and Related Air Cells

CORONAL GRAPHICS

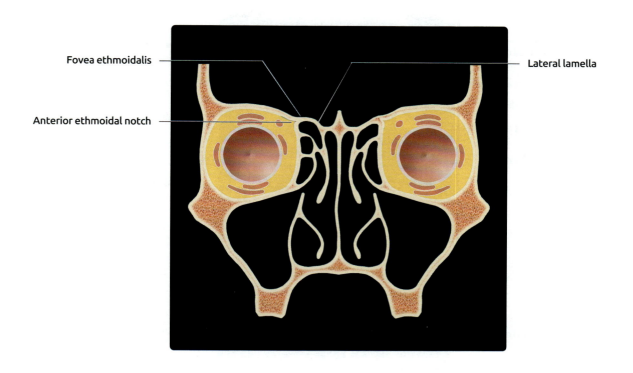

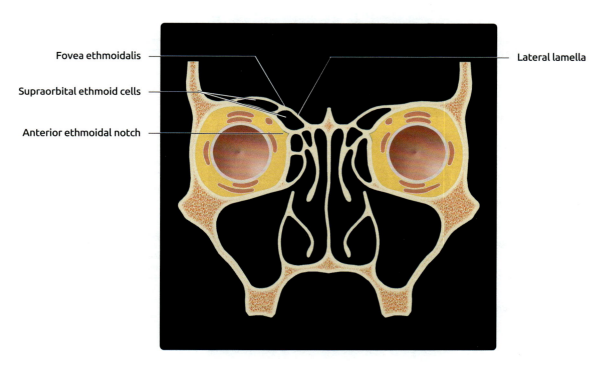

(Top) Graphic shows the anterior ethmoidal notch (containing the anterior ethmoid artery) abutting the fovea ethmoidalis/lateral lamella of the cribriform plate. The anterior ethmoid artery is considered relatively protected during FESS with this anatomy. (Bottom) Graphic shows SOEC immediately above the anterior ethmoidal notch. This anatomy predisposes anterior ethmoid artery injury risk during FESS, since the artery travels freely within the air cells, ethmoid sinus/suprabullar recess. SOEC are anterior ethmoid air cells that extend superolaterally over the orbit from the FR and are seen posterolateral to the FR. They are formed by pneumatization of the orbital plate of the frontal bone posterior to the frontal sinus and posterolateral to FR. SOECs drain into the lateral aspect of the FR; SOEC ostium is seen just anterior to the anterior ethmoidal artery canal in sequential coronal CT images. The ostium can be mistaken for the frontal sinus ostium during FESS.

Frontal Recess and Related Air Cells

SAGITTAL AND CORONAL BONE CT

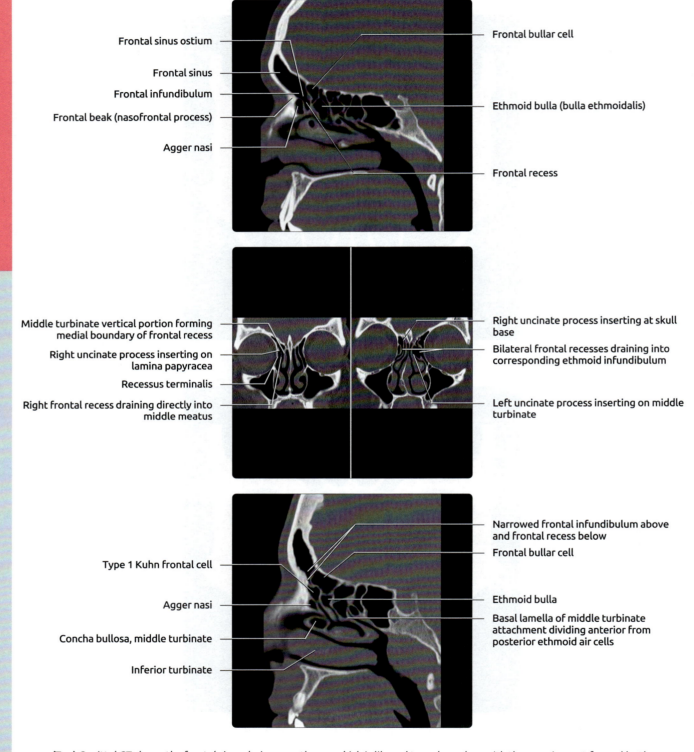

(Top) Sagittal CT shows the frontal sinus drainage pathway, which is likened to an hourglass with the superior part formed by the funnel-shaped posteroinferomedial frontal sinus and inferior part by the inverted funnel-shaped FR; the waist of the hourglass is at frontal sinus ostium level. The frontal beak (the nasofrontal process) is the anterior landmark of the frontal sinus ostium. The FR is bordered anterolaterally by agger nasi and Kuhn cells (no Kuhn cells are present here). (Middle) Coronal CT images show inferior drainage of the FR. If uncinate process (UP) turns laterally to insert on lamina papyracea, the FR drains into the middle meatus directly, and the ethmoid infundibulum is closed superiorly by a blind-ending pouch called "recessus terminalis" (labeled on right side of 1st patient). If UP runs superiorly to insert on the skull base (labeled on right side of 2nd patient, not labeled on left side of 1st patient) or turns medially to insert on middle turbinate (labeled on left side of 2nd patient), the FR drains into the ethmoid infundibulum and then the middle meatus. (Bottom) Sagittal CT shows a type 1 Kuhn cell, a single cell above agger nasi.

Frontal Recess and Related Air Cells

SAGITTAL BONE CT

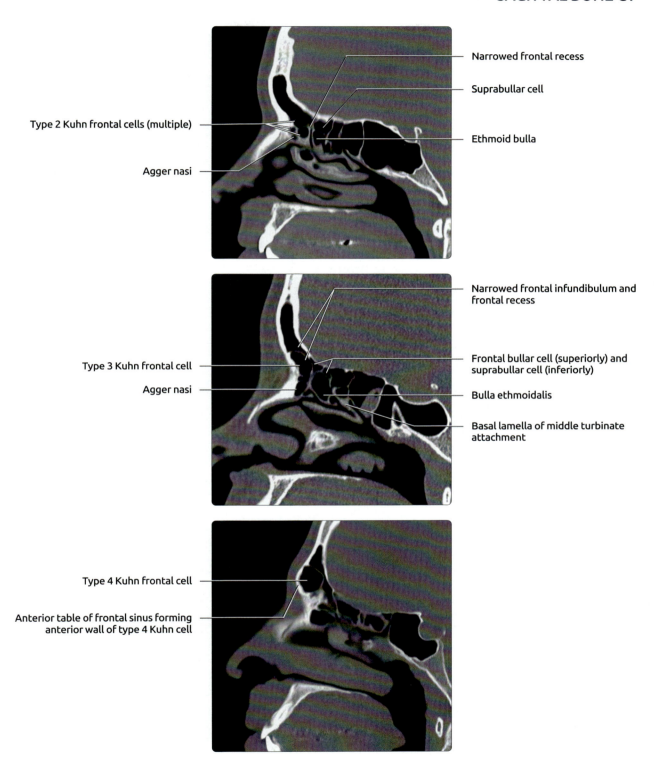

(Top) Sagittal CT shows type 2 Kuhn frontal cells. Kuhn cells form anterior and lateral boundary of the superior aspect of FR. Types 1-3 Kuhn cells are FR air cells just above agger nasi, but type 4 is a single, isolated cell within frontal sinus not abutting agger nasi. Type 1 is single and type 2 are multiple cells in FR, whereas a type 3 cell is a single air cell in FR extending superiorly into frontal infundibulum/frontal sinus proper. (Middle) Sagittal CT shows a type 3 Kuhn frontal cell. Its posterior wall is a free partition in FR and frontal infundibulum/frontal sinus and can narrow these structures from anterior aspect. In contrast, frontal bullar cell narrows FR and frontal infundibulum/frontal sinus from its posterior aspect; suprabullar cell narrows only FR from posterior aspect. (Bottom) Sagittal CT shows a type 4 Kuhn cell, a rare isolated cell in frontal sinus. Its anterior/inferior margin is anterior table/floor of frontal sinus; the posterior wall is a free partition in sinus. Note: "Modified Kuhn classification" defines type 3 cells as extending up from FR above frontal beak but < 50% of vertical height of frontal sinus, whereas type 4 cells extends from FR into frontal sinus > 50% of its height.

Frontal Recess and Related Air Cells

CORONAL, AXIAL, AND SAGITTAL BONE CT

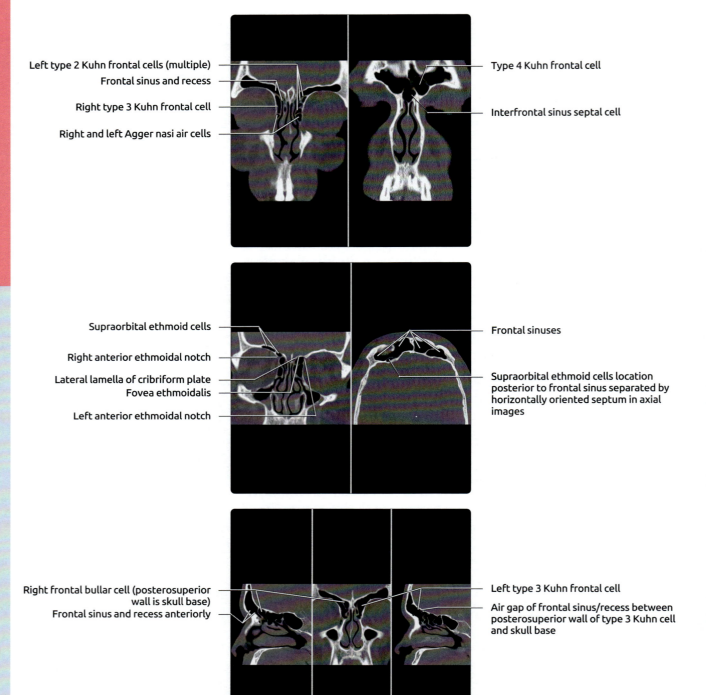

(Top) Coronal CT on the right shows types 1-3 Kuhn cells lie lateral to FR, just above Agger nasi. Coronal CT on the left shows interfrontal sinus septal cell; it can extend into crista galli when extensive. It drains into medial aspect of FR and can obstruct frontal sinus ostium. Also shown is a left type 4 Kuhn cell. **(Middle)** Coronal CT shows SOECs immediately above anterior ethmoidal notch on right; this predisposes anterior ethmoid artery injury at FESS. Anterior ethmoid artery is relatively safer on left without SOECs, where anterior ethmoidal notch abuts fovea ethmoidalis/lateral lamella. SOECs can mimic a septated frontal sinus in coronal CT, but axial CT shows its location posterior to frontal sinus separated by a horizontally oriented septum. **(Bottom)** Coronal and sagittal CT images show a right frontal bullar cell and a larger left type 3 Kuhn cell. Both extend from FR into frontal sinus and cannot be differentiated on coronal CT. In sagittal images, posterosuperior wall of frontal bullar cell (posterior to FR) is skull base; whereas that of a type 3 Kuhn cell (anterior to FR) is a free partition in FR and frontal sinus with an air gap of frontal sinus/recess between it and skull base.

Frontal Recess and Related Air Cells

CORONAL, AXIAL, AND SAGITTAL BONE CT

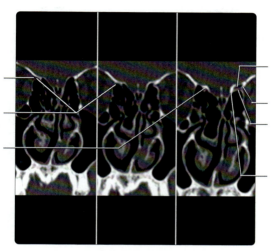

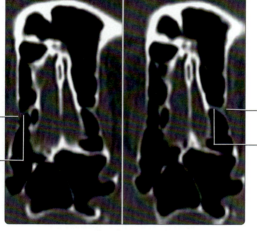

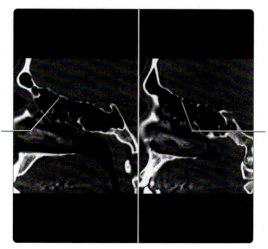

(Top) Coronal CT images from posterior to anterior show the course of anterior ethmoid arteries that run in anterior ethmoidal notch along medial orbital wall, crossing anterior ethmoid cells in anteromedial oblique bony canal called the anterior ethmoidal canal and then entering anterior cranial fossa at a point in lateral lamella of the cribriform plate (near its junction with fovea ethmoidalis) called the ethmoidal sulcus. Anterior ethmoid cell is ~ 8 mm long, with 40% showing some bony dehiscence, and lies ~ 11 mm (range: 6-15 mm) behind posterior wall of the FR (in suprabullar recess in 85%). It is usually in contact with skull base (right side), but is sometimes 1-3 mm below skull base within a bony mesentery (left side). Anterior ethmoid artery usually lies well posterior to anterior wall of the ethmoid bulla, so "intact bulla" technique for FR surgery can protect it to some extent. (Middle) Axial CT images (same patient) show bilateral anterior ethmoidal notches and canals containing anterior ethmoidal arteries. (Bottom) Sagittal CT images show right anterior ethmoidal canal in contact with skull base and the left canal hanging down a few mm below skull base within a bony mesentery.

SECTION 5
Suprahyoid and Infrahyoid Neck

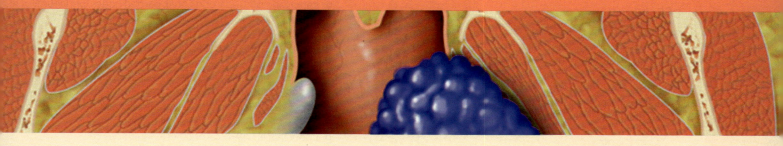

Suprahyoid and Infrahyoid Neck Overview	**272**
Parapharyngeal Space	**290**
Pharyngeal Mucosal Space	**298**
Masticator Space	**310**
Parotid Space	**320**
Carotid Space	**332**
Retropharyngeal Space	**340**
Perivertebral Space	**348**
Posterior Cervical Space	**356**
Visceral Space	**364**
Larynx	**372**
Hypopharynx	**392**
Thyroid and Parathyroid Anatomy	**402**
Cervical Trachea and Esophagus	**416**
Cervical Lymph Nodes	**426**
Facial Muscles and Superficial Musculoaponeurotic System	**440**

Suprahyoid and Infrahyoid Neck Overview

TERMINOLOGY

Abbreviations
- Suprahyoid neck (SHN); infrahyoid neck (IHN)

Definitions
- SHN: Spaces from skull base to hyoid bone (excluding orbit, sinuses, & oral cavity) including parapharyngeal (PPS), pharyngeal mucosal (PMS), masticator (MS), parotid (PS), carotid (CS), buccal (BS), retropharyngeal (RPS), & perivertebral (PVS)
- IHN: Spaces below level of hyoid bone with some continuing into mediastinum including visceral space (VS), posterior cervical space (PCS), anterior cervical space (ACS), CS, RPS, & PVS

IMAGING ANATOMY

Overview
- **Key** to understanding SHN & IHN spaces is **fascia**
- 3 layers of deep cervical fascia cleave neck into spaces
  - **Superficial layer, deep cervical fascia (SL-DCF)**
    - SHN: Around MS & PS; part of carotid sheath
    - IHN: Invests neck by surrounding strap, sternocleidomastoid & trapezius muscles
  - **Middle layer, deep cervical fascia (ML-DCF)**
    - SHN: ML-DCF defines PMS deep margin; contributes to carotid sheath
    - IHN: Circumscribes VS; part of carotid sheath
  - **Deep layer, deep cervical fascia (DL-DCF)**
    - SHN & IHN: Surrounds perivertebral space
    - SHN & IHN: Contributes to carotid sheath
    - SHN & IHN: **Alar fascia** is slip of DL-DCF forming posterior wall of RPS separating true RPS from DS

Spaces of Suprahyoid & Infrahyoid Neck
- **Parapharyngeal space**
  - Location: SHN from skull base to posterior submandibular space
  - Contents: Fat, veins of pharyngeal & pterygoid plexuses
  - Importance: Pattern of displacement helps define SHN mass space of origin
- **Pharyngeal mucosal space**
  - Location: SHN space medial to PPS, anterior to RPS
  - Contents: Mucosa, minor salivary glands, PMS lymphatic ring, constrictor muscles
    - Nasopharyngeal, oropharyngeal, & hypopharyngeal mucosal surfaces
    - PMS of nasopharynx: Torus tubarius, adenoids, superior constrictor, & levator palatini muscles
    - PMS of oropharynx: Anterior & posterior tonsillar pillars, palatine & lingual tonsils, soft palate
  - Fascia: ML-DCF on nonairway side of PMS
  - Importance: Squamous cell carcinoma & NHL here
- **Masticator space**
  - Location: Anterolateral to PPS in SHN
  - Contents: Ramus & condyle of mandible, CNV3, masseter, medial & lateral pterygoid & temporalis muscles, pterygoid venous plexus
  - Fascia: MS surrounded by SL-DCF
  - Importance: Perineural tumor on CNV3; sarcoma
- **Parotid space**
  - Location: Lateral to PPS in SHN
  - Contents: Parotid gland, extracranial CNVII, nodes, retromandibular vein, external carotid artery
  - Fascia: PS surrounded by SL-DCF
  - Importance: Intraparotid CNVII; parotid nodes; perineural tumor on CNVII
- **Carotid space**
  - Location: Posterior to PPS in SHN; lateral to VS & RPS in IHN
    - Begins at inferior jugular foramen & carotid canal of skull base; extends to aortic arch
  - Contents: CNIX-XII, internal jugular vein, carotid artery
  - Fascia: All 3 layers, deep cervical fascia
  - Importance: CNX & carotid here; squamous cell carcinoma nodes along superficial margin
- **Retropharyngeal space**
  - Location: Posterior to PMS in SHN & VS in IHN
    - Begins at clivus; traverses SHN-IHN to T3 (variable C6-T6) level where alar fascia fuse to ML-DCF
  - Contents: Nodes & fat in SHN; no nodes in IHN
  - Fascia: Anterior fascia is ML-DCF, posterior fascia is DL-DCF (alar fascia)
  - Importance: Inferior communication with DS allows infection access to mediastinum
- **Danger space**
  - Posterior to RPS in SHN & IHN; continues inferiorly into mediastinum & to level of diaphragm
- **Perivertebral space**
  - Location: Behind RPS & around spine in SHN & IHN
    - Defined from skull base above to clavicle below
  - Contents: Prevertebral & paraspinal components
    - Prevertebral: Vertebral body, veins & arteries, prevertebral & scalene muscles, brachial plexus, & phrenic nerve
    - Paraspinal: Posterior elements of vertebra, levator scapulae, & paraspinal muscles
  - Fascia: Surrounded by DL-DCF
    - Divided by DL-DCF slip into prevertebral & paraspinal components
  - Importance: PVS malignancy may be epidural
- **Visceral space**
  - Location: IHN only; extends into mediastinum
  - Contents: Thyroid & parathyroids, paratracheal nodes, esophagus, trachea, recurrent laryngeal nerve
  - Fascia: VS surrounded by ML-DCF
  - Importance: Trachea & esophagus traverse VS
- **Posterior cervical space**
  - Location: SHN PCS begins at mastoid tip, extends to clavicle; most PCS volume in IHN
  - Contents: Fat, CNXI, spinal accessory nodes
  - Fascia: Between SL- & DL-DCF
  - Importance: Spinal accessory nodal diseases

Key Spatial Relationships
- **SHN spaces surrounding PPS**
  - Medial is PMS: PMS mass displaces PPS laterally
  - Anterior is MS: MS mass displaces PPS posteriorly
  - Lateral is PS: PS mass displaces PPS medially
  - Posterior is CS: CS mass displaces PPS anteriorly
  - Posteromedial is lateral RPS: Lateral RPS nodal mass displaces PPS anterolaterally

Suprahyoid and Infrahyoid Neck Overview

GRAPHICS

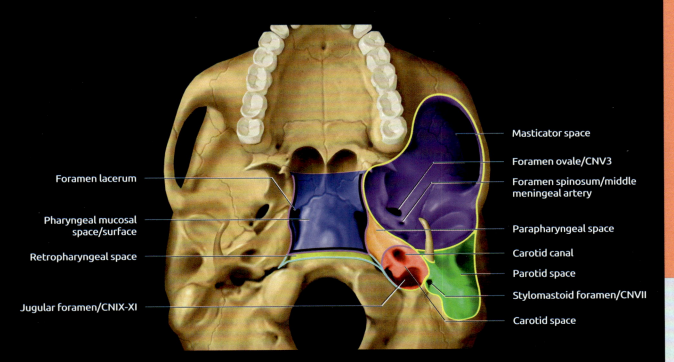

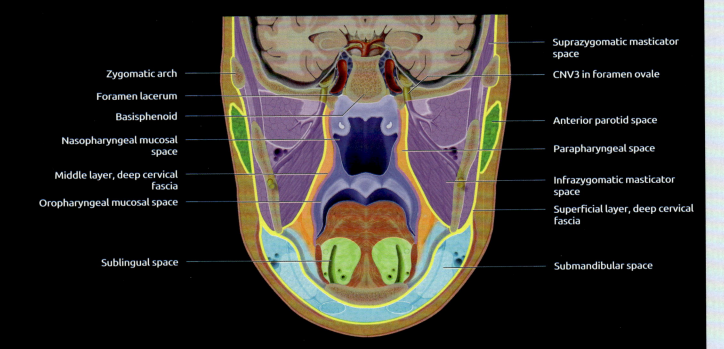

(Top) *Graphic of skull base from below shows spaces of suprahyoid neck with relationship to skull base. Four spaces have key interactions with skull base: Masticator (MS), parotid (PS), carotid (CS), and pharyngeal mucosal spaces (PMS). PS (green) malignancy can follow CNVII into stylomastoid foramen. MS (purple) receives CNV3 while CNIX-XII enter the CS (red). The PMS abuts the foramen lacerum, which is covered by fibrocartilage in life. Also note that the superficial layer of deep cervical fascia (yellow line) surrounds the MS and PS, and middle layer is on nonairway side of PMS (pink line).* **(Bottom)** *Coronal graphic shows suprahyoid neck spaces as they interact with the skull base. The MS has the largest area of abutment with the skull base, including CNV3. The PMS abuts the basisphenoid and foramen lacerum.*

Suprahyoid and Infrahyoid Neck Overview

GRAPHICS

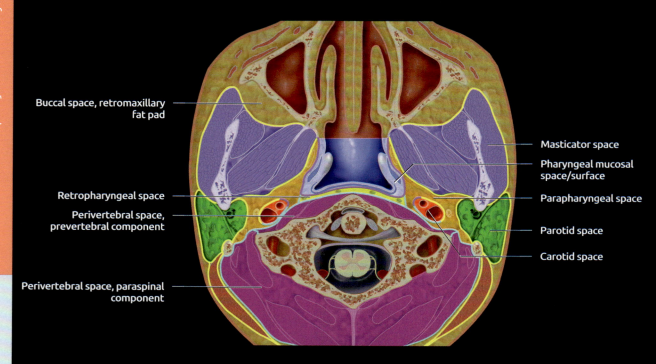

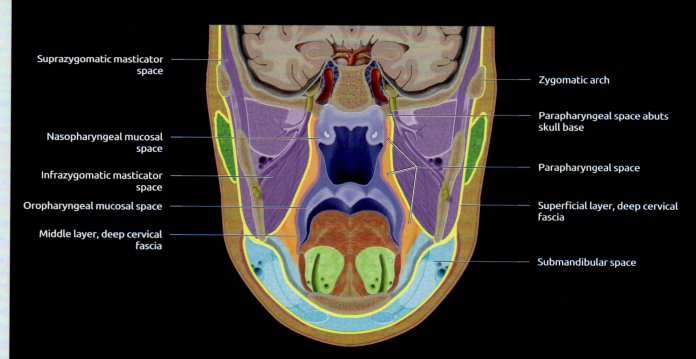

(Top) Axial graphic depicts the spaces of the suprahyoid neck. Surrounding the paired fat-filled parapharyngeal spaces (PPSs) are the 4 critical paired spaces of this region: The PMS, MS, PS, and CS. The retropharyngeal and perivertebral spaces are the midline nonpaired spaces. A PMS mass pushes the PPS laterally; MS mass pushes PPS posteriorly; PS mass pushes PPS medially; CS mass pushes PPS anteriorly. (Bottom) Coronal graphic shows the PPS. The PPSs are paired, fat-filled spaces in the more lateral aspect of the suprahyoid neck. This space abuts the skull base between the MS and PMS. There are no important structures at the point of intersection between the PPS and the skull base. Inferiorly, the PPS communicates with the posterior submandibular space.

Suprahyoid and Infrahyoid Neck Overview

GRAPHICS

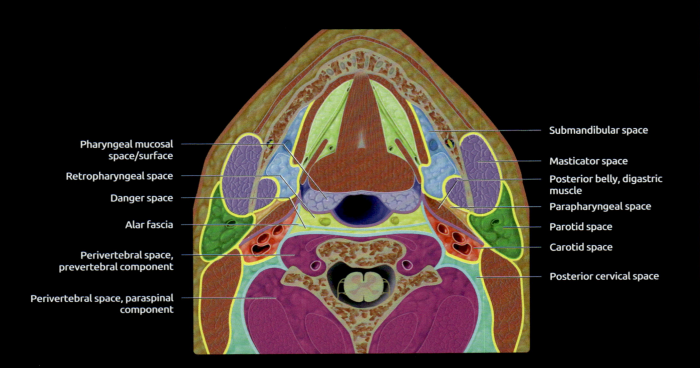

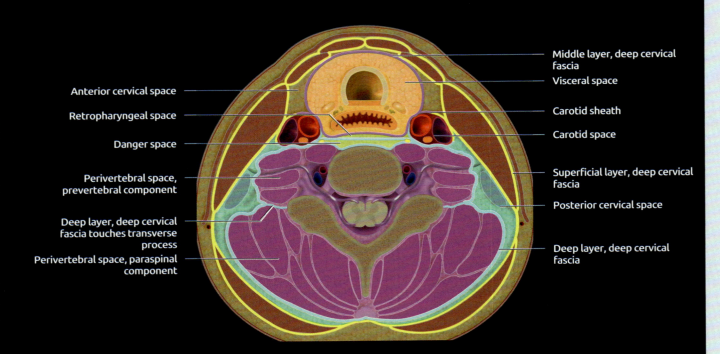

(Top) Axial graphic shows the suprahyoid neck spaces at the level of the oropharynx. The superficial (yellow line), middle (pink line), and deep (turquoise line) layers of deep cervical fascia outline the suprahyoid neck spaces. Notice the alar fascia separates the retropharyngeal and danger spaces and represents a slip of the deep layer of deep cervical fascia. (Bottom) Axial graphic depicts the fascia and spaces of the infrahyoid neck. The 3 layers of deep cervical fascia are present in the suprahyoid and infrahyoid neck. The carotid sheath is made up of all 3 layers of deep cervical fascia (tricolor line around CS. Notice the deep layer completely circles the perivertebral space, diving in laterally to divide it into prevertebral and paraspinal components.

Suprahyoid and Infrahyoid Neck Overview

GRAPHICS

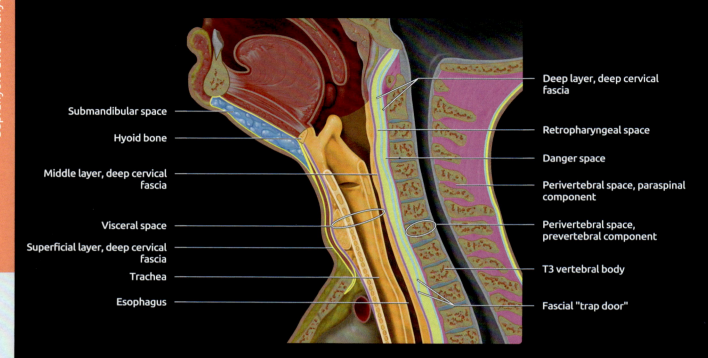

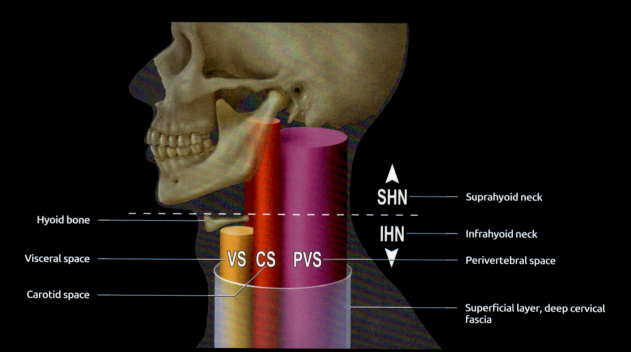

(Top) Sagittal graphic depicting longitudinal spatial relationships of the infrahyoid neck is shown. Anteriorly, the visceral space is seen surrounded by a middle layer of deep cervical fascia. Just anterior to the vertebral column, the retropharyngeal and danger spaces run inferiorly toward the mediastinum. Notice the fascial "trap door" found at the approximate level of T3 vertebral body that serves as a conduit from the retropharyngeal to the danger space. Retropharyngeal space infection or tumor may access the mediastinum via this route of spread. (Bottom) Lateral graphic of extracranial head and neck show the spaces as "tubes" as they traverse the area. This is particularly true of the CSs, which reach from the skull base to the aortic arch. Both the visceral and perivertebral spaces continue inferiorly into the thorax.

Suprahyoid and Infrahyoid Neck Overview

AXIAL CECT OF SUPRAHYOID NECK

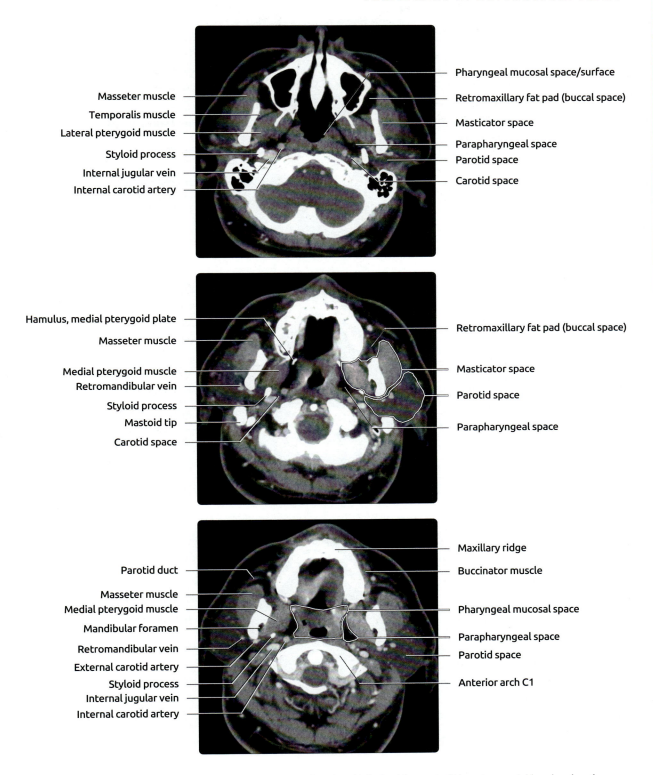

(Top) First of 12 axial contrast-enhanced CT images of both the suprahyoid and infrahyoid aspect of the extracranial head and neck presented from superior to inferior is shown. This image at the level of the nasopharynx shows the 4 key spaces surrounding the PPS: PMS, MS, PS, and CS. (Middle) In this image at level of inferior maxillary sinus, the styloid process is seen anterolateral to the CS. The superficial layer of deep cervical fascia defines the MS and PS. The more anterior buccal space (BS) has no fascial definition. (Bottom) At the level of the maxillary ridge, the area of the PMS is outlined between the paired, fat-filled PPSs. Posterior to the PMS are the tightly packed retropharyngeal and perivertebral spaces.

Suprahyoid and Infrahyoid Neck Overview

AXIAL CECT OF SUPRAHYOID NECK

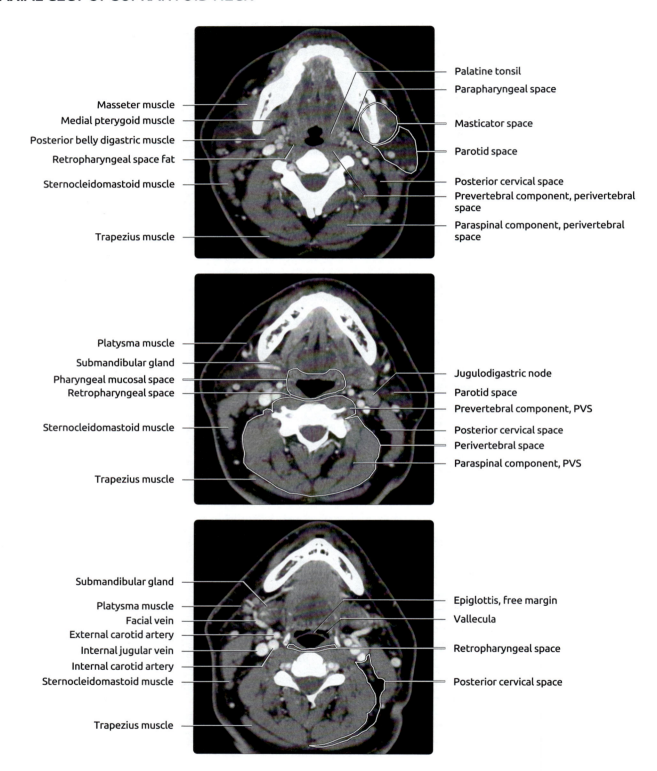

(Top) In this image at the level of the mandibular body, the posterior belly of the digastric muscle can be seen dividing the parotid tail from the CS. The direction of displacement of this muscle can define whether a lesion is in the PS (posteromedial displacement) or in the CS (anterolateral displacement). (Middle) In this image through the low oropharynx, the PMS has been outlined anterior to the perivertebral space. The space between them is the retropharyngeal space that includes an anterior true retropharyngeal space in front of alar fascia and a posterior danger space behind it. The very thin alar fascia that separates these compartments of the retropharyngeal space is not usually visualized and may be identified in patients with retropharyngeal space edema in situations like postradiation therapy. (Bottom) At the level of the free margin of epiglottis, the retropharyngeal space is outlined behind the PMS. The posterior cervical space contains fat, accessory cranial nerve (CNXI), and the spinal accessory nodal chain (level 5 nodes).

Suprahyoid and Infrahyoid Neck Overview

AXIAL CECT OF INFRAHYOID NECK

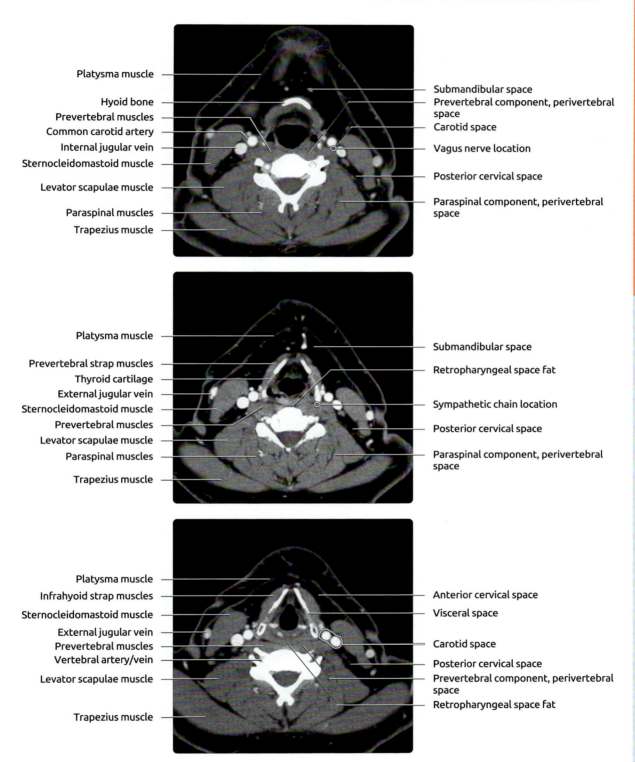

(Top) Axial CT image at the level of the hyoid bone shows the CS now contains the common carotid artery, internal jugular vein, and vagus nerve only. The large, fat-filled submandibular space is seen anteriorly. (Middle) In this image at the level of the supraglottis of the larynx, the large sternocleidomastoid and trapezius muscles are seen in the lateral neck. Both muscles are innervated by the accessory cranial nerve. (Bottom) In this image at the level of the glottis of the larynx, the visceral space contains the hypopharynx, larynx, and infrahyoid strap muscles. Just behind the hypopharynx is the RPS, which contains only fat in the infrahyoid neck. Notice that the inferior extension of the submandibular space into the infrahyoid neck is the anterior cervical space.

Suprahyoid and Infrahyoid Neck Overview

AXIAL CECT OF INFRAHYOID NECK

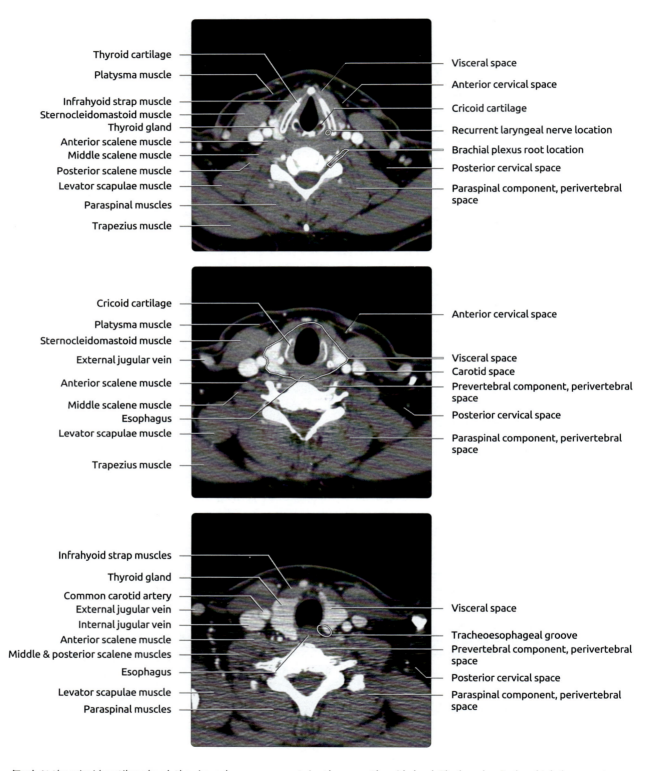

(Top) At the cricoid cartilage level, the visceral space now contains the upper thyroid gland. The low-density brachial plexus root projects anterolaterally from the neural foramen to pass between the anterior and middle scalene muscles in the prevertebral component of perivertebral space. (Middle) In this image, the visceral space contains the high-density thyroid gland, the upper cervical esophagus, and the cricoid cartilage. The middle layer of the deep cervical fascia circumscribes the visceral space. (Bottom) At the level of the upper cervical trachea, the visceral space is filled with the thyroid gland, parathyroid glands (not visible), trachea, and cervical esophagus. The area of tracheoesophageal groove contains the recurrent laryngeal nerve and the paratracheal nodal chain. It is via the paratracheal nodal chain that differentiated thyroid carcinoma accesses the mediastinum.

Suprahyoid and Infrahyoid Neck Overview

AXIAL CECT OF CERVICOTHORACIC JUNCTION

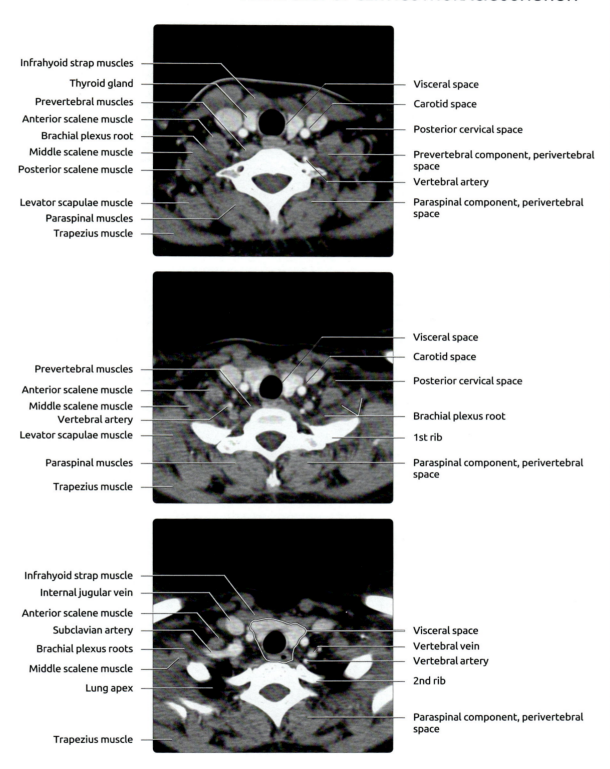

(Top) First of 3 axial CECT images through the lower cervical neck and cervicothoracic junction presented from superior to inferior shows the anterior, middle, and posterior scalene muscles in the prevertebral component of the perivertebral space. Notice the brachial plexus roots between the anterior and middle scalene muscles. (Middle) At the level of the 1st thoracic vertebral body and 1st rib, the anterior scalene is clearly visibile anterior to the roots of the brachial plexus. The visceral space contains the thyroid gland, parathyroid glands (not visible on CT), the cervical esophagus, and trachea. (Bottom) In this image at the level of the lung apices, the visceral space is outlined by the middle layer of deep cervical fascia. The right subclavian artery passes between the anterior and middle scalene muscles along with the brachial plexus roots.

Suprahyoid and Infrahyoid Neck Overview

AXIAL T1 MR

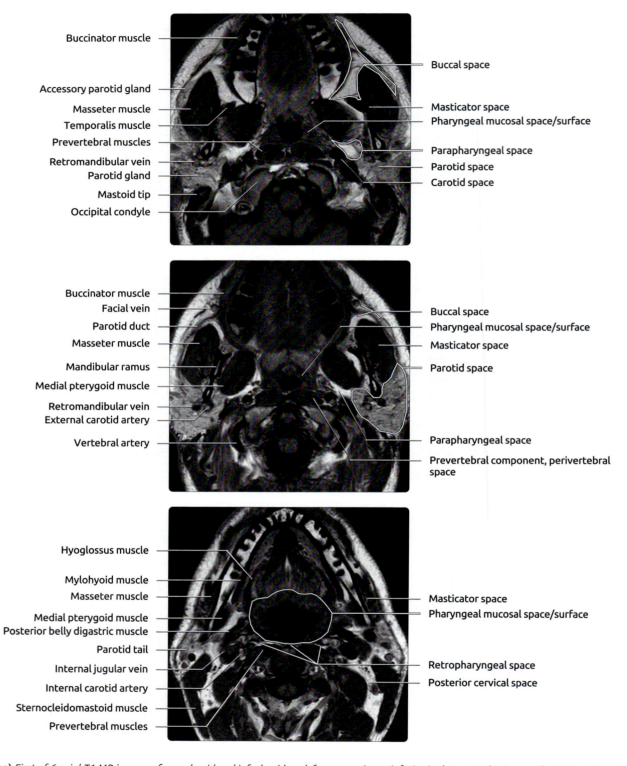

(Top) First of 6 axial T1 MR images of suprahyoid and infrahyoid neck from superior to inferior is shown. In this image, the BS is outlined on the left. The BS is bounded medially by buccinator muscle, posteriorly by MS, laterally by PS, & anteriorly by superficial muscles of the facial expression & investing fascia. Inferiorly, it blends imperceptibly with the submandibular space. The BS does not have complete fascial coverings separating it from adjacent spaces, allowing disease to spread easily. The BS contents are fat, minor salivary glands, parotid duct, lymph nodes, facial vein, facial, angular & buccal arteries, & buccal branches of facial & mandibular nerves. The PPS is seen as a fat-filled region bordered by the PMS, MS, PS, and CS. (Middle) In this image at the mandibular teeth level, the PS is seen posterior to the MS. Both are surrounded by the superficial layer of deep cervical fascia. (Bottom) In this image, the PMS is made up of the anterior lingual & lateral palatine tonsils. The fat stripe behind the PMS is the retropharyngeal space; behind that is the prevertebral component of the perivertebral space. The posterior belly of digastric muscle separates carotid from the PS.

Suprahyoid and Infrahyoid Neck Overview

AXIAL T1 MR

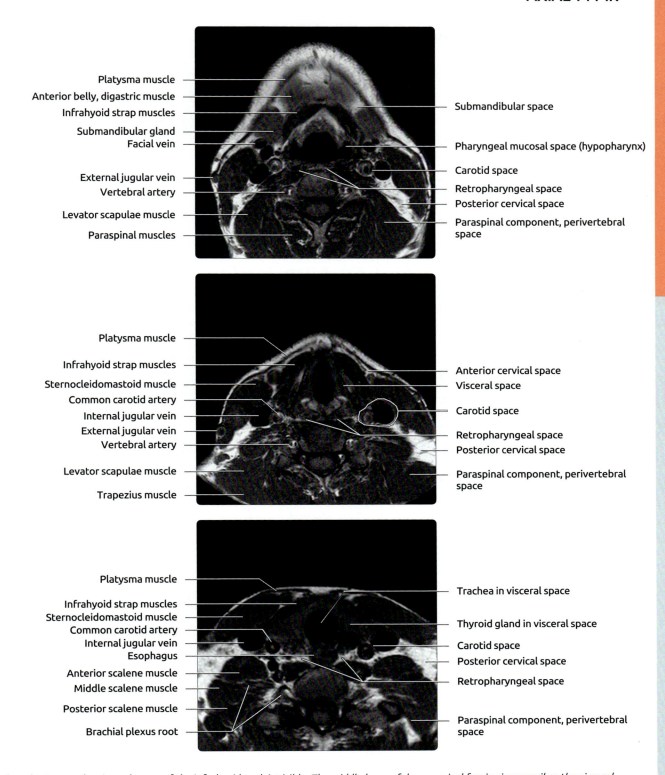

(Top) In this image, the visceral space of the infrahyoid neck is visible. The middle layer of deep cervical fascia circumscribes the visceral space. The visceral space at this level contains the infrahyoid strap muscles, pyriform sinuses, and epiglottis. (Middle) At the level of true vocal cords, both the anterior and posterior cervical spaces are seen. Note the anterior cervical space is a direct extension of the submandibular space into the infrahyoid neck. The CS is surrounded by the carotid sheath. The common carotid artery, internal jugular vein, and vagus nerve are found in the infrahyoid CS. (Bottom) At the level of the upper trachea, the thyroid gland is now the largest structure in the visceral space. The parathyroid glands, cervical trachea and esophagus, paratracheal nodes, and recurrent laryngeal nerve are all in the visceral space.

Suprahyoid and Infrahyoid Neck Overview

AXIAL T2 MR

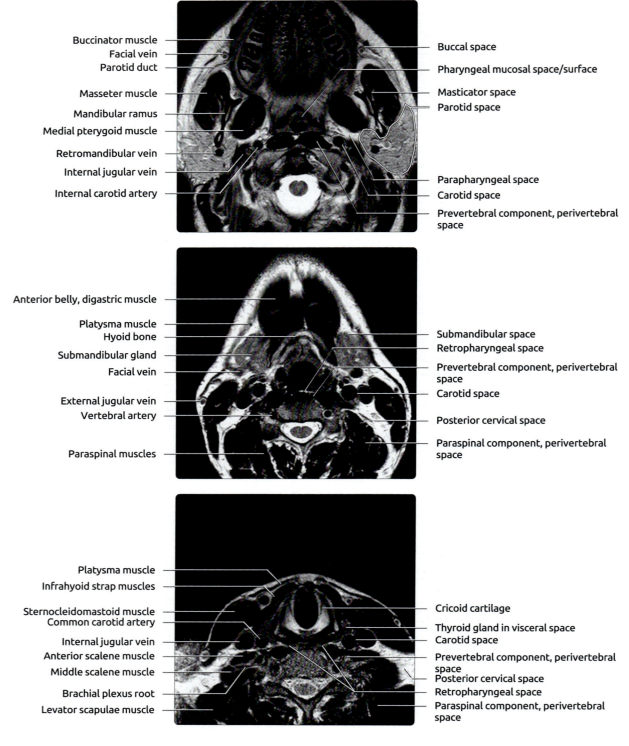

(Top) First of 3 axial T2 MR images of the neck at the level of the maxillary alveolar ridge shows the 4 key spaces surrounding the fat-filled PPS. These important 4 spaces are the PMS, MS, PS, and CS. The PS and MS are circumscribed by a superficial layer of deep cervical fascia. *(Middle)* In this image at the level of hyoid bone, the large submandibular glands are visible in the submandibular space deep to the platysma muscle. *(Bottom)* At the level of the cricoid cartilage, the prevertebral and paraspinal components of the perivertebral space can be seen. The brachial plexus roots exit the prevertebral component between the anterior and middle scalene muscles to enter the posterior CS fat on their way to the axilla.

Suprahyoid and Infrahyoid Neck Overview

CORONAL T1 MR

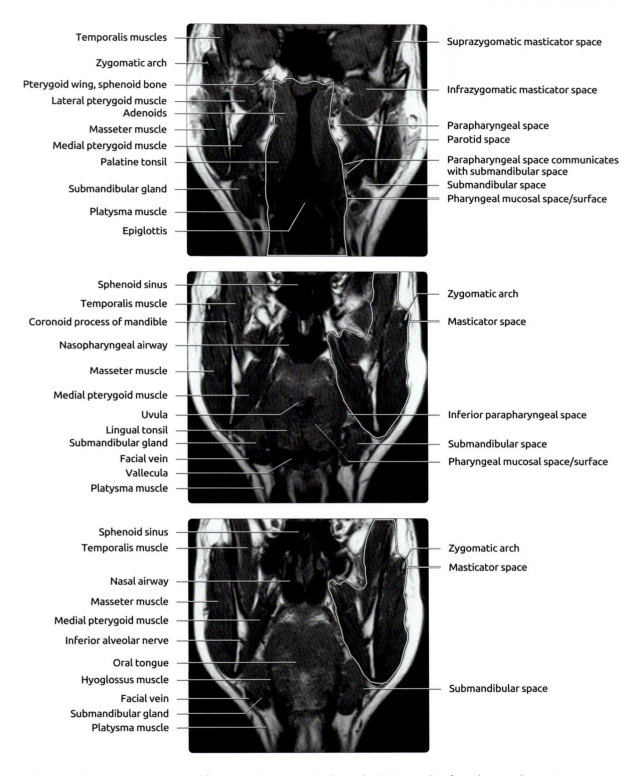

(Top) First of 3 coronal T1 MR images presented from posterior to anterior shows the PMS extending from the nasopharynx to hypopharynx. It is from the PMS that the most common malignancies of the head and neck arise, squamous cell carcinoma from the mucosa, non-Hodgkin lymphoma from the tonsils, and minor salivary gland malignancy from the minor salivary glands. **(Middle)** In this image, the MS has been outlined. Remember this space has a suprazygomatic and an infrazygomatic component. Since there is no "horizontal fascia" between the zygomatic arch, diseases may spread within the MS between the suprazygomatic and infrazygomatic components. **(Bottom)** In this image through the posterior nose, 3 of the major muscles of mastication are visible, the masseter, medial pterygoid, and temporalis muscles.

Suprahyoid and Infrahyoid Neck Overview

TRANSVERSE ULTRASOUND

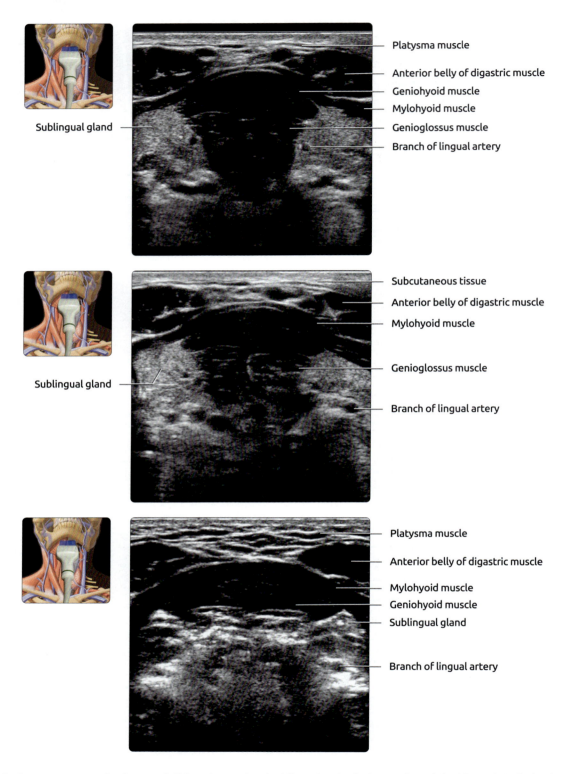

(Top) Anterior transverse grayscale ultrasound of the submental and sublingual region is shown. The mylohyoid muscle is the landmark for division of the sublingual space (deep to the mylohyoid plane) and submandibular space (superficial to the muscle plane). The sublingual gland appears as homogeneous, hyperechoic structure lateral to the geniohyoid/genioglossus muscle. Branches of lingual artery can be easily picked up on transverse plane. The submandibular duct sits alongside the lingual vessels, and a submandibular calculus may impact at this site. (Middle) Slightly more posterior transverse grayscale ultrasound allows the clear depiction of extrinsic muscles of the tongue at the root. (Bottom) Transverse grayscale ultrasound shows the submental region in a more posterior location.

Suprahyoid and Infrahyoid Neck Overview

POWER DOPPLER ULTRASOUND AND TRANSVERSE ULTRASOUNDS

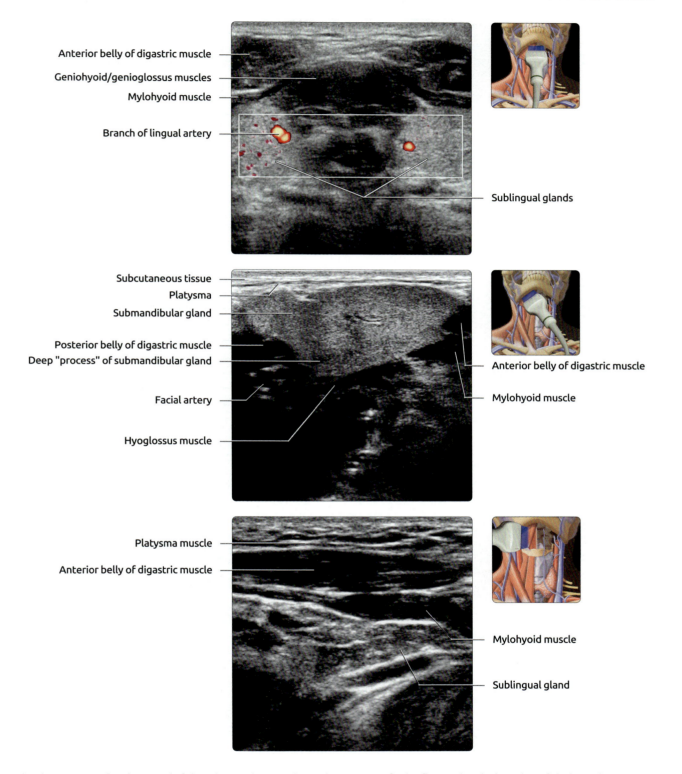

(Top) Power Doppler ultrasound of the submental region shows the presence of color flow within the branches of the lingual artery. The use of Doppler examination aids in differentiation from the dilated submandibular duct. (Middle) Transverse grayscale ultrasound of the submandibular region taken more laterally shows the submandibular gland. The submandibular gland is the key structure in this region and is easily recognized by its homogeneous echotexture. The gland sits astride the mylohyoid and posterior belly of the digastric muscles. (Bottom) Parasagittal longitudinal grayscale ultrasound shows the submental region. The sublingual gland is visualized within the sublingual space (deep to the mylohyoid muscle) underneath the anterior belly of the digastric and mylohyoid muscles.

Suprahyoid and Infrahyoid Neck Overview

TRANSVERSE ULTRASOUND

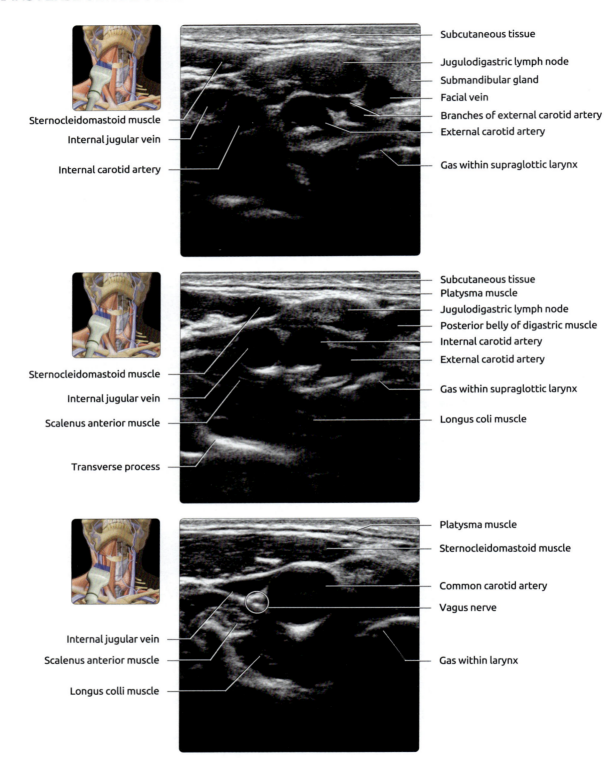

(Top) First image in a series of consecutive transverse grayscale ultrasound images of the upper cervical level clearly identifies key vascular landmarks, including the internal and external carotid arteries and the internal jugular vein. The uppermost and largest deep cervical lymph node (i.e., the jugulodigastric lymph node) is consistently seen in the upper cervical level superficial to the carotid artery. It is usually elliptical, hypoechoic, and demonstrates echogenic hilum. (Middle) Second image shows the carotid bifurcation in the transverse plane. The external carotid artery is usually more medial and smaller than the internal carotid artery. (Bottom) Third image below the level of carotid bifurcation clearly shows the common carotid artery, internal jugular vein, and vagus nerve to be major structures within the carotid sheath.

Suprahyoid and Infrahyoid Neck Overview

TRANSVERSE ULTRASOUND

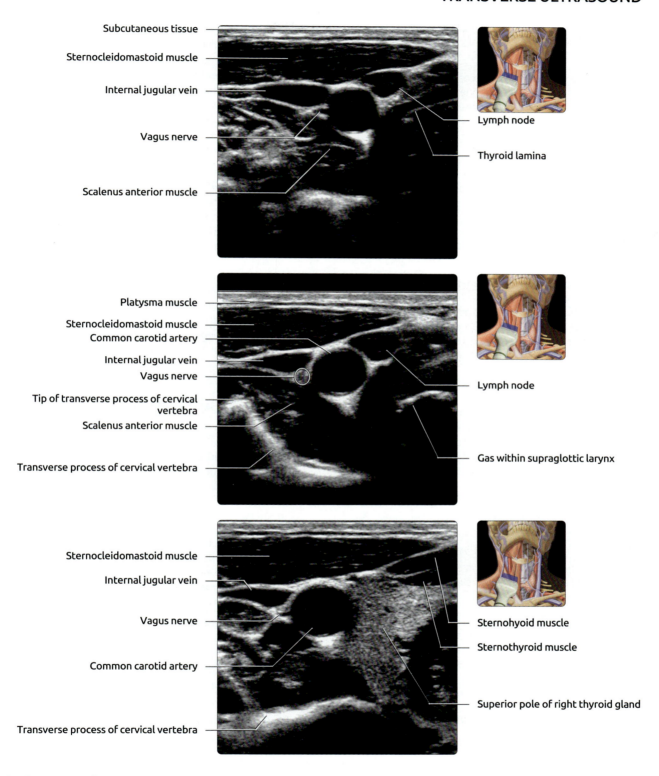

(Top) First image shows consecutive transverse grayscale ultrasound of midcervical level. Deep cervical lymph nodes are commonly found along and anterior to the major vessels of the carotid sheath. These are commonly hypoechoic and elliptical with a normal echogenic hilum and hilar vascularity. (Middle) Second image shows midcervical level in transverse plane. At this level, the common carotid artery, internal jugular vein, and vagus nerve are the main structures within the carotid sheath. The vagus nerve is usually located between the common carotid artery and the internal jugular vein and appears as a small, round, hypoechoic nodule with a central echogenic dot. (Bottom) Third image shows the midcervical level. The cricoid cartilage may not be routinely seen on ultrasound, but visualization of the superior pole of the thyroid gland approximately coincides with this level.

Parapharyngeal Space

TERMINOLOGY

Abbreviations
- Parapharyngeal space (PPS)

Synonyms
- Some authors define PPS more broadly, separating it into prestyloid and poststyloid components
- In this text, **PPS** preferred over prestyloid PPS and **carotid space** (CS) over poststyloid PPS

Definitions
- **PPS**: Central, fat-filled space in lateral suprahyoid neck (SHN) around which most of important spaces are located
  - These surrounding important spaces are pharyngeal mucosal space (PMS), masticator space (MS), parotid space (PS), and CS

IMAGING ANATOMY

Overview
- PPS contents are limited; therefore few lesions actually originate in this location
  - Diseases of PPS usually arise in adjacent spaces (PMS, MS, PS, CS), spreading secondarily into PPS
- Importance of PPS is its conspicuity on CT and MR as well as its direction of displacement by mass lesions of surrounding spaces
  - **PPS displacement pattern helps define actual space of origin**
    - PMS mass lesion pushes PPS laterally
    - MS mass lesion pushes PPS posteriorly
    - PS mass lesion pushes PPS medially
    - CS mass lesion pushes PPS anteriorly
    - Lateral retropharyngeal space mass (nodal) pushes PPS anterolaterally
  - Combining center of mass lesion with displacement direction of PPS yields strong impression of "space of origin" of SHN mass lesion

Extent
- Crescent-shaped, fat-filled space in craniocaudal dimension extends from skull base above to superior cornu of hyoid bone inferiorly

Anatomy Relationships
- As fatty tube separating other SHN spaces from one another, PPS functions as "elevator shaft" through which infection and tumor from these adjacent spaces may travel from skull base to hyoid bone
- Inferiorly there is **no fascia** separating inferior PPS from submandibular space (SMS)
  - Open communication between inferior PPS and posterior SMS therefore exists
- Superiorly, PPS interacts with skull base in bland triangular area on inferior surface of petrous apex
  - **No exiting skull base foramina** are found in this area of attachment
- Surrounding spaces include
  - PMS medially
  - MS anterolaterally
  - PS laterally
  - CS posteriorly
  - RPS posteromedially

Internal Contents
- PPS has **no** mucosa, muscle, bone, nodes, or major salivary gland tissue within its boundaries
  - Consequently few things primarily begin in PPS
- **Critical PPS contents**
  - **Fat**: Key constituent making PPS easily identifiable even with larger SHN mass lesions
  - Minor salivary glands (ectopic, rare)
  - Internal maxillary artery
  - Ascending pharyngeal artery
  - Pterygoid venous plexus (small portion, mostly MS)

Fascial of Parapharyngeal Space
- Fascial margins of PPS are complex; made up of different layers of deep cervical fascia
  - Medial fascial margin of PPS
    - Made up of middle layer, deep cervical fascia as it curves around lateral margin of PMS
  - Lateral fascial margin of PPS
    - Formed by medial slip of superficial layer of deep cervical fascia along deep border of MS and PS
  - Posterior fascial margin of PPS
    - Formed by deep layer of deep cervical fascia on anterolateral margin of retropharyngeal space and anterior part of carotid sheath (made up of components of all 3 layers of deep cervical fascia)

ANATOMY IMAGING ISSUES

Questions
- Because of limited normal anatomic contents of PPS, few lesions primarily arise in PPS
  - Rare lesions found in PPS include benign mixed tumor (from minor salivary gland rests in PPS), lipoma, and atypical second branchial cleft cyst
  - To say lesion is primary to PPS, it must be completely surrounded by PPS fat
  - In most cases where lesion is thought to be primary to PPS, careful observation will find connection to one of surrounding spaces (usually PS)
- **PPS fat displacement** is **key imaging relationship** used in evaluation of SHN mass lesions

Imaging Recommendations
- MR better delineates skull base, meningeal, and perineural lesions
  - Fat-saturated contrast-enhanced T1 MR may make PPS fat difficult to see

Imaging Pitfalls
- Remember most lesions of PPS arise from adjacent SHN spaces

CLINICAL IMPLICATIONS

Clinical Importance
- Since PPS empties inferiorly into SMS, PPS lesion may present as "angle of mandible" mass
- However, most lesions within PPS cannot be evaluated by physical examination

Parapharyngeal Space

GRAPHICS

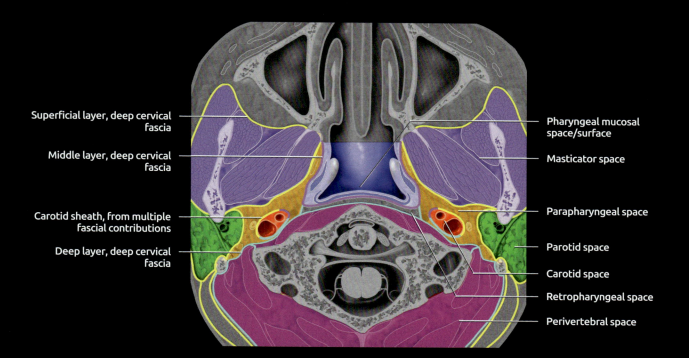

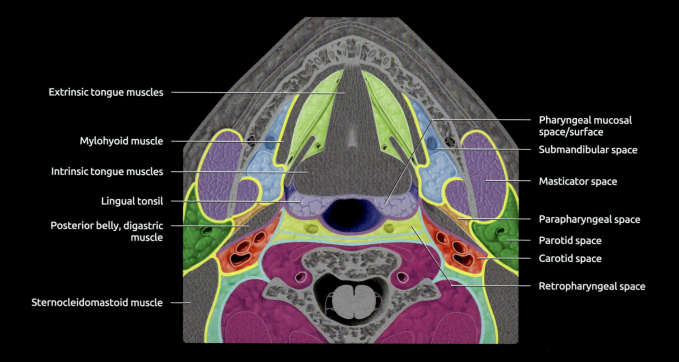

(Top) *Axial graphic of the normal parapharyngeal space at the level of the nasopharynx demonstrates the complex fascial margins and the fat-only contents. The surrounding pharyngeal mucosal, masticator, parotid, and carotid spaces when affected by mass lesions push into the parapharyngeal space. The resulting displacement pattern of the parapharyngeal space may be helpful in defining the space of origin of a mass in the suprahyoid neck.* (Bottom) *Axial graphic at the level of the low oropharynx shows the slip of parapharyngeal space fat is just anterolateral to the posterior belly of the digastric muscle. Inferior to this level, the parapharyngeal space communicates anteriorly with the submandibular space. Yellow lines in the drawing represent superficial layer, pink lines middle layer, and aquamarine lines deep layer of deep cervical fascia.*

Parapharyngeal Space

GRAPHICS

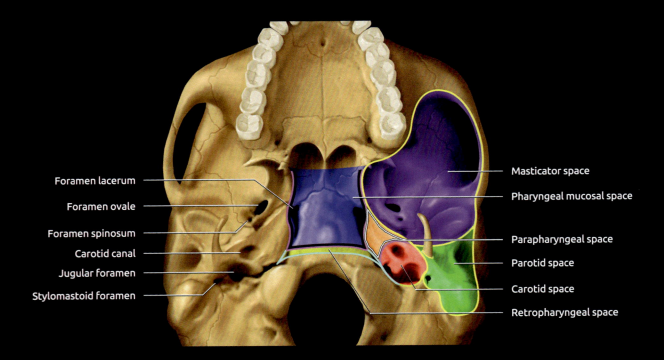

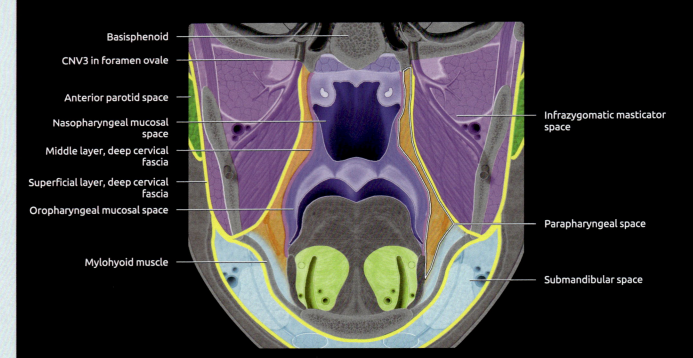

(Top) Axial graphic of the suprahyoid neck spaces interaction with the skull base highlighting the parapharyngeal space is shown. Notice that the parapharyngeal space abuts the inferior surface of the skull base in an area with no critical structures. (Bottom) Coronal graphic of suprahyoid neck spaces as they interact with the skull base superiorly and submandibular space inferiorly is shown. The parapharyngeal space interacts with no critical structures as it abuts the skull base. Inferiorly it "empties" into the posterior submandibular space along the posterior margin of the mylohyoid muscle. As a consequence of this anatomic arrangement, it is possible for an infection or a malignant tumor that breaks into the parapharyngeal space to present inferiorly as an "angle of mandible" mass.

Parapharyngeal Space

AXIAL CECT

Suprahyoid and Infrahyoid Neck

Top image labels (left): Medial pterygoid plate; Lateral pterygoid plate; Coronoid process, mandible; Masseter muscle; Lateral pterygoid muscle; Mandibular condyle; Parotid gland; Styloid process; Eustachian tube opening; Torus tubarius

Top image labels (right): Retromaxillary fat pad (buccal space); Masticator space; Parapharyngeal space; Parotid space; Carotid space; Pharyngeal mucosal space/surface

Middle image labels (left): Medial pterygoid plate; Lateral pterygoid plate; Masseter muscle; Medial pterygoid muscle; Prevertebral muscle; Deep lobe, parotid gland; Styloid process; Internal jugular vein; Internal carotid artery

Middle image labels (right): Retromaxillary fat pad (buccal space); Masticator space; Parapharyngeal space; Parotid space; Carotid space; Pharyngeal mucosal space/surface

Bottom image labels (left): Buccinator muscle; Palatine tonsil; Mandibular ramus; Masseter muscle; Medial pterygoid muscle; Retromandibular vein; Deep lobe, parotid gland; Styloid process; Internal jugular vein; Internal carotid artery

Bottom image labels (right): Buccal space; Masticator space; Parapharyngeal space; Parotid space; Carotid space; Pharyngeal mucosal space/surface

(Top) *First of 6 contrast-enhanced axial CT images of the suprahyoid neck presented from superior to inferior shows the superior end of the parapharyngeal space just before it abuts the skull base. Notice the 4 major spaces surrounding the parapharyngeal space, the pharyngeal mucosal, masticator, parotid, and carotid spaces.* **(Middle)** *In this image at the level of the inferior maxillary sinus, the complex shape of the parapharyngeal space is visible. Notice the lateral margin of the parapharyngeal space is the deep lobe of the parotid gland.* **(Bottom)** *In this midoropharynx image, the parapharyngeal space has the palatine tonsil on its entire medial border. It is easy to see that a squamous cell carcinoma of the palatine tonsil that is deeply invasive would immediately enter the parapharyngeal space fat, pushing it from medial to lateral.*

293

Parapharyngeal Space

AXIAL CECT

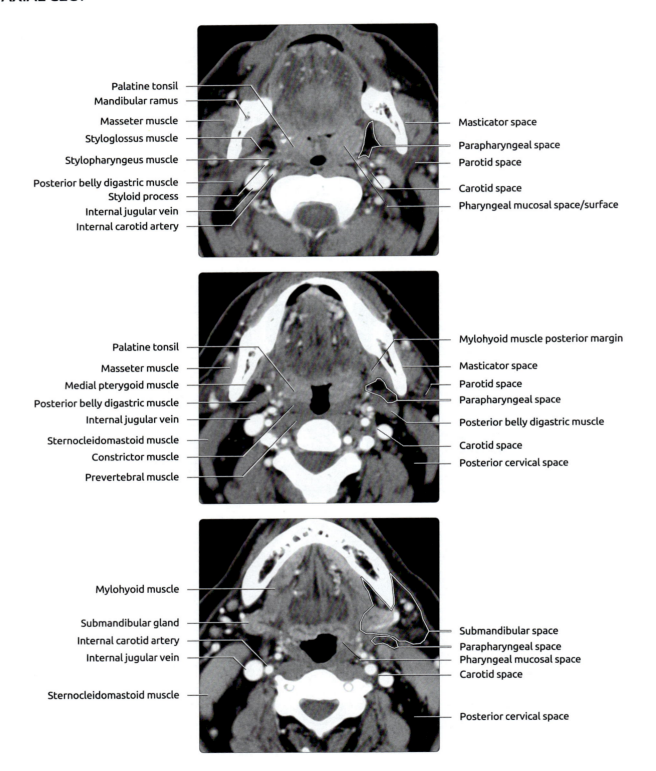

(Top) In this image the parapharyngeal space points anteriorly toward the submandibular space. On more inferior images, it will communicate with the posterosuperior submandibular space in this area. Notice the stylopharyngeus and styloglossus muscle on the posterior margin of the parapharyngeal space. (Middle) At the level of the mandibular body, the parapharyngeal space is seen entering the superior submandibular space just anterior to the posterior belly of the digastric muscles and just posterior to the mylohyoid muscle. (Bottom) In this image through the superior submandibular space, it is possible to see the most inferior parapharyngeal space merging with the submandibular space. Remember there is no fascia separating the inferior parapharyngeal, posterior submandibular, and sublingual spaces at the posterior margin of the mylohyoid muscle.

Parapharyngeal Space

AXIAL T1 MR

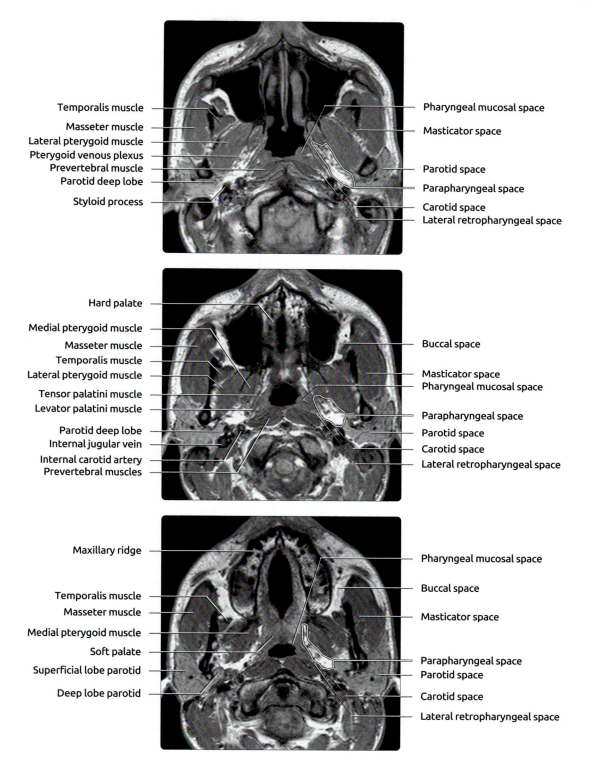

(Top) First of 6 axial T1 MR images of the suprahyoid neck presented from superior to inferior shows the parapharyngeal space at the level of the nasopharynx. Here the surrounding spaces include the pharyngeal mucosal, masticator, parotid, and carotid spaces. Notice the lateral retropharyngeal space is on the posteromedial aspect of the parapharyngeal space. (Middle) In this image at the level of the hard palate, the posterior margins of the tensor and levator palatini muscles are visible along the anteromedial margin of the parapharyngeal space on the right. (Bottom) At the level of the maxillary ridge, the parapharyngeal space on the left is surrounded in clockwise order by the medial pterygoid muscle, deep lobe of parotid, internal carotid artery, lateral pharynx, and the soft palate.

Parapharyngeal Space

AXIAL T1 MR

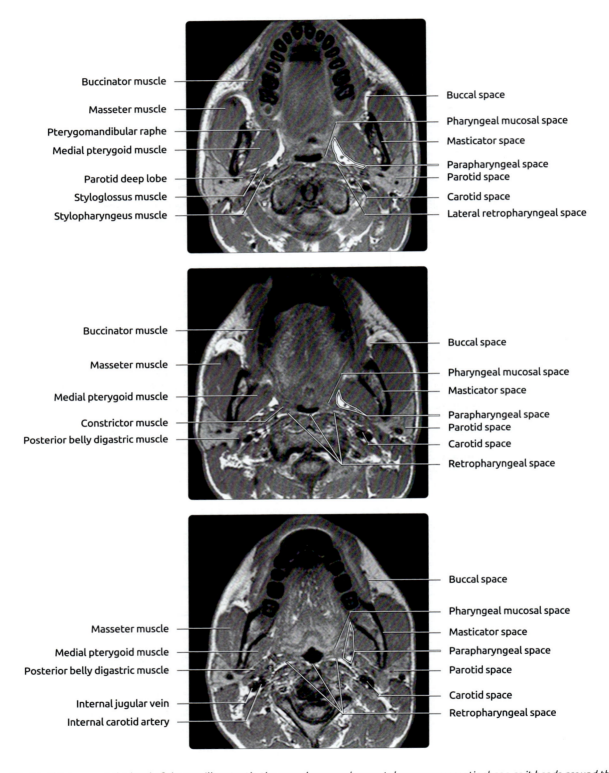

(Top) In this image at the level of the maxillary teeth, the parapharyngeal space takes on a crescentic shape as it bends around the medial pterygoid muscle of the masticator space. The pharyngeal mucosal space makes up the medial border of the parapharyngeal space. Posteromedially, the lateral retropharyngeal space is found while the carotid space makes up the parapharyngeal space posterolateral border. The deep lobe of the parotid gland makes up the lateral margin of the parapharyngeal space. **(Middle)** In this image at the level of the midoropharynx, the parapharyngeal space becomes smaller along its inferior margin. **(Bottom)** In this image at the level of the mandibular teeth, the parapharyngeal space is visible "pointing" anteriorly where it joins the posterosuperior margin of the submandibular space. Parapharyngeal abscess and tumor may access the submandibular space via this route.

Parapharyngeal Space

CORONAL T1 MR

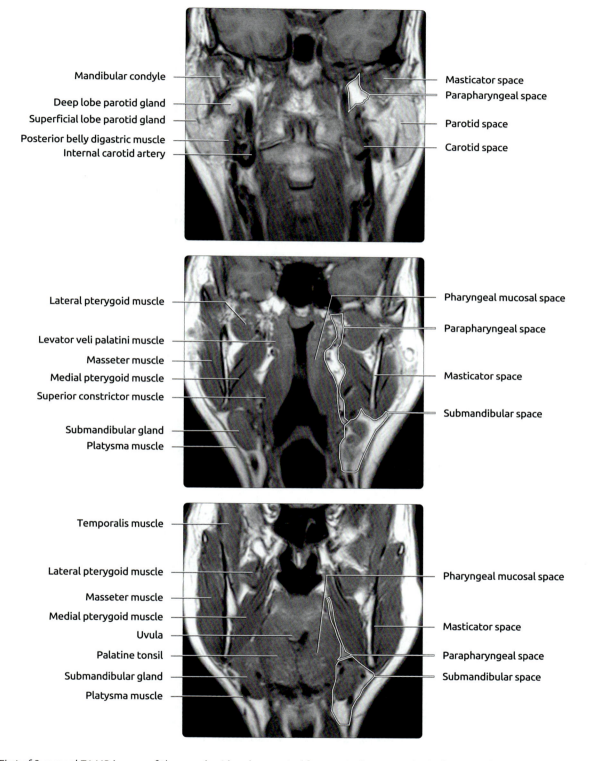

(Top) First of 3 coronal T1 MR images of the suprahyoid neck presented from posterior to anterior is shown. In this image through the mandibular condyles, the posterior parapharyngeal space is seen medial to the deep lobe of the parotid gland. (Middle) In this image, the parapharyngeal space is visible from its superior area of skull base abutment to its inferior area merging with the submandibular space. Note the site of abutment with the skull base contains no vital structures. Remember that there is no fascia present between the inferior parapharyngeal space and the posterior submandibular space. (Bottom) In this image through the anterior parapharyngeal space, the connection between the parapharyngeal space and submandibular space is seen. Submandibular space disease, especially abscess, may at times spread superiorly into the parapharyngeal space via this connection.

Pharyngeal Mucosal Space

TERMINOLOGY

Abbreviations
- Pharyngeal mucosal space (PMS)

Definitions
- **PMS**: Nasopharyngeal, oropharyngeal, & hypopharyngeal surface structures on airway side of middle layer of deep cervical fascia (ML-DCF)

IMAGING ANATOMY

Overview
- PMS is conceptual construct to complete map of spaces of suprahyoid neck
  - PMS alternative term: Pharyngeal mucosal surface
- There is **no fascia on surface of PMS**, so it is not true fascia-enclosed space

Extent
- PMS is continuous mucosal sheet defined from nasopharynx to hypopharynx (includes soft palate)
- Nasopharyngeal, oropharyngeal, & hypopharyngeal mucosal space components
  - See larynx anatomy for hypopharynx anatomy

Anatomy Relationships
- Airway side of PMS has no fascial border
- Posterior to PMS is retropharyngeal space
- Lateral to PMS is parapharyngeal space (PPS)
- Skull base relationship to PMS
  - Broad area of attachment to skull base present
  - Attachment area includes posterior basisphenoid (sphenoid sinus floor), anterior basiocciput (anterior clivus)
  - Also includes **foramen lacerum**
    - Foramen lacerum: Cartilaginous floor of anterior horizontal petrous internal carotid artery
    - Represents perivascular route for nasopharyngeal carcinoma to access intracranial structures

Internal Contents
- **Mucosal surface of pharynx**
- **PMS lymphatic ring**: Lymphatic ring of tissue of PMS that declines in size with advancing age
  - Synonym: Waldeyer ring
  - Nasopharynx: **Adenoids**
  - Oropharynx, lateral wall: **Palatine (faucial) tonsil**
  - Oropharynx, base of tongue: **Lingual tonsil**
- **Minor salivary glands**
  - Soft palate mucosa has highest concentration
- **Pharyngobasilar fascia**
  - Tough aponeurosis that connects superior constrictor muscle to skull base
  - Posterosuperior margin notch = **sinus of Morgagni**
    - Levator palatini muscle & eustachian tube pass through this notch on way from skull base to PMS
- **PMS muscles**
  - Superior, middle, & inferior constrictor muscles
  - Salpingopharyngeus muscle
  - Levator palatini muscle, distal end
- **Torus tubarius**: Cartilaginous end of eustachian tube

Fascia of Pharyngeal Mucosal Space
- **ML-DCF** represents deep margin of PMS
  - In nasopharynx, ML-DCF encircles lateral & posterior margins of pharyngobasilar fascia
  - In oropharynx, ML-DCF on deep margin of superior & middle constrictor muscles
  - In hypopharynx, ML-DCF on deep margin of inferior constrictor muscle

ANATOMY IMAGING ISSUES

Questions
- What imaging findings define lesion as primary to PMS?
  - Lesion is designated primary to PMS under following circumstances
    - Lesion center is **medial to PPS**
    - PMS mass **pushes PPS fat from medial to lateral**
    - PMS mass **disrupts normal PMS mucosal & submucosal architecture**

Imaging Recommendations
- CECT or MR can both successfully image PMS
- If skull base invasion or perineural tumor suspected, T1 C+ fat-saturated MR best
- Bone CT may then be added to delineate skull base bone changes & tumor matrix

Imaging Approaches
- If malignant tumor of PMS suspected, remember to stage primary tumor & cervical nodes in neck

Imaging Pitfalls
- Most common error in interpreting images of PMS is labeling normal asymmetry as tumor
- Lateral pharyngeal recess (fossa of Rosenmüller) is notoriously asymmetric & may have fluid within it
- Variable amounts of lymphoid tissue or lymphoid hypertrophy in Waldeyer ring can also create misimpression of tumor
- Retropharyngeal course of carotid may cause asymmetry of posterior pharynx

CLINICAL IMPLICATIONS

Clinical Importance
- Referring MD can see PMS surface either directly or with endoscopy
  - Use clinical impressions as part of imaging report
- Most common lesion of PMS is squamous cell carcinoma (SCCa)
  - Become familiar with routes of spread of SCCa by specific primary tumor site
  - Become familiar with staging criteria for each specific primary tumor site
- **Differential diagnosis of PMS mass**
  - From mucosa: SCCa
  - From lymphoid tissue: Non-Hodgkin lymphoma
  - From minor salivary glands: Minor salivary gland malignancies (uncommon)

Pharyngeal Mucosal Space

GRAPHICS

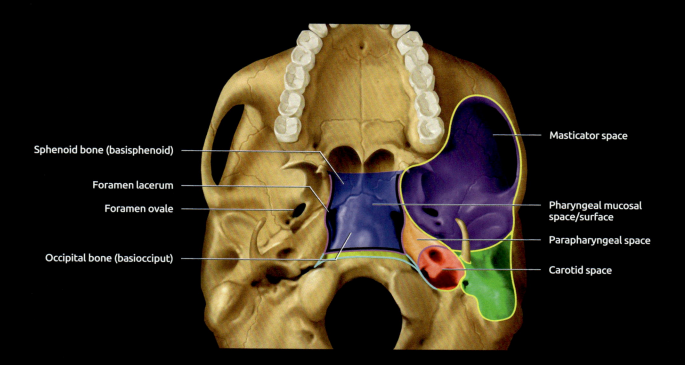

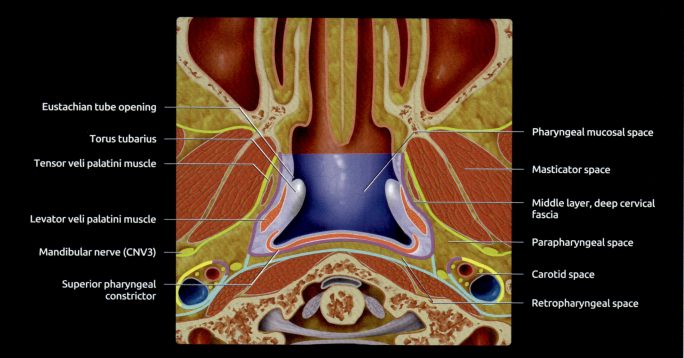

(Top) Graphic of skull base from below shows the relationships of the spaces of the suprahyoid neck and the skull base, with an emphasis on the pharyngeal mucosal space. Notice the pharyngeal mucosal space abuts a broad area of the sphenoid and occipital bones. The foramen lacerum, the cartilaginous floor to the anteromedial horizontal petrous internal carotid artery canal, is within this abutment area. Malignant tumors of the nasopharyngeal mucosal space can access the intracranial compartment via the foramen lacerum. (Bottom) Axial graphic of the nasopharyngeal mucosal space (in blue) shows the superior pharyngeal constrictor and levator veli palatini muscles are within the space. The middle layer of the deep cervical fascia provides a deep margin to the space. The retropharyngeal space is behind, and the parapharyngeal space is lateral to the pharyngeal mucosal space.

Pharyngeal Mucosal Space

GRAPHICS

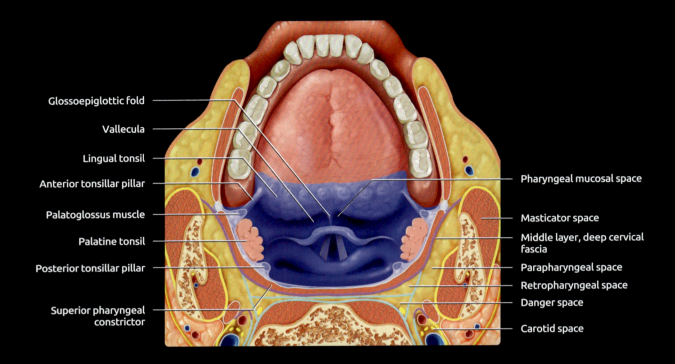

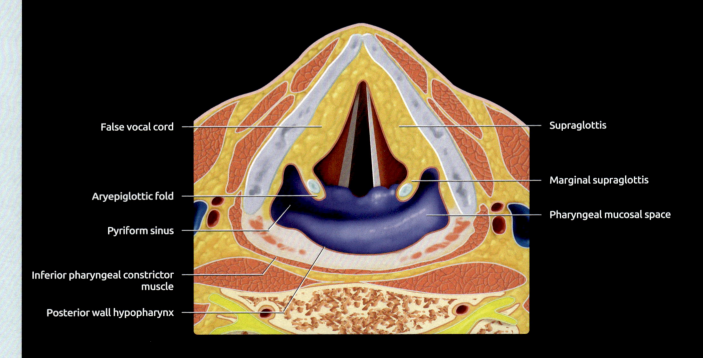

(Top) Axial graphic of the oropharyngeal mucosal space (in blue) viewed from above reveals the superior pharyngeal constrictor; the tonsillar pillars along with the palatine and lingual tonsils are all occupants of this space. The middle layer of the deep cervical fascia provides a deep margin to the space. The retropharyngeal space is behind, and the parapharyngeal space is lateral to the pharyngeal mucosal space. (Bottom) Axial graphic of the hypopharyngeal aspect of the pharyngeal mucosal space is shown. At the level of the supraglottis, the hypopharynx is made up of the pyriform sinus and posterior wall. Notice that the posterior wall of the aryepiglottic fold is in the hypopharynx, while the anterior wall is in the supraglottic larynx. For this reason, this area is commonly referred to as the "marginal supraglottis."

Pharyngeal Mucosal Space

GRAPHICS

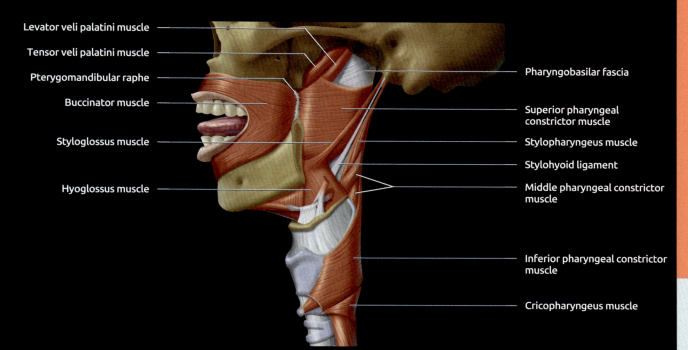

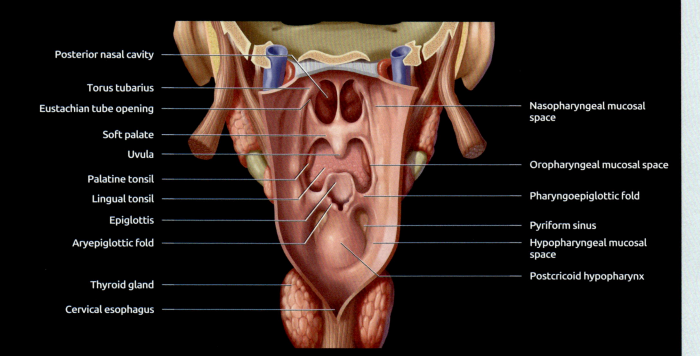

(Top) Lateral graphic shows the major muscles of the pharyngeal mucosal space. Notice the superior, middle, and inferior pharyngeal constrictor muscles are in the posterior wall of the pharyngeal mucosal space from the nasopharynx through the oropharynx to the hypopharynx. The pharyngobasilar fascia attaches the superior pharyngeal constrictor to the skull base. The distal end of the levator veli palatini muscle is on the airway side of the middle layer of deep cervical fascia, making it a part of the pharyngeal mucosal space. (Bottom) Graphic of the pharyngeal mucosal space/surface seen from behind shows this space can be divided into nasopharyngeal, oropharyngeal, and hypopharyngeal areas. The lymphatic ring of the pharyngeal mucosal space contains the nasopharyngeal adenoids and the oropharyngeal palatine and lingual tonsils.

Pharyngeal Mucosal Space

GENERIC PHARYNGEAL MUCOSAL SPACE MASS

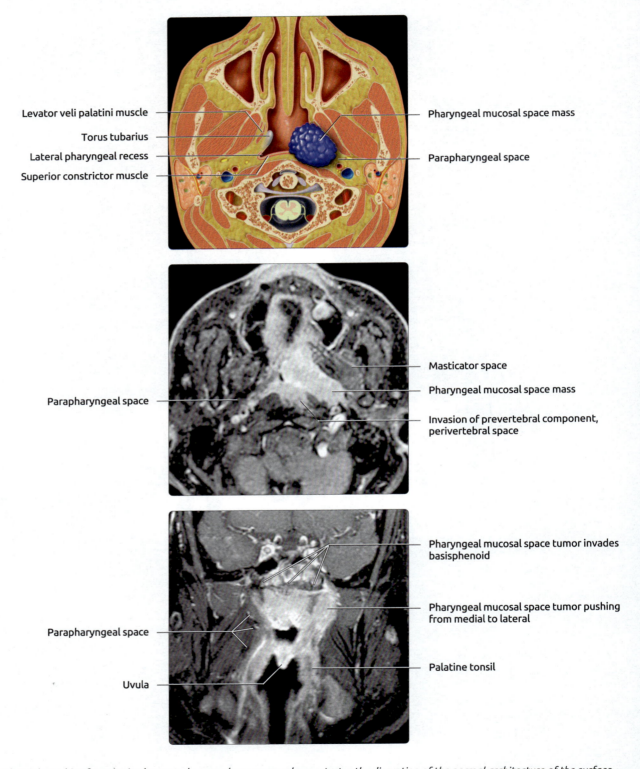

(Top) Axial graphic of a generic pharyngeal mucosal space mass demonstrates the disruption of the normal architecture of the surface of the pharynx with bulging of the mass into the pharyngeal airway. Also notice the deep margin of the mass is displacing the parapharyngeal space fat from medial to lateral. (Middle) In this illustrative case of squamous cell carcinoma of the nasopharyngeal aspect of the pharyngeal mucosal space, the tumor can be seen disrupting the mucosal surface of the nasopharynx while pushing into the parapharyngeal space from medial to lateral. The parapharyngeal space is more difficult to see because this is a fat-saturated T1-enhanced MR. (Bottom) In this coronal fat-saturated T1 C+ MR of nasopharyngeal carcinoma, the area of abutment and invasion of the skull base by this pharyngeal mucosal space tumor are clearly visible.

Pharyngeal Mucosal Space

BARIUM SWALLOW

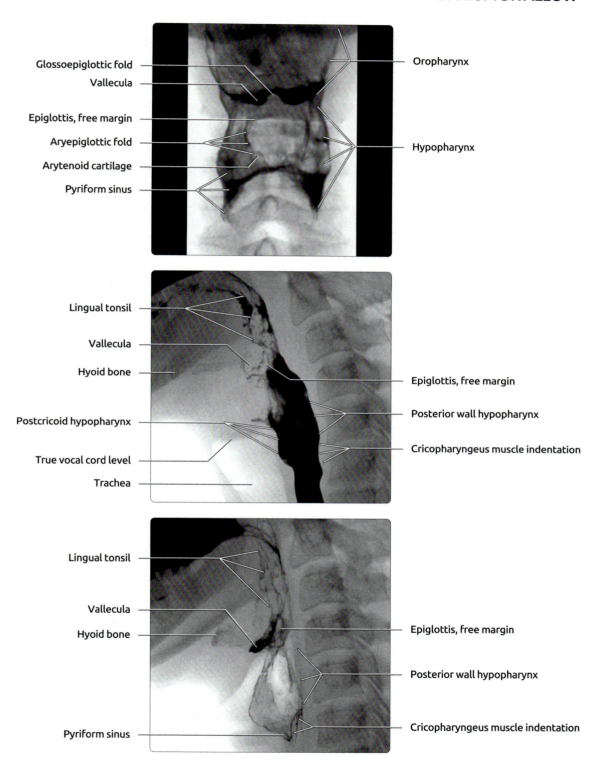

(Top) Anteroposterior barium swallow image focused on the low oropharyngeal and hypopharyngeal mucosal space surfaces is shown. Notice the hypopharynx extends from the level of the vallecula and glossoepiglottic fold superiorly to the inferior margin of the pyriform sinus. (Middle) In this lateral view of a barium swallow, the irregular surface of the lingual tonsil is recognized along the posterior margin of the tongue. The postcricoid area and the posterior wall of the hypopharynx make up 2 of the 3 major subsites within the hypopharynx. The 3rd subsite is the pyriform sinus. (Bottom) In this lateral barium swallow image, the indentation of the cricopharyngeus muscle is particularly well seen. Remember, the inferior margin of the vallecula marks the transition from oropharynx to hypopharynx.

Pharyngeal Mucosal Space

AXIAL T1 MR

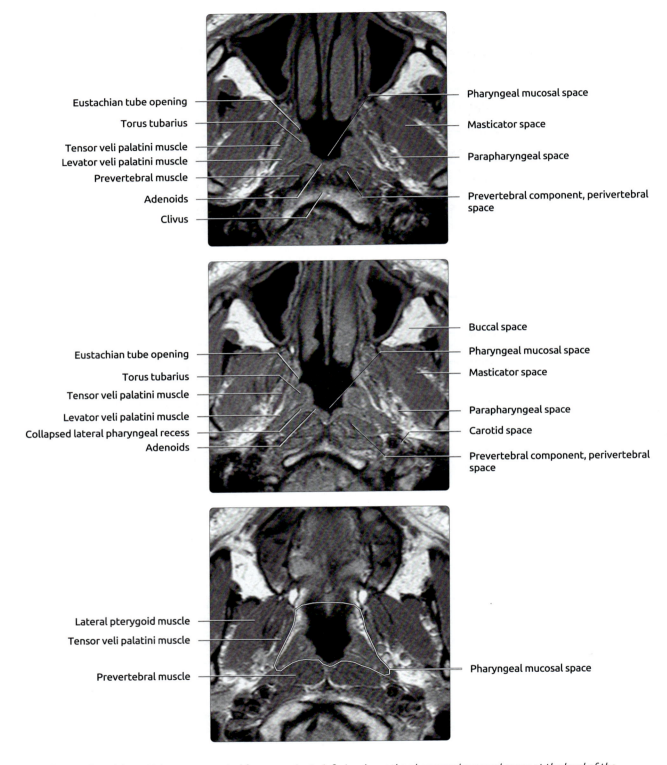

(Top) *First of 6 axial T1 MR images presented from superior to inferior shows the pharyngeal mucosal space at the level of the nasopharynx. Notice the torus tubarius (distal cartilaginous eustachian tube) and nasopharyngeal adenoids. The lateral pharyngeal recess is collapsed and therefore not visible on imaging.* (Middle) *In this image, the levator veli palatini muscle is seen transitioning to the pharyngeal side of the middle layer of deep cervical fascia (not seen). It does so over the superior margin of the pharyngobasilar fascia in the sinus of Morgagni. The tensor veli palatini muscle does not enter the pharyngeal mucosal space.* (Bottom) *In this image through the inferior maxillary sinuses, the area of the pharyngeal mucosal space is outlined. Remember, the middle layer of deep cervical fascia forms the lateral and posterior deep margins of the pharyngeal mucosal space.*

Pharyngeal Mucosal Space

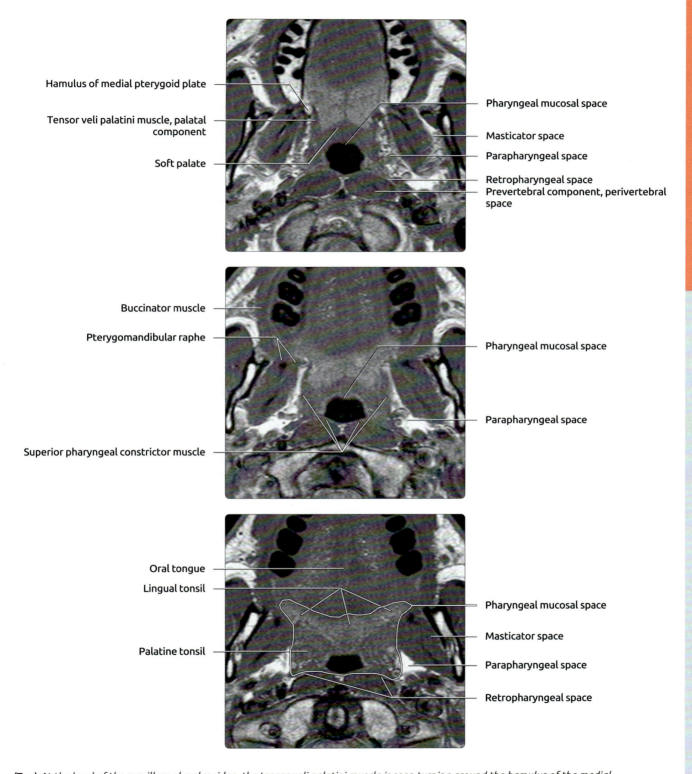

(Top) At the level of the maxillary alveolar ridge, the tensor veli palatini muscle is seen turning around the hamulus of the medial pterygoid plate to enter the anterolateral soft palate. Notice that posterior to the pharyngeal mucosal space, the thin fat stripe of the retropharyngeal space is just visible in front of the prevertebral component of the perivertebral space. (Middle) At the level of the maxillary teeth, the pharyngeal mucosal space of the superior oropharynx is seen. Note the superior margin of the palatine tonsil along with the soft palate itself. The superior pharyngeal constrictor muscle is present along the margins of the pharyngeal mucosal space just inside the middle layer of deep cervical fascia, which cannot be seen with imaging. (Bottom) In the midoropharynx, the lingual and palatine tonsils of the pharyngeal mucosal space lymphatic ring fill the pharyngeal mucosal space.

Pharyngeal Mucosal Space

AXIAL T2 MR

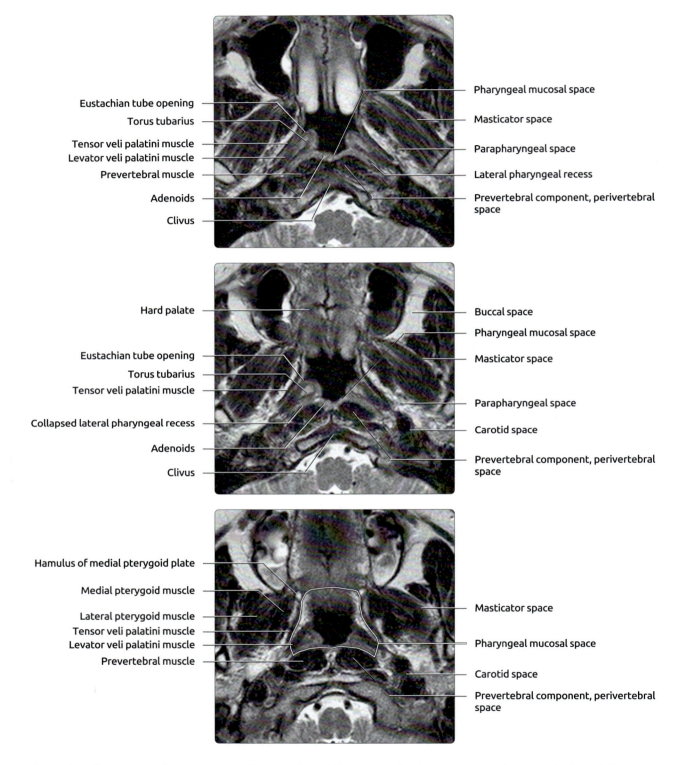

(Top) *First of 9 axial T2 MR images presented from superior to inferior shows the pharyngeal mucosal space at the level of the nasopharynx. Notice the torus tubarius (distal cartilaginous eustachian tube) and nasopharyngeal adenoids. The lateral pharyngeal recess is collapsed and therefore not visible on imaging.* (Middle) *In this image, the levator veli palatini muscle is seen transitioning to the pharyngeal side of the middle layer of deep cervical fascia (not seen). It does so over the superior margin of the pharyngobasilar fascia in the sinus of Morgagni. The tensor veli palatini muscle does not enter the pharyngeal mucosal space.* (Bottom) *In this image through the inferior maxillary sinuses, the area of the pharyngeal mucosal space is outlined.*

Pharyngeal Mucosal Space

AXIAL T2 MR

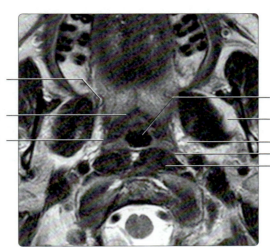

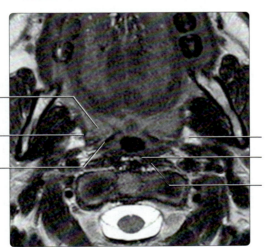

(Top) At the level of the soft palate, the pharyngeal mucosal space is seen with the parapharyngeal space along its lateral borders. The retropharyngeal space is very thin at this level, but it is present between the posterior pharyngeal mucosal space and the prevertebral component of the perivertebral space. (Middle) At the level of the maxillary teeth, the pharyngeal mucosal space of the superior oropharynx is visible. Note the superior margin of the palatine tonsil. The superior pharyngeal constrictor muscle is present along the margins of the pharyngeal mucosal space just inside the middle layer of deep cervical fascia, which cannot be seen with imaging. (Bottom) In this image through the midoropharynx, the palatine tonsil is the main occupant of the pharyngeal mucosal space. The retropharyngeal space fat stripe is seen posteriorly, while the parapharyngeal spaces are lateral.

Pharyngeal Mucosal Space

AXIAL T2 MR

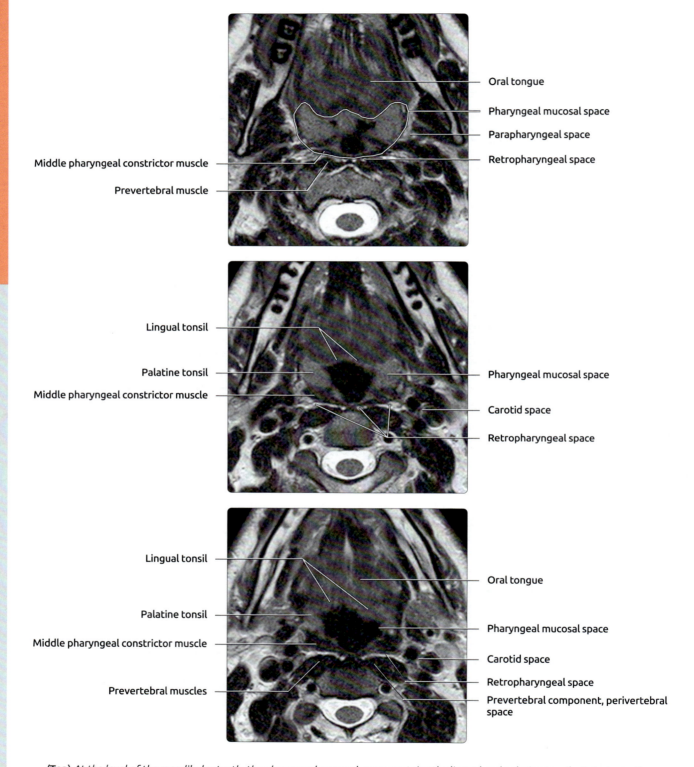

(Top) At the level of the mandibular teeth, the pharyngeal mucosal space contains the lingual and palatine tonsils. Anterior to the lingual tonsil is the oral tongue of the oral cavity. (Middle) In this image, the retropharyngeal space fat stripe is clearly seen posterior to the pharyngeal mucosal space. Behind the retropharyngeal space is the prevertebral component of the perivertebral space. A posterior pharyngeal wall squamous cell carcinoma may directly invade the retropharyngeal space or spread via lymphatics to the retropharyngeal nodes. (Bottom) Low in the oropharynx, thicker lingual tonsillar tissue can be seen along with an attenuated palatine tonsil. Remember the lingual tonsil is located in the oropharynx, not the oral cavity.

Pharyngeal Mucosal Space

GRAPHIC & CORONAL T1 C+ MR

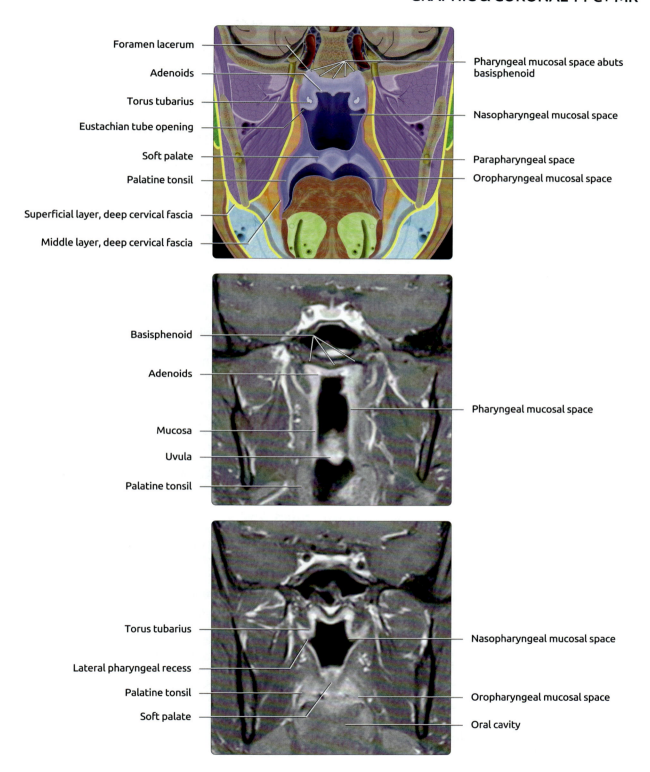

(Top) Coronal graphic of the nasopharyngeal and oropharyngeal mucosal space is shown. Notice the middle layer of deep cervical fascia defining the lateral margin of the pharyngeal mucosal space. The parapharyngeal spaces are paired fatty spaces lateral to the pharyngeal mucosal space. (Middle) Coronal T1 C+ FS MR shows the pharyngeal mucosal space surface enhances. Notice that the roof of the nasopharyngeal mucosal space abuts the basisphenoid. Remember that a nasopharyngeal carcinoma that begins in the roof of the nasopharynx will often have invaded the sphenoid sinus at the time of presentation. (Bottom) Coronal T1 C+ FS MR reveals the enhancing sheet of mucosa with the torus tubarius (cartilaginous eustachian tube) and lateral pharyngeal recess.

Masticator Space

TERMINOLOGY

Abbreviations
- Masticator space (MS), lateral pterygoid (LP), medial pterygoid (MP), foramen ovale (FO)

Definitions
- Large, paired anterolateral spaces of suprahyoid neck containing muscles of mastication, posterior body & ramus of mandible, maxillary artery, & CNV3
- Surgical terms
  - Temporal fossa: Suprazygomatic MS
  - Infratemporal fossa: Infrazygomatic MS

IMAGING ANATOMY

Overview
- **Suprazygomatic MS**: Contains only belly of temporalis muscle
- **Infrazygomatic MS**: MS "proper"; deep to zygomatic arch & superficial to pterygomaxillary fissure; contains masseter, MP, LP, maxillary artery, CNV3, mandible ramus/posterior body

Extent
- Craniocaudal extent of MS is more extensive than commonly recognized; reaches parietal bone at top
- Superior limit of muscular origin of temporalis muscle is "inferior temporal line," anteroposteriorly arched line crossing middle of parietal bone; temporal fascia covering muscle attaches to "superior temporal line" just above it
- Medially, MS fascia attaches to central skull base, medial to FO & foramen spinosum

Internal Contents
- **Muscles of mastication**
  - **Masseter**: Origin from zygomatic arch; inserts on lateral surface of ramus/angle of mandible
  - **Temporalis**: Origin from parietal bone; inserts on medial surface of coronoid process & anterior surface of mandibular ramus
  - **LP**: Origin from greater wing of sphenoid (superior head) & lateral surface of LP plate (inferior head); inserts on capsule & articular disk of TMJ (superior head) & neck of mandible (inferior head)
  - **MP**: Origin from medial surface LP plate & palatine bone pyramidal process; inserts on medial surface mandibular ramus
- **Mandibular division, trigeminal nerve (V3)**
  - **Relationship to skull base**: As main trunk of V3 exits FO, it is considered to be within MS; located just medial to LP & lateral to tensor veli palatini (TVP) muscle, surrounded by perineural venous plexus & trigeminal fat pad
  - **Masticator motor nerve branches** (proximal V3 motor to muscles of mastication)
  - **Mylohyoid nerve branch** (motor to anterior belly of digastric & mylohyoid muscles)
  - **Inferior alveolar nerve branch** (V3 sensory to mandible & chin)
  - **Lingual nerve** (V3 sensory to anterior 2/3 tongue, floor of mouth)
  - **Auriculotemporal nerve** (V3 sensory to external auditory canal/TMJ)

- **Ramus & posterior body of mandible**
  - Coronoid process: Temporalis muscle inserts here
  - Condylar process: Mandibular condyle neck & head
  - Temporomandibular joint is within MS
- **Maxillary artery** arises behind neck of mandible as larger terminal branch of external carotid artery & passes through MS; 3 parts
  - 1st (mandibular): Originates in retromandibular location & passes medial to mandibular neck, below auriculotemporal nerve, & along inferior margin of LP; 5 branches, most important is middle meningeal artery (MMA)
  - 2nd (pterygoid): Passes anteriorly, superficial to (or sometimes deep to or through) inferior head of LP
  - 3rd (pterygopalatine): Passes between 2 heads of LP → then through pterygomaxillary fissure → into pterygopalatine fossa, most important is sphenopalatine artery (artery of epistaxis)
- **Pterygoid venous plexus** along posterior border of LP & parapharyngeal space

Fascia of Masticator Space
- **Superficial layer, deep cervical fascia** (SL-DCF) splits along inferior mandible, creating "sling" enclosing MS
  - **Medial fascial slip** runs along deep surface of pterygoid muscles; inserts skull base undersurface medial to FO
  - **Lateral slip SL-DCF** covers surface of masseter muscle, attaching to zygomatic arch; continues cephalad covering temporalis muscle to top of suprazygomatic MS
  - **No horizontal fascia** exists deep to zygomatic arch; MS lesions pass freely craniocaudally under zygomatic arch
    - MS lesions pass freely in cranial-caudal directions under zygomatic arch

ANATOMY IMAGING ISSUES

Questions
- What imaging features define lesion as primary to MS?
  - Center of MS lesion must be in muscles of mastication or mandibular ramus
  - MS lesions displace parapharyngeal space fat from anterior to posterior

Imaging Recommendations
- CECT & MR are complimentary
- CT best delineates osseous involvement of mandible, skull base, pterygoid plates
- Enhanced multiplanar MR best for evaluating soft tissue, marrow involvement, & perineural tumor spread of V3
- If MS lesion affects **CNV3**, entire course of lesion should be imaged; from mental foramen anteriorly to nerve insertion at pons

Imaging Pitfalls
- MS pseudolesions
  - Pterygoid venous plexus variable & asymmetric; may appear as infiltrating lesion or perineural tumor spread
  - Unilateral V3 motor atrophy of muscles of mastication can be confusing depending on acuity of denervation
  - Asymmetric accessory parotid tissue may appear as a unilateral "mass" over surface of masseter muscle

Masticator Space

GRAPHICS

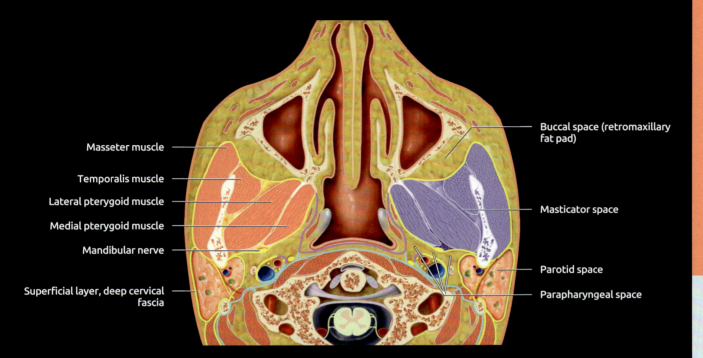

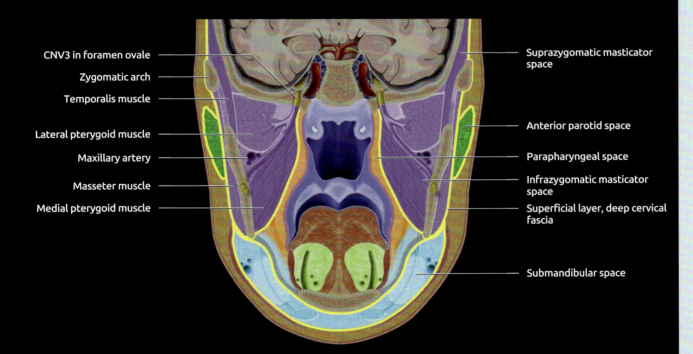

(Top) Axial graphic shows the masticator space enclosed by a superficial layer, deep cervical fascia (yellow line). The muscles of mastication from medial to lateral are the medial & lateral pterygoid, temporalis, & masseter muscles. The buccal space is anterior, while the parapharyngeal & parotid space are posterior to the masticator space. Masticator space frequently communicates posteriorly with the buccal space because the parotidomasseteric fascia is sometimes incomplete medially where it joins the buccopharyngeal fascia. (Bottom) Coronal graphic of the masticator space reveals a suprazygomatic & infrazygomatic component. Notice the superficial layer of deep cervical fascia attaches to the skull base just medial to the foramen ovale. There is no "horizontal fascia" beneath the zygomatic arch preventing spread of masticator space disease superiorly into the suprazygomatic masticator space.

Masticator Space

GRAPHICS

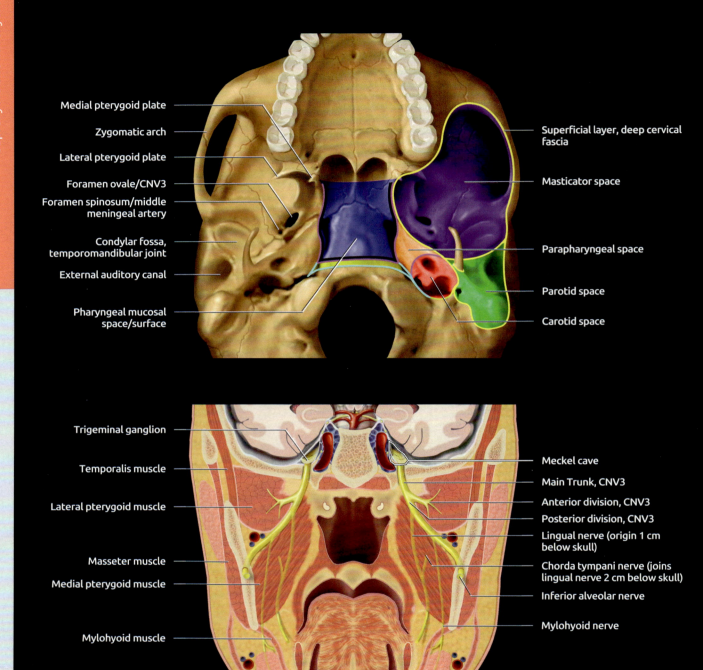

(Top) Graphic of skull base viewed from below shows masticator space abutting the sphenoid & temporal bones. Masticator space (purple) has a broad abutment with skull base. CNV3 enters masticator space through foramen ovale, while foramen spinosum conveys middle meningeal artery into intracranial compartment. Notice the temporomandibular joint is within the confines of masticator space. (Bottom) Coronal graphic shows mandibular division of trigeminal nerve. CNV3 exits skull base through foramen ovale without entering cavernous sinus. The motor branch from CNV3 main trunk is nerve to medial pterygoid, which also supplies tensor veli palatini & tensor tympani muscles. Anterior division motor branches are masseteric nerve, 2 deep temporal nerves to temporalis, & nerve to lateral pterygoid. The mylohyoid nerve (branch of inferior alveolar nerve), which supplies mylohyoid & anterior belly of digastric muscles, contains all motor fibers of posterior division. Main sensory branches are the meningeal branch (from main trunk), buccal nerve (from anterior division) & auriculotemporal nerve, & terminal lingual & inferior alveolar nerves (branches of posterior division).

Masticator Space

GENERIC MASTICATOR SPACE MASS

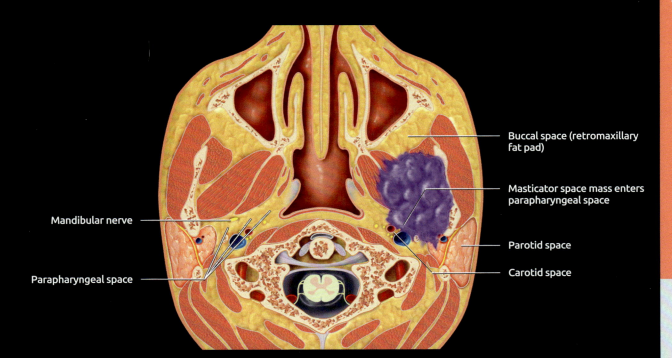

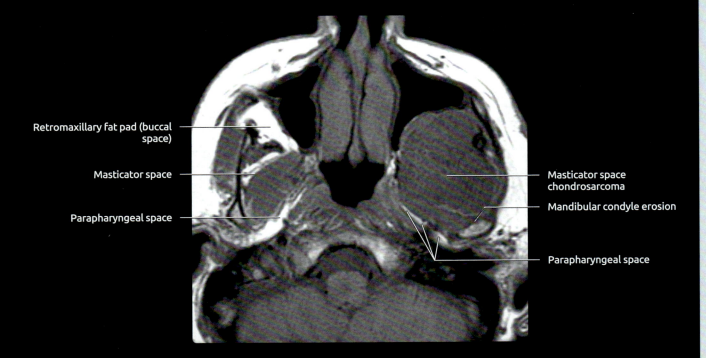

(Top) *Axial graphic at the level of the low nasopharynx demonstrates a generic masticator space mass invading the parapharyngeal space from anterior to posterior. Notice the mandibular nerve is engulfed by the tumor. Masticator space masses invade the masticator muscles & erode the posterior body, ramus, or condylar process of the mandible.* (Bottom) *Axial T1 MR through the nasopharynx shows a large mass of the masticator space that displaces the parapharyngeal space from anterior to posterior, invades the muscles of mastication, & erodes the mandibular condyle. The differential diagnosis of primary tumors of the masticator space includes sarcoma & non-Hodgkin lymphoma. In this case, the tumor was a chondrosarcoma.*

Masticator Space

PERINEURAL CNV3 MALIGNANCY

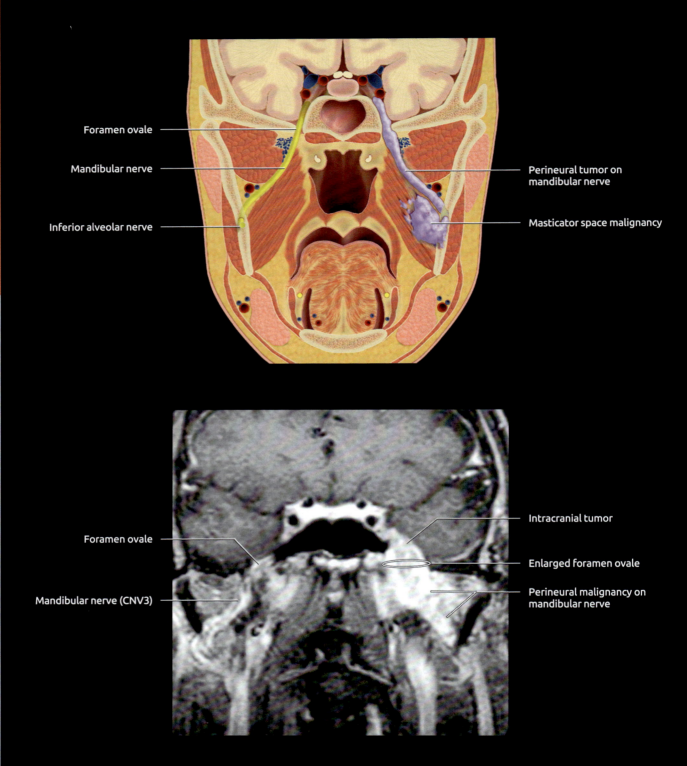

(Top) Coronal graphic of the suprahyoid neck focused on the masticator space & mandibular nerve is shown. In this drawing, a generic masticator space malignancy is visible invading the lower masticator space, invading the adjacent mandible, & spreading via a perineural route up the mandibular nerve through the foramen ovale into the intracranial compartment. Both primary masticator space malignancy & squamous cell carcinoma of the oral cavity can access the intracranial compartment in this manner. (Bottom) Coronal T1 C+ FS MR through the foramen ovale shows an enhancing perineural malignant tumor spreading superiorly from the left masticator space along the mandibular nerve. Notice the enlarged left foramen ovale & intracranial tumor. In this case, the tumor came from a primary melanoma on the skin of the chin.

Masticator Space

AXIAL CECT

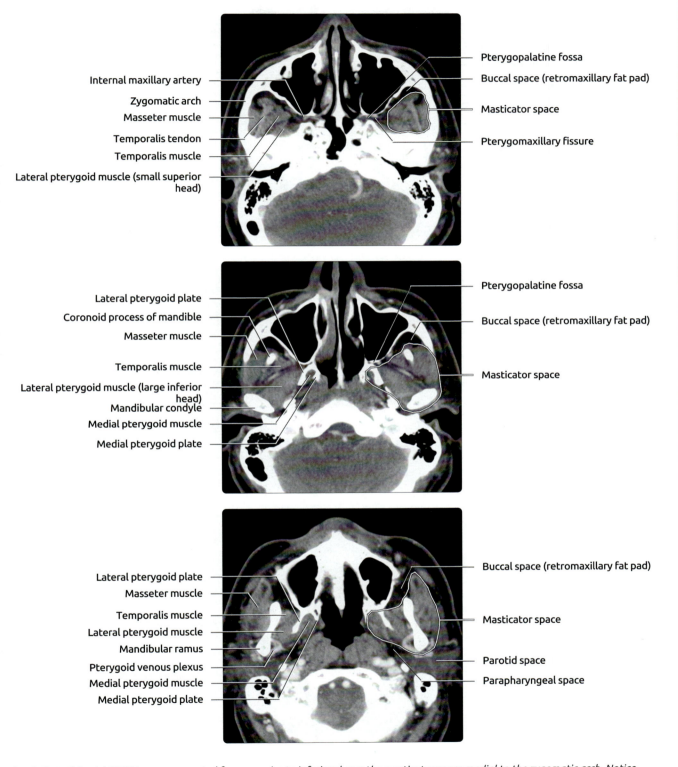

(Top) First of 6 axial CECT images presented from superior to inferior shows the masticator space medial to the zygomatic arch. Notice the masseter muscle arising from the inferior margin of the zygomatic arch. Also note the superior head of the lateral pterygoid muscle. The 3rd (pterygopalatine) part of the maxillary artery enters the pterygopalatine fossa through the pterygomaxillary fissure, after passing between 2 heads of the lateral pterygoid muscle. (Middle) At the level of the mandibular condyles, the masticator space contains the muscles of mastication & temporomandibular joint. Note the inferior head of the lateral pterygoid muscle arising from the lateral surface of the lateral pterygoid plate. The medial pterygoid muscle arises from the pterygoid fossa. (Bottom) In this image through the low maxillary sinuses, the masticator space is seen between the more anterior buccal space & the more posterior parapharyngeal & parotid spaces. Notice the pterygoid venous plexus as the enhancing area along the posterolateral margin of the masticator space.

Masticator Space

AXIAL CECT

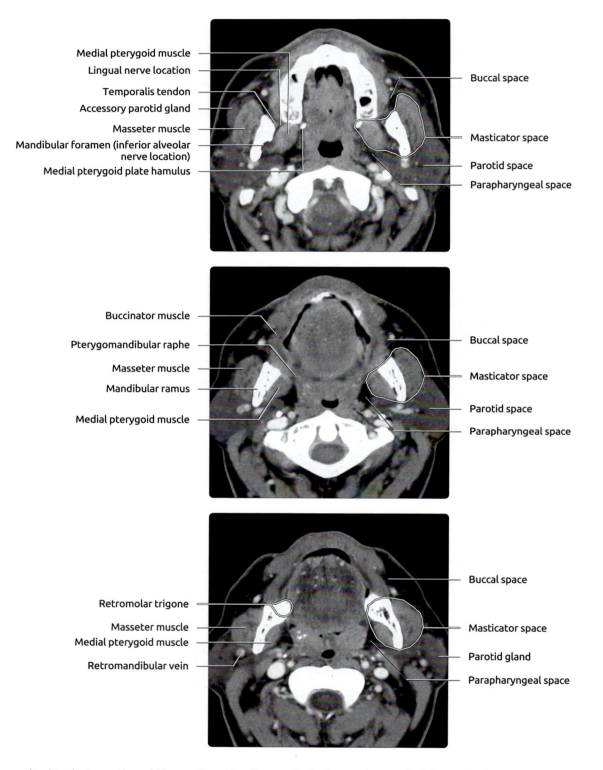

(Top) *In this image through the maxillary ridge, the mandibular foramen is seen. The inferior alveolar nerve enters the mandible in this location. Lingual nerve is located along the anterior margin of the medial pterygoid muscle at this level. Note the hamulus of the medial pterygoid plate, which acts as a pulley for the tendon of the tensor veli palatini muscle & is the site of superior attachment of the pterygomandibular raphe.* (Middle) *In this image, the attachment of the medial pterygoid is visible along the medial ramus. Remember, the pterygomandibular raphe is the tendinous point of junction between the buccinator muscle & the superior constrictor muscle.* (Bottom) *In this image, the retromolar triangle is seen. Notice the retromolar trigone sits on the anterior surface of the masticator space. If a squamous cell carcinoma arises in the retromolar trigone, the masticator space may be directly invaded. From there, perineural tumor spread on CNV3 may occur.*

Masticator Space

AXIAL T1 MR

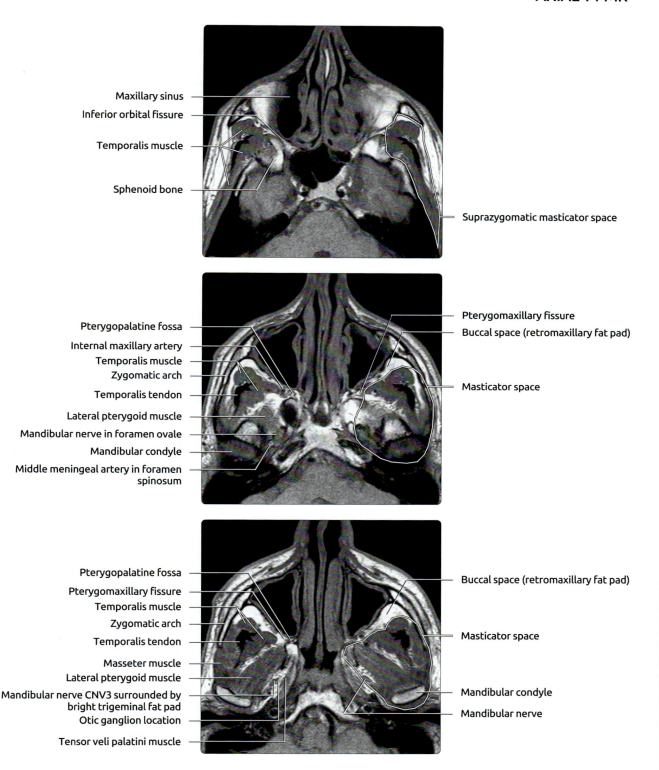

(Top) First of 6 axial T1 MR images from superior to inferior shows that above zygomatic arch, the suprazygomatic masticator space is seen. Notice temporalis muscle & fat are only occupants of this portion of masticator space. (Middle) The mandibular nerve (CNV3) can be visualized within foramen ovale. Middle meningeal artery can be seen posterolateral to foramen ovale within foramen spinosum. Auriculotemporal nerve, which arises by 2 roots of proximal posterior division of CNV3, runs backward, encircling middle meningeal artery & forms a single trunk. Pterygopalatine fossa opens laterally through pterygomaxillary fissure into masticator space. (Bottom) Mandibular nerve is visible along posteromedial border of lateral pterygoid muscle. Temporalis muscle & its hypointense tendon fill anterolateral masticator space. Lateral pterygoid muscle inferior head originates from lateral surface of lateral pterygoid plate. Main trunk of mandibular nerve is located near skull base medial to lateral pterygoid & lateral to tensor veli palatini muscle, within T1-hyperintense trigeminal fat pad. Otic ganglion (not visualized) lies just below skull base between CNV3 & tensor veli palatini.

Masticator Space

AXIAL T1 MR

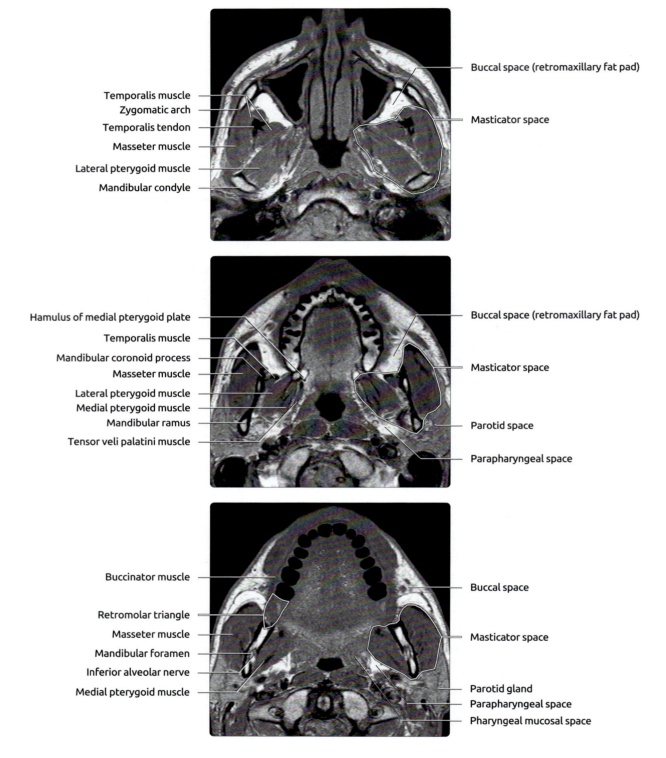

(Top) The masseter muscle is seen arising from the inferior surface of the zygomatic arch. The retromaxillary fat pad (superior buccal space) is visible anterior to the masticator space. (Middle) In this image at the level of the maxillary ridge, the temporalis muscle is seen inserting on the medial surface of the coronoid process of the mandible. The tensor veli palatini muscle approaches the hamulus of the medial pterygoid plate where it will turn medially to the soft palate. (Bottom) In this image at the level of the mandibular teeth, the inferior alveolar nerve can be seen entering the mandibular foramen. The retromolar triangle represents the mucosal surface behind the 3rd mandibular molar & in front of the anterior mandibular ramus. Squamous cell carcinoma of the retromolar triangle, when invasive, readily involves the masticator space.

Masticator Space

CORONAL T1 MR

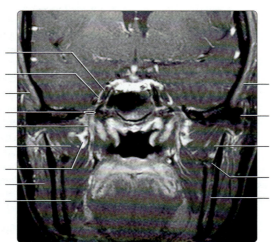

- Meckel cave
- Trigeminal ganglion
- Temporalis muscle
- Foramen ovale
- Mandibular nerve
- Lateral pterygoid muscle
- Pterygoid venous plexus
- Masseter muscle
- Medial pterygoid muscle
- Suprazygomatic masticator space
- Zygomatic arch
- Infrazygomatic masticator space
- Mandibular foramen
- Mandibular ramus

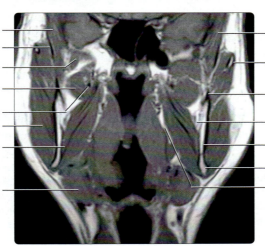

- Temporalis muscle
- Temporalis tendon
- Lateral pterygoid muscle, superior head
- Lateral pterygoid muscle, inferior head
- Internal maxillary artery
- Masseter muscle
- Medial pterygoid muscle
- Submandibular gland
- Suprazygomatic masticator space
- Zygomatic arch
- Mandibular coronoid process
- Infrazygomatic masticator space
- Mandibular ramus
- Angle of mandible
- Parapharyngeal space

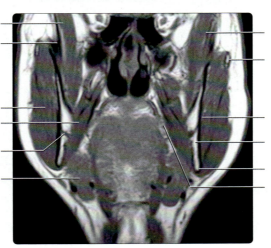

- Temporalis muscle
- Temporalis tendon
- Masseter muscle
- Medial pterygoid muscle
- Inferior alveolar nerve
- Submandibular gland
- Suprazygomatic masticator space
- Zygomatic arch
- Infrazygomatic masticator space
- Mandibular ramus
- Angle of mandible
- Parapharyngeal space

(**Top**) Coronal T1 FS MR shows mandibular nerve (main trunk CNV3) descending through foramen ovale. Although not seen in CT/MR, note secretomotor supply to parotid gland via auriculotemporal branch of CNV3 functionally comes from parasympathetic fibers of glossopharyngeal nerve (CNIX), relaying in otic ganglion; ganglion is only topographically related to CNV3. Also note chorda tympani nerve joining lingual nerve ~ 2 cm below skull base is a branch of the facial nerve (CNVII), which senses taste from anterior 2/3 of tongue & provides secretomotor supply to submandibular/sublingual salivary glands via its preganglionic parasympathetic supply to submandibular ganglion functionally through CNVII; ganglion is only topographically related to lingual nerve (CNV3) in sublingual space. (**Middle**) Coronal T1-unenhanced MR reveals superior & inferior heads of lateral pterygoid muscles. Also note medial pterygoid muscle arises from pterygoid fossa above & inserts on medial ramus & angle of mandible. (**Bottom**) Coronal T1-unenhanced MR through posterior nose shows masseter muscle arising from inferior surface of zygomatic arch & inserting on lateral ramus & angle of mandible. Note inferior alveolar nerve as focal low-signal focus within high-signal fatty marrow of mandible.

Parotid Space

Suprahyoid and Infrahyoid Neck

TERMINOLOGY

Abbreviations

- Parotid space (PS)

Definitions

- **PS**: Paired lateral suprahyoid neck spaces enclosed by superficial layer deep cervical fascia containing parotid glands, nodes, and extracranial facial nerve branches

IMAGING ANATOMY

Extent

- PS extends from external auditory canal (EAC) and mastoid tip superiorly to below angle of mandible (parotid tail)
  - Parotid tail inserts inferiorly between platysma and sternocleidomastoid muscle in area of posterior submandibular space

Anatomy Relationships

- Parapharyngeal space (PPS) is directly medial to PS
- Masticator space is anterior to PS
- Buccal space (BS) is anterolateral to PS superficially
- Carotid space (CS) is posteromedial to PS; posterior belly of digastric muscle separates upper PS from CS

Internal Contents

- **Parotid gland**
  - Superficial lobe represents ~ 2/3 of PS
  - Deep lobe projects medially, abuts PPS
- **Extracranial facial nerve (CNVII)**
  - Exits stylomastoid foramen as single trunk; ramifies within PS lateral to retromandibular vein
  - Ramifying intraparotid facial nerve creates surgical plane between superficial and deep lobes
  - Intraparotid facial nerve **not visible** with CT or MR except proximally with high-resolution 3T MR
  - Divides into 2 branches, temporofacial (divides into temporal and zygomatic branches) and cervicofacial (divides into buccal, marginal mandibular, and cervical branches)
  - Auriculotemporal nerve (CNV3 branch) crosses through body of parotid gland at right angles to facial nerve and usually has direct communications with CNVII here; parotid perineural tumor spread can occur to CNV
  - Facial nerve does not supply parotid; gland nerve supply from auriculotemporal nerve (parasympathetic secretomotor and sensory); parotid fascia and skin sensory supply from great auricular nerve (C2, C3)
- **External carotid artery (ECA)**
  - Medial, smaller vessel of 2 seen just behind mandibular ramus in PS
- **Retromandibular vein**
  - Lateral, larger of 2 vessels seen just behind mandibular ramus in parotid
  - Intraparotid facial nerve branches course just lateral to retromandibular vein
- **Intraparotid lymph nodes**
  - ~ 20 lymph nodes found in each parotid gland
  - Parotid nodes are 1st-order drainage for EAC, pinna, surrounding deep face and scalp
  - PS undergoes **late encapsulation** in embryogenesis resulting in intraparotid lymph nodes
- **Parotid duct (Stensen duct)**
  - ~ 5 cm long, emerges from anterior PS, runs along surface of masseter muscle in BS
  - Duct then arches through BS to pierce buccinator muscle at level of upper 2nd molar
- **Accessory parotid glands**
  - Project over surface of masseter muscles, along parotid duct (facial process of parotid)
  - Present in ~ 20% of normal anatomic dissections
  - Have their own blood supply and secondary duct emptying into Stensen duct
  - Other small processes are glenoid process (superior extension between EAC and TMJ), pterygoid process (between medial pterygoid and mandible ramus), and poststyloid process

Fascia of Parotid Space

- Superficial layer of deep cervical fascia surrounds PS
- Superficial lamina (parotidomasseteric fascia) thick and adherent to gland; parotid swellings very painful due to unyielding nature of fascia
- Stylomandibular ligament is portion of deep lamina; separates parotid tail from submandibular salivary gland; ligament pierced by ECA

ANATOMY IMAGING ISSUES

Imaging Recommendations

- CECT or MR can both readily image PS; T1 C+ fat-saturated axial and coronal MR better for perineural CNVII spread
- Small, superficial lobe PS lesions need no imaging; needle aspiration to confirm benign mixed tumor with superficial parotidectomy sufficient
- If inflammation-infection of PS suspected, 2- to 3-mm slice thickness CECT best; angle gantry to avoid dental amalgam and visualize parotid duct looking for cause of obstruction
- If tumor suspected, T1 C+ fat-saturated MR best, temporal bone CT helps for bony changes; look for perineural facial nerve tumor along intratemporal segments CNVII

Imaging Pitfalls

- Parotid ~ soft tissue in children, progressively fatty with age
- Parotid tail mass must be identified as intraparotid or excision may injure facial nerve
- Facial nerve plane in parotid can only be estimated

CLINICAL IMPLICATIONS

Clinical Importance

- In cases of tumor, assess relationship of lesion to estimated facial nerve plane and evaluate for perineural spread
- Facial nerve horizontal within parotid, blood vessels vertical; parotid abscess best drained by horizontal incision/small holes (Hilton method) below angle of mandible
- If larger mass lesion of deep lobe, mass displaces PPS from lateral to medial with widening of stylomandibular gap
- Parotid tumors: Benign mixed tumor (75%), Warthin tumor (5%), adenoid cystic carcinoma (5%), mucoepidermoid carcinoma (5%), other (10%)

Parotid Space

GRAPHICS

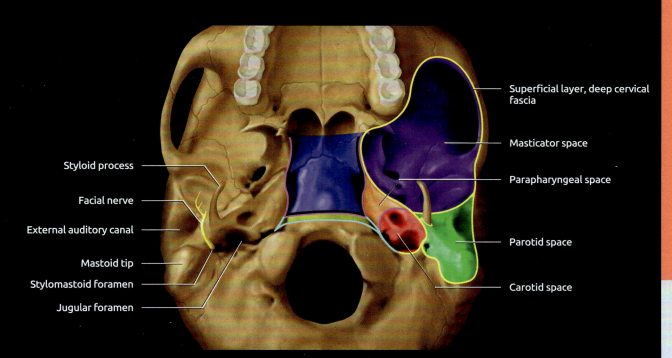

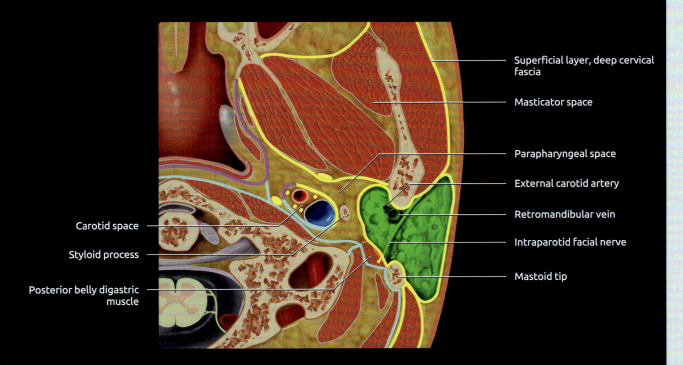

(Top) Axial graphic of the skull base viewed from below illustrates the interaction between the parotid space and the skull base. CNVII exits through the stylomastoid foramen at the skull base, just posterior to the styloid process and lateral to the jugular foramen. The parotid space is the most lateral space in the nasopharyngeal and oropharyngeal area, extending from the external auditory canal above to the level of the mandibular angle below. (Bottom) Axial graphic of the parotid space at the level of C1 vertebral body is shown. The parotid space contains the external carotid artery, retromandibular vein, and facial nerve, from medial to lateral. The intraparotid CNVII creates a surgical plane that divides the gland into superficial and deep lobes. Parotid masses arising in the deep lobe will displace the parapharyngeal space fat medially. The parotid space is enclosed by the superficial layer of the deep cervical fascia.

Parotid Space

GRAPHICS

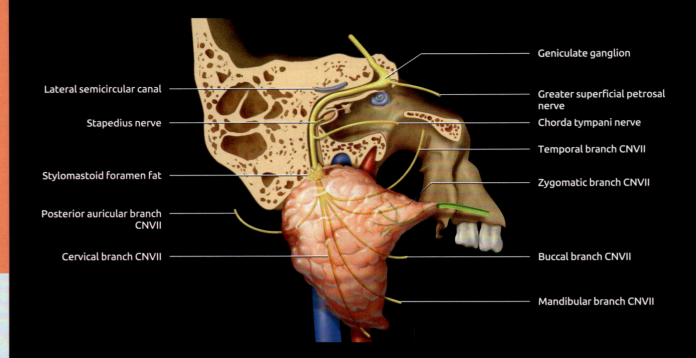

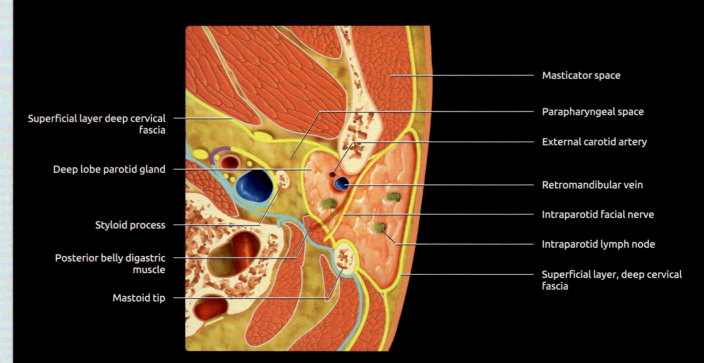

(Top) Sagittal graphic of the parotid gland and facial nerve is shown. The facial nerve exits the skull base at the stylomastoid foramen, and then enters the parotid gland where it ramifies into 6 major branches. The plane of the facial nerve branches within the parotid gland is used by the surgeons to define a superficial and deep lobe of the parotid. This is a surgically defined, not a radiologically defined, delineation. (Bottom) Axial graphic of the parotid space at the level of C1 vertebral body is shown. The intraparotid course of the facial nerve extends from just medial to the mastoid tip to a position just lateral to the retromandibular vein. Late embryologic encapsulation of the parotid gland accounts for intraparotid lymph nodes, which serve as 1st-order drainage for malignancies of the deep face, scalp, and external ear. The normal parotid gland contains ~ 20 nodes.

Parotid Space

GENERIC PAROTID SPACE MASS

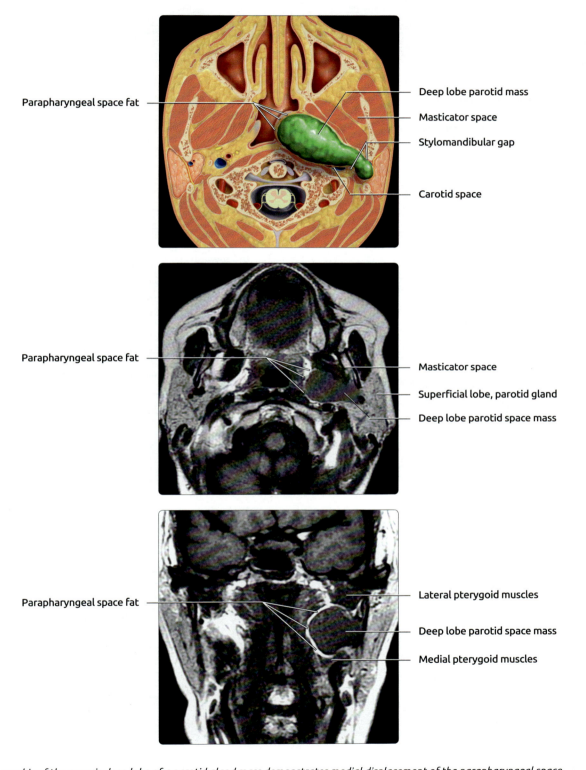

(Top) Axial graphic of the generic deep lobe of a parotid gland mass demonstrates medial displacement of the parapharyngeal space fat. Also notice the slight enlargement of the stylomandibular gap. Smaller lesions of the superficial lobe of the parotid gland are easily identified as intraparotid. Larger deep lobe lesions may be more difficult to identify as parotid space in origin. (Middle) Axial T1 MR through the maxillary ridge reveals a pear-shaped mass arising from the deep lobe of the parotid gland. This benign mixed tumor enlarges medially, displacing the parapharyngeal space from lateral to medial. (Bottom) Coronal T1 MR of a large benign mixed tumor enlarging medially from its origin in the deep lobe of the parotid gland is shown. Note the crescent of parapharyngeal space fat arching medially and still visible despite the large size of this deep lobe tumor.

PERINEURAL PAROTID SPACE MALIGNANCY

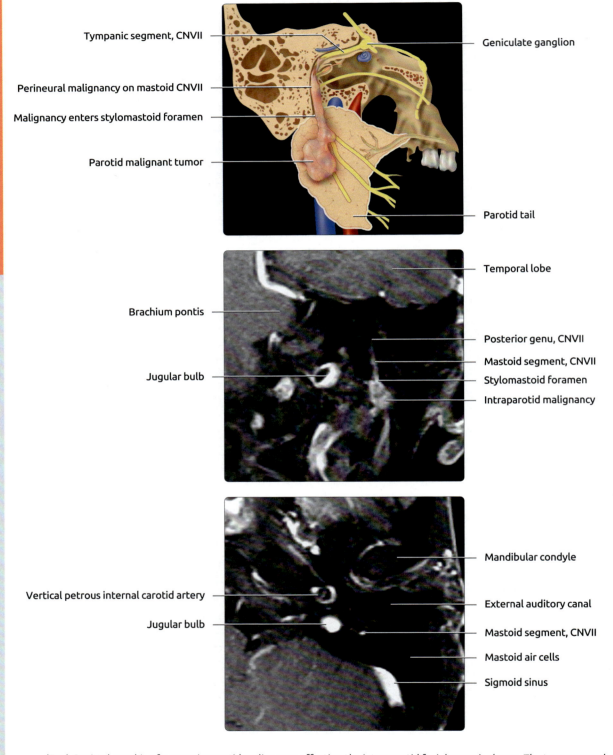

(Top) Sagittal graphic of a generic parotid malignancy affecting the intraparotid facial nerve is shown. The tumor spreads along CNVII through the stylomastoid foramen to the proximal mastoid segment within the temporal bone. If left untreated, such a perineural malignant tumor will eventually access the intracranial compartment via the internal auditory canal. (Middle) Coronal T1 C+ FS MR of the left temporal bone shows an enhancing adenoid cystic carcinoma of the parotid gland spreading into the lower flared portion of the stylomastoid foramen. This malignant tumor then spreads in a perineural fashion up the mastoid segment of the facial nerve to the posterior genu. (Bottom) Axial T1 C+ FS MR reveals an enlarged enhancing mastoid segment of CNVII as a result of perineural spread of adenoid cystic carcinoma from the parotid space.

Parotid Space

AXIAL CECT

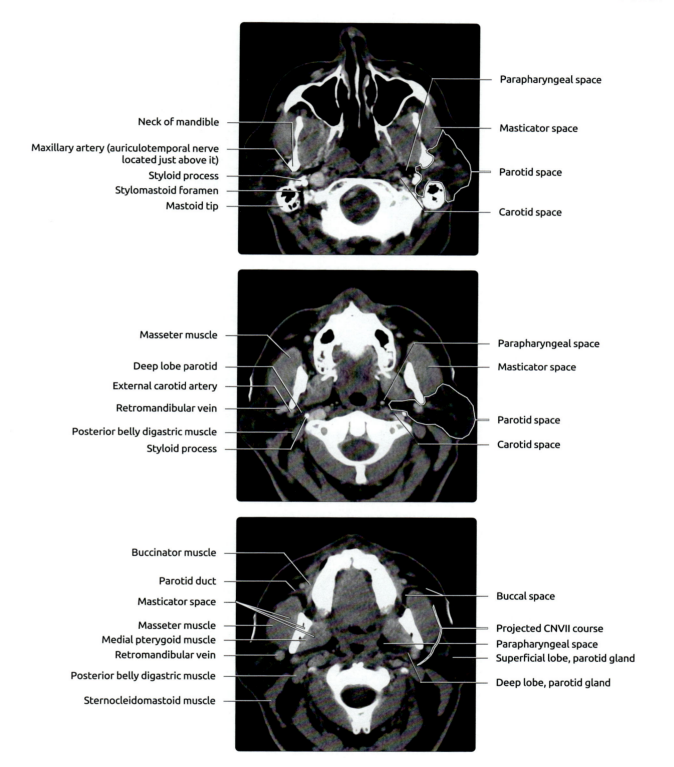

(Top) First of 6 axial CECT images from superior to inferior shows right stylomastoid foramen with low-attenuation fat contained within. Facial nerve is not visualized on CT images. If a perineural tumor is present, stylomastoid foramen fat will be replaced by tumor. Note maxillary artery, which is 1 of 2 terminal branches of external carotid artery within parotid, leaving the gland at its anteromedial aspect. Auriculotemporal nerve (CNV3 branch) is situated just above maxillary artery at this level posterior to neck of mandible. Auriculotemporal nerve crosses through body of parotid gland at right angles to facial nerve & usually has direct communications with CNVII here with chances for facial to trigeminal perineural tumor spread. (Middle) Image shows deep lobe of parotid gland projecting through stylomandibular gap to abut parapharyngeal space. Note medial external carotid artery & more lateral retromandibular vein. (Bottom) Image shows parotid duct (in buccal space) piecing buccinator muscle just lateral to 2nd maxillary molar. Projected course of extracranial CNVII lateral to retromandibular vein & over surface of masseter muscle is drawn. Note large size of superficial lobe compared to deep lobe of parotid.

Parotid Space

AXIAL CECT

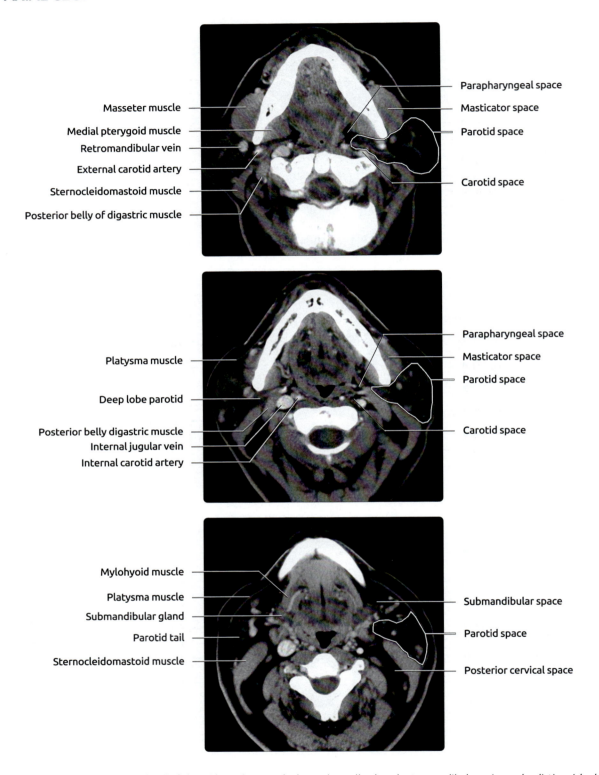

(Top) In this image at the level of the mid oropharynx, the larger laterally placed retromandibular vein can be distinguished from the more medial external carotid artery. Remember that the intraparotid facial nerve cannot be seen on CECT, but its path can be projected along a line just lateral to the retromandibular vein and out over the surface of the masseter muscle. (Middle) At the level of the mandibular angle, the parotid space is now separated from the carotid space by the posterior belly of the digastric muscle. Note the platysma muscle is now visible over the surface of the parotid gland. (Bottom) Just below the mandible, the parotid tail is visible projecting into the posterior aspect of the submandibular space. Excisional biopsy of a low-lying mass, unrecognized as being in the parotid tail, may result in facial nerve injury.

Parotid Space

AXIAL T1 MR

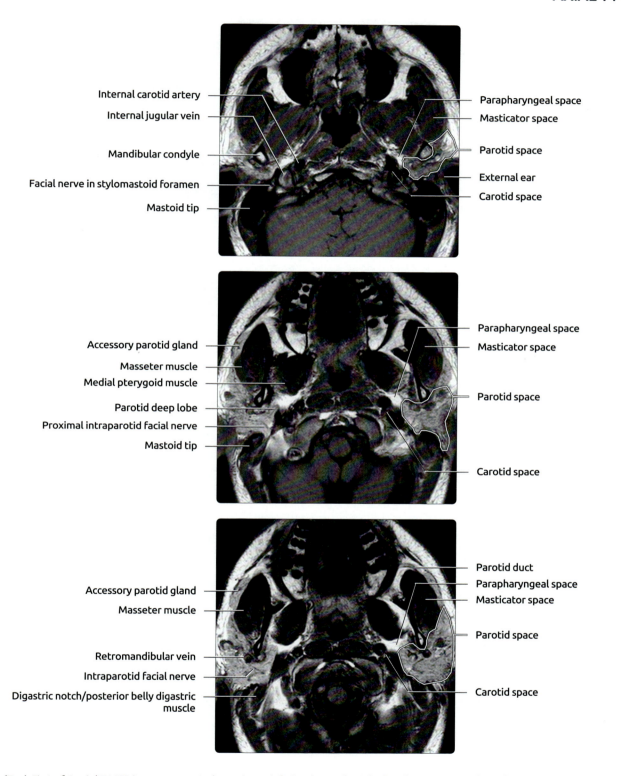

(Top) First of 6 axial T1 MR images presented superior to inferior shows the right facial nerve exiting the stylomandibular foramen. There is fat in the lower flared aspect of the stylomastoid foramen so the main trunk of the facial nerve is visible. (Middle) In this image, the proximal intraparotid facial nerve is seen on the right. Note the accessory parotid gland overlying the right masseter muscle bilaterally. (Bottom) At the level of the maxillary ridge, a branch of the intraparotid facial nerve is seen projecting anterolaterally around the lateral margin of the retromandibular vein. Usually not visible on routine imaging, the intraparotid facial nerve and its branches follow a predictable course anterolaterally around the lateral margin of the retromandibular vein, and from there anteriorly along the lateral surface of the masseter muscle. Frey syndrome (auriculotemporal syndrome) is gustatory sweating as a result of injury to the auriculotemporal nerve, which carries parasympathetic fibers to the parotid and overlying skin sweat glands. Inappropriate regeneration of parasympathetic nerve fibers may switch course resulting in sweating in anticipation of eating, instead of normal salivatory response.

Parotid Space

AXIAL T1 MR

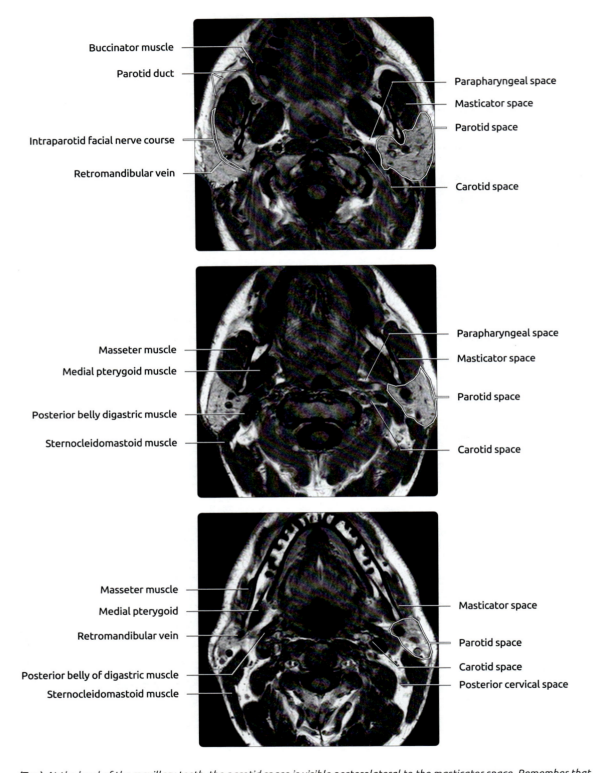

(Top) At the level of the maxillary teeth, the parotid space is visible posterolateral to the masticator space. Remember that both the masticator and parotid spaces are circumscribed by the superficial layer of the deep cervical fascia. Note the projected intraparotid facial nerve course drawn on the right. *(Middle)* In this image, the posterior belly of the digastric muscle is seen on the posteromedial boundary of the parotid space, separating the parotid space from the carotid space. The posterior belly of the digastric muscle is innervated by a branch of the facial nerve. *(Bottom)* In this image, the parotid gland is seen at the mandibular angle. The posterior belly of the digastric muscle is seen between the parotid tail and the carotid space on the left. When a parotid space mass is present, the medial displacement of the posterior belly of the digastric muscle helps define its location.

Parotid Space

AXIAL T2 FS MR

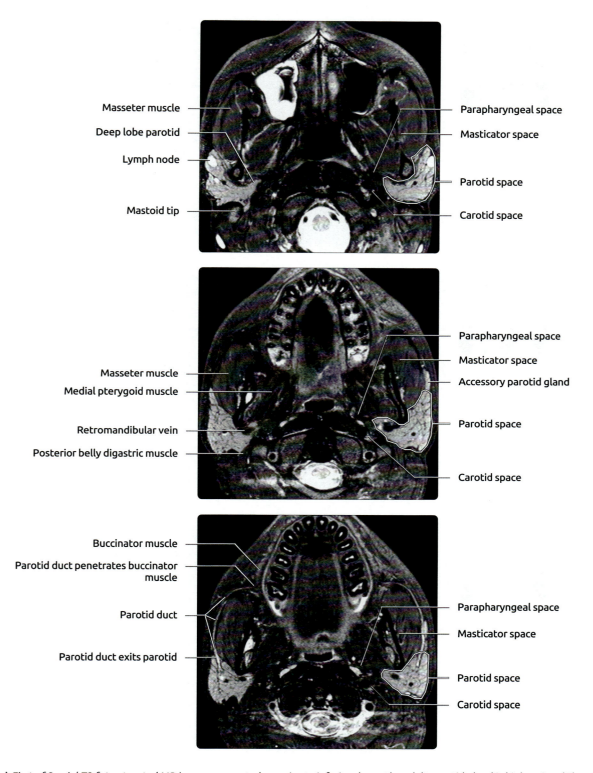

(Top) First of 3 axial T2 fat-saturated MR images presented superior to inferior shows the adult parotid gland is higher signal than the surrounding muscles of the suprahyoid neck. A few sporadic high-signal intraparotid nodes are present at this level. The parapharyngeal space fat is low signal because of the fat-saturation MR sequence. (Middle) The parotid space often abuts the accessory parotid gland that may be seen over the surface of the masseter muscle. Both are within the superficial layer of deep cervical fascia. (Bottom) In this image at the level of the maxillary teeth, the high-signal linear parotid duct is easily visualized extending anteriorly from the parotid gland along the surface of the masseter muscle to penetrate the buccinator muscle.

Parotid Space

TRANSVERSE ULTRASOUND

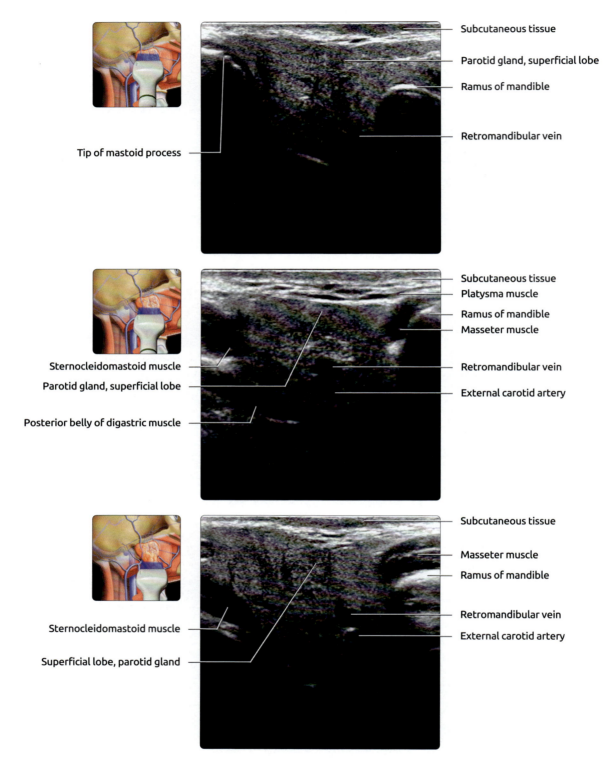

(Top) Transverse grayscale ultrasound shows the parotid region. Note its relationship to the mastoid process and the mandibular ramus. The glandular parenchyma shows a homogeneous, hyperechoic pattern. The retromandibular vein is visualized as a round, anechoic structure within the parotid gland (partially obscured in this image). *(Middle)* Transverse grayscale ultrasound shows the parotid tail region. The sternocleidomastoid muscle and the posterior belly of the digastric muscle are related to the posterior margin of the parotid tail. The retromandibular vein and external carotid artery serve as markers to infer the location of CNVII. *(Bottom)* Transverse grayscale ultrasound shows the parotid gland. The retromandibular vein is usually larger and lateral to the external carotid artery within the parotid gland. Note that the deep lobe is obscured by shadowing from the mandibular ramus.

Parotid Space

LONGITUDINAL ULTRASOUND

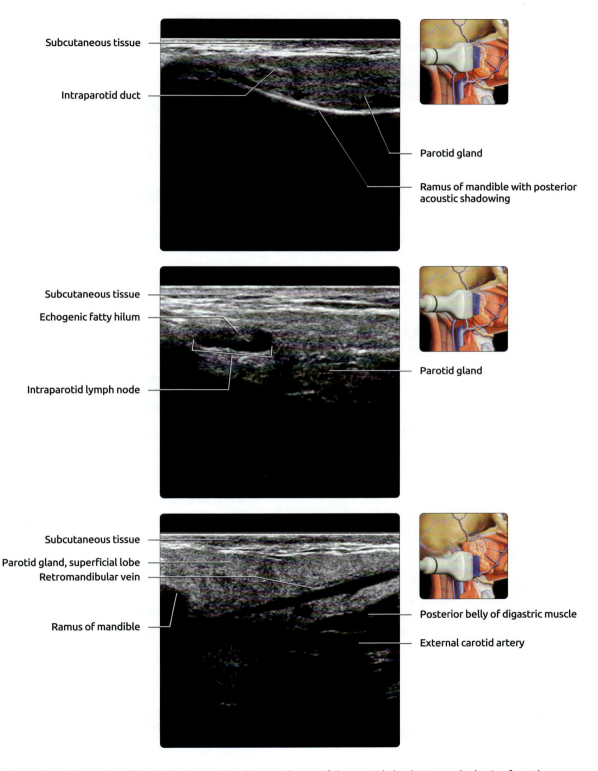

(Top) This is the 1st image in a series of longitudinal grayscale ultrasound scans of the parotid gland. Intense shadowing from the ramus of the mandible precludes visualization of deeper structures, including the deep lobe of the parotid gland. (Middle) Second image shows a normal intraparotid lymph node in the superficial lobe of the parotid gland. On high-resolution ultrasound, normal nodes are invariably seen in the parotid tail and in the pretragal parotid gland. The elliptical shape and normal internal architecture with echogenic hilum suggest its benign nature. (Bottom) Third image at the plane of the retromandibular vein is shown. Such anatomy is best seen in children and young adults where there is not much fat deposition in the gland.

Carotid Space

TERMINOLOGY

Abbreviations

- Carotid space (CS)
- Suprahyoid neck (SHN) and infrahyoid neck (IHN)

Definitions

- Paired, tubular spaces surrounded by carotid sheath that contain carotid arteries, internal jugular veins (IJVs), and **cranial nerves (CNs) IX-XII (SHN) and CNX (IHN)**

IMAGING ANATOMY

Overview

- CS travels from inferior margins of jugular foramen-carotid canal above to aortic arch below
- SHN CS contains CNIX-XII, internal carotid artery (ICA), and IJV
- IHN CS contains CNX only, common carotid artery (CCA), IJV; internal jugular nodal chain is closely associated with its outer surface

Extent

- CS defined from skull base (carotid canal and jugular foramen) to aortic arch below
- CS can be divided into its major segments
  - Nasopharyngeal, oropharyngeal, cervical, and mediastinal

Anatomy Relationships

- **SHN CS adjacent spaces**
  - Retropharyngeal space (RPS) medial; perivertebral space posterior; parapharyngeal space (PPS) anterior; and parotid space lateral
    - Posterior belly of digastric muscle separates CS from deep lobe of parotid gland
- **IHN CS adjacent spaces**
  - Visceral space and RPS medial; perivertebral space posterior; anterior cervical space anterior; and posterior cervical space lateral

Internal Contents

- **SHN CS**
  - **Vessels: ICA and IJV**
  - **CNIX-XII in nasopharyngeal CS**
  - Only CNX remains in CS from oropharyngeal CS inferiorly
  - CNX located in posterior notch formed by ICA and IJV
  - **Sympathetic plexus** lies outside carotid sheath posterior to it or between medial CS and lateral RPS, plastered to prevertebral fascia
- **IHN CS**
  - **Vessels: CCA and IJV**
  - **Vagus nerve**
  - **Ansa cervicalis** embedded in anterior wall of carotid sheath
  - Superior root (descendens hypoglossi) descending over ICA and CCA is continuation of descending branch of hypoglossal nerve; fibers are from C1 spinal nerve; supplies superior belly of omohyoid
  - Inferior root (descending cervical nerve) descends winding around IJV; fibers are from C2, C3 spinal nerves; supplies inferior belly of omohyoid; and joins superior root anteroinferiorly in front of CCA to form ansa cervicalis, which supplies sternohyoid and sternothyroid
  - Internal jugular nodes closely associated but **not** in CS

Fascia of CS

- **Carotid sheath** made from components of **all 3 layers of deep cervical fascia**
  - Suprahyoid CS: Carotid sheath incomplete or less substantial
  - Infrahyoid CS: Carotid sheath well-defined, tenacious fascia

ANATOMY IMAGING ISSUES

Questions

- What imaging features define lesion as primary to CS?
- **Lesion in SHN CS**
  - Center of lesion is within area of ICA-IJV, posterior to PPS
  - Lesion displaces PPS fat anteriorly; pushes posterior belly of digastric muscle laterally; and, if in nasopharyngeal CS, pushes styloid process anterolaterally
  - When mass begins in posterior SHN CS (vagal schwannoma, neurofibroma, paraganglioma), ICA is pushed anteromedially and IJV posterolaterally as mass enlarges
  - **Sympathetic schwannoma** does not separate ICA and IJV (unlike vagal schwannoma); instead, it **displaces both ICA and IJV together anteriorly** or anterolaterally
- **Lesion in IHN CS**
  - May engulf CCA and IJV on MR imaging or push them apart
  - May splay external carotid artery and ICA (carotid body paraganglioma)

Imaging Recommendations

- CECT or MR can easily identify normal CS anatomy and lesions
- If using MR, remember to acquire unenhanced T1 (to look for high velocity flow voids of paraganglioma)
- MRA and MRV for defining normal and diseased vessels of CS (ICA dissection; pseudoaneurysm; IJV thrombosis)

Imaging Approaches

- Remember that CS runs from jugular foramen-carotid canal of skull base above to aortic arch below
- If imaging CS because of **left** vagal neuropathy, must reach aortopulmonic window inferiorly

Imaging Pitfalls

- Normal vascular flow phenomenon of IJV may mimic schwannoma or thrombosis

CLINICAL IMPLICATIONS

Clinical Importance

- **CNIX-XII** and **carotid artery** are vital structures in CS

Function Dysfunction

- **Injury to nasopharyngeal CS** may result in complex cranial neuropathy involving some combination of **CNIX-XII**
- **Vagus nerve injury**: Vocal cord paralysis

Carotid Space

GRAPHICS

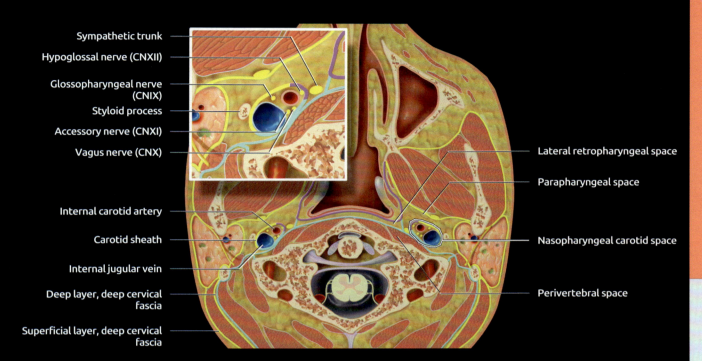

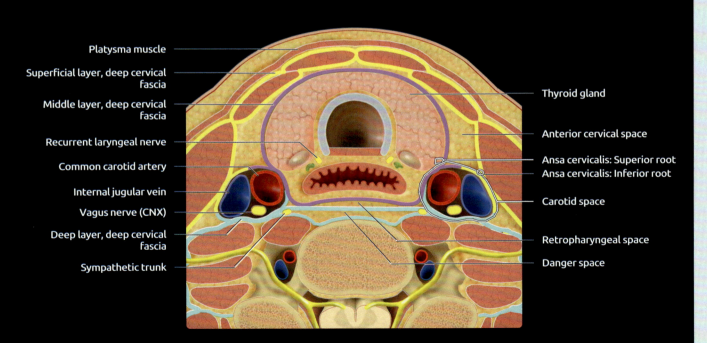

(Top) Axial graphic shows the suprahyoid neck at the level of C1 vertebral body with insert showing magnified carotid space (CS). The suprahyoid CS contains CNIX-XII, the internal carotid artery, and the internal jugular vein. The carotid sheath is made up of components of all 3 layers of deep cervical fascia (tricolor line around CS). In the suprahyoid neck, the carotid sheath is less substantial than it is in the infrahyoid neck. The sympathetic trunk runs just medial to the CS. (Bottom) Axial graphic shows the CS in the infrahyoid neck. Note that the carotid sheath contains all 3 layers of the deep cervical fascia (tricolor line). In the infrahyoid neck, the carotid sheath is tenacious throughout its length. The infrahyoid CS contains the common carotid artery, internal jugular vein, and only the vagus cranial nerve. Note that the sympathetic plexus lies outside the carotid sheath posterior to it and the ansa cervicalis lies embedded in the anterior wall of the carotid sheath.

Carotid Space

GRAPHICS

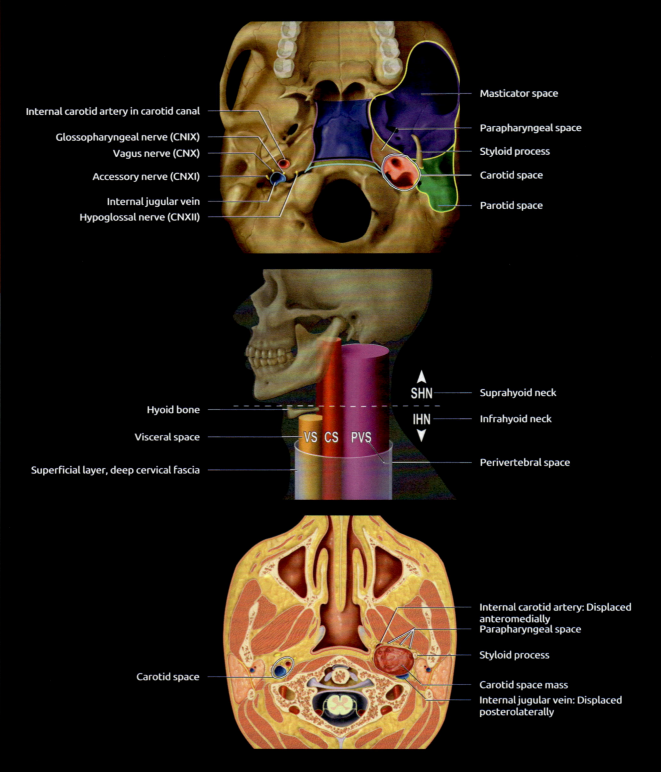

(Top) Axial graphic shows the skull base viewed from below, illustrating the interaction between the CS and the skull base. The nasopharyngeal CS is an inferior continuation of the carotid canal, jugular foramen, and hypoglossal canal. The internal carotid artery, internal jugular vein, and CNIX-XII are found within the CS. The carotid sheath is depicted as a tricolor line because it is formed from all 3 layers of deep cervical fascia. (Middle) Lateral oblique graphic of the neck shows the CS as a tube running from the skull base to the aortic arch. The CS is divided at the hyoid bone level into suprahyoid and infrahyoid portions. Suprahyoid CS has CNIX-XII within it and the infrahyoid CS has only a vagus nerve inside. (Bottom) Axial graphic shows a generic CS mass. A CS mass displaces the parapharyngeal space fat anteriorly as well as lifts the styloid process anterolaterally. A typical example is a vagal schwannoma lying sandwiched between the anteromedially displaced internal carotid artery and posterolaterally displaced internal jugular vein as shown.

Carotid Space

CECT & MRA OF CAROTID SPACE VESSELS

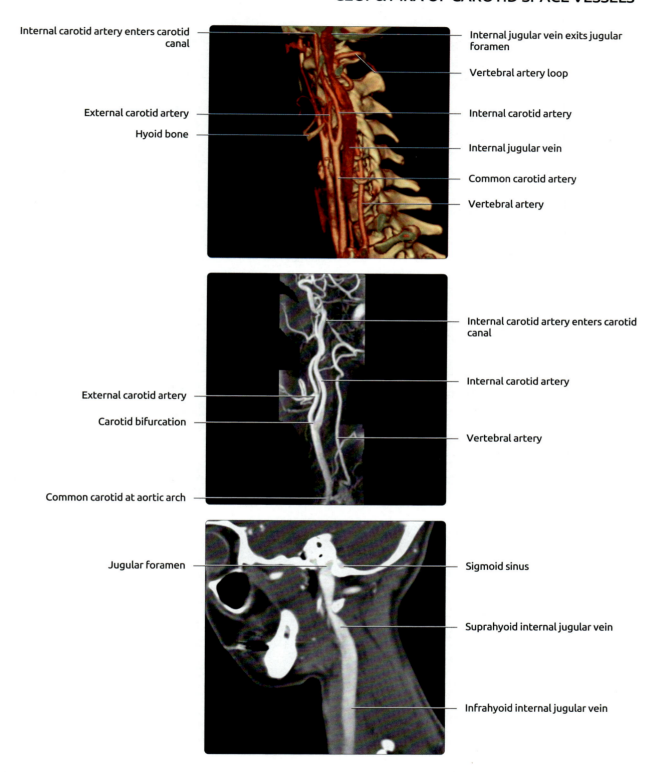

(Top) Lateral view 3D-VRT CECT reconstruction shows the major vessels of the neck. The hyoid bone is approximately at the level of the carotid bifurcation with the internal carotid artery found in the suprahyoid CS and the common carotid artery found within the infrahyoid CS. (Middle) Lateral view of an extracranial MRA shows the carotid artery from the arch below to the supraclinoid area above. Remember that the carotid artery extends in the CS throughout this entire distance. (Bottom) Sagittal reformation of CECT of the extracranial head and neck shows the internal jugular vein from its emergence from the jugular foramen above to the clavicle level below. Thrombosis of this vessel can mimic infection (acute thrombophlebitis) or tumor (chronic thrombosis).

Carotid Space

AXIAL CECT

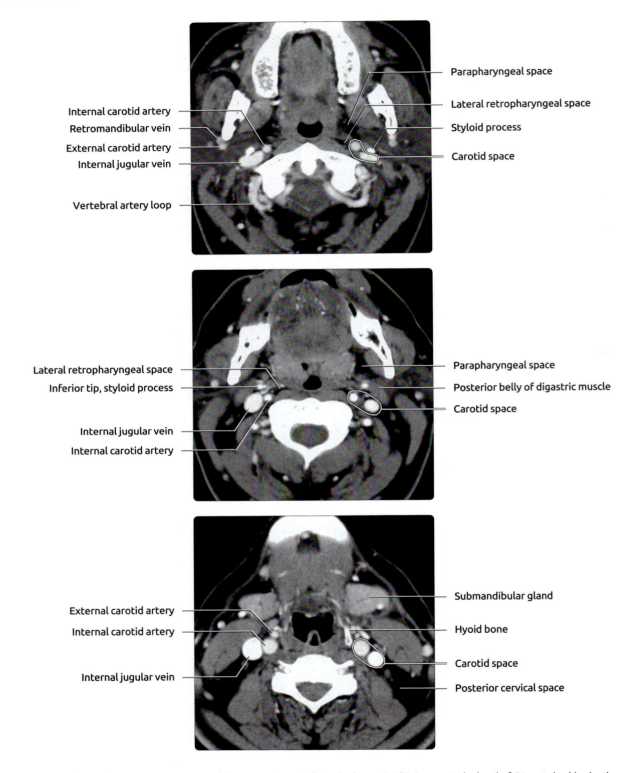

(Top) First of 6 axial CECT images presented from superior to inferior is shown. In this image at the level of C1 vertebral body, the nasopharyngeal CS contains the internal carotid artery, internal jugular vein, and CNIX-XII. Notice that the CS is posterior to the styloid process. At the level of the nasopharynx, a CS mass will push from posterior to anterior into the parapharyngeal space and displace the styloid process anterolaterally. (Middle) In this image at the level of the mid oropharynx, the posterior belly of the digastric muscle is visible anterolateral to the CS. A CS mass here would push this muscle anterolaterally and the parapharyngeal space anteriorly. (Bottom) At the level of the hyoid bone, the carotid bifurcation can be seen. At this level, only the vagus nerve is left within the CS.

Carotid Space

AXIAL CECT

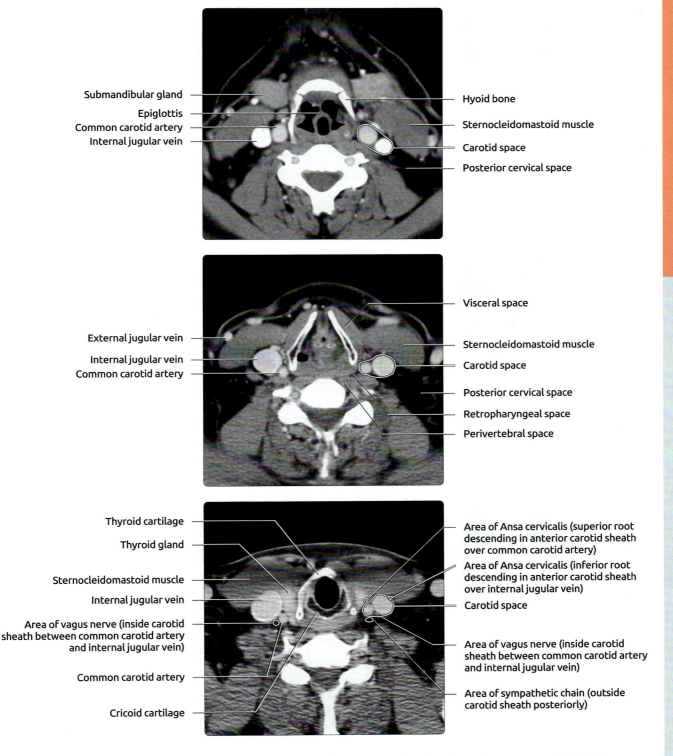

(Top) At the level of the hyoid bone, the CS has only the common carotid artery, internal jugular vein, and vagus nerve within it. Notice that, despite the high-resolution nature of this CT image, it is not possible to see the vagus nerve or the carotid sheath. (Middle) In this image through the infrahyoid aspect of the CS, the surrounding deep tissue anatomy can be seen. Posterolateral to the CS, the large fat-filled posterior cervical space is visible. Posteromedially, the perivertebral space is found. Medial to the CS are the visceral space and the retropharyngeal space. Anteriorly the sternocleidomastoid muscle resides. (Bottom) At the level of the cricoid cartilage, the infrahyoid CS contains the common carotid artery, internal jugular vein, and vagus nerve. Despite its large size, the vagal trunk cannot be visualized in its location between the common carotid artery and internal jugular vein within the carotid sheath. The sympathetic chain lies outside the carotid sheath posterior to it, and the ansa cervicalis lies embedded in the anterior wall of carotid sheath. These are also not demonstrated (expected locations are marked).

Carotid Space

COMMON CAROTID ARTERY ULTRASOUND

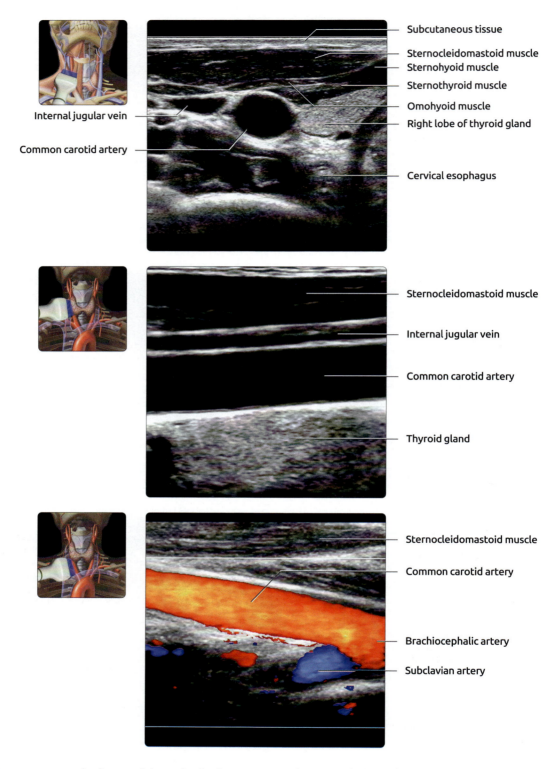

(Top) Transverse grayscale ultrasound shows the distal common carotid artery at the level of the upper pole of the thyroid gland. Note that the artery wall in a normal individual is smooth with no intimal thickening or atherosclerotic plaque. The lumen is circular in cross section. There is no major named branch of the common carotid proximal to the bifurcation. (Middle) Longitudinal grayscale ultrasound of the common carotid artery shows the smooth outline of the intimal layer. (Bottom) Color Doppler ultrasound of the proximal common carotid artery at the root of the neck in the longitudinal plane demonstrates the normal antegrade arterial flow in the cranial direction. Its origin along with the subclavian artery from the right brachiocephalic artery is also well demonstrated.

Carotid Space

VAGUS NERVE ULTRASOUND

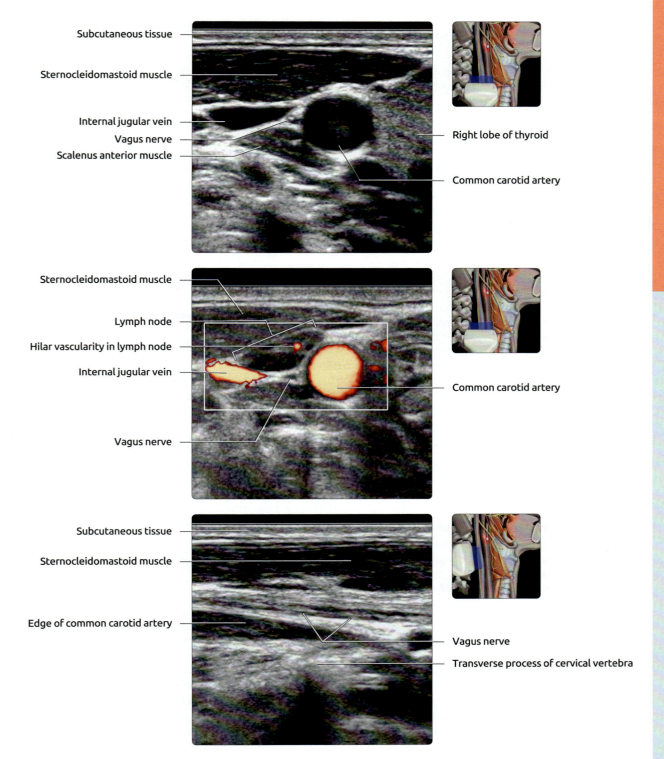

(Top) Transverse grayscale ultrasound of the lower cervical level at the thyroid gland level shows the vagus nerve as a small, round, hypoechoic structure that exhibits central echogenicity within the carotid sheath and is located between the common carotid artery and the internal jugular vein. (Middle) Power Doppler ultrasound of the midcervical level in the transverse plane demonstrates the avascular nature of the vagus nerve adjacent to the common carotid artery and internal jugular vein. Note the presence of hilar vascularity in the adjacent normal deep cervical lymph node. (Bottom) Longitudinal grayscale ultrasound shows the vagus nerve, which appears as a long, thin, tubular, hypoechoic structure with a central echogenic fibrillary pattern. On ultrasound, the vagus nerve is readily seen from the carotid bifurcation to the lower cervical region.

Retropharyngeal Space

TERMINOLOGY

Abbreviations
- Retropharyngeal space (RPS); danger space (DS)

Definitions
- RPS: Midline space just posterior to pharynx and cervical esophagus running from skull base to mediastinum

IMAGING ANATOMY

Extent
- **True RPS**: Skull base to T3 vertebral body level in upper mediastinum (variable C6-T6) where alar fascia fuses to middle layer of deep cervical fascia
- **DS**: Directly posterior to RPS; continues inferiorly into mediastinum to diaphragm

Anatomy Relationships
- **Suprahyoid neck (SHN) RPS**
  - Pharyngeal mucosal space (PMS) is anterior
  - DS is directly posterior to RPS
- **Infrahyoid neck (IHN) RPS**
  - Hypopharynx and cervical esophagus are anterior
  - RPS empties via "fascial trap door" inferiorly into DS inferiorly at ~ T3 level (variable C6-T6) where **alar fascia** fuses to middle layer of deep cervical fascia
  - Fascial trap-door serves as **inferior entry point into DS** for infection from true RPS and then into mediastinum
  - Carotid space (CS) is lateral to RPS in SHN and IHN

Internal Contents
- **SHN RPS** (skull base to hyoid bone)
  - Fat is primary occupant of SHN RPS
  - **RPS lymph nodes: Lateral group**: Nodes of Rouvière; **medial group**: Less often visible on imaging
- **IHN RPS** (hyoid bone to T3 vertebral body in mediastinum)
  - **Fat only** in IHN RPS; no RPS nodes in IHN

Fascia of Retropharyngeal Space
- **Anterior wall fascia**: Middle layer, deep cervical fascia (a.k.a. "buccopharyngeal fascia," especially superiorly)
  - Fascia is just behind constrictor muscle of PMS
- **Alar fascia**: Slip of deep layer, deep cervical fascia forming posterior wall of true RPS, separating it from posterior DS
- Extension of alar fascia to base of skull is controversial
- Classic teaching is that uppermost RPS (nasopharyngeal portion) is "tight," and in RPS abscess, path of least resistance is inferiorly
- Recent study found that alar fascia begins at C1 level, and loose fibroareolar connective tissue fills space between inferior nuchal line and skull base; this transitional level may be alternative **superior entry point into DS** for infection
- Alar fascia comparable in thickness and integrity to buccopharyngeal and prevertebral fasciae
- Lateral fibers of alar fascia are large contributor to medial aspect of carotid sheath and may be factor in spread of infection into CS
- **Posterior wall fascia**: Deep layer, deep cervical fascia forming posterior wall of DS
  - Fascia is just anterior to prevertebral muscles of perivertebral space
- **Median raphe** divides RPS into 2 halves

- Relatively weak fascial slip that is present more consistently in superior RPS

ANATOMY IMAGING ISSUES

Questions
- What radiologic findings define lesion as primary to RPS?
- **Unilateral-nodal SHN mass**
  - Centered posteromedial to parapharyngeal space (PPS) and directly medial to CS
  - Encroaches on PPS from posteromedial to anterolateral (mimics CS mass)
- **"Extranodal" mass in SHN or IHN** (pus or tumor filling RPS)
  - Rectangular-shaped mass centered behind PMS
  - Mass anterior to prevertebral muscles; flattens and remains anterior to prevertebral muscles as it enlarges (whereas perivertebral space mass elevates prevertebral muscles as it enlarges)
- **SHN RPS lesion imaging appearances**
  - Lesion begins most commonly in RPS nodes; seen on CT or MR as unilateral RPS mass
  - If extranodal disease (edema, infection, or tumor), will fill RPS from side to side
- **IHN RPS lesion imaging appearances**
  - Originates in SHN RPS, spreads inferiorly into IHN; fills entire IHN RPS from side to side
  - Remember to look at SHN RPS, if IHN RPS disease seen

Imaging Approaches
- **CECT best** imaging tool in evaluation of **RPS infection**
- **MR** far more sensitive to detect **RPS tumor/adenopathy**

Imaging Pitfalls
- RPS and DS indistinguishable on CT/MR imaging; consider DS as conduit for RPS disease into mediastinum only
  - Otherwise, describe lesions in RPS only and ignore DS from imaging perspective
- Lateral RPS nodal mass may mimic CS mass
  - Look for mass medial to CS
  - Mass displacement of CS is posterolaterally
  - Both RPS and CS displace PPS anteriorly
- Not all fluid in RPS is abscess: Nonabscess fluid: No enhancement of wall; minimal mass effect
  - Internal jugular vein thrombosis, superior vena cava syndrome (transudate), recent chemo-/radiotherapy (lymphedema), pharyngitis, sinusitis, dental infection, angioedema, and longus colli tendonitis (cellulitis or transudate) all can cause RPS edema

CLINICAL IMPLICATIONS

Clinical Importance
- RPS nodes are seeded by pharyngitis
  - Once seeded they react, suppurate, and eventually rupture to create RPS abscess
- Squamous cell carcinoma of nasopharynx and posterior wall of oropharynx and hypopharynx drain into RPS nodal chain

Retropharyngeal Space

GRAPHICS

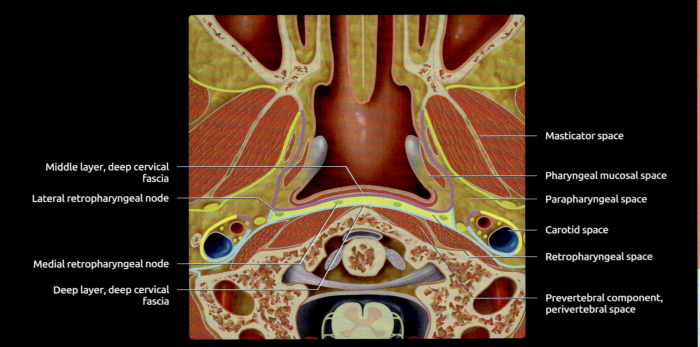

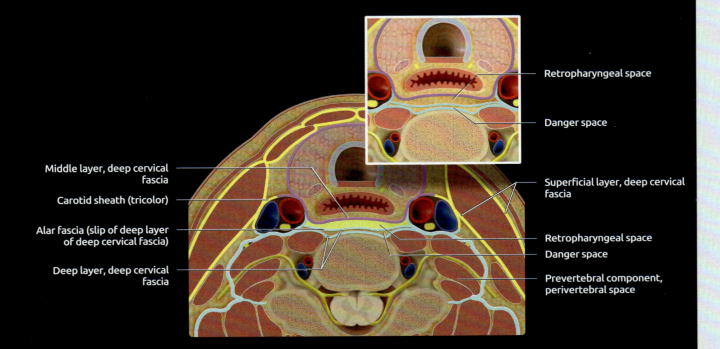

(Top) Axial graphic shows the retropharyngeal space in suprahyoid neck. In the suprahyoid neck, the retropharyngeal space has medial and lateral retropharyngeal nodes. Notice the middle layer of deep cervical fascia (called buccopharyngeal fascia here) is the anterior border of the retropharyngeal space, while the alar fascia, a slip of the deep layer of deep cervical fascia, is the posterior border. (Bottom) Axial graphic depicts the fascia that make up the borders of the retropharyngeal and danger spaces in the infrahyoid neck. Alar fascia is a slip of the deep layer of deep cervical fascia forming the posterior wall of the anteriorly located true retropharyngeal space, separating it from the posteriorly located danger space. Posterior wall of danger space is also formed by the deep layer of deep cervical fascia, separating it from the prevertebral space. Notice that there is only fat in the infrahyoid retropharyngeal space. Nodes are only present above the hyoid bone.

Retropharyngeal Space

GRAPHICS

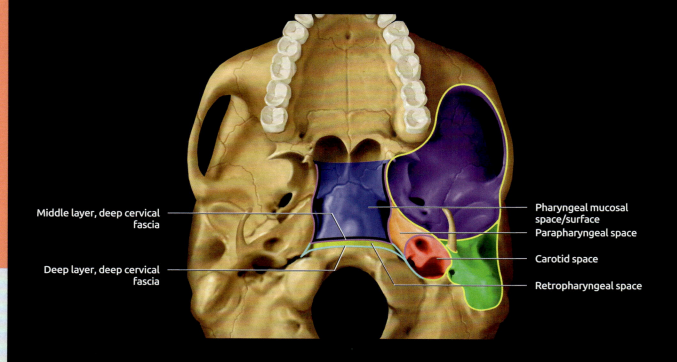

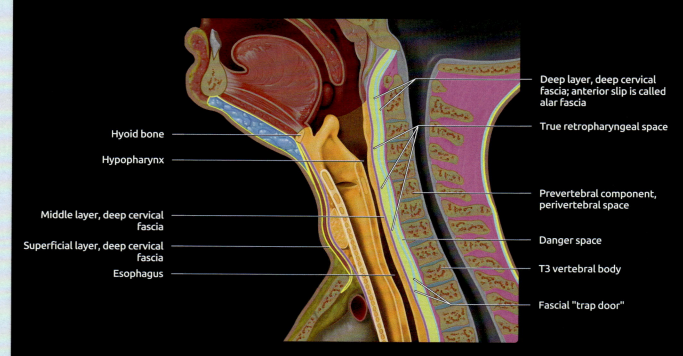

(Top) Axial graphic of the skull base from below shows the abutment of the retropharyngeal space with the skull base. Notice that the retropharyngeal space abuts the external surface of the basiocciput in an area where there are no foramina. (Bottom) Sagittal graphic depicts longitudinal spatial relationships of the infrahyoid neck with emphasis on the retropharyngeal and danger spaces. Seen just anterior to the vertebral column, the retropharyngeal and danger spaces run inferiorly from the skull base toward the mediastinum. Notice the fascial "trap door" found at the approximate level of T3 vertebral body that serves as an inferior conduit from the retropharyngeal to the danger space. Retropharyngeal space infection or tumor may access the mediastinum via this route of spread. Note that the extension of alar fascia to the base of skull is controversial; a recent cadaveric study found that the alar fascia begins at C1 level, and loose fibroareolar connective tissue fills the space between inferior nuchal line and skull base; this transitional level may be an alternative superior entry point into danger space for infection.

Retropharyngeal Space

AXIAL SHN RPS GENERIC MASS

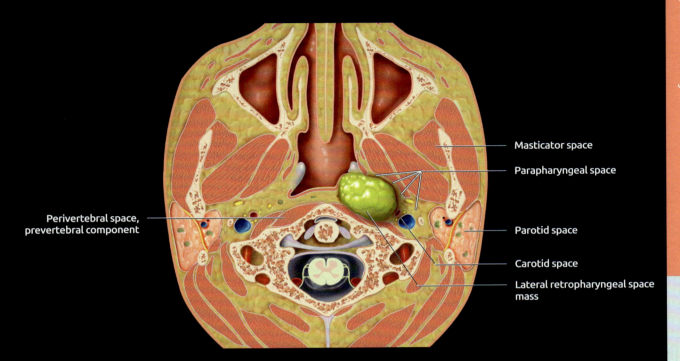

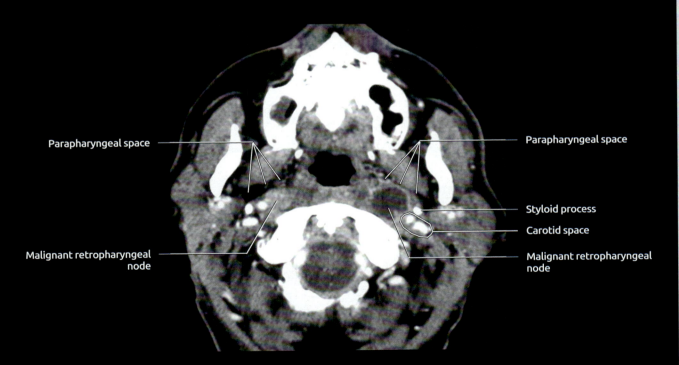

(Top) Axial graphic depicts a generic mass beginning in the lateral retropharyngeal nodal group of the retropharyngeal space. Notice that the lateral retropharyngeal space mass displaces the carotid space posterolaterally and the parapharyngeal space anteriorly. This mass lesion can be mistaken for a carotid space mass if the imager is not cognizant of its more medial location. (Bottom) Axial CECT at the level of the low nasopharynx reveals bilateral malignant lateral retropharyngeal lymph nodes from a posterior oropharyngeal wall squamous cell carcinoma (not shown). The larger left-sided necrotic node displaces the parapharyngeal space anteriorly and the carotid space posterolaterally. The smaller right-sided node has not yet caused significant mass effect on either the parapharyngeal or carotid spaces.

Retropharyngeal Space

AXIAL IHN RPS GENERIC MASS

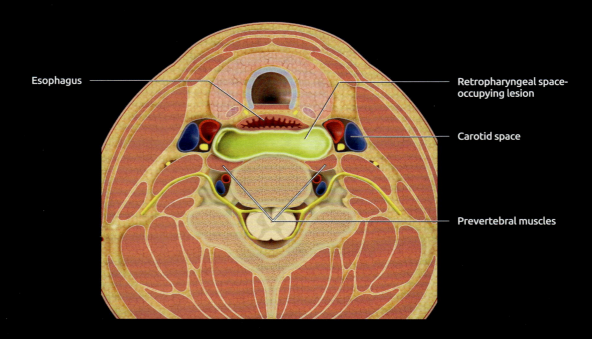

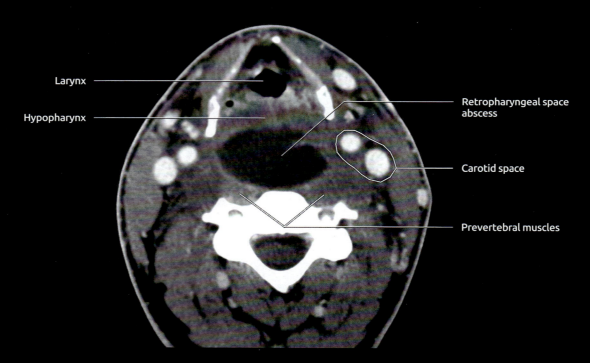

(Top) Axial graphic of a generic retropharyngeal space lesion in the infrahyoid neck is shown. Note the anterior displacement of the visceral space and the lateral displacement of the carotid spaces. The prevertebral muscles are flattened, not elevated. **(Bottom)** Axial CECT at the level of the infrahyoid neck supraglottic larynx demonstrates an abscess filling the retropharyngeal space. This ovoid-shaped abscess displaces the visceral space (hypopharynx/larynx) anteriorly and the carotid spaces laterally. The prevertebral muscles are posterior to the abscess cavity.

Retropharyngeal Space

AXIAL CECT

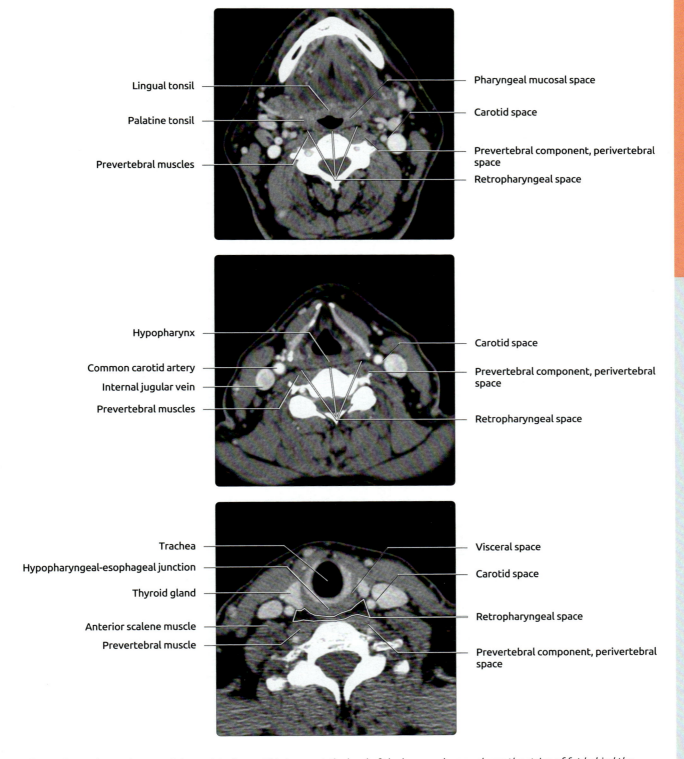

(Top) First of 3 axial CECT images of the neck is shown. This image at the level of the low oropharynx shows the stripe of fat behind the pharyngeal mucosal space that represents the retropharyngeal space. Posterior to the retropharyngeal space is the prevertebral portion of the perivertebral space. Lateral to it are the carotid spaces. (Middle) In this image at the level of the supraglottis, the stripe of fat behind the larynx and hypopharynx is the retropharyngeal space. The carotid spaces are at the lateral margin of the retropharyngeal space bilaterally. (Bottom) At the level of the midinfrahyoid neck, the retropharyngeal space is larger and more obvious than in the suprahyoid neck. Anterior is the visceral space with the hypopharyngeal-esophageal junction abutting the retropharyngeal space. The prevertebral component of the perivertebral space is posterior to the retropharyngeal space.

Retropharyngeal Space

AXIAL T1 MR

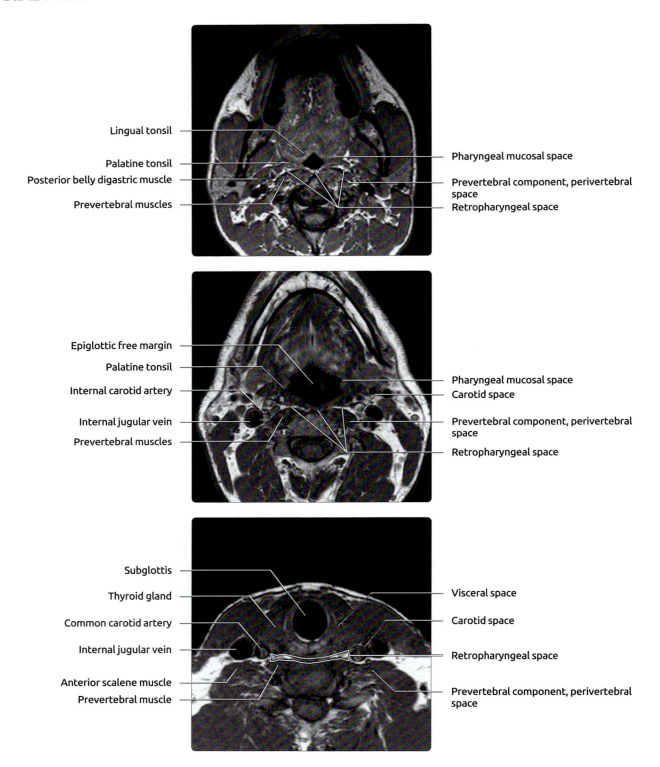

(Top) First of 3 axial T1 MR images of the extracranial head and neck is shown. This image at the level of the oropharynx shows a thin stripe of high-signal fat behind the pharyngeal mucosal space that represents the retropharyngeal space. Posterior to the retropharyngeal space is the prevertebral portion of the perivertebral space. (Middle) In this image at the level of the low oropharynx, the high-signal stripe of fat behind the oropharyngeal mucosal space is the retropharyngeal space. The carotid spaces are at the lateral margin of the retropharyngeal space bilaterally. The prevertebral muscles in the perivertebral space are directly posterior to the retropharyngeal space. (Bottom) In this image at the level of the midinfrahyoid neck, the retropharyngeal space is easily seen between the carotid spaces. The visceral space is anterior and the prevertebral component of the perivertebral space posterior to the retropharyngeal space.

Retropharyngeal Space

AXIAL BONE CT AND T2 MR

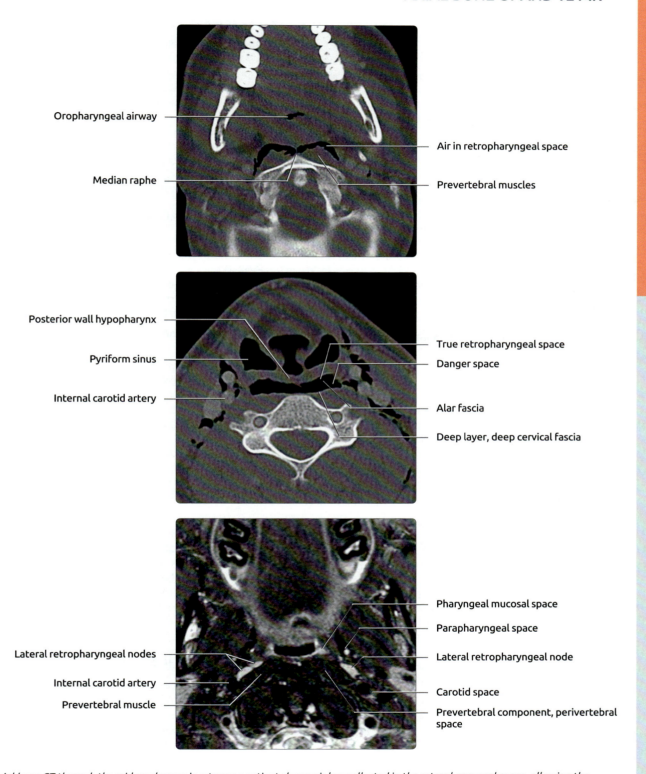

(Top) Axial bone CT through the midoropharynx in a trauma patient shows air has collected in the retropharyngeal space, allowing the median raphe to be seen. The median raphe functions as an attachment of the constrictor muscles. In addition, it provides an initial barrier to the spread of disease from side to side in the retropharyngeal space. (Middle) Axial bone CT at level of the supraglottis in a trauma patient shows air in the true retropharyngeal and danger spaces. Air allows identification of the alar fascia that separates these 2 spaces. (Bottom) Axial fat-saturated T2 MR through the low nasopharynx in a young adolescent reveals normal lateral retropharyngeal space nodes bilaterally. Notice these nodes are positioned just medial to the internal carotid artery and posteromedial to the fat-saturated parapharyngeal space.

Perivertebral Space

Suprahyoid and Infrahyoid Neck

TERMINOLOGY

Abbreviations

- Perivertebral space (PVS)

Definitions

- "Perivertebral" is inclusive term to include all tissues within cylindrical space surrounding vertebral column and bounded by deep layer of deep cervical fascia (DL-DCF)
- PVS subdivided into anterior **prevertebral** and posterior **paraspinal** components

IMAGING ANATOMY

Extent

- For practical purposes, anterior **prevertebral** component extends from skull base to T4, where ventral component of DL-DCF attaches to 4th thoracic vertebra
  - Some anatomists contend that prevertebral space exists as potential space between vertebrae and DL-DCF and therefore extends inferiorly to coccyx
- Posterior **paraspinal** component continues inferiorly to sacrum

Anatomy Relationships

- **PVS consists of 2 major components**, separated at level of transverse processes (TPs)
  - Prevertebral portion or space
  - Paraspinal portion or space
- **Prevertebral-PVS** sits directly behind retropharyngeal and danger space in extracranial head and neck
  - Carotid space is anterolateral to prevertebral-PVS
  - Anterior aspect of posterior cervical space is lateral to prevertebral-PVS
- **Paraspinal-PVS** is deep to posterior cervical space and posterior to cervical spine TPs

Internal Contents

- **Prevertebral-PVS or prevertebral space**
  - Vertebral bodies
  - Prevertebral muscles (longus colli and capitis)
    - Longus capitis: Origin (O): C3-C6 TPs; insertion (I): Basilar occipital bone
    - Longus colli: O: C3-5 TPs, C5-T3 vertebral bodies; I: Anterior arch C1, C2-4 vertebral bodies
  - Scalene muscles (anterior, middle, and posterior)
    - O: C3-C6 TPs (anterior), C2-C7 TPs (middle), C5-C7 TPs (posterior)
    - I: Scalene tubercle 1st rib (anterior), upper surface 1st rib (middle), lateral surface 2nd rib (posterior)
  - Brachial plexus (BP) roots
  - Phrenic nerve (C3-C5)
  - Vertebral artery and vein
- **Paraspinal-PVS or paraspinal space**
  - Paraspinal muscles (include splenius capitis, splenius cervicis, semispinalis capitis, longissimus capitis, levator scapulae, multifidus, interspinales)
  - Posterior elements, vertebral column
- **BP**, proximal aspect
  - BP has complex spatial anatomy
  - C5-T1 roots leave neural foramina, pass between anterior and middle scalene of prevertebral-PVS
  - BP roots pass through sleeves in DL-DCF, into posterior cervical space on their way to axilla

Fascia of PVS

- **DL-DCF completely circumscribes PVS**
  - Anterior portion arches from cervical spine TP across prevertebral muscles to opposite TP
    - Anterior DL-DCF called "**carpet**" by surgeons
    - Pharynx slides up and down on this smooth, carpet-like surface
    - Carpet is tenacious, acting as barrier to disease spread from pharynx to PVS and vice-versa
  - Posterior portion DL-DCF arches over surface of paraspinal muscles to attach to nuchal ligament of spinous process of vertebral body

ANATOMY IMAGING ISSUES

Questions

- What imaging findings localize mass lesion to prevertebral-PVS?
  - Mass centered in prevertebral muscles or vertebral body
  - Mass lifts or pushes prevertebral muscles anteriorly (retropharyngeal space mass pushes them posteriorly)

Imaging Approaches

- Lateral plain film
  - Assess for prevertebral soft tissue swelling and integrity of cervical vertebral bodies
  - Prevertebral soft tissue: Adults: < 7 mm at C2 and < 22 mm at C6; child: < 14 mm at C6
- CECT (soft tissue and bone algorithm and sagittal reformation)
  - Most practical evaluation of cervical soft tissue and bones
- Complete cervical MR with gadolinium and fat-saturation images best to assess for marrow process and epidural disease

Imaging Pitfalls

- **Hypertrophic levator scapulae muscle** (LSM): Mistaken for enhancing mass or recurrent tumor
  - Secondary to CNXI injury (during neck dissection)
    - Sternocleidomastoid (SCM) and trapezius atrophy
    - LSM hypertrophies to help lift arm
  - Imaging: LSM enlarges and may enhance, SCM and trapezius small, fatty infiltrated

CLINICAL IMPLICATIONS

Clinical Importance

- Important structures: Proximal BP, phrenic nerve, vertebral arteries
- Most PVS lesions originate in vertebral body or disc space (infection or metastatic tumor)
- Prevertebral-PVS disease may involve epidural space
  - If infection or malignancy extend from cervical vertebral body into prevertebral-PVS, 1st obstruction to spread is DL-DCF
  - Path of least resistance of spreading pus or tumor is deep through neural foramen into epidural space
  - When prevertebral PVS disease is found on imaging, **always check for epidural space extension**

Perivertebral Space

GRAPHICS

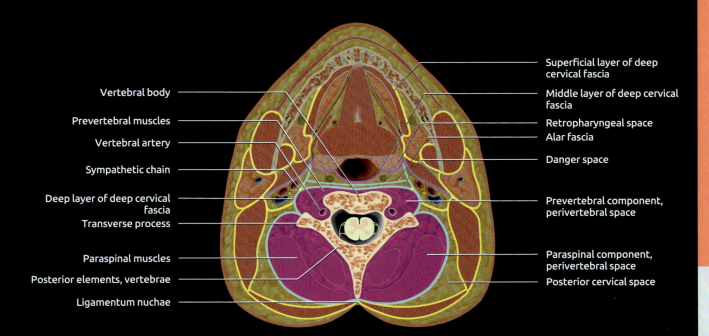

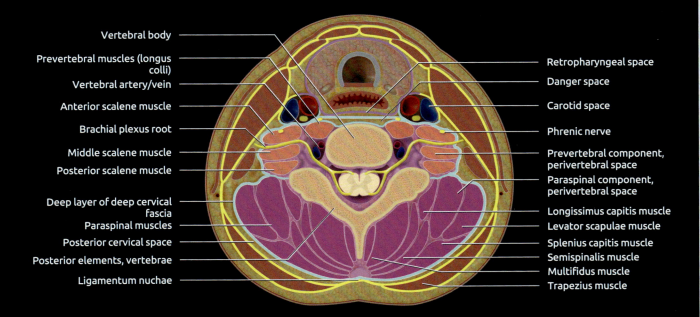

(Top) Axial graphic through the level of the oropharynx shows prevertebral and paraspinal components of the perivertebral space beneath the deep layer of deep cervical fascia. Notice this fascia curves medially to touch the transverse processes of the vertebra, dividing the perivertebral space into prevertebral and paraspinal components. The danger and retropharyngeal spaces are anterior to the perivertebral space, while the posterior cervical space is lateral and posterior. (Bottom) Axial graphic through the thyroid bed shows prevertebral and paraspinal components of the perivertebral space beneath the deep layer of deep cervical fascia. Notice this fascia curves medially to touch the transverse processes of the vertebra, dividing the perivertebral space into prevertebral and paraspinal components. The prevertebral component is key, as it contains brachial plexus roots.

Perivertebral Space

GRAPHICS

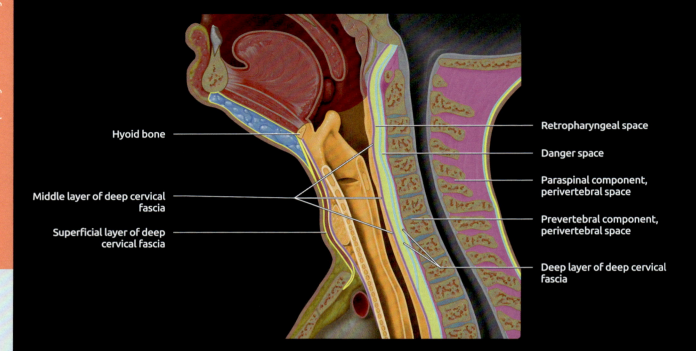

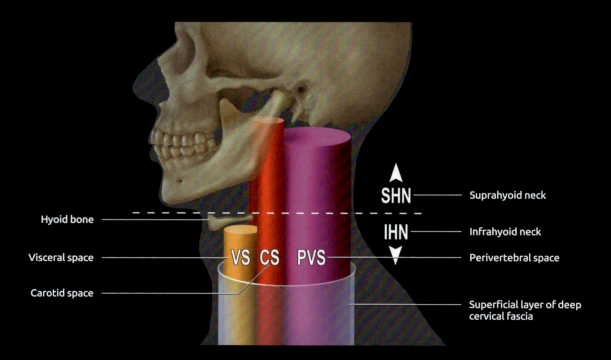

(Top) Sagittal graphic depicting midline longitudinal spatial relationships of the infrahyoid neck is shown. In the midline, only the vertebral body is seen in the prevertebral component of the perivertebral space. Just anterior to the vertebral column, the retropharyngeal and danger spaces run inferiorly toward the mediastinum. In the midline paraspinal component of the perivertebral space, only the spinous processes are visible. (Bottom) Lateral graphic of the extracranial head and neck shows the spaces as "tubes" as they traverse the area. The perivertebral space is shown as a tube of tissue that projects from the skull base inferiorly into the thorax. Notice the superficial layer of deep cervical fascia envelops all the spaces of the extracranial head and neck below the hyoid bone.

Periverbetral Space

GENERIC PERIVERTEBRAL SPACE SUPRAHYOID MASS

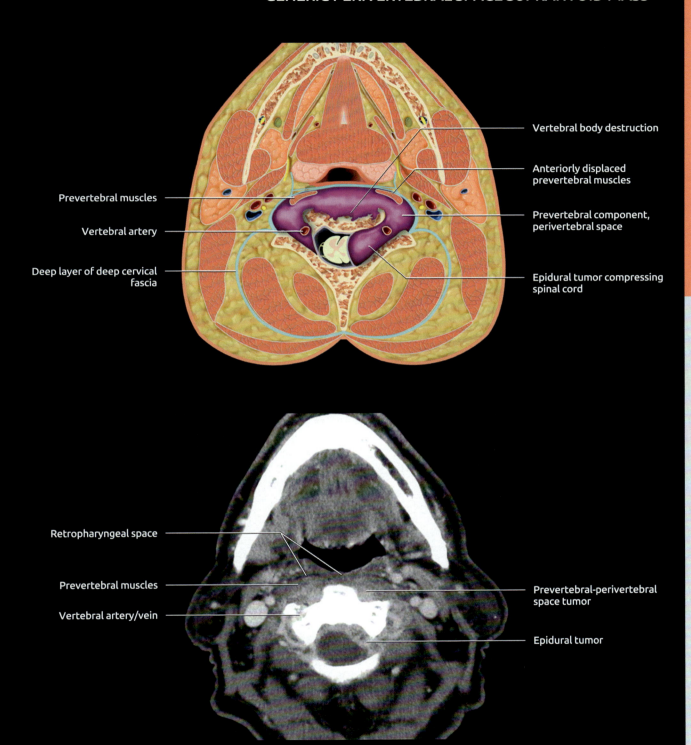

(Top) Axial graphic through the oropharynx reveals a generic suprahyoid neck perivertebral space mass involving the vertebral body. Notice the vertebral body destruction and the elevation of the prevertebral muscles. The vertebral arteries are engulfed by tumor. In addition, the tumor is confined by the deep layer of deep cervical fascia, forcing it centrally into the epidural space where it is causing spinal cord compression. (Bottom) Axial contrast-enhanced CT demonstrates an enhancing malignant tumor involving the prevertebral component of the perivertebral space. The tumor remains confined to the perivertebral space by the deep layer of deep cervical fascia. Consequently, the tumor spreads centrally into the epidural space where it may cause cord compression.

Perivertebral Space

GENERIC PERIVERTEBRAL SPACE INFRAHYOID MASS

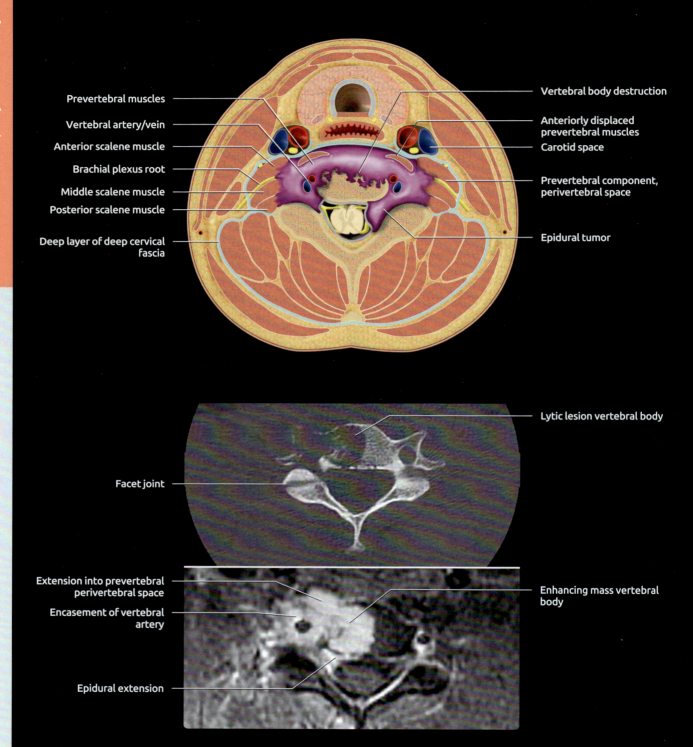

(Top) Axial graphic through the thyroid bed shows a generic infrahyoid neck perivertebral space mass arising out of the vertebral body. Notice the vertebral body destruction and the elevation of the prevertebral muscles. The vertebral artery and vein as well as the brachial plexus roots are engulfed by the tumor. In addition, the tumor is confined by the deep layer of deep cervical fascia, forcing it centrally into the epidural space. (Bottom) Axial bone CT and axial MR with gadolinium and fat saturation show a tumor arising from the cervical vertebra and extending into the epidural space, neural foramen, and prevertebral component of the perivertebral space. CT imaging best shows the lytic changes of bone; MR imaging best shows the soft tissue components with marrow space involvement.

Perivertebral Space

AXIAL CECT

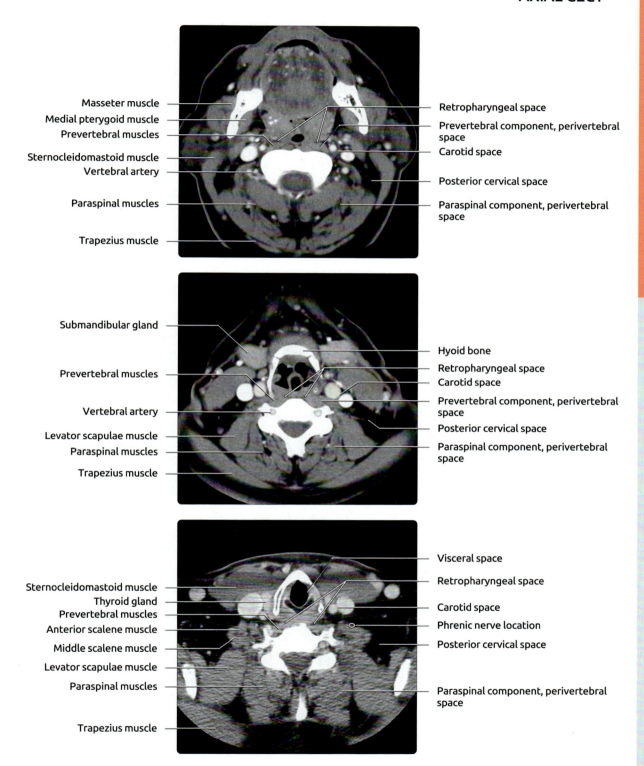

(Top) First of 6 axial CECT images through the extracranial head and neck show the normal features of the perivertebral space. This image at the level of the C2 vertebral body shows the prevertebral component of the perivertebral space contains the prevertebral muscles, vertebral body, and vertebral artery only. The retropharyngeal space fat stripe is visible anteriorly. (Middle) In this image at the level of the hyoid bone, the levator scapulae muscles and the paraspinal muscles along with the posterior elements of the vertebral body are the principal occupants of the paraspinal component of the perivertebral space. (Bottom) At the level of the cricoid cartilage, the scalene muscles are visible. The phrenic nerve location is marked on the left, although it is not visible on imaging.

Periverbral Space

Suprahyoid and Infrahyoid Neck

AXIAL CECT

Sternocleidomastoid muscle

Anterior scalene muscle
Middle scalene muscle
Posterior scalene muscle

Levator scapulae muscle

Trapezius muscle

Brachial plexus root

Prevertebral component, perivertebral space

Paraspinal component, perivertebral space

Sternocleidomastoid muscle

Posterior cervical space

Anterior scalene muscle
Middle scalene muscle

Posterior scalene muscle
Levator scapulae muscle

Prevertebral muscles
Vertebral artery/vein

Brachial plexus roots

Paraspinal component, perivertebral space

Esophagus
Prevertebral muscles
Anterior scalene muscle
Middle scalene muscle

Levator scapulae muscle

Retropharyngeal space

Vertebral artery/vein

Brachial plexus roots

Paraspinal component, perivertebral space

(Top) *At the level of the upper thyroid bed, the scalene muscles are seen in the prevertebral component of the perivertebral space. The anterior band of the deep layer of deep cervical fascia is referred to as the "carpet."* (Middle) *In this image at the level of the mid thyroid bed, the low-density ovoid brachial plexus roots can be seen emerging from the cervical neural foramina to pass anterolaterally between the anterior and middle scalene muscles in the prevertebral component of the perivertebral space.* (Bottom) *At the level of the low thyroid bed, the low-density brachial plexus roots are visible passing anterolaterally between the anterior and middle scalene muscles in the prevertebral component of the perivertebral space. These roots continue through openings in the deep layer of deep cervical fascia into the posterior cervical space on their way to the axillary apex.*

Perivertebral Space

AXIAL T2 FS AND CORONAL STIR MR

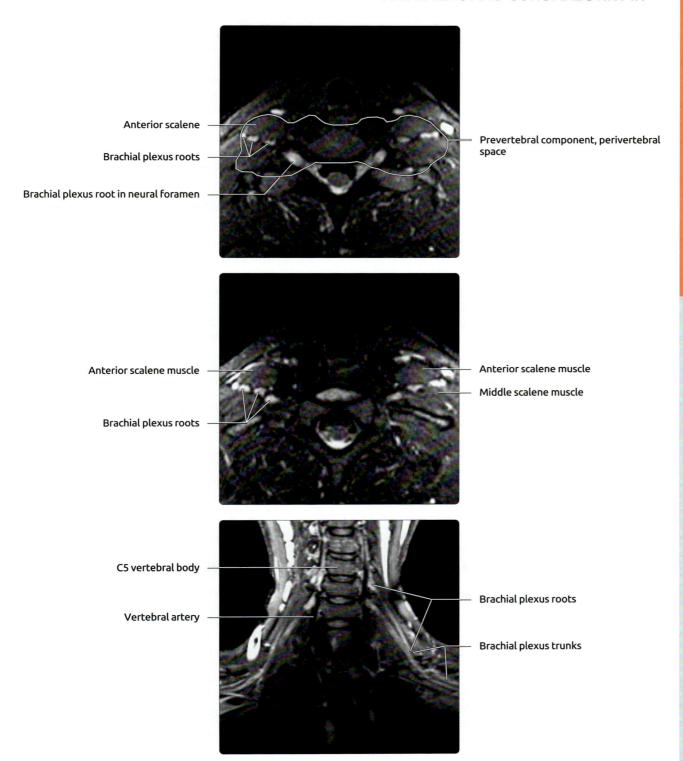

(Top) Axial T2 fat-saturated MR at the level of the thyroid gland shows the normal high-signal brachial plexus roots between the anterior and middle scalene muscles. Notice a single root passes through the neural foramen bilaterally. The brachial plexus arises from the ventral rami of C5 through T1. **(Middle)** In this axial T2 fat-saturated MR image, the anterior and middle scalene muscles can be seen on the anterior and posterior sides of the high-signal brachial plexus roots. Distally, the 5 roots become 3 trunks (upper, middle, and lower) as they emerge from their interscalene muscle location. **(Bottom)** Coronal STIR MR through the lower cervical vertebral bodies shows both the 5 brachial plexus roots and the 3 trunks in the same plane. The brachial plexus transitions from roots to trunks to divisions to cords to end in branches.

Posterior Cervical Space

TERMINOLOGY

Abbreviations

- Posterior cervical space (PCS)

Definitions

- Radiologically defined as posterolateral fat-containing space in neck with complex fascial boundaries; extends from posterior mastoid tip to clavicle
- Encompasses major portion of what clinicians & surgeons refer to as posterior triangle

IMAGING ANATOMY

Overview

- Posterolateral fat-filled space just deep & posterior to sternocleidomastoid (SCM) muscle
- Lesions of PCS arise from **spinal accessory nodal (SAN) chain**
  - Infection, inflammation, & tumor involving these nodes constitute vast majority of lesions in PCS

Extent

- PCS extends from small superior component near mastoid tip to broader base at level of clavicle

Anatomy Relationships

- SCM anterolateral to PCS
- Deep to PCS is perivertebral space
  - Anterior PCS is superficial to **prevertebral component of perivertebral space**
  - Posterior PCS is superficial to **paraspinal component of perivertebral space**
- Anteromedial to PCS is carotid space

Internal Contents

- **Fat** is primary occupant of PCS
- **Spinal accessory nerve (CNXI)**
- **Spinal accessory nodal (SAN) chain**
  - In node level numbering system, this is **level V**
  - Level VA lymph nodes are above inferior margin of cricoid cartilage, & level VB nodes are below this
- **Preaxillary brachial plexus**
  - Segment of brachial plexus emerging from scalene triangle passes through PCS
- **Dorsal scapular nerve**
  - Arises from ventral ramus of CNV
  - Motor innervation to rhomboid & levator scapulae muscles

Fascia of Posterior Cervical Space

- Complex fascial boundaries surround PCS
  - Superficial: Superficial layer of deep cervical fascia
  - Deep: Deep layer of deep cervical fascia
  - Anteromedial: Carotid sheath (all 3 layers, deep cervical fascia)

Surgical Triangles

- **Posterior triangle**
  - Region of cervical neck posterolateral to SCM & anteromedial to trapezius muscle
  - Subdivided by inferior belly of omohyoid muscle into **occipital & subclavian triangles**

- **Occipital triangle**
  - Boundaries: Anteromedial SCM; posterolateral trapezius muscle; inferior is inferior belly of omohyoid muscle
  - Contents: Fat, accessory nerve (CNXI), dorsal scapular nerves, & SAN chain
  - Includes majority of PCS
- **Subclavian triangle**
  - Boundaries: Superior inferior belly of omohyoid muscle; anteromedial SCM muscle; posterolateral trapezium muscle
  - Contents: 3rd portion of subclavian artery, cervical brachial plexus
  - Subclavian triangle is lower, smaller portion of posterior triangle

ANATOMY IMAGING ISSUES

Questions

- What are criteria for defining cervical neck mass lesion as primary to PCS?
  - Lesion must be **centered within fat of PCS**
  - Lesion displaces carotid space anteromedially
  - Lesion elevates SCM muscle
  - Lesion flattens deeper perivertebral space structures
- How can you tell internal jugular node from SAN?
  - Lower PCS
    - Jugular chain nodes abut carotid space
    - SANs (level VB) are separated from carotid space by fat & are lateral to oblique line drawn from posterior edge of SCM to posterior edge of anterior scalene muscle
  - Upper PCS
    - Internal jugular & SAN chain converge cephalad toward jugulodigastric group
    - Nodes that abut anterior, lateral, or posterior carotid space, consider internal jugular nodes
    - If node has fat slip separating it from carotid space, or is posterior to coronal line along posterior margin of SCM, consider SAN (level VA)

CLINICAL IMPLICATIONS

Clinical Importance

- Most common adult pathology is malignant lymphadenopathy from primary head & neck malignancy or lymphoma
- Less common: Nerve sheath tumors, lipoma, congenital lymphatic malformation, 3rd branchial cleft cyst
- Pseudomasses include cervical ribs, prominent transverse processes, & levator scapulae muscle hypertrophy

Function Dysfunction

- Spinal accessory cranial neuropathy results when CNXI injured
  - Most commonly injured during neck dissection for malignant squamous cell carcinoma nodes
  - Dysfunction: Sternomastoid & trapezius muscle paresis
    - Acute denervation: Muscles may swell & enhance
    - Chronic denervation: Muscles atrophy & fatty infiltrate
    - Levator scapulae muscle hypertrophies
    - Patient has difficulty lifting arm

Posterior Cervical Space

GRAPHICS

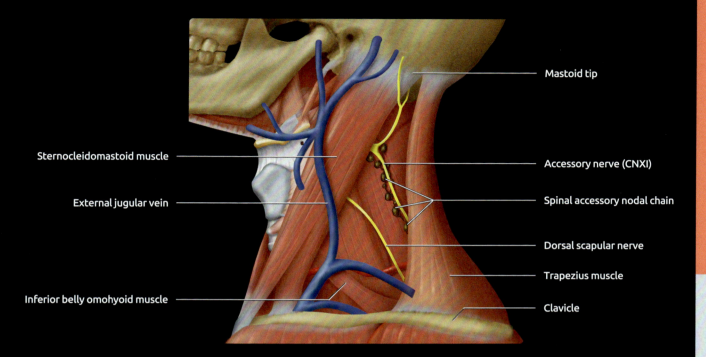

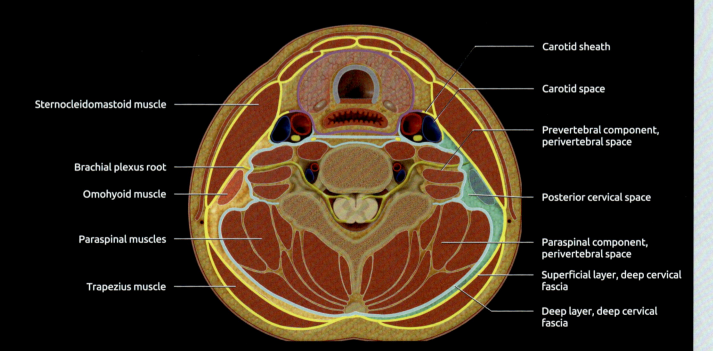

(Top) Lateral graphic of extracranial head and neck shows the posterior cervical space as a "tilting tent" with its superior margin at the level of the mastoid tip and its inferior border at the clavicle. Notice it has 2 main nerves in its floor, the spinal accessory nerve (CNXI) and the dorsal scapular nerve. The spinal accessory nodal chain is its key occupant with regards to the kind of lesions found in the posterior cervical space. (Bottom) Axial graphic through the thyroid bed of the infrahyoid neck depicts the posterior cervical space with its complex fascial borders. The superficial layer of the deep cervical fascia is its superficial border, while the deep layer of the deep cervical fascia is its deep border. Note the tricolored carotid sheath is its anteromedial border. The brachial plexus roots travel through the posterior cervical space on their way to the axillary apex.

Posterior Cervical Space

POSTERIOR CERVICAL SPACE NODAL STATIONS/DISEASES

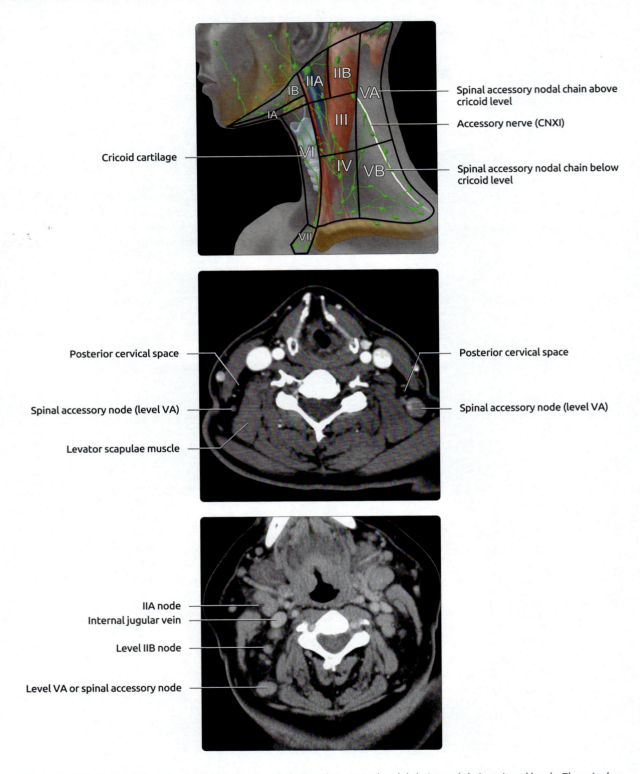

(Top) Oblique graphic of the extracranial head and neck depicts the principal nodal chains and their assigned levels. The spinal accessory chain (level V) is divided at the axial level of the cricoid cartilage into the upper level VA and lower level VB groups. Levels II, III, and IV nodes are in the internal jugular chain. (Middle) Axial CECT of the cervical neck at the level of the supraglottis shows bilateral level VA nodes in the posterior cervical space of the neck. They are considered VA because they are in the posterior cervical space above the cricoid cartilage. (Bottom) CECT demonstrates an enlarged spinal accessory nerve chain lymph node level VA in the posterior cervical space. The lymph nodes anterior to the carotid sheath or in contact with the carotid sheath are level IIA nodes, and lymph nodes posterior to the carotid sheath are level IIB nodes.

Posterior Cervical Space

GENERIC MASS IN POSTERIOR CERVICAL SPACE

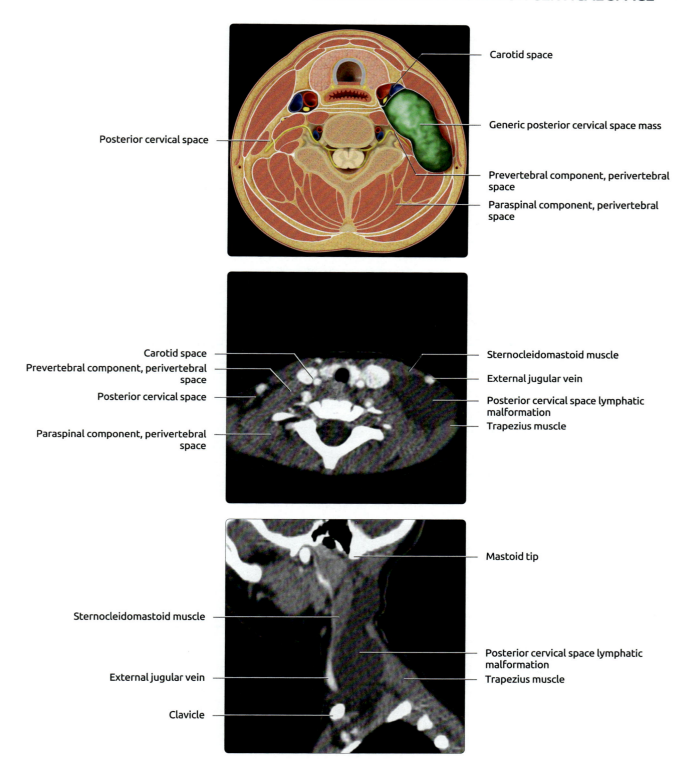

(Top) Axial graphic in the infrahyoid neck shows a generic mass in the posterior cervical space on the left. Notice the lesion is centered within fat of the posterior cervical space. A posterior cervical space mass typically displaces the carotid space anteromedially, elevates the sternocleidomastoid muscle, and flattens the deeper perivertebral space structures. (Middle) In this axial CECT at the level of the thyroid bed, a lymphatic malformation is seen filling the left posterior cervical space. (Bottom) Sagittal CECT reformation reveals a posterior cervical space lymphatic malformation. The image is presented to show the "tilted tent" shape of the posterior cervical space from its superior margin at the mastoid tip to its inferior margin at the clavicle.

Posterior Cervical Space

AXIAL CECT

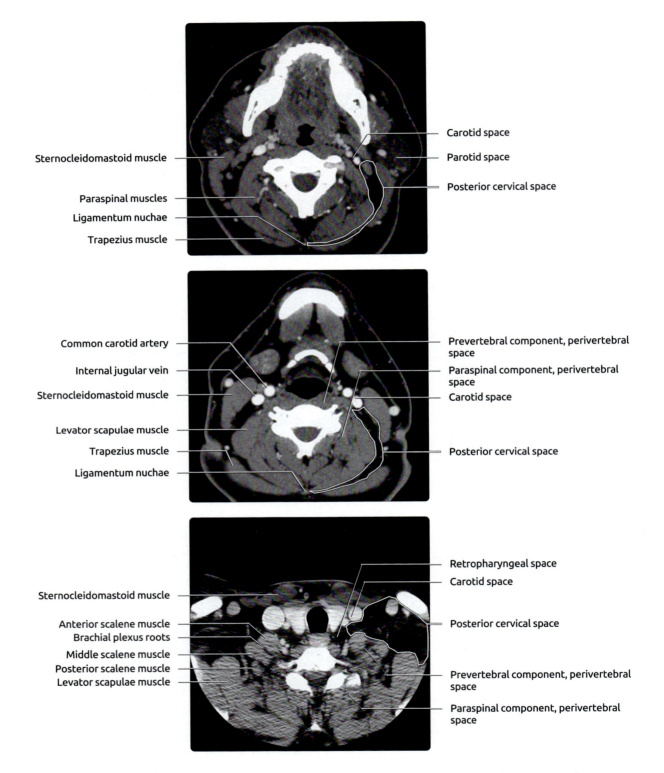

(Top) First of 3 axial CECT images at the level of the mid oropharynx shows the fat-filled posterior cervical space. Notice the posteromedial extension of the posterior cervical space between the paraspinal muscles and the trapezius where it reaches as far as the ligamentum nuchae. (Middle) In this CECT at the level of the hyoid bone, the anteromedial border of the posterior cervical space abuts the carotid space. Deep to the posterior cervical space is the paraspinal component of the perivertebral space. The lateral-most muscle in the paraspinal muscle group is the levator scapulae muscle. (Bottom) At the level of the clavicle, the posterior cervical space is visible enlarging in the inferolateral direction to meet the axillary apex. Notice the brachial plexus roots must traverse the posterior cervical space as they emerge from between the anterior and middle scalene muscles.

Posterior Cervical Space

CORONAL T1 MR

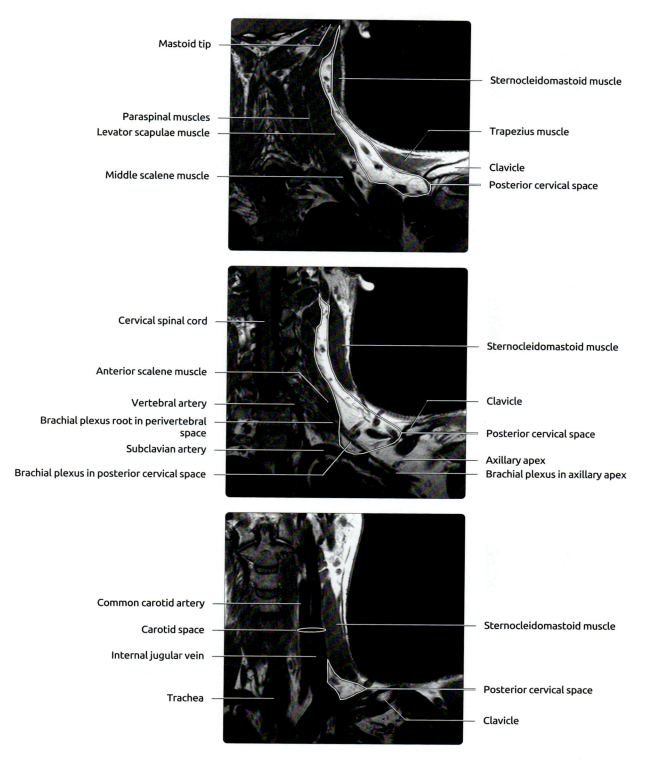

(Top) First of 3 coronal T1 MR images of the extracranial head and neck presented from posterior to anterior emphasizing the anatomy of the posterior cervical space is shown. In this image, the posterior cervical space is seen spanning the distance between the mastoid tip superiorly and the axillary apex inferolaterally. A few scattered level V spinal accessory lymph nodes are seen in the high-signal fat of the posterior cervical space. (Middle) In this image through the cervical spinal cord, the brachial plexus roots are visible exiting the perivertebral space into the posterior cervical space on their way to the axillary apex. Lymph node disease of the lower spinal accessory chain in the posterior cervical space can affect the brachial plexus. (Bottom) In this image through the carotid space, the most anteroinferior aspect of the posterior cervical space is seen.

Posterior Cervical Space

TRANSVERSE ULTRASOUND

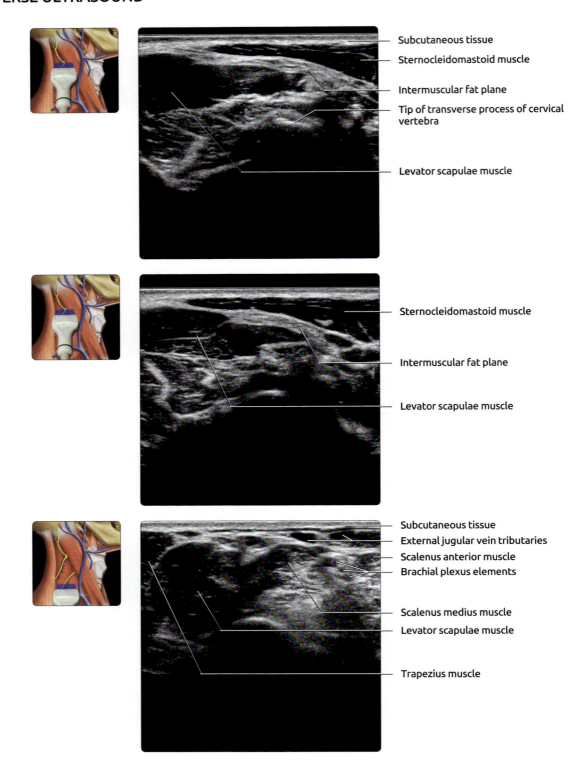

(Top) First of 3 transverse grayscale ultrasound images shows the posterior triangle. The sternocleidomastoid muscle marks the anterior border of the posterior triangle. Muscles form the floor of the posterior triangle. Note the accessory nerve and nodes lie in the intermuscular fat plane. (Middle) Standard transverse grayscale ultrasound shows the intermuscular fat plane, which is best screened in this plane. Once pathology is detected, further examination, particularly Doppler, is best done longitudinally. (Bottom) Lower level of the posterior triangle is shown. The trapezius muscle marks the posterior margin of the posterior triangle. The main bulk of the levator scapulae muscle forms the muscular floor.

Posterior Cervical Space

LONGITUDINAL AND TRANSVERSE ULTRASOUND

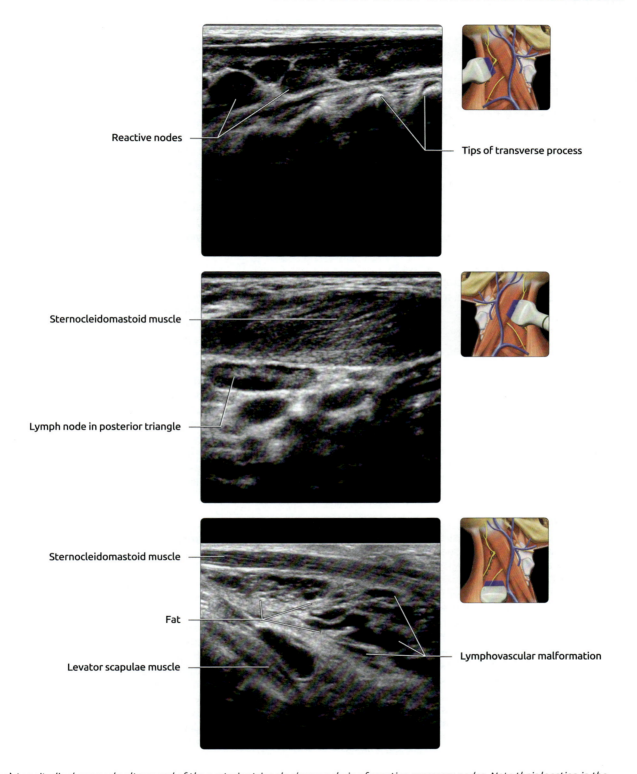

(Top) Longitudinal grayscale ultrasound of the posterior triangle shows a chain of reactive accessory nodes. Note their location in the intermuscular fat plane. Do not mistake the tips of the transverse processes with calcified nodes. (Middle) Longitudinal grayscale ultrasound shows hypertrophy of the sternocleidomastoid muscle (pseudotumor) in an infant with torticollis. Note the internal muscular striations are preserved helping to identify this as a muscle and not a mass. (Bottom) Oblique transverse grayscale ultrasound of a child who underwent 2 treatments of ultrasound-guided sclerotherapy for a large, multiloculated lymphovascular malformation is shown. Note that small cystic locules persist; however, much of the lymphatic malformation has been replaced by fatty tissue. Ultrasound safely guides intralesional injection and readily monitors posttreatment change in size and appearance.

Visceral Space

TERMINOLOGY

Abbreviations
- Visceral space (VS)

Definitions
- **VS**: Cylindrical space in midline infrahyoid neck (IHN) enclosed by middle layer of deep cervical fascia (ML-DCF)

IMAGING ANATOMY

Overview
- Cylindrical space containing central contents of IHN; extends from hyoid bone to upper mediastinum
- **Critical contents**: Larynx, trachea, hypopharynx (HP), esophagus, thyroid and parathyroid glands

Anatomy Relationships
- VS is largest space of IHN with multiple important anatomic subunits
- Lateral to VS are paired anterior cervical spaces
- Posterolateral to VS are paired carotid spaces (CS)
- Posterior to VS is retropharyngeal space (RPS)

Internal Contents
- **Larynx**
  - Hollow, mucosal-lined, muscular, and cartilaginous organ within VS of neck
  - Involved in several important respiratory and airway functions: Breathing, phonation, and protection against aspiration
  - **Supraglottis** extends from top of epiglottis to laryngeal ventricle below
  - **Glottis** consists of true vocal cords (TVCs), anterior and posterior commissures, and central air space created by these structures
  - **Subglottis** extends from undersurface of TVC to inferior cricoid
- **Cervical trachea**
  - Trachea is semiflexible tube comprised of cartilage, smooth muscle, connective tissue, and mucosal lining that serves as protected airway from larynx to main bronchi of lungs
  - Provides humidification and warming of inspired air, also functions in mucociliary clearance
  - Extends from C6 vertebra to carina at T5
  - Total length of trachea contains 15-20 hyaline cartilages; each cartilage is horseshoe-shaped "incomplete ring" surrounding anterior 2/3 of trachea
  - Posterior wall of trachea is formed by fibromuscular tissue and devoid of cartilage
  - Smooth muscle fibers in posterior membrane (trachealis muscle) attach to free ends of tracheal cartilages and can alter cross-sectional area of airway
  - Mucosa consists of pseudostratified ciliated columnar epithelium interspersed with goblet cells with both lying on basal lamina
  - Measurement is variable: Anterior-posterior dimension ~10-25 mm; transverse dimension ~ 10-25 mm
  - At thyroid level, trachea is bordered anteriorly and bilaterally by thyroid gland; above this, cervical trachea is bordered anteriorly by fat plane and strap muscles

- Thin layer of fatty tissue separates posterior wall of trachea from esophagus
- **Hypopharynx**
  - Inferior continuation of oropharynx
  - Begins at level of pharyngoepiglottic folds, at ~ horizontal level of hyoid bone and merges with esophagus below at esophageal verge
  - Complex mucosal and muscular tube consisting of 5 principal layers
    - **Mucosa**: Stratified squamous epithelium that lines lumen
    - **Submucosa**: Loose stroma that can contain fat and can be identified on cross-sectional imaging as thin fat plane
    - Fibrous layer that represents limited inferior continuation of **pharyngobasilar fascia** (pharyngeal aponeurosis)
    - **Muscular layer** consisting of middle and inferior constrictors
    - Outer fascial layer originating from buccopharyngeal fascia
  - Consists of 3 major regions
    - **Pyriform sinuses (PS)**
      - □ Anterolateral recesses of HP
      - □ Each PS has shape of inverted pyramid with base of pyramid positioned superiorly at level of pharyngoepiglottic fold and inferior tip (PS apex) positioned at level of true cord
      - □ Majority of hypopharyngeal squamous cell carcinomas (2/3) originate in PS
    - **Posterior wall**
      - □ Inferior continuation of posterior oropharyngeal wall, from approximate level of hyoid bone to inferior tip of cricoid cartilage
      - □ Muscular layer formed by middle and inferior constrictor muscles
      - □ Posterior wall separated from **perivertebral space** by **RPS**
    - **Postcricoid region**
      - □ Anterior wall of lower HP
      - □ Mucosa of postcricoid region faces posteriorly and is normally directly apposed to mucosa of posterior wall during routine cross-sectional imaging
      - □ Anterior-posterior dimension of postcricoid soft tissue should be < 1 cm normally
- **Cervical esophagus**
  - HP merges with esophagus below at esophageal verge
  - Esophageal verge is best defined by cricopharyngeus muscle that encircles junction, but this muscle cannot be identified easily on cross-sectional imaging
  - Cricopharyngeus muscle is located at approximate level of inferior margin of cricoid cartilage
  - Descends posterior to trachea and thyroid, lying in front of lower cervical vertebrae
  - Positioned slightly to left in lower cervical neck and upper mediastinum
  - Nonkeratinized stratified squamous epithelium
  - Thin layer of fatty tissue separates posterior wall of trachea from esophagus
  - Thin fat planes are generally present on lateral margins of cervical esophagus

Visceral Space

- o Esophageal diameter is variable, depends upon degree of distension
- o Esophageal wall is generally < 5 mm thick
- **Recurrent laryngeal nerves**
  - o Positioned within tracheoesophageal grooves bilaterally
  - o Arise from vagus nerves, innervate all intrinsic muscles of larynx except cricothyroid muscle
  - o Left: Recurs at level of arch where it passes through aortopulmonic window
  - o Right: Recurs in most inferior IHN around right subclavian artery
- **Thyroid gland**
  - o Shield-shaped endocrine organ in lower neck that produces thyroid hormones (T3 and T4) that are involved in many functions, including metabolism (cardiac rate and output) and protein synthesis (growth); also produces calcitonin
  - o Lies anterior and lateral to trachea in VS of IHN, at C5-T1 level
  - o 2 lobes connected by isthmus
- **Parathyroid glands**
  - o Small glands in VS of neck, intimately associated with posterior margin of thyroid gland, that produce parathormone, hormone that regulates calcium concentration in serum and interstitial fluids
  - o 4 glands, 2 pairs behind upper and lower poles of thyroid gland
  - o Superior 2 glands consistent in location
  - o Inferior 2 glands less reliable in location
    - May be normally found in cervicothoracic junction or superior mediastinum
- **VS lymph nodes**
  - o Considered **level VI nodal group**
  - o Paratracheal lymph node group
    - **1st-order drainage for thyroid malignancy**
    - Serves as primary conduit for nodal spread into superior mediastinum
  - o Prelaryngeal nodal group
  - o Pretracheal nodal group

Fascia

- **ML-DCF** completely encloses VS
- ML-DCF also referred to as "visceral fascia"

ANATOMY IMAGING ISSUES

Imaging Approaches

- Imaging approach is determined by clinical symptoms and anatomic subunit under investigation
- **Thyroid**
  - o **Ultrasound** ± needle aspiration biopsy is **1st-line approach** to lesions of thyroid gland
  - o If differentiated thyroid carcinoma, total thyroidectomy performed, and nuclear medicine (I-131) diagnostic study is then done 6 weeks after surgery
  - o If suspected nodes from clinical examination or I-131 study or significant residual uptake remaining in thyroid bed, therapeutic I-131 dose is administered
  - o MR is preferred imaging tool to stage superior mediastinum as it prevents iodine load delaying iodine-based nuclear medicine therapy

- o If suspect VS malignancy, image to carina to include level VI (paratracheal, prelaryngeal, and pretracheal) nodes and superior mediastinal nodes (level VII)
- o Most common symptom is palpable thyroid mass or adenopathy
- **Parathyroid**
  - o Ultrasound is best first-line approach
  - o Tc-99m sestamibi useful for localizing parathyroid adenoma (PTA)
  - o CT, CTA, and MR useful in challenging cases, especially ectopic PTA cases
  - o Searching for PTA includes upper mediastinal search
  - o Symptoms associated with hypercalcemia produced by excessive parathyroid hormone
- **HP and cervical esophagus**
  - o CECT is best overall modality for evaluating soft tissue masses of HP and cervical esophagus
  - o MR is useful in problem-solving, especially evaluation of local invasion
  - o Barium swallow can evaluate for motility disorder, obstruction, aspiration
  - o Symptoms include dysphagia, intolerance to solid foods
- **Larynx and cervical trachea**
  - o CECT is best overall approach for evaluating lesion of larynx and proximal trachea
  - o Symptoms include cough, stridor, aspiration, hoarseness
  - o Recurrent laryngeal nerve: Distal vagal neuropathy with isolated vocal cord paralysis; hoarseness

Imaging Pitfalls

- Patulous esophagus may project from behind left tracheal margin, mimicking PTA
- Ending VS cross-sectional imaging at cervicothoracic junction is significant imaging mistake
  - o **Multiple VS lesions require imaging to carina**
    - When staging VS tumor, especially differentiated thyroid carcinoma, must evaluate upper mediastinal nodes (level VII)
    - Distal vagal neuropathy requires continuing to carina if on **left**
- Small lymph nodes in VS can be mistaken for PTAs on cross-sectional imaging; hypervascularity on arterial-phase CTA can help distinguish PTA, but sestamibi scan is more specific for identifying PTAs

Visceral Space

GRAPHICS

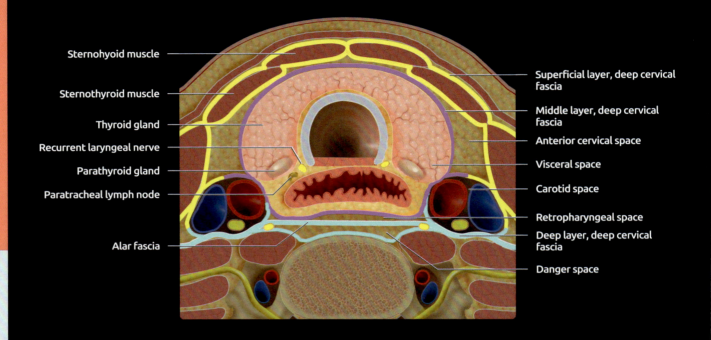

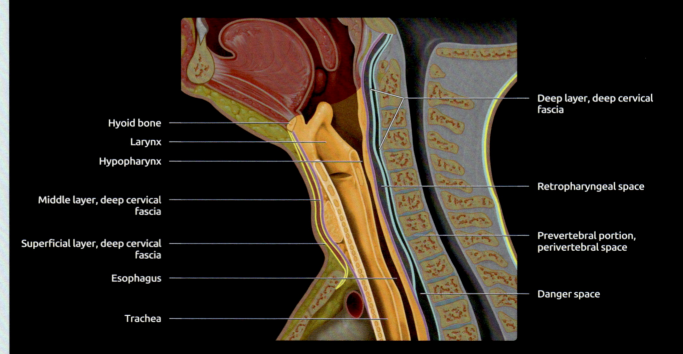

(Top) Axial graphic shows the visceral space defined by the middle layer of the deep cervical fascia (pink). Middle layer of the deep cervical fascia, also called "visceral fascia," runs along deep surface of strap muscles, merges anteriorly with superficial layer of deep cervical fascia (yellow), and splits to encapsulate thyroid gland. Middle layer of the deep cervical fascia also forms the anterior margin of the retropharyngeal space and contributes to the carotid sheath. Recurrent laryngeal nerve lies in the tracheoesophageal groove, and injury results in vocal cord paralysis and hoarseness. **(Bottom)** Sagittal graphic shows longitudinal relationships of the infrahyoid neck. Note the visceral space (orange) is the only space unique to the infrahyoid neck extending from the hyoid bone to the superior mediastinum. Visceral space is the cylindrical space in the anterior midline neck surrounded by the middle layer of the deep cervical fascia (pink).

Visceral Space

AXIAL CECT

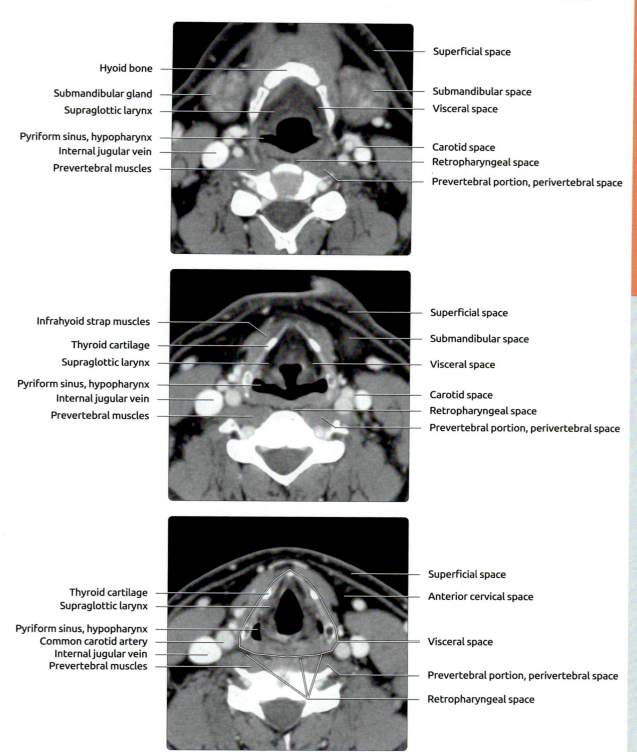

(Top) First of 6 axial CECT images of the visceral space presented from superior to inferior shows the hyoid bone, which represents the superior extent of the visceral space. This cylindrical space in the midline infrahyoid neck is enclosed by the middle layer of the deep cervical fascia and extends to the superior mediastinum. Submandibular space is continuous with the anterior cervical space. *(Middle)* This image shows the visceral space contains the larynx and hypopharynx at this level. It is bordered posteriorly by the retropharyngeal space and posterolaterally by carotid spaces. *(Bottom)* This image shows the visceral space is completely enclosed by the middle layer of the deep cervical fascia, represented by line drawing. Paired anterior cervical spaces are lateral to the visceral space and are continuous with submandibular spaces superiorly. Retropharyngeal space is seen as stripe of fat between the posterior hypopharynx and prevertebral muscles.

Visceral Space

AXIAL CECT

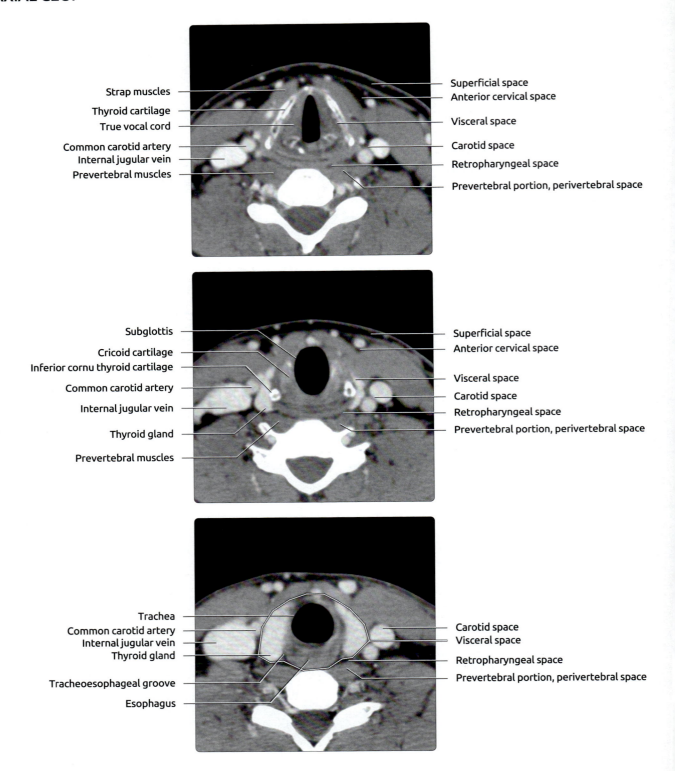

(Top) Image at level of the glottis shows the visceral space in the anterior midline surrounded by the anterior cervical space, carotid space, and retropharyngeal space. Recurrent laryngeal nerve is located in the tracheoesophageal groove but cannot be seen on conventional imaging. Injury of this nerve results in vocal cord paralysis, and imaging should extend to the carina in patients with left-sided injury. (Middle) Image at the subglottic larynx level shows the upper thyroid lobes. (Bottom) Image at the thyroid gland level shows the inferior visceral space, which includes the esophagus and trachea. Thyroid disease is one of the most common lesions of the visceral space and is often best evaluated by ultrasound. If differentiated thyroid disease is present, nuclear medicine I-131 study is next best study. CECT may delay therapy in patients planned for iodine-based nuclear medicine therapy.

Visceral Space

THYROID MASS GRAPHIC & CORONAL CECT

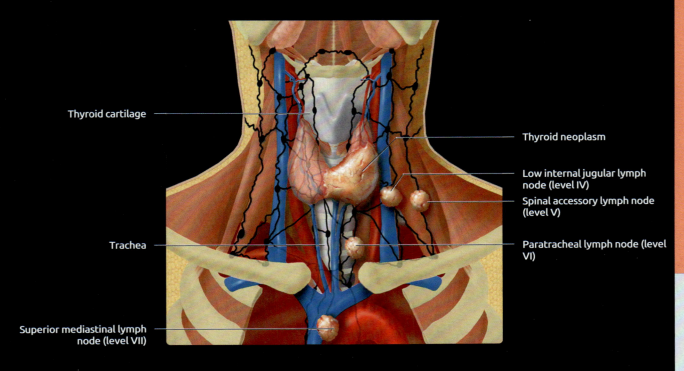

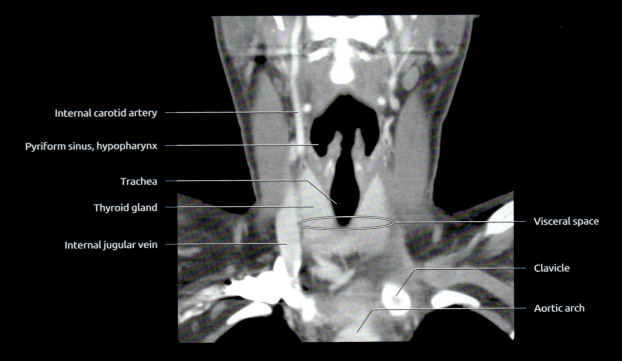

(Top) Coronal graphic shows a typical visceral space mass, differentiated thyroid carcinoma, within the left lobe of the thyroid gland. Several metastatic lymph nodes are seen, including paratracheal lymph nodes (within visceral space), superior mediastinal, low internal jugular, and spinal accessory chain lymph nodes. Paratracheal lymph node group is 1st-order drainage for thyroid malignancy and serves as main conduit for nodal spread into superior mediastinum. (Bottom) Coronal CECT shows the chevron shape of the thyroid gland to best advantage. Visceral space contents includes larynx, hypopharynx, trachea, esophagus, thyroid, and parathyroid glands. Recurrent laryngeal nerves and paratracheal (level VI) lymph nodes are other important visceral space structures. Ending imaging at cervicothoracic junction is an important imaging mistake. Many visceral space lesions require imaging to the carina.

Visceral Space

GENERIC VISCERAL SPACE MASS GRAPHIC & SAGITTAL ANATOMY

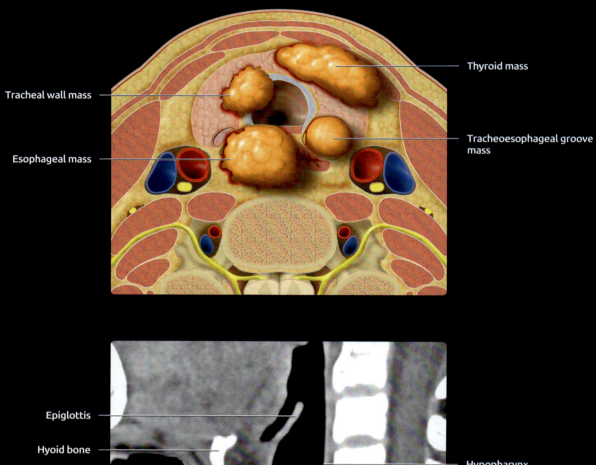

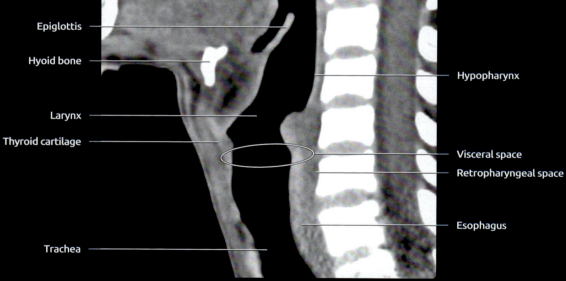

(Top) Axial graphic shows 4 distinct generic visceral space mass locations. Thyroid mass is defined by a mass at least partially surrounded by thyroid tissue. A mass involving the tracheoesophageal groove typically results in recurrent laryngeal nerve injury. Differential considerations for a tracheoesophageal groove lesion include a malignant paratracheal lymph node (often from differentiated thyroid carcinoma), parathyroid adenoma, traumatic dislocation of cricothyroid joint, recurrent laryngeal nerve schwannoma, or patulous esophagus. Tracheal wall mass is centered in the tracheal wall and displaces the thyroid gland laterally and esophagus posteriorly. An esophageal mass is typically midline and displaces the trachea and thyroid anteriorly. (Bottom) Sagittal NECT reformation shows the visceral space in the midline infrahyoid neck, anterior to the retropharyngeal space.

Visceral Space

VISCERAL SPACE: RADIOLOGIC CORRELATION

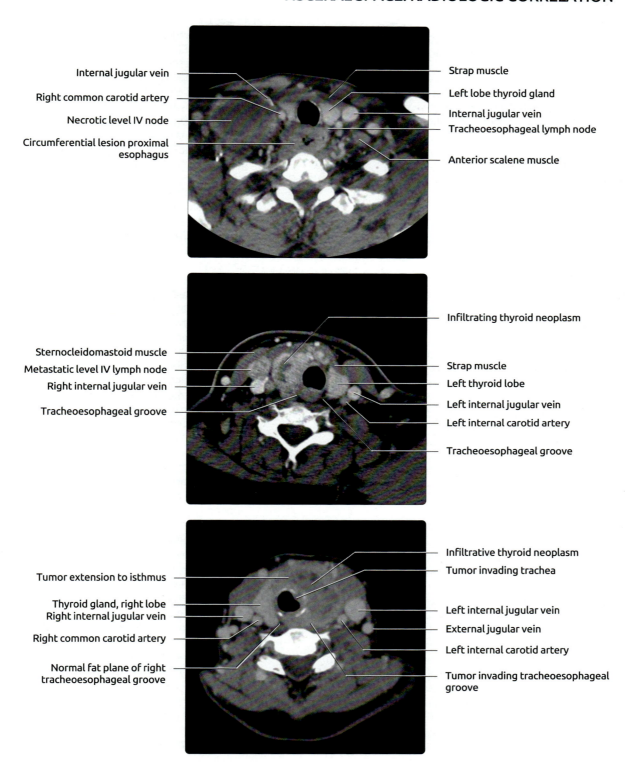

(Top) Axial CECT through level of thyroid gland shows a large circumferential lesion involving cervical esophagus consistent with SCCa. There is a large necrotic level IV lymph node (that demonstrates peripheral enhancement & central low density) on patient's right. Air density in central lumen of esophagus is present. (Middle) Axial CECT through level of thyroid gland in a patient with right vocal cord paralysis & hoarseness shows there is a heterogeneously enhancing tumor (medullary thyroid cancer) that infiltrates right side of thyroid lobe with enlargement of lobe & extracapsular extension of tumor to right tracheoesophageal groove. Tumor extends medially to involve thyroid isthmus. There is a heterogeneous level IV lymph node on the right consistent with nodal metastasis. (Bottom) Axial CECT through thyroid gland demonstrates a large infiltrative & invasive lesion involving left lobe of thyroid gland (biopsy proven anaplastic thyroid carcinoma). Medially, the lesion extends into isthmus of thyroid. Tumor extends beyond medial capsular margin of thyroid itself & tumor extends through tracheal wall. Nodular soft tissue tumor can be seen along left lateral lumen of trachea. Tumor obliterates normal fat plane of left tracheoesophageal groove.

Larynx

TERMINOLOGY

Abbreviations
- True vocal cord (TVC); false vocal cord (FVC)
- Hypopharynx (HP); aryepiglottic fold (AEF)

Definitions
- Larynx: Hollow, mucosal-lined, muscular and cartilaginous organ within ventral neck involved in several important respiratory functions: Breathing, phonation, and protection against aspiration

IMAGING ANATOMY

Extent
- Located in ventral aspect of neck, suspended from hyoid bone, and extending superiorly to inferiorly between ~ C3 and C6
- Continuous inferiorly with trachea, opens superiorly into pharynx

Internal Contents
- **Laryngeal cartilages**
  - Thyroid, cricoid, and base of arytenoid (hyaline cartilage) ossify after 25 years age
  - Epiglottis, corniculate, cuneiform, and processes of arytenoid (elastic cartilage) do not ossify
  - **Thyroid cartilage**: Largest cartilage; "shields" larynx
    - 2 lateral laminae meet anteriorly at acute angle; with superior notch
    - Superior cornua elongated and narrow, attach to lateral thyrohyoid ligament
    - Inferior cornua are short and thick, articulating medially with sides of cricoid cartilage
    - Thyrohyoid membrane extends from superior margin of thyroid cartilage to hyoid bone
      - Focal midline thickening of membrane called median thyrohyoid ligament
      - Thickened lateral margins of membrane = lateral thyrohyoid ligament
      - Triticeous cartilage is small, occasionally calcified cartilage located centrally within lateral thyrohyoid ligament
      - Small aperture in lateral thyrohyoid membrane allows passage of superior laryngeal artery and internal branch of superior laryngeal nerve
  - **Cricoid cartilage**: Only complete ring in endolarynx
    - Broad posterior "lamina" and narrow anterior "arch"
    - Lower border of cricoid cartilage is junction between larynx above and trachea below
  - **Arytenoid cartilage**: Paired pyramidal cartilages that sit atop posterior cricoid cartilage
    - Vocal and muscular processes are at level of TVC
    - Vocal processes: Anterior projections of arytenoids where posterior margins of TVC attach
  - Corniculate cartilage: Rests on top of superior process of arytenoid cartilage, within AEF
  - Cuneiform cartilage: Within AEF just ventral to corniculate cartilage
- **Supraglottis of endolarynx**
  - Supraglottis extends from top of epiglottis to laryngeal ventricle below

- Contains epiglottis, preepiglottic fat, AEFs, FVCs, paraglottic space, laryngeal ventricles, and upper arytenoid cartilages
  - **Laryngeal aperture** = superior opening of larynx formed by epiglottis, AEFs, and interarytenoid space; **laryngeal vestibule** represents superior airway of larynx that extends from aperture superiorly to TVCs inferiorly
  - **Epiglottis**: Leaf-shaped cartilage, larynx lid with free margin (suprahyoid), fixed portion (infrahyoid)
    - Petiole is "stem" of leaf, which attaches epiglottis to thyroid lamina via thyroepiglottic ligament
    - Hyoepiglottic ligament attaches epiglottis to hyoid; glossoepiglottic fold is midline mucous membrane covering superior aspect of hyoepiglottic ligament
  - **Preepiglottic space**: Fat-filled space between hyoid bone anteriorly and epiglottis posteriorly
    - Devoid of lymph nodes
  - **AEFs**: Projects from cephalad tip of arytenoid cartilages to inferolateral margin of epiglottis
    - Represents superolateral margin of supraglottis, dividing it from pyriform sinus (HP)
  - **FVCs (also called vestibular folds)**: Symmetric medially bulging mucosal surfaces of larynx that create mild narrowing of lower vestibule
    - Mucosa covers supportive vestibular ligament (= inferior margin of quadrangular membrane)
    - Deep to vestibular ligament is paraglottic fat
    - Airway opening between FVCs called rima vestibuli
  - **Quadrangular membrane**: Fibrous membrane extending from upper arytenoid and corniculate cartilages posteriorly to lateral margin epiglottis anteriorly; forms medial margin of paraglottic space; part of AEF
    - Free lower margin is vestibular ligament, under FVC
  - **Paraglottic space**: Paired fat-containing spaces lateral/deep to FVC and TVCs
    - Superiorly, paraglottic space merges with preepiglottic space
    - Bound by conus elasticus inferomedially
    - At level of false cords, space is easily recognized by abundant fat
    - At level of true cords, fat lateral to thyroarytenoid muscles (TAMs) is very thin and can be imperceptible
    - Authors disagree as to whether vocalis muscle and thyroarytenoid muscles are within paraglottic space or medial to it
  - Epithelium composed of respiratory pseudostratified columnar epithelium with abundance of mucous glands and lymphatic vessels
  - Main blood supply is superior laryngeal artery
  - Internal branch of superior laryngeal nerve provides main sensory afferent to supraglottic laryngeal mucosa
  - **Laryngeal ventricles**: Lateral outpouchings situated between false vocal folds above and true vocal folds (cords) below
    - Along anterior roof of each ventricle is small outpouching called laryngeal saccule that functions to lubricate ipsilateral cord
    - Saccule projects superiorly within paraglottic space fat
    - Dilatation of saccule can lead to laryngocele formation
- **Glottis of endolarynx**

Larynx

- o Consists of TVCs, anterior and posterior commissures, and central air space created by these structures
- o **TVC**
  - – Also referred to as true vocal fold
  - – **Complex microanatomy**: TVC consists of multilayered arrangement of tissues
    - □ **Squamous epithelium** is most superficial layer, supported by basement membrane; can give rise to squamous cell carcinoma of TVC
    - □ **Superficial lamina propria**: Soft gelatinous tissue with loose elastic and collagenous tissue; Reinke space is potential space between superficial lamina propria and intermediate lamina propria
    - □ **Intermediate lamina propria and deep lamina propria**
    - □ These 2 layers of densely packed collagen and elastin fibers combine to form thin linear band of tissue, called vocal ligament, that provides both strength and elasticity to TVC
    - □ Vocal ligaments course anteriorly from vocal process of arytenoid cartilage to thyroid cartilage
    - □ Vocal ligament merges inferiorly with conus elasticus
  - – Airway opening/space in between TVCs called rima glottidis
- o **Anterior commissure**
  - – Midline, anterior meeting point of TVC ≤ 1-mm thickness
  - – Broyle ligament (BL) consists of dense connective tissue at insertion of vocal ligaments to thyroid cartilage
    - □ Above glottic plane, BL resists tumor invasion from glottic carcinoma
    - □ Just caudal to glottic plane, BL is replaced by thin layer of connective tissue and is more vulnerable to tumor invasion
    - □ At point of attachment of BL to thyroid cartilage, cartilage is devoid of perichondrium, making region more vulnerable to tumor invasion
- o **Posterior commissure**
  - – Essentially represents fixed midline posterior wall of glottis
- • **Subglottis of endolarynx**
  - o Extends from undersurface of TVC to inferior cricoid
  - o Mucosal surface closely applied to cricoid cartilage
  - o **Conus elasticus**: Fibroelastic supporting membrane extends from medial margin of TVC above to cricoid below; continuous with cricothyroid membrane anteriorly
    - – Free upper margin merges with vocal ligament
- • **Laryngeal muscles**
  - o Extrinsic muscles function to raise and lower larynx; includes digastric, mylohyoid, geniohyoid, stylohyoid, sternothyroid, sternohyoid, thyrohyoid, and omohyoid muscles
  - o **Intrinsic muscles**
    - – AE: Lies within AEF, extends from side of epiglottis, and attaches to ipsilateral arytenoid cartilage

- – Oblique arytenoid: Extends from muscular process of 1 arytenoid cartilage to contralateral AE muscle and corniculate cartilage; paired muscles crisscross each other, creating X-shaped configuration superficial to transverse arytenoid muscle
- – Thyroepiglottic: From upper border thyroid lamina to side of epiglottis
- – TAM: From anterior inner thyroid cartilage to arytenoid cartilage, paralleling vocal ligament; medial component is referred to as vocalis muscle; TAM makes up bulk of tissue of TVC
- – Posterior cricoarytenoid: From posterior cricoid cartilage to muscular process of arytenoid; abduction of TVCs
- – Lateral cricoarytenoid: Lateral cricoid to lateral muscular process of arytenoid, adduction
- – Transverse arytenoid: Fibers connect posterior arytenoid cartilages together, adduction
- – Cricothyroid: Inner margin of thyroid lamina to anterior cricoid cartilage, tensor of TVC

- • **Innervation of larynx**
  - o Vagus nerve (CNX) provides sensory and motor innervation to larynx
  - o **Superior laryngeal nerve** arises from inferior ganglion of vagus nerve and descends toward larynx
    - – Internal branch: Perforates thyrohyoid membrane posteriorly, enters larynx, and supplies sensory innervation to laryngeal mucosa
    - – External branch: Remains external to larynx, supplies motor innervation to cricothyroid muscle
  - o **Recurrent laryngeal nerve (RLN)**: Branch of vagus nerve that initially descends, then ascends lower neck in tracheoesophageal groove, returning to larynx
    - – Left RLN loops around aorta inferiorly
    - – Right RLN loops around right subclavian artery
    - – RLN innervates all intrinsic muscle of larynx except cricothyroid muscles

- • **Embryology**
  - o Supraglottic larynx from primitive buccopharyngeal anlage and has rich lymphatics
  - o Glottic and subglottic larynx from tracheobronchial buds and has few lymphatics
  - o Clinical implication: Supraglottic squamous cell carcinoma have much higher incidence of nodal metastases at presentation than glottic and subglottic

Larynx

GRAPHICS

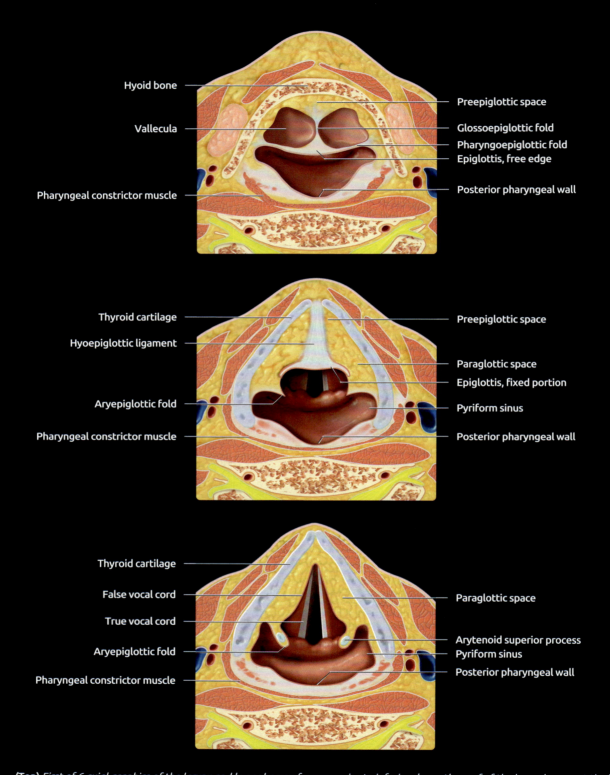

(Top) First of 6 axial graphics of the larynx and hypopharynx from superior to inferior shows the roof of the hypopharynx at the hyoid bone level and high supraglottic structures. The free edge of the epiglottis is attached to the hyoid bone via the hyoepiglottic ligament, which is covered by a glossoepiglottic fold, a ridge of mucous membrane. (Middle) Graphic at the mid supraglottic level shows the hyoepiglottic ligament dividing the lower preepiglottic space. No fascia separates the preepiglottic space from the paraglottic space. These 2 endolaryngeal spaces are submucosal locations where tumors hide from clinical detection. Aryepiglottic fold (marginal supraglottis) represents the junction between the larynx and hypopharynx. (Bottom) Graphic at the low supraglottic level shows false vocal cords formed by mucosal surfaces of the laryngeal vestibule. The paraglottic space is beneath false vocal cords, a common location for submucosal tumor spread.

Larynx

GRAPHICS

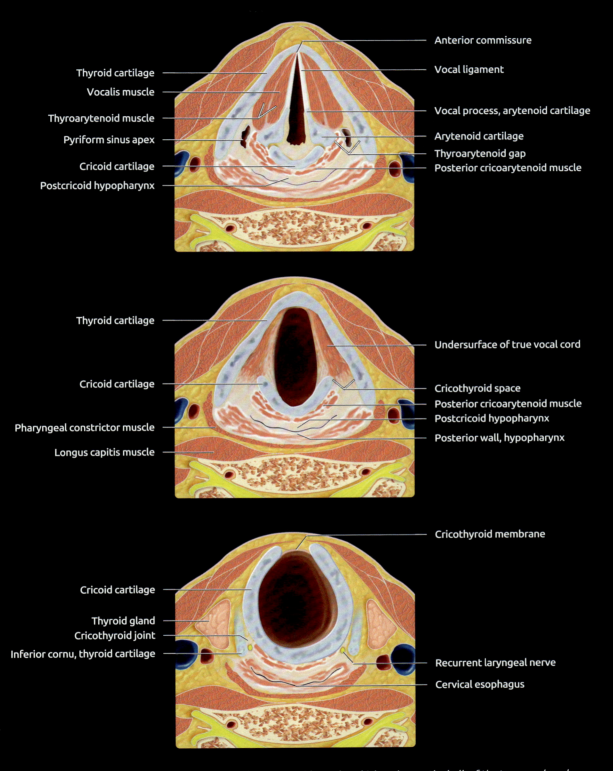

(Top) Graphic at the glottic, true vocal cord level shows the thyroarytenoid muscle, which makes up the bulk of the true vocal cord. Medial fibers of the thyroarytenoid muscle are known as the vocalis muscle. The pyriform sinus apex is seen at the glottic level. The thyroarytenoid gap is the location where tumors may spread between the larynx and hypopharynx. (Middle) Graphic at the level of the undersurface of the true vocal cord shows posterior lamina of cricoid cartilage. The postcricoid hypopharynx represents the anterior wall of the lower hypopharynx and extends from the cricoarytenoid joints to the lower edge of cricoid cartilage at the cricopharyngeus muscle. The posterior wall of the hypopharynx represents inferior continuation of the posterior oropharyngeal wall and extends to the cervical esophagus. (Bottom) Graphic at subglottic level shows the cricothyroid joint immediately adjacent to the recurrent laryngeal nerve, located in the tracheoesophageal groove. Life-saving emergency laryngotomy procedure is done by inserting a needle through the cricothyroid membrane.

Larynx

GRAPHICS

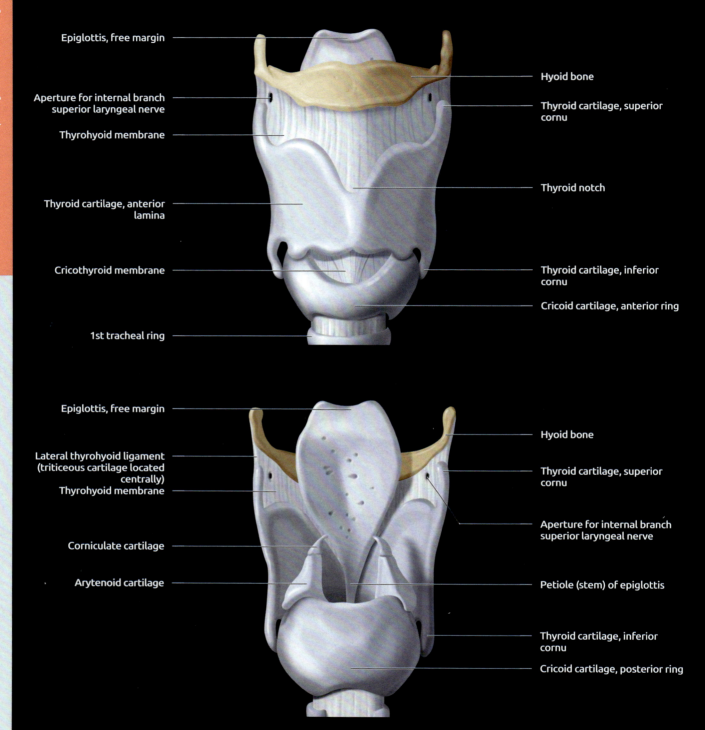

(Top) Anterior view of the laryngeal cartilages is shown. Note 2 large anterior laminae of the thyroid cartilage that "shield" the larynx. The thyrohyoid membrane contains an aperture through which the internal branch of superior laryngeal nerve and associated vessels course. Internal laryngeal nerve then passes beneath mucosa of the pyriform sinus; removal of foreign bodies from the sinus may damage this nerve, leading to supraglottic anesthesia and impaired protective cough reflex. Mixed (external) laryngoceles herniate through the thyrohyoid membrane to extend into the submandibular space. (Bottom) Posterior view shows arytenoid cartilage sitting on top of the posterior cricoid cartilage. The true vocal cord attaches to the vocal process of arytenoid cartilage and forms the glottis. The epiglottis is a leaf-shaped cartilage, which forms the lid of larynx and contains fixed and free margins. Cricoid cartilage is the only complete ring in the endolarynx and provides structural integrity. Calcified triticeous cartilage could be mistaken for a foreign body in radiographs.

Larynx

GRAPHICS

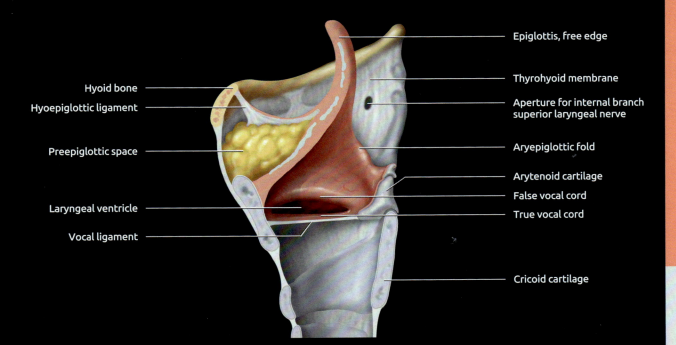

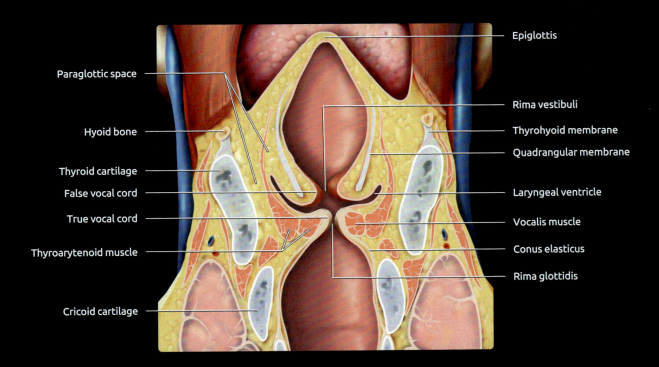

(Top) Sagittal graphic of the midline larynx shows the laryngeal ventricle, air-space that separates false vocal cords above with true vocal cords below. Aryepiglottic folds project from the tip of arytenoid cartilage to the inferolateral margin of the epiglottis. Aryepiglottic folds represent the junction between the supraglottis and hypopharynx. The medial wall of the aryepiglottic fold is endolaryngeal, while the posterolateral wall is the anteromedial margin of the pyriform sinus. (Bottom) Coronal graphic posterior view shows false and true vocal cords separated by the laryngeal ventricle. The quadrangular membrane is a fibrous membrane, which extends from the upper arytenoid and corniculate cartilages to the lateral epiglottis. The conus elasticus is a fibroelastic membrane, which extends from the vocal ligament of the true vocal cord to the cricoid. Their membranes represent a relative barrier to tumor spread but are not seen on conventional imaging.

Larynx

GRAPHIC AND REFORMATTED CT

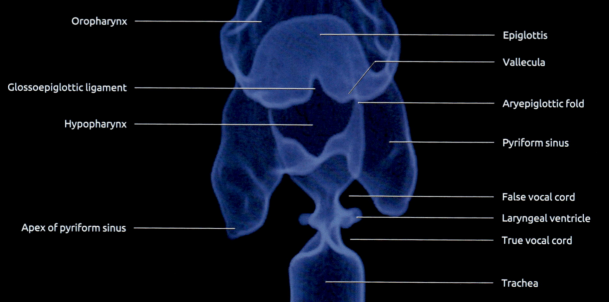

(Top) Multiple graphics demonstrate the internal laryngeal muscles. The posterior cricoarytenoid muscle is the only muscle directly functioning to abduct (separate) the vocal cords. The recurrent laryngeal nerves innervate all of the internal laryngeal muscles except the cricothyroid muscle (external branch of the superior laryngeal nerve). The thyroarytenoid muscle makes up much of the bulk of the vocal fold and includes the medial component, the vocalis muscle. *(Bottom)* Coronal 3D reformatted CT shows mucosal surfaces of the larynx and hypopharynx. The pyriform sinus represents the anterolateral recess of the hypopharynx and is the most common location for hypopharyngeal tumors. The pyriform sinus apex (inferior tip) lies at the level of the true vocal cord, which allows pyriform sinus tumors access to true vocal cords. (Courtesy C. Glastonbury, MBBS.)

Larynx

AXIAL CECT CORDS ABDUCTED (APART)

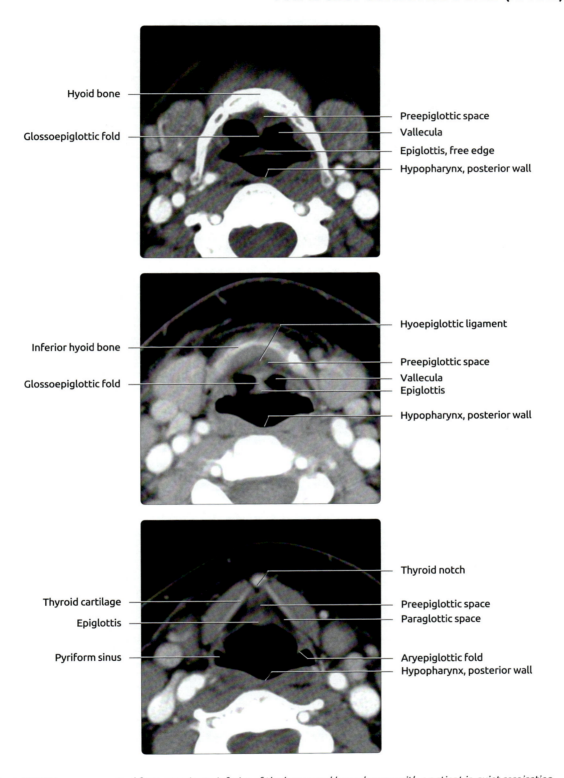

(Top) First of 9 axial CECT images presented from superior to inferior of the larynx and hypopharynx with a patient in quiet respiration is shown. The hyoid bone represents the level of the roof of the larynx and hypopharynx. The glossoepiglottic and pharyngoepiglottic folds represent transition from the oropharynx above to the larynx and hypopharynx below. (Middle) Image of the high supraglottic level of the larynx shows a C-shaped preepiglottic space, a common location for tumors to hide. If supraglottic tumor extends to the preepiglottic space, it becomes a T3 tumor. (Bottom) Image of the high supraglottic level shows that the preepiglottic and paraglottic spaces are continuous, with no intervening fascia. This allows tumors to spread submucosally in these locations. The aryepiglottic fold, part of the larynx, represents transition between the larynx and the hypopharynx. The posterolateral wall of the aryepiglottic fold is the anteromedial margin of the pyriform sinus.

Larynx

AXIAL CECT CORDS ABDUCTED (APART)

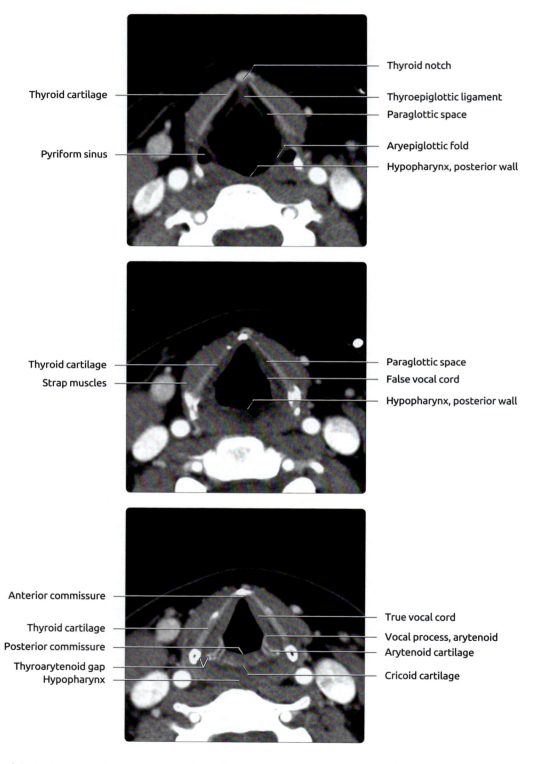

(Top) Image of the mid supraglottic level shows the thyroepiglottic ligament dividing the preepiglottic space. Aryepiglottic folds are at the margin of the pyriform sinus and larynx; a tumor primary to the aryepiglottic fold is considered a "marginal supraglottic" tumor. (Middle) Image of the low supraglottic level shows the false vocal cord level. The paraglottic space represents the deep fatty space beneath the false vocal cords. Tumors that cross the laryngeal ventricle and involve false and true vocal cords are considered transglottic. (Bottom) Image at the glottic level shows true vocal cords in abduction in quiet respiration. The true vocal cord level is identified on CT when arytenoid and cricoid cartilages are seen and muscle fills the inferior paraglottic space. Anterior and posterior commissures of true vocal cords should be < 1 mm in normal patients. The postcricoid hypopharynx is typically collapsed.

Larynx

AXIAL CECT CORDS ABDUCTED (APART)

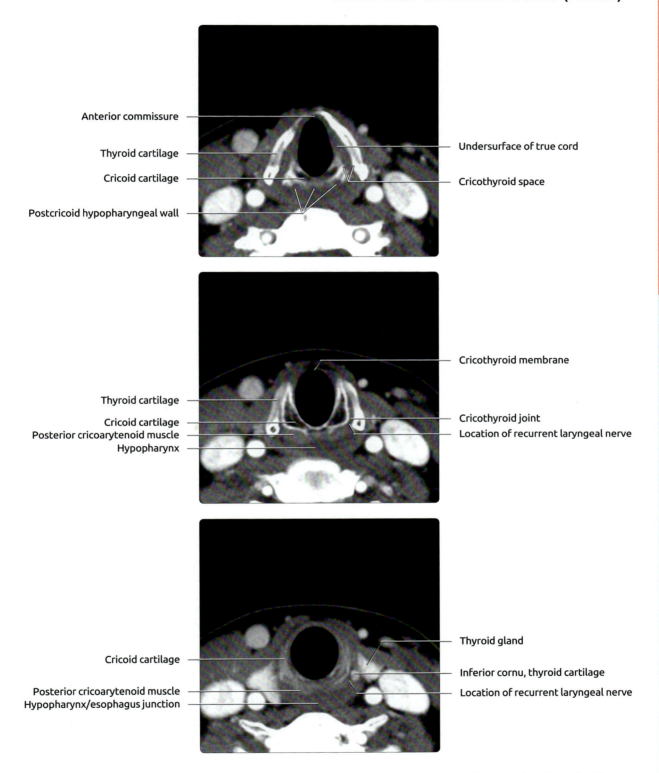

(Top) *In this image through the undersurface of the true cord level, the cricothyroid space is seen. Lack of arytenoid cartilage identifies the undersurface of the true cord level.* (Middle) *Image more inferior shows the subglottic level with the cricoid ring nearly complete. Cricoid is the only complete cartilage ring in the larynx and provides structural integrity. Dislocations of the cricothyroid joint may result in vocal cord paralysis secondary to recurrent laryngeal nerve injury. There may be associated atrophy of the posterior cricoarytenoid muscle on the involved side of vocal cord paralysis. Posterior cricoarytenoid is the only abductor of the vocal cord and could be seen to be slightly hypermetabolic physiologically in F-18 FDG PET/CT scans.* (Bottom) *At the level of the inferior cricoid cartilage, the inferior margin of the larynx and hypopharynx are transitioning to the trachea and cervical esophagus. Mucosa along the subglottis should be no more than 1 mm in normal patients. Thickened mucosa raises concern for tumor.*

Larynx

AXIAL CECT CORDS ADDUCTED (TOGETHER)

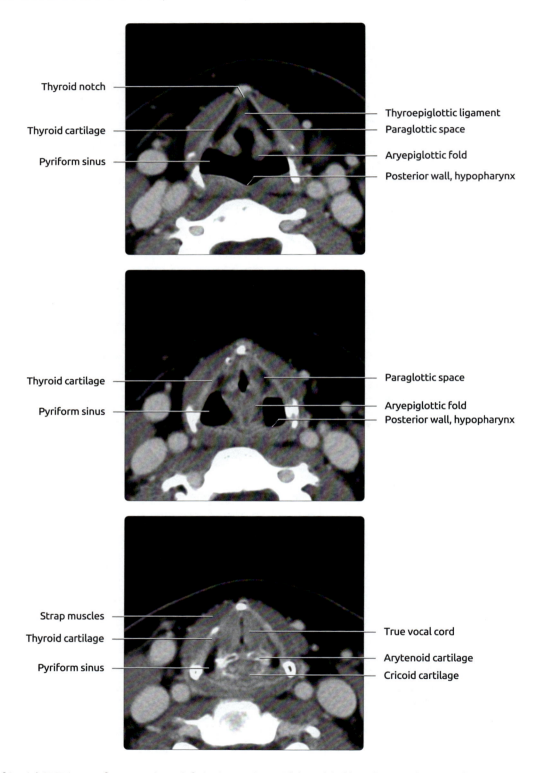

(Top) First of 3 axial CECT images from superior to inferior in a patient with breath holding shows adduction of false and true vocal cords as well as aryepiglottic folds. (Middle) Image at the low supraglottic level shows the level of false vocal cords in adduction. Note the mucosa of the aryepiglottic folds contacts the posterior hypopharyngeal wall. (Bottom) Image at the glottic level shows adduction of the true vocal cords. With breath holding, true vocal cords oppose in the midline. A cord that remains paramedian is either paralyzed or mechanically fixed. Vocal cord paralysis typically results in paramedian true vocal cords with associated abnormal location of arytenoid cartilage, which is fixed in an anterior-medial position. With breath holding, the paralyzed cord remains fixed, while the opposite normal cord crosses the midline in attempt to close the glottis. There may be an associated patulous pyriform sinus.

Larynx

CORONAL NECT

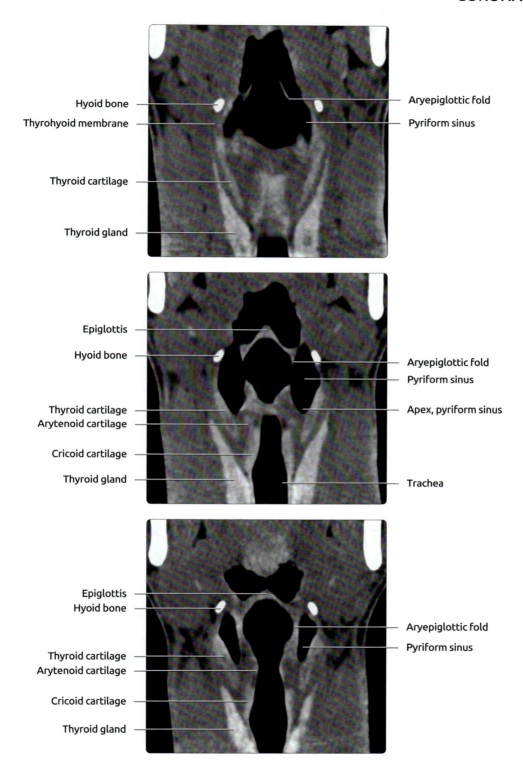

(Top) First of 6 NECT coronal reformation images of the larynx and hypopharynx presented from posterior to anterior shows the hyoid bone, which represents the level of the roof of the larynx and hypopharynx. CT is particularly good for evaluation of patients with diseases of the larynx and hypopharynx, as these patients often have difficulty with secretions, coughing, and swallowing, making a short exam time vital. (Middle) Image more anterior shows laryngeal cartilages. These cartilages are variably ossified in adults, which makes pathologic conditions, such as cartilage invasion, difficult to diagnose with certainty. Apex of the pyriform sinus extends inferiorly to the level of true vocal cord. (Bottom) In this image, aryepiglottic folds are well seen as they extend from the lateral epiglottis to arytenoid cartilage. The pyriform sinus is the most common location for tumors of the hypopharynx.

Larynx

CORONAL NECT

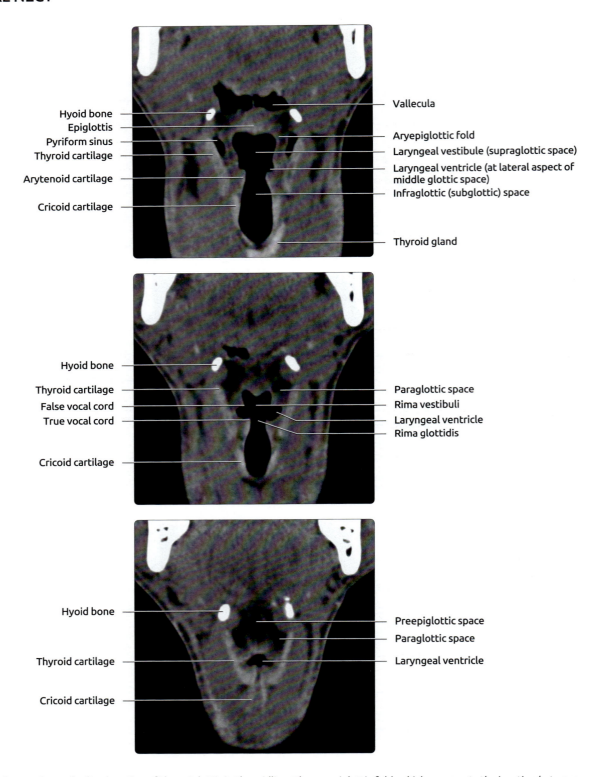

(Top) *This image shows the fixed portion of the epiglottis in the midline. The aryepiglottic fold, which represents the junction between the larynx anteriorly and hypopharynx posteriorly, is noted. The supraglottic, middle glottic, and subglottic spaces are also demarcated.* (Middle) *In this image, the laryngeal ventricle is visible as an air space between false vocal cords above and true vocal cords below. When a tumor crosses the laryngeal ventricle to involve true and false cords, it is transglottic, which has important treatment implications. Coronal imaging is particularly useful for evaluation of transglottic disease. The rima vestibuli is the opening between false vocal cords. The rima glottidis is the opening between true vocal cords and is the narrowest part of laryngeal cavity.* (Bottom) *This image reveals preepiglottic fat to be continuous with paraglottic fat. These are the most important spaces of the endolarynx, as they allow submucosal spread of tumors, which is undetectable by clinical exam.*

Larynx

SAGITTAL NECT

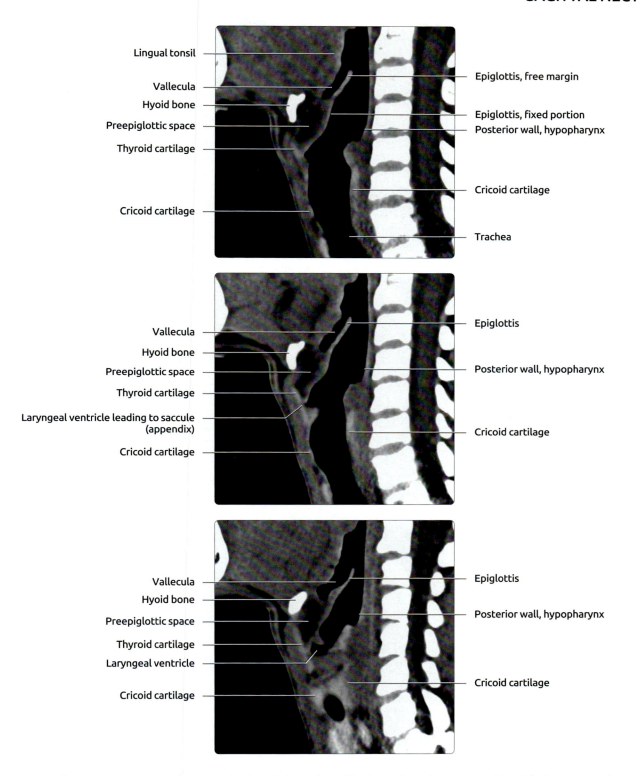

(Top) First of 3 sagittal NECT images from medial to lateral shows the midline larynx/hypopharynx. Preepiglottic fat is seen posterior and inferior to the hyoid bone. Posterior hypopharyngeal wall pathology is well seen on sagittal images and also helps define the craniocaudal extent of lesions. (Middle) A more lateral image shows the laryngeal ventricle, the lateral air space of the middle glottic cavity separating false vocal cords above from true cords below. The laryngeal ventricle can have an anterosuperior tubular extension between the vestibular fold and thyroid cartilage, called the laryngeal saccule or ventricular appendix. They have mucous glands to lubricate vocal folds that are termed "oil can of larynx." Laryngoceles are dilated air or fluid-filled laryngeal saccules. (Bottom) More lateral image shows laryngeal cartilages, variably ossified in adults, making pathology difficult to evaluate, particularly cartilage invasion from tumors and traumatic injury. Cricoid cartilage, the only complete ring in the larynx, has a signet ring shape with the larger signet portion projecting posteriorly.

Larynx

AXIAL T1 MR

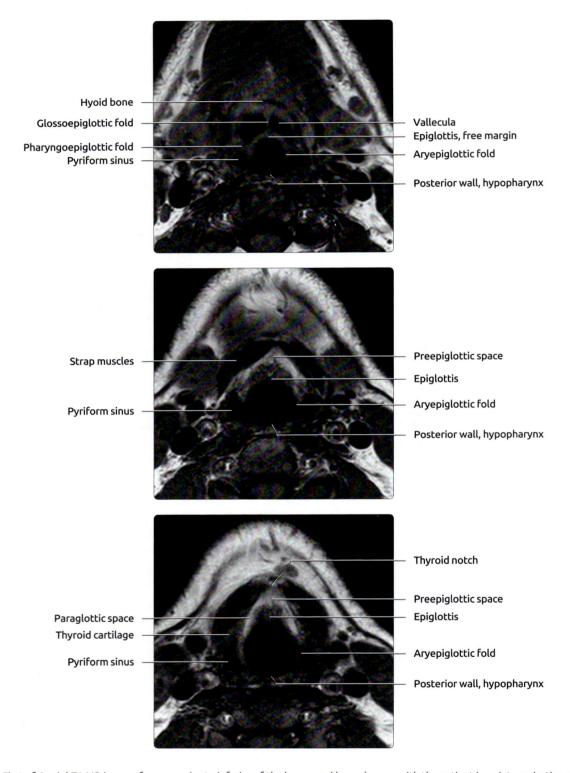

(Top) First of 6 axial T1 MR images from superior to inferior of the larynx and hypopharynx with the patient in quiet respiration shows the roof of the larynx, which is defined by the epiglottis, glossoepiglottic, and pharyngoepiglottic folds. MR is typically reserved for answering specific questions, such as cartilage invasion rather than as a 1st imaging study of a patient with larynx or hypopharynx disease. (Middle) Image at the level of the high supraglottis shows a C-shaped, fat-filled preepiglottic space and fixed portion of the epiglottis. Cartilage is variably ossified, which makes it somewhat difficult to visualize on T1 MR images. (Bottom) Image at the mid supraglottic level shows fat of the preepiglottic space continuous with fat of the paraglottic space. Lack of fascia between these 2 submucosal spaces allows tumor to travel from one to the other and hide from clinical detection.

Larynx

AXIAL T1 MR

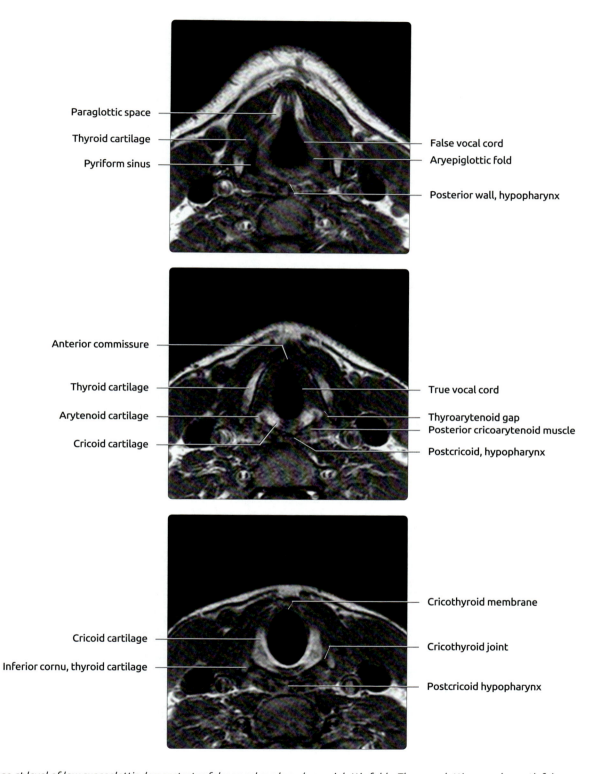

(Top) Image at level of low supraglottis demonstrates false vocal cords and aryepiglottic folds. The paraglottic space beneath false vocal cords is primarily fat-filled. Aryepiglottic folds often contact the posterior wall of the hypopharynx in normal patients. (Middle) Image at the glottic level shows muscle in the paraglottic space beneath the true vocal cords. Both cricoid and arytenoid cartilage are seen at the true vocal cord level. The thyroarytenoid muscle makes up the bulk of true vocal cords. The posterior cricoarytenoid muscle is often atrophied in patients with vocal cord paralysis. (Bottom) Image at the subglottic level shows large, broad posterior cricoid cartilage. The cricothyroid joint is where the recurrent laryngeal nerve is located. Dislocation of this joint is associated with recurrent laryngeal nerve injury. The postcricoid hypopharynx extends from the cricoarytenoid joints to the lower cricoid cartilage.

Larynx

SAGITTAL T1 MR

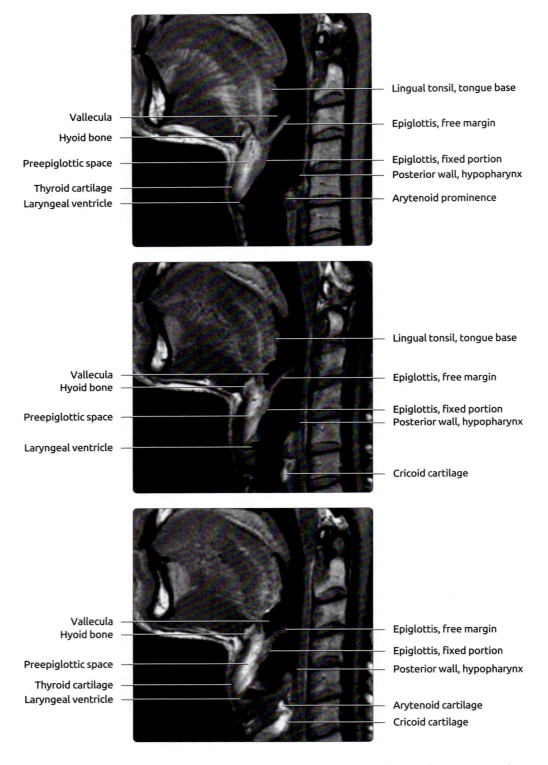

(Top) First of 3 sagittal T1 MR images from medial to lateral of the larynx and hypopharynx shows midline structures. The preepiglottic space is T1 hyperintense as it is primarily fat-filled. The free margin (suprahyoid) and fixed portion (infrahyoid) of the epiglottis is well visualized, making sagittal imaging useful for evaluation of epiglottic lesions. (Middle) Image just lateral to the midline shows the laryngeal ventricle, which is important as it is the air space that separates false vocal cords above from true vocal cords below. Knowing if a tumor crosses the laryngeal ventricle is vital for surgical planning. (Bottom) Paramedial image through the cricoarytenoid joint shows arytenoid cartilage sitting on top of posterior cricoid cartilage. Traumatic dislocation of arytenoid cartilage may mimic vocal cord paralysis clinically and on imaging. Posterior arytenoid dislocation may occur during withdrawal of the endotracheal tube with an incompletely deflated cuff, whereas the mechanism of anterior dislocation is the arytenoid tip being caught on the distal opening of the tube lumen during intubation.

Larynx

CLINICAL CORRELATES

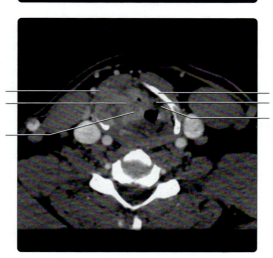

(Top) Axial CT through the vocal cords in a case of left vocal cord paralysis shows that left arytenoid cartilage is rotated medially and slightly inferior to normal. The laryngeal ventricle on the left is also widened slightly and comes into view anteriorly. The right vocal cord is in normal position during quiet respiration and its soft tissue is primarily of thyroarytenoid muscle (including the vocalis muscle). Note very little, if any, paraglottic space fat at the true cord level. Superior cricoid cartilage supports the posterior midline wall of the glottis that is called the posterior commissure. (Middle) Axial CECT through the false cord shows invasive neoplasm on the left. Enhancing tumor encroaches upon the airway medially and extends into left paraglottic space fat. Note the superior tip of arytenoid cartilage and fat in the right paraglottic space. Tumor involved the false and true cords (not shown), making it a "transglottic" tumor. (Bottom) Large invasive supraglottic carcinoma on the right extends from mucosa medially, through paraglottic fat, destroys thyroid cartilage lamina, and extends into extralaryngeal soft tissues.

Larynx

TRANSVERSE ULTRASOUND

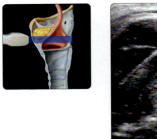
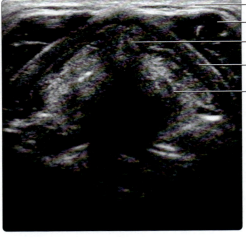

- Subcutaneous tissue
- Strap muscles
- Preepiglottic space
- Thyroid lamina
- Paraglottic space

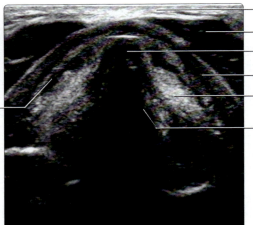

Intrinsic muscles of larynx at supraglottic level

- Subcutaneous tissue
- Strap muscles
- Preepiglottic space
- Thyroid lamina
- Paraglottic space
- False vocal cord

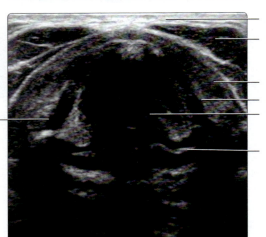

Intrinsic muscles of larynx at glottic larynx level

- Subcutaneous tissue
- Strap muscles
- Thyroid cartilage
- Paraglottic space
- True vocal cord
- Cricoarytenoid joint

(Top) Axial grayscale ultrasound of the larynx at the supraglottic larynx level shows that the thyroid laminae are the largest cartilaginous structures of the larynx and appear as thin, hypoechoic bands that join at the midline anteriorly. The hyperechoic, fat-filled paraglottic and preepiglottic spaces are important surgical landmarks for the staging of laryngeal carcinoma. (Middle) Transverse grayscale ultrasound of the larynx at the level of the false vocal cords shows abundant fat in the paraglottic spaces. The echo-poor intrinsic muscles of the larynx are embedded within the echogenic paraglottic fat. (Bottom) Transverse grayscale ultrasound of the larynx at the level of the true vocal cords shows that the arytenoid cartilage appears as echogenic foci posteriorly with attachments to the true vocal cords, which have distinct echo-poor appearances.

Larynx

LONGITUDINAL ULTRASOUND

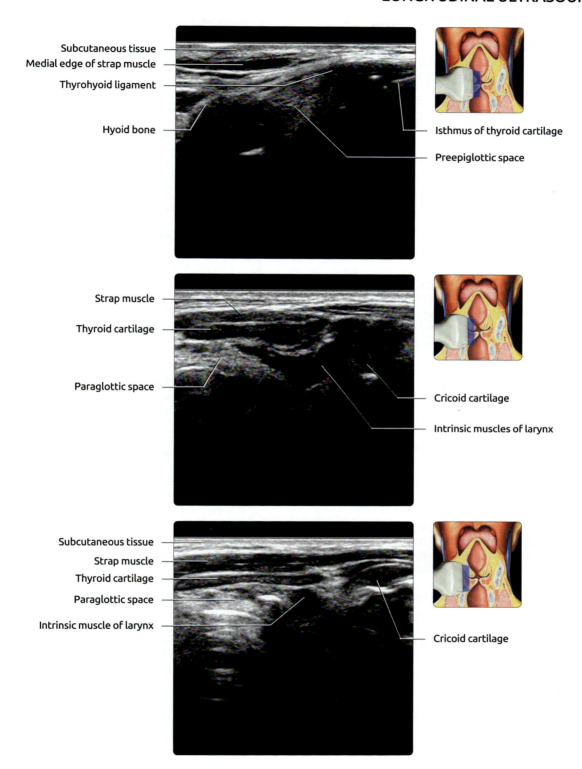

(Top) Midline sagittal longitudinal grayscale ultrasound of the supraglottic larynx shows the fat-filled, echogenic, preepiglottic space underneath the thyrohyoid membrane. Tumor spread at this location is readily assessed by ultrasound. (Middle) Parasagittal longitudinal grayscale ultrasound of the larynx shows sonolucent thyroid and cricoid cartilages with no laryngeal calcification/ossification in a young adult. The paraglottic space is fat-filled and appears echogenic. The intrinsic muscles of the larynx are embedded within the paraglottic space and are hypoechoic on ultrasound. (Bottom) Parasagittal longitudinal grayscale ultrasound shows the larynx further lateral. Gas within the laryngeal lumen appears highly echogenic, casting posterior acoustic shadowing.

Hypopharynx

TERMINOLOGY

Abbreviations

- Hypopharynx (HP)

Definitions

- Caudal continuation of pharyngeal mucosal space, between oropharynx and esophagus

IMAGING ANATOMY

Extent

- From inferior margin of oropharynx to esophagus at esophageal verge

Anatomy Relationships

- HP is inferior continuation of oropharynx
- HP begins at level of pharyngoepiglottic folds, at ~ horizontal level of hyoid bone
- HP merges with esophagus below at esophageal verge
- Esophageal verge is best defined by cricopharyngeus muscle that encircles junction, but this muscle cannot be identified easily on cross-sectional imaging
- Cricopharyngeus muscle is located at approximate level of inferior margin of cricoid cartilage
- Relative to cervical vertebrae, HP extends from ~ C3 level to C6 level
- HP is posterior to larynx, medial to carotid spaces bilaterally, and ventral to retropharyngeal space

Internal Contents

- **HP** consists of 3 regions starting with letter P
- **Pyriform sinuses (PS)**
  - Anterolateral recesses of HP
  - Each PS has shape of inverted pyramid with base of pyramid positioned superiorly at level of pharyngoepiglottic fold and inferior tip (**PS apex**) positioned at level of true cord
  - PS bounded anteromedially by **aryepiglottic (AE) fold**; AE fold separates PS from laryngeal airway
  - Bounded laterally by lateral pharyngeal wall and inner surface of thyrohyoid membrane (above) and thyroid cartilage (below)
  - Posterior boundary is posterior wall of HP
  - Majority of hypopharyngeal squamous cell carcinomas (SCCas) (2/3) originate in PS
  - During swallowing, nasopharynx and laryngeal vestibule are sealed and food is usually deviated laterally away from larynx into PS by epiglottis and AE folds
- **Posterior wall**
  - Inferior continuation of posterior oropharyngeal wall, from approximate level of hyoid bone to inferior tip of cricoid cartilage
  - Muscular layer formed by middle and inferior constrictor muscles
    - On CT and MR, bulk of soft tissue we identify as posterior wall of HP represents constrictor muscle layer
  - Posterior wall separated from **perivertebral space** by **retropharyngeal space**
- **Postcricoid region**
  - Anterior wall of lower HP

- Extends from cricoarytenoid joints to esophageal verge at ~ level of lower edge of cricoid
  - Mucosa of postcricoid region faces posteriorly and is normally directly apposed to mucosa of posterior wall during routine cross-sectional imaging
- **Layers**: In general, pharynx is complex mucosal and muscular tube consisting of 5 principal layers; these layers, or their derivations, are present in HP
  - **Mucosa**: Stratified squamous epithelium that lines lumen
  - **Submucosa**: Loose stroma that can contain fat and can be identified on cross-sectional imaging as thin fat plane
  - Fibrous layer that represents limited inferior continuation of **pharyngobasilar fascia** (pharyngeal aponeurosis)
  - **Muscular layer** consisting of middle and inferior constrictors
  - Outer fascial layer originating from **buccopharyngeal fascia**
    - Pharyngeal plexuses of veins and nerves lies between muscular coat (mainly middle constrictor) and buccopharyngeal fascia
- **Muscles and relationships**
  - Middle constrictor muscles arise bilaterally from hyoid bone and insert into midline tendinous raphe posteriorly
  - Inferior constrictors arise bilaterally from ventral thyroid and cricoid cartilages and insert into midline raphe
  - Inferior constrictor muscle has 2 parts; thyropharyngeus with oblique fibers and cricopharyngeus with transverse fibers continuous with circular fibers of esophagus; between these 2 is potential gap, Killian dehiscence
  - Stylopharyngeus muscle and glossopharyngeal nerve pass through gap between superior and middle constrictors
  - Internal laryngeal nerve and superior laryngeal vessels pierce thyrohyoid membrane in gap between middle and inferior constrictors and run through piriform sinus to reach larynx
  - Recurrent laryngeal nerve and inferior laryngeal vessels pass through gap between inferior constrictor and esophagus
- **Nerve supply**
  - Pharyngeal plexus (CNIX-X branches and sympathetic fibers of superior cervical ganglion)
  - Motor fibers in plexus from pharyngeal branch of vagus carrying cranial accessory nerve fibers and supply all pharyngeal and soft palate muscles except stylopharyngeus (by CNIX) and tensor veli palatini (by CNV)
  - Sensory fibers in plexus are from glossopharyngeal nerve and supply all 3 parts of pharynx
- **Blood supply**: HP by branches of external carotid (ascending pharyngeal) and subclavian (inferior thyroid) arteries; venous plexus at posterolateral aspect of pharynx receives blood from pharynx, soft palate, and prevertebral region and drain to internal jugular vein

ANATOMY IMAGING ISSUES

Imaging Recommendations

- CECT is best overall modality for evaluating soft tissue masses of HP

Hypopharynx

- MR is useful in problem solving, especially evaluation of laryngeal cartilage and prevertebral soft tissue invasion by HP tumor
- CT/PET study can be useful especially in identifying occult PS primary tumor

Imaging Sweet Spots

- **PS tumor evaluation**
  - Small tumor in PS can be occult and represent clinical and radiologic blind spot, could be primary etiology in some cases of metastatic SCCa of unknown primary
  - Tumors of PS can extend in multiple directions given anatomic location
    - Anterior: Larynx
    - Lateral: Thyrohyoid membrane, thyroid cartilage
    - Posterior: Prevertebral invasion
    - Inferior: Postcricoid subsite of HP and to esophagus
    - Superior: Oropharynx extension common
  - Majority hypopharyngeal SCCas (2/3) originate in PS
- **Posterior wall tumor evaluation**
  - Given paucity of fat in retropharyngeal space in lower neck, it may be difficult to identify tissue plane between posterior wall of HP and prevertebral musculature
  - Mucosal SCCa involving posterior wall can invade prevertebral soft tissues and prevent complete surgical resection
  - Accuracy for CT and MR in predicting prevertebral invasion and fixation is limited
  - However, identification of intact retropharyngeal fat plane on MR between tumor of posterior wall and prevertebral space provides reasonably good negative predictor for tumor invasion
- **Postcricoid tumor evaluation**
  - With conventional cross-sectional imaging, HP is typically nondistended, and postcricoid mucosa is normally directly apposed to mucosa of posterior wall
  - Distinguishing postcricoid soft tissue components can be difficult on CT or MR but can be differentiated with optimal mucosal enhancement and presence of visible intramural fat planes
  - Soft tissue posterior to cricoid cartilage region consists of posterior cricoarytenoid muscles, postcricoid region mucosal space, posterior wall mucosal space, and longus colli muscles
  - **AP dimension of postcricoid soft tissue should be < 1 cm normally**
  - Increased soft tissue width in this region should raise concern for neoplasm
- **Referred otalgia**
  - Referred otalgia (ear pain) occurs in patients with pathology outside temporal bone, due to complex interconnections of neural pathways in temporal bone and neck
  - Sensory nerves from superior laryngeal nerve and pharyngeal plexus can ultimately communicate with Arnold nerve (sensory to ear) at level of jugular foramen
  - Hypopharyngeal carcinoma can be source of referred otalgia
  - When no source of otalgia is found in temporal bone, further clinical and radiologic evaluation with CECT or CT/PET is recommended to exclude another source of referred pain in head and neck, including HP

- **Esophagopharyngeal diverticulum (Zenker)**
  - Killian dehiscence (or Killian triangle) is triangular area of muscular weakness formed between oblique (thyropharyngeus) and transverse orientated muscle fibers (cricopharyngeus muscle) of inferior pharyngeal constrictor muscle
  - Esophagopharyngeal diverticulum is formed by outpouching of Killian dehiscence as result of neuromuscular incoordination between thyropharyngeus and cricopharyngeus parts of inferior constrictor
  - If sphincteric cricopharyngeus (supplied by recurrent laryngeal nerve) fails to relax when propulsive thyropharyngeus (supplied by pharyngeal plexus) contracts, then food bolus is pushed backward and tends to form diverticulum
  - Barium esophagram is best imaging tool
    - Confirms diagnosis and shows diverticular neck
    - Evaluates associated reflux and hiatal hernia

EMBRYOLOGY

Embryologic Events

- Pharynx develops from most cranial aspect of foregut, buccopharyngeal anlage
- Endodermal pouches are formed in relation to lateral wall of foregut here, and most of them lose contact with pharyngeal wall
- Floor of foregut gives rise to midline tracheobronchial diverticulum from which entire respiratory system develops later
- Site of midline respiratory diverticulum becomes inlet of larynx
- Pharynx subdivides into nasopharynx, oropharynx, and HP with establishment of palate and mouth
- Pharyngeal wall muscles develop from 3rd and subsequent pharyngeal arches

Hypopharynx

GRAPHICS

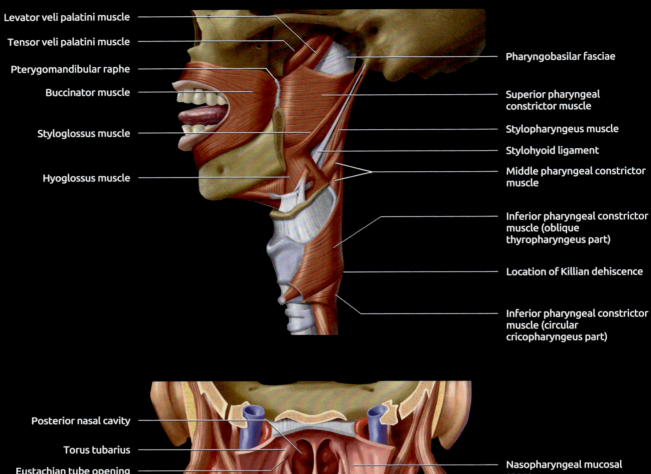

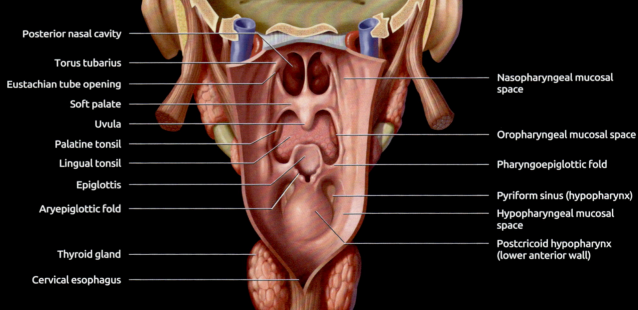

(Top) Lateral graphic shows major muscles of pharyngeal mucosal space (PMS). Note superior (naso/oropharynx), middle, & inferior pharyngeal constrictor (hypopharynx) muscles are in posterior wall of PMS from nasopharynx through oropharynx to hypopharynx. Note inferior constrictor muscle has 2 parts: Thyropharyngeus with oblique fibers & cricopharyngeus with transverse fibers continuous with circular fibers of esophagus; between these 2 is a potential gap called the Killian dehiscence. The pharyngobasilar fascia (at nasopharyngeal level) attaches the superior pharyngeal constrictor to the skull base. The distal end of the levator veli palatini muscle is on the airway side of the middle layer of deep cervical fascia, making it a part of the PMS. (Bottom) Graphic of PMS/surface seen from behind shows this space can be divided into nasopharyngeal, oropharyngeal, & hypopharyngeal areas. The lymphatic ring of PMS contains nasopharyngeal adenoids, oropharyngeal palatine, & lingual tonsils. Anterior wall of hypopharynx is formed by the inlet of larynx above & the posterior surfaces of cricoid & arytenoid cartilages below.

Hypopharynx

GRAPHICS

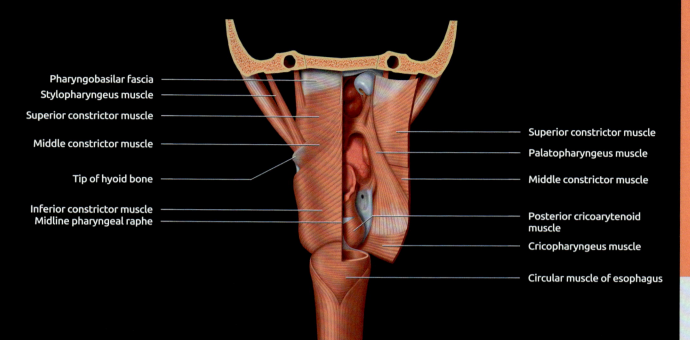

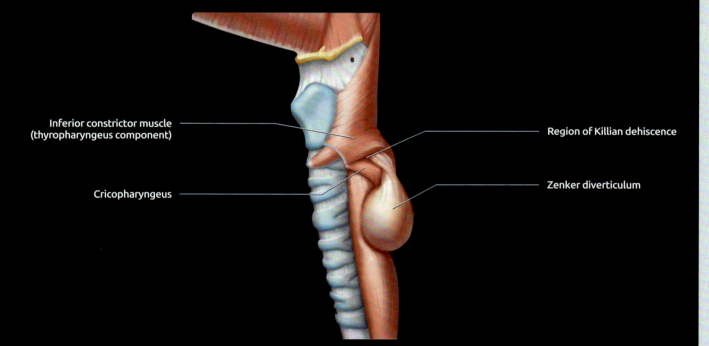

(Top) Posterior view of the pharynx demonstrates the overlapping appearance of the pharyngeal musculature. The thickened fibrous attachment at the skull base is the pharyngobasilar fascia. The constrictor muscles arise from bone and cartilage and attach posteriorly along the midline pharyngeal raphe. (Bottom) Graphic depicts a Zenker diverticulum with herniation at the Killian dehiscence between the thyropharyngeal and cricopharyngeal fibers of the inferior constrictor muscle.

Hypopharynx

GRAPHICS

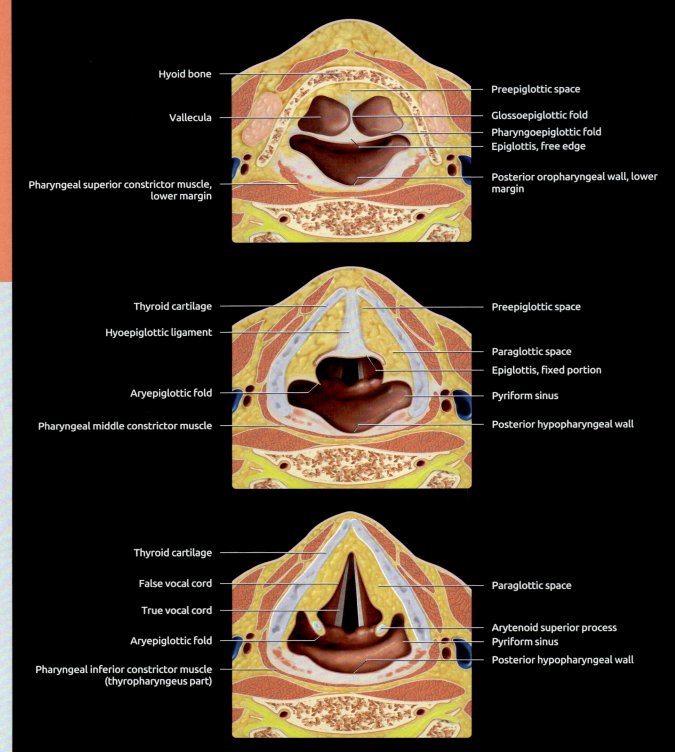

(Top) First of 6 axial graphics of larynx & hypopharynx from superior to inferior shows roof of hypopharynx/lower margin of oropharynx junction at hyoid bone level & high supraglottic structures. Free edge of epiglottis is attached to hyoid bone via hyoepiglottic ligament, covered by a glossoepiglottic fold, a ridge of mucous membrane. Hypopharynx (laryngopharynx) extends from level of glossoepiglottic & pharyngoepiglottic folds superiorly (inferior margin of vallecula, at hyoid bone level) to cricoid cartilage (cricopharyngeus muscle) inferiorly. (Middle) Graphic at midsupraglottic shows hyoepiglottic ligament dividing lower preepiglottic space. Fascia does not separate preepiglottic space from paraglottic space. These 2 endolaryngeal spaces are submucosal locations where tumors hide from clinical detection. Aryepiglottic fold represents junction between larynx & hypopharynx. Middle constrictor muscle is now seen deep to upper posterior hypopharyngeal wall. Middle constrictor originates from stylohyoid ligament & greater & lesser horns of hyoid bone. (Bottom) Graphic at low supraglottic shows false vocal cords. Inferior constrictor muscle (upper thyropharyngeus part) is seen in deep midposterior hypopharyngeal wall.

Hypopharynx

GRAPHICS

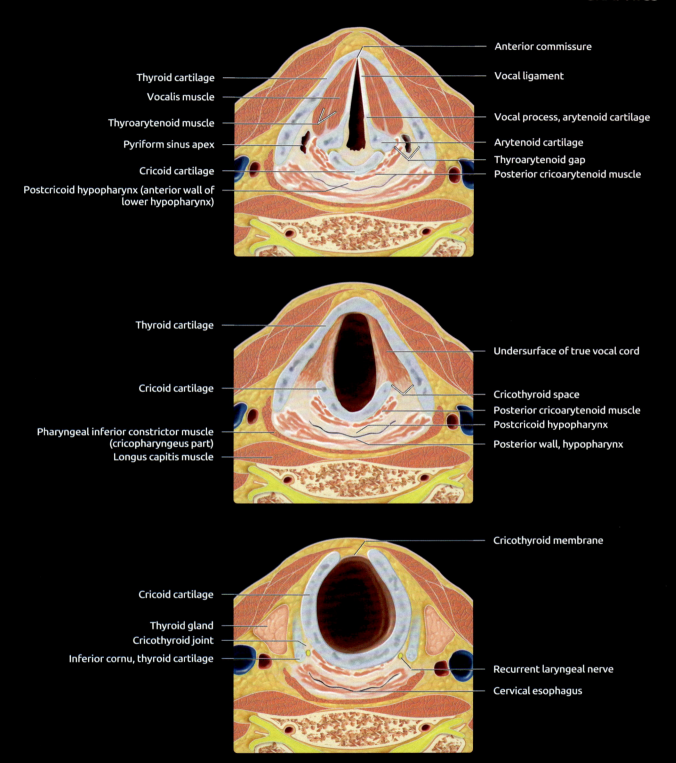

(Top) Graphic at glottic, true vocal cord level shows thyroarytenoid muscle; this makes up bulk of true vocal cord. Medial fibers of thyroarytenoid muscle are known as the vocalis muscle. Pyriform sinus apex (hypopharynx) is seen at glottic level. Thyroarytenoid gap is location where tumors may spread between larynx & hypopharynx. Postcricoid region is anterior wall of lower hypopharynx. (Middle) Graphic at undersurface level of true vocal cord shows posterior lamina of cricoid cartilage. Postcricoid hypopharynx represents anterior wall of lower hypopharynx & extends from cricoarytenoid joints to lower edge of cricoid cartilage at cricopharyngeus muscle. Posterior wall of lower hypopharynx at this level is formed by inferior circular cricopharyngeus part of inferior constrictor muscle. Unlike other pharyngeal constrictors, fibers in this lower part of inferior constrictor muscle bypasses pharyngeal raphe & inserts itself into circular fibers of esophagus to serve as a superior esophageal sphincter. (Bottom) Subglottic level graphic shows upper cervical esophagus. Note cricothyroid joint immediately adjacent to recurrent laryngeal nerve, located in tracheoesophageal groove.

Hypopharynx

AXIAL CECT

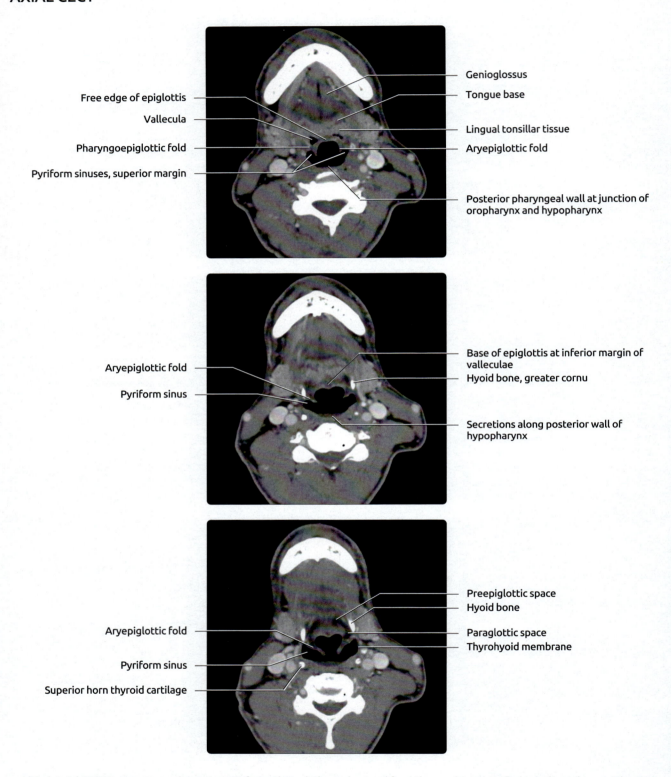

(Top) Axial CECT images proceed superior to inferior through the neck extend from the oropharynx to the lower hypopharynx. The 1st axial image is at the level of the oropharynx. The tongue base and free edge of the epiglottis are identified. The upper aspects of the aryepiglottic folds begin to form as curvilinear folds along the lateral margins of the epiglottis. (Middle) Axial image at the floor of the valleculae demonstrate the base of the epiglottis is indistinguishable from the tongue base. The hyoid bone is becoming visible bilaterally. (Bottom) The preepiglottic and paraglottic spaces are continuous with no intervening fascia. This allows tumors to spread submucosally in these locations. Aryepiglottic fold, part of larynx, represents transition between the larynx and hypopharynx. Posterolateral wall of the aryepiglottic fold is the anteromedial margin of the pyriform sinus. The lateral wall of the the pyriform sinus is just medial to the thyrohyoid membrane. Tumors can extend laterally from the pyriform sinus through the thyrohyoid membrane into lateral neck.

Hypopharynx

AXIAL CECT

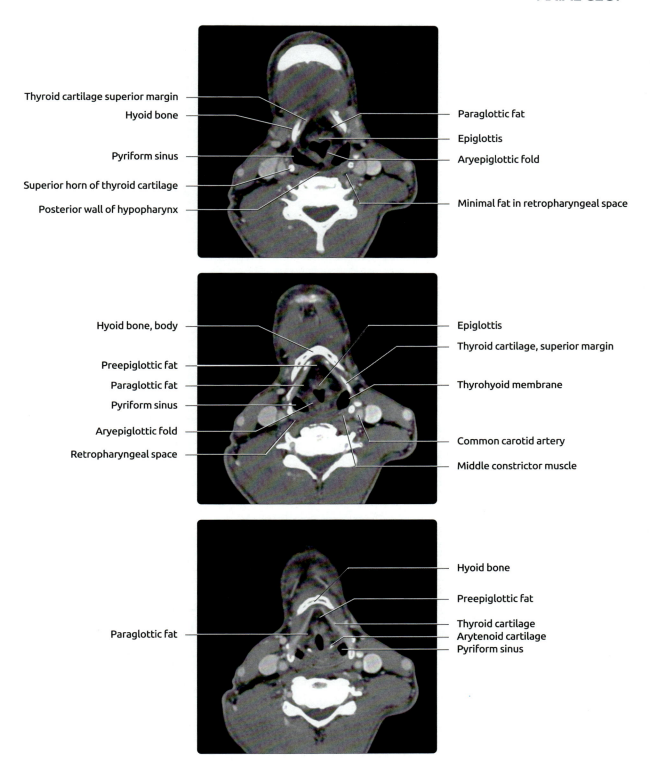

(Top) The hypodensity of the preepiglottic and paraglottic space fat is easily identified. The aryepiglottic folds continue to form the funnel-shaped vestibule to the larynx and further define the larynx from the hypopharynx. (Middle) Axial CECT image at body of hyoid bone level shows epiglottis beginning to narrow inferiorly. (Bottom) Axial CECT image through the larynx/hypopharynx at the level of the upper arytenoid cartilage is shown. The pyriform sinus extends inferiorly. Notice the relationship of the pyriform sinus with the posterior margin of the paraglottic fat and the medial margin of the thyroid cartilage. Tumor in the pyriform sinus can invade the paraglottic space and invade thyroid cartilage readily.

Hypopharynx

AXIAL CECT

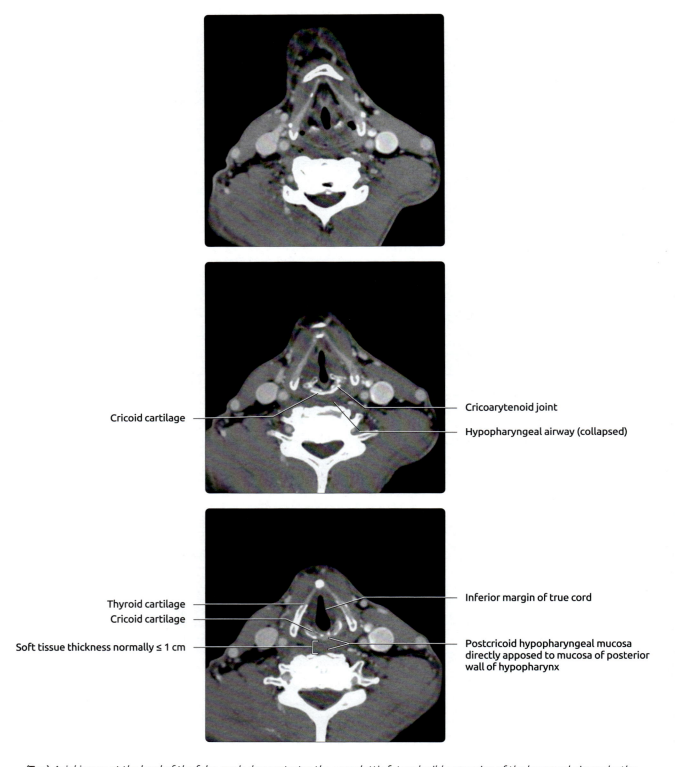

(Top) Axial image at the level of the false cords demonstrates the paraglottic fat and mild narrowing of the laryngeal airway by the false cords. (Middle) Axial CECT at the level of the true cords is shown. The vocalis muscle represents the bulk of soft tissue of the true vocal cord. At this level, the pyriform sinuses are not discernible anymore, and the entire hypopharynx is nondistended (collapsed), making it difficult to identify the individual mucosal layers of the postcricoid hypopharynx and the mucosa or the posterior wall. (Bottom) Axial image at the level of the upper cricoid cartilage is shown. From anterior to posterior, the soft tissue posterior to the cricoid cartilage includes the posterior cricoarytenoid muscles, postcricoid mucosa, posterior wall mucosa, including the middle/inferior constrictor muscles, and longus colli muscles of the prevertebral space. The soft tissue between the anterior vertebral body margin and the cricoid cartilage should normally measure ≤ 1 cm in AP thickness.

Hypopharynx

AXIAL CECT

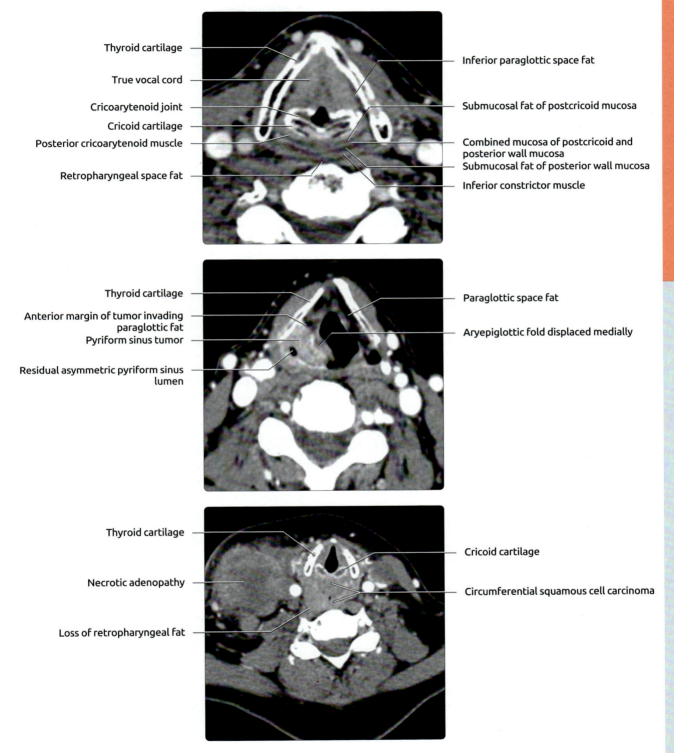

(Top) Axial CECT through normal hypopharynx/larynx at level of cricoarytenoid joints demonstrates laminated appearance of multiple tissue layers dorsal to cricoid cartilage. Individual intramural fat planes help distinguish normal components of hypopharynx at this level in relationship to larynx & retropharynx. In routine cross-sectional imaging, hypopharyngeal lumen at this level is nondistended & mucosa of postcricoid mucosa is directly apposed to mucosa of posterior wall. (Middle) Axial CECT through false cords & hypopharynx level demonstrates enhancing lesion of patient's right pyriform sinus, primarily involving anterior & medial walls. Lesion pushes anteriorly into posterior margin of ipsilateral paraglottic space fat & contacts thyroid cartilage laterally. (Bottom) Axial CECT in patient with circumferential hypopharyngeal tumor & bulky adenopathy on right is shown. Axial image through cricoid cartilage level demonstrates circumferential soft tissue thickening posterior to cricoid cartilage, obliterating normal tissue planes, & increasing width between posterior cricoid margin & anterior margin of vertebral body. There is loss of retropharyngeal fat plane on patient's right, raising concern for prevertebral invasion. However, CT cannot reliably predict presence of prevertebral invasion.

Thyroid and Parathyroid Anatomy

TERMINOLOGY

Abbreviations
- Parathyroid gland (PTG)

Definitions
- Thyroid gland: Shield-shaped endocrine organ in lower neck that produces thyroid hormones (T3 and T4) that are involved in many functions, including metabolism (cardiac rate and output) and protein synthesis (growth); also produces calcitonin
- PTGs: Small glands in visceral space of neck, intimately associated with posterior margin of thyroid gland, that produce parathormone (PTH), which is hormone that regulates calcium concentration in serum and interstitial fluids

THYROID

Imaging Anatomy
- **Overview**
  - Thyroid is shield-shaped or U-shaped gland in anterior neck
  - 2 elongated lateral lobes with superior and inferior poles connected by median isthmus
- **Anatomy relationships**
  - Thyroid gland lies anterior and lateral to trachea in visceral space of infrahyoid neck, at C5-T1 level
  - Posteromedially is tracheoesophageal groove (paratracheal nodes, recurrent laryngeal nerve, PTGs)
  - Posterolaterally are carotid spaces
  - Anteriorly are infrahyoid strap muscles
  - Anterolaterally are sternocleidomastoid muscles
  - PTGs are closely applied to deep surface of the thyroid
- **Internal contents**
  - **Thyroid gland** (average: 25 grams)
  - **Right and left lobes** ~ 5.0 x 2.5 x 2.5 cm each, larger in females, commonly asymmetric
    - Each lobe has apex, base and lateral, medial and posterior surfaces; anterior and posterior borders
    - Apex is limited superiorly by sternothyroid strap muscle attachment to oblique line of thyroid cartilage medial to it
  - Lateral lobes joined by midline **isthmus**, at 2nd-4th tracheal ring level
  - Pyramidal lobe present in 40% of cases; ascends in midline from isthmus or rarely from one of lobes
    - Levator glandulae thyroidea: Fibromuscular band from hyoid body to isthmus or pyramidal lobe
  - Zuckerkandl tubercle: Protuberance from posterior aspect of gland to tracheoesophageal groove
    - Surgeons use as landmark for superior PTG and recurrent laryngeal nerve
    - Seen in 70% patients; R > L, may be bilateral
- **Histology**
  - Thyroid follicles consist of rim of cells surrounding core of colloid that consists primarily of thyroid hormone precursor proteins (thyroglobulin), iodinated glycoprotein
  - Follicular cells: Cuboid to columnar cells aligned along margins of follicle; secrete thyroid hormones (T3 and T4) in response to thyroid stimulating hormone
  - Parafollicular cells are scattered between follicles and secrete calcitonin
- **Arterial supply to thyroid**
  - Superior thyroid arteries
    - Superior thyroid artery is 1st anterior branch of external carotid artery
    - Proximal course closely associated with external (superior) laryngeal nerve
    - Anterior branch descends on anterior border of thyroid lobe, sending branch deep into gland before curving along upper border of isthmus where it anastomoses with contralateral anterior branch
    - Posterior branch descends on posterior border of thyroid lobe and anastomose with ascending branch of inferior thyroid artery and supply PTG
    - Anastomosis good guide to PTG, usually lie near it
  - Inferior thyroid arteries
    - Arises from thyrocervical trunk, branch of subclavian artery
    - Ascends vertically, then curves medially to enter tracheoesophageal groove in plane posterior to carotid space
    - Most of its branches penetrate posterior aspect of thyroid lobe; one ascending branch anastomose with superior thyroid artery
    - Terminal part near thyroid closely associated with recurrent laryngeal nerve, while proximal part is away from nerve
    - Inferior thyroid artery ligated away from gland during thyroidectomy to protect recurrent laryngeal nerve; whereas superior thyroid artery ligated close to gland to protect external laryngeal nerve
  - Thyroidea ima occasionally present (3%)
    - Single vessel originating from aortic arch or innominate artery
    - Enters thyroid gland at inferior border of isthmus
- **Venous drainage from thyroid**
  - 3 pairs of veins arise from venous plexus on surface of thyroid gland
  - Superior and middle thyroid veins drain into internal jugular vein
  - Inferior thyroid veins end in left brachiocephalic vein
- **Lymphatic drainage**
  - Lymphatic drainage is extensive and multidirectional
  - Drainage initially into periglandular nodes **(level VI)**
    - Prelaryngeal (Delphian), pretracheal, and paratracheal nodes
    - Regional drainage to internal jugular chain (levels II-IV) and spinal accessory chain (level V)
- **Fascia**
  - **Middle layer of deep cervical fascia** surrounds visceral space and ensheaths thyroid and PTG
  - Thyroid gland **inner true capsule** formed by peripheral condensed connective tissue of gland
    - Dense capillary plexus deep to true capsule, so thyroid is removed along with true capsule
  - **Outer false capsule** from pretracheal layer of deep cervical fascia, thick medially and forms suspensory ligament of Berry connecting thyroid lobe to cricoid cartilage

Thyroid and Parathyroid Anatomy

Embryology: Thyroid

- **Embryologic events**
  - Thyroid is 1st endocrine gland to develop (24th gestational day)
  - Originates from 1st and 2nd pharyngeal pouches (medial anlage)
  - Originates as proliferation of endodermal cells on median surface of developing pharyngeal floor, called **foramen cecum**
  - Bilobed thyroid gland descends anterior to pharyngeal gut along **thyroglossal duct**
    - Tubular duct later solidifies and ultimately obliterated (gestational weeks 7-10)
  - Inferior descent of thyroid gland carries it anterior to hyoid bone and laryngeal cartilages, ultimately to pretracheal location
- **Practical implications**
  - **Thyroglossal duct cyst** results from failure of involution of portion of thyroglossal duct
    - Occurs anywhere along course of thyroglossal duct from foramen cecum at tongue base to just anterior to thyroid lobes
    - Most occur in midline at/near hyoid bone
    - When infrahyoid, most commonly paramedian, dorsal to lateral thyroid lobe
    - Often have thyroid tissue in wall
  - **Thyroid tissue remnants** from sequestration of thyroid tissue along thyroglossal duct
    - Seen along course of thyroglossal duct
    - Pyramidal lobe of thyroid is midline normal variant remnant
    - Ectopic thyroid occurs from incomplete descent of thyroid
      - □ Seen anywhere from tongue base to superior mediastinum
      - □ Most common location: Deep to foramen cecum in tongue base = **lingual thyroid**

Imaging Approaches

- Ultrasound best 1st-line approach
- CT and MR can evaluate thyroid lesion, its relationship to other structures and adenopathy
- If thyroid neoplasia is suspected, iodinated contrast should not be given; will delay therapeutic iodine I-131 treatment

PARATHYROID

Imaging Anatomy

- **Anatomy relationships**
  - PTG closely applied to posterior surface of thyroid lobes within visceral space
  - Extracapsular (outside thyroid capsule) in most cases, vicinity of tracheoesophageal groove
- **Histology**
  - Composed of chief cells & oxyphil cells embedded within fibrous capsule and mixed with adipose tissue
  - **Chief cells** manufacture PTH
    - PTH regulates concentration of calcium in interstitial fluids
    - Serum calcium levels regulate secretion of PTH
- **Internal contents**

- Small lentiform glands posterior to thyroid glands in visceral space
- ~ 6 mm length, 3-4 mm transverse, and 1-2 mm in anteroposterior diameter
- **Normal number = 4**, 2 superior and 2 inferior
  - May be as many as 12 total PTGs
- **Superior PTG normal locations**
  - Lie on posterior border of middle 1/3 of thyroid 75% of time
  - 25% found behind upper or lower 1/3 of thyroid
  - 7% found below inferior thyroidal artery
  - Rarely found behind pharynx or esophagus
- **Inferior PTG normal locations**
  - Inferior glands lie lateral to lower pole of thyroid gland (50%)
  - 15% lie within 1 cm of inferior thyroid poles
  - 35% position is variable, residing anywhere from angle of mandible to lower anterior mediastinum
  - Intrathyroidal PTG are rare
- **Arterial supply**
  - Superior PTG supplied by superior thyroid artery
  - Inferior PTG supplied by **inferior thyroid artery**
- **Fascia**: Visceral space and its contents, including PTGs, are surrounded by **middle layer of deep cervical fascia**

Embryology

- **Superior PTG** develop from 4th branchial pouch along with primordium of **thyroid gland**
  - < 2% of superior PTG are **ectopic**
- **Inferior PTG** develop from 3rd branchial pouch along with anlage of **thymus**
  - Descend variable distance with thymic anlage in thymopharyngeal duct tract
  - May descend into anterior mediastinum as far as pericardium
- Abnormal PTG descent may cause inferior PTG to occupy "ectopic" sites
  - May be of critical importance when searching for parathyroid adenoma
  - In cases where surgical exploration for primary thyroid adenoma (PTA) is done without imaging, no PTA may be found if PTG is ectopic
  - **Most frequent ectopic site** is just **below inferior thyroid pole**
  - Less commonly, PTG may migrate into superior mediastinum with thymus creating ectopic mediastinal PTA
  - Rarely, PTG does not descend significantly, which creates ectopic in upper cervical neck PTA
  - Rarest reported locations include retropharyngeal, retroesophageal, and posterior mediastinal PTA

Imaging Approaches

- Primary hyperparathyroidism with hypercalcemia is most commonly secondary to **PTA**
- Imaging of PTG is primarily to find PTA
- US is best 1st examination for localizing most PTA
- Tc-99m sestamibi concentrates in PTA and is useful for locating ectopic PTA
- CT, CTA, and MR useful in challenging cases, especially ectopic cases

Thyroid and Parathyroid Anatomy

GRAPHICS

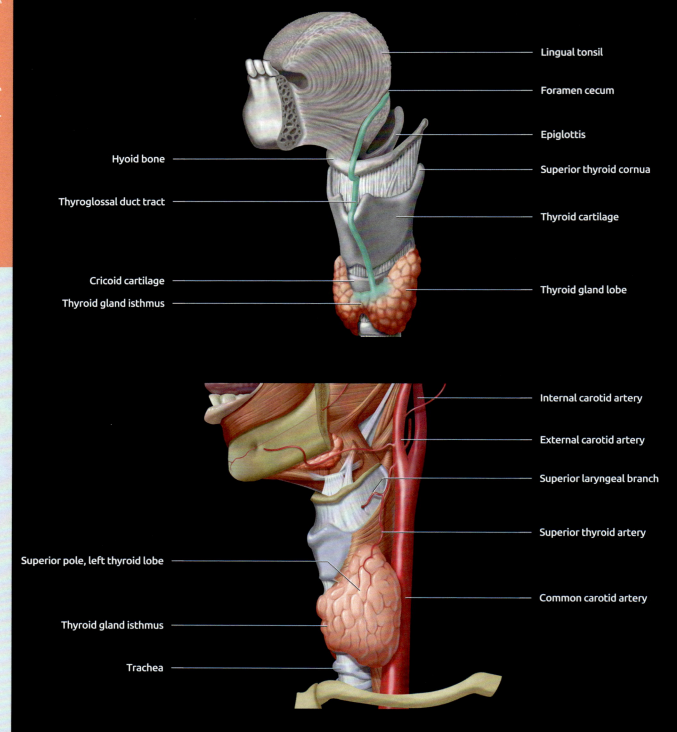

(Top) Sagittal oblique graphic displays thyroglossal duct tract as it traverses cervical neck from its origin at foramen cecum to its termination in anterior & lateral visceral space of infrahyoid neck. The thyroid is 1st endocrine gland in the body to develop. At ~ day 24 of gestation, it develops from a median endodermal thyroid diverticulum, the medial anlage, arising from paramedian aspect of 1st & 2nd branchial pouches (foramen cecum of tongue area). The lower end of diverticulum enlarges to form gland & the rest remains narrow (called thyroglossal duct). It descends through tongue base, floor of mouth, around & in front of hyoid bone, & through an area of infrahyoid strap muscles to a final position in thyroid bed of visceral space. Thyroglossal duct begins to involute by 7-10 weeks of gestation; its lower end often persists as pyramidal lobe. Lateral thyroid lobes may form from 4th & 6th branchial pouches (lateral anlagen). Fetal thyroid becomes functional during 3rd month of gestation. (Bottom) Oblique graphic of neck shows superior thyroid artery as 1st branch of external carotid artery. Its proximal course is closely associated with superior laryngeal nerve.

Thyroid and Parathyroid Anatomy

GRAPHICS

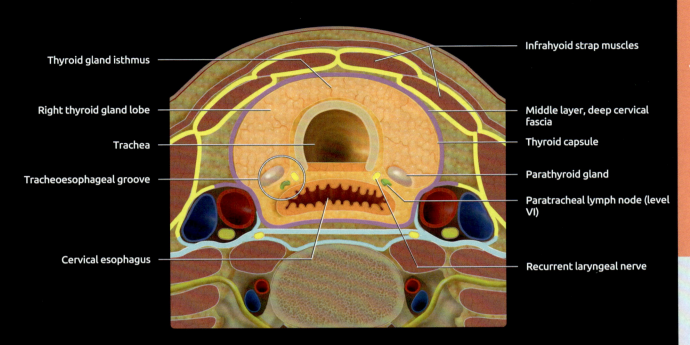

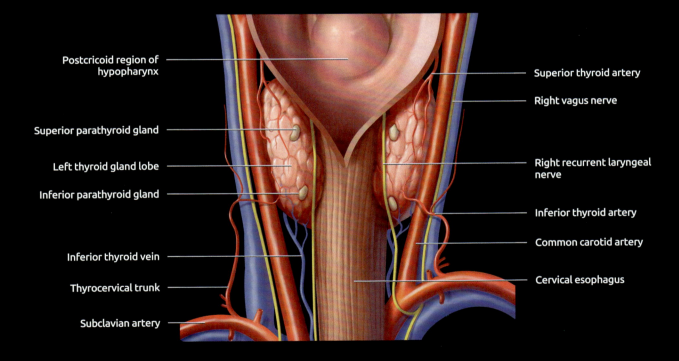

(**Top**) *Axial graphic at the thyroid level depicts the thyroid lobes and isthmus in the anterior visceral space wrapping around the trachea. Notice that there are 3 key structures found in the area of the tracheoesophageal groove: The recurrent laryngeal nerve, paratracheal lymph node chain, and parathyroid gland (PTG). The PTGs may be inside or outside of the thyroid capsule.* (**Bottom**) *Coronal graphic shows the thyroid and PTGs from behind. The drawing depicts the typical anatomic relationships of the paired superior and inferior PTGs closely applied to the posterior lobes of the thyroid gland. Note the arterial supply to superior and inferior thyroid lobes and the superior and inferior thyroid arteries, respectively.*

Thyroid and Parathyroid Anatomy

AXIAL CECT

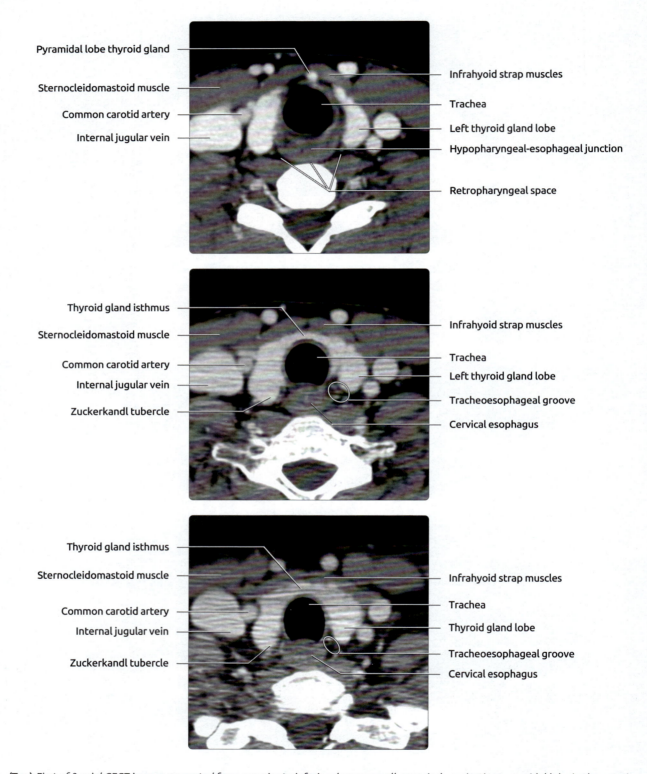

(Top) First of 3 axial CECT images presented from superior to inferior shows a small, superiorly projecting pyramidal lobe in the anterior midline just beneath the infrahyoid strap muscles. Notice the retropharyngeal space fat stripe extends posterior to the thyroid lobes and esophagus. **(Middle)** In this image, the thyroid lobes are found along the lateral margin of the trachea. A more prominent right posterior thyroid protuberance is described as the Zuckerkandl tubercle, which is a landmark for surgeons for the location of the recurrent laryngeal nerve and superior PTG. Nodularity in this gland portion can mimic a tracheoesophageal groove node or enlarged PTG. **(Bottom)** The thyroid gland isthmus is prominent on this image. The tracheoesophageal groove has been circled. Remember that the recurrent laryngeal nerve, paratracheal nodes, and PTGs can all be normally found in this location. None of these structures are typically visible on routine enhanced CT images.

Thyroid and Parathyroid Anatomy

CORONAL CECT

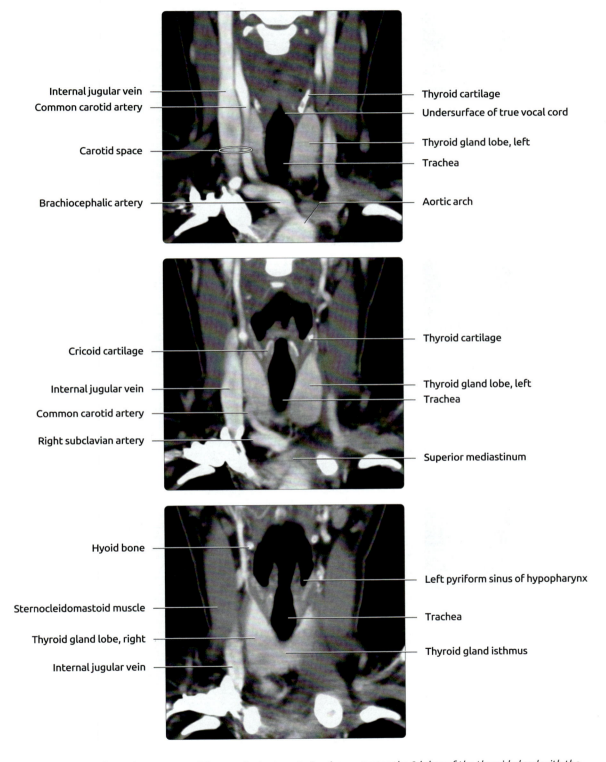

(Top) First of 3 coronal CECT reformations presented from posterior to anterior demonstrates the 2 lobes of the thyroid gland with the trachea on their medial borders. Lateral to each of the thyroid lobes are the carotid spaces containing the vagus nerve, common carotid artery, and internal jugular vein. (Middle) In this image, the chevron-shaped lobes of the thyroid gland are particularly well seen. Notice the intimate relationship between the superomedial thyroid gland and the larynx. Remember that thyroid gland malignancy 1st-order nodes are the paratracheal nodes. The paratracheal nodes drain inferiorly into the superior mediastinum. Consequently, it is important for the radiologist to image to the aortic arch in cases of thyroid gland malignancy. (Bottom) The isthmus of the thyroid gland is visible just anterior to the trachea in this image.

Thyroid and Parathyroid Anatomy

TRANSVERSE ULTRASOUND

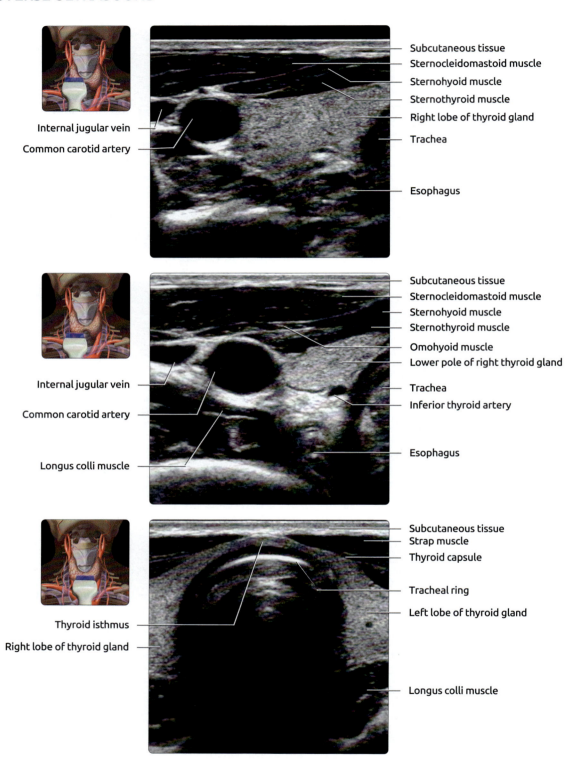

(Top) Transverse grayscale ultrasound of the right lobe of the thyroid gland shows the homogeneous, hyperechoic echo pattern of the glandular parenchyma. Note its close anatomical relationship with the major vessels of the carotid sheath (internal jugular vein and common carotid artery) laterally, the trachea medially, and the cervical esophagus posteromedially. (Middle) Transverse grayscale ultrasound shows the level of the inferior pole of the thyroid gland. The inferior thyroid artery is a consistent finding related to and supplying the inferior pole. (Bottom) Midline transverse grayscale ultrasound shows the thyroid isthmus connecting the 2 lobes. The isthmus lies on the anterior surface of the trachea. In view of the intimate anatomical relationship between the thyroid gland and the trachea, a local tumor invasion into the trachea from malignant thyroid carcinoma can occur, rendering surgical excision more extensive than total thyroidectomy.

Thyroid and Parathyroid Anatomy

LONGITUDINAL ULTRASOUND

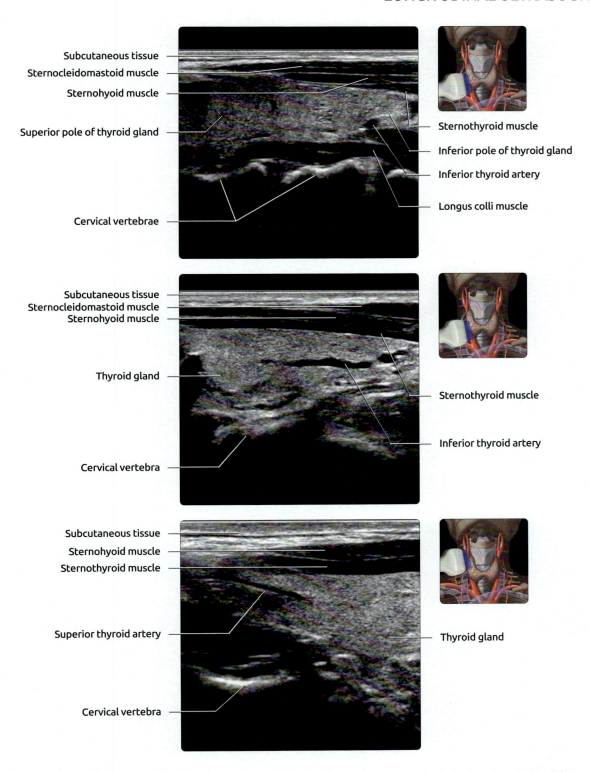

(Top) Parasagittal longitudinal grayscale ultrasound shows the thyroid gland. The homogeneous, hyperechoic echo pattern of the glandular parenchyma is better assessed on longitudinal scans. Part of the tortuous course of the inferior thyroid artery is seen in relation to the lower pole. (Middle) Parasagittal longitudinal grayscale ultrasound shows the inferior thyroid artery coursing superiorly from the inferior pole within the glandular parenchyma. (Bottom) Parasagittal longitudinal grayscale ultrasound shows the superior thyroid artery, the 1st anterior branch of the external carotid artery, running inferiorly within and supplying the upper pole of the thyroid gland. Longitudinal scans best evaluate the glandular parenchyma and vascularity.

Thyroid and Parathyroid Anatomy

GRAPHICS OF THYROID LESION

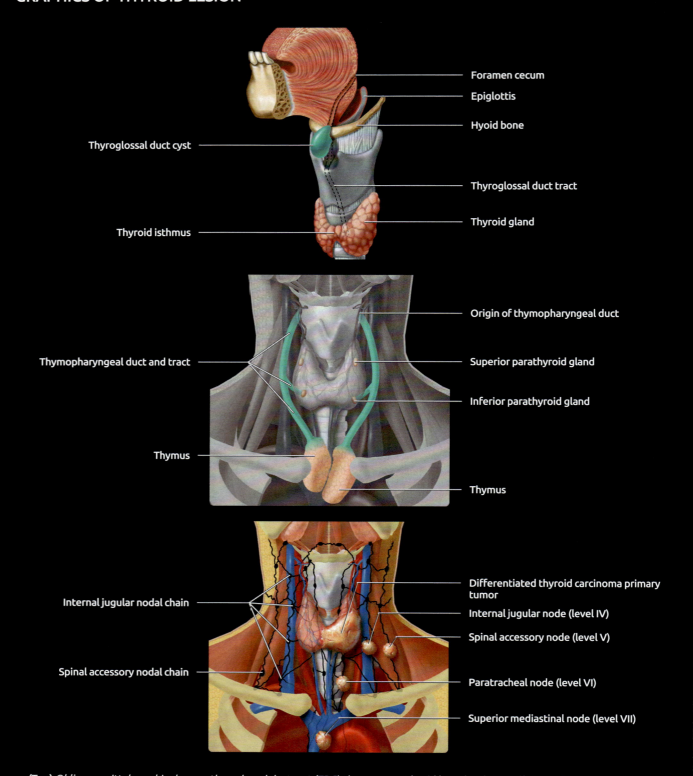

(Top) Oblique sagittal graphic shows a thyroglossal duct cyst (TDC) that occurs at hyoid bone level. TDCs (failure of involution of duct) or thyroid tissue remnants may be found anywhere along its tract from foramen cecum at tongue base to just anterior to thyroid lobes. Most TDCs are located near hyoid bone with 50% at hyoid bone & 20-25% in suprahyoid neck, often in midline. Remaining 25% are located in infrahyoid neck, in midline, or within strap muscles in paramidline location. Most common thyroid ectopia is the lingual thyroid. (Middle) AP graphic of cervical neck shows course of inferomedial migration of thymic primordia & inferior PTGs along paired thymopharyngeal duct tracts. Note tracts extend from lateral hypopharyngeal area to anterior mediastinum. Variable descent of inferior PTGs may result in ectopic locations along thymopharyngeal ducts. (Bottom) Coronal graphic of infrahyoid neck & superior mediastinum shows left thyroid lobe & isthmus differentiated thyroid carcinoma primary. Notice that in addition to nodal metastases in internal jugular & spinal accessory chains, there are also nodal metastases in paratracheal & superior mediastinal nodal groups.

Thyroid and Parathyroid Anatomy

GENERIC TRACHEOESOPHAGEAL GROOVE MASS

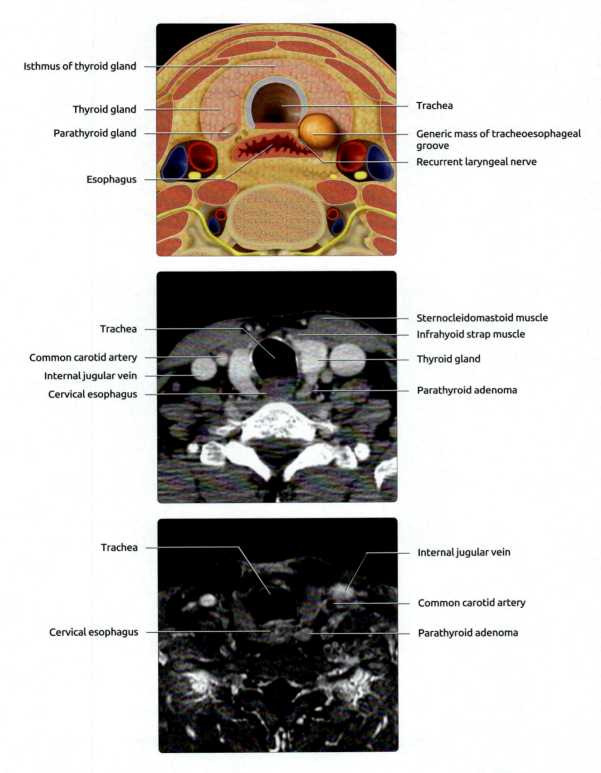

(Top) Axial graphic shows a well-circumscribed generic mass in the left tracheoesophageal groove, causing mass effect on the recurrent laryngeal nerve, esophagus, trachea, and left thyroid lobe. Parathyroid adenoma (PTA), recurrent laryngeal nerve schwannoma, and nodal disease in the paratracheal nodal chain all could cause such an appearance. (Middle) Axial CECT at the level of the thyroid gland shows an enhancing PTA in the left tracheoesophageal groove, posterior to the left thyroid lobe. In a patient with hypercalcemia and elevated parathormone, this location and appearance is diagnostic. (Bottom) Axial T1 contrast-enhanced fat-saturated MR at the level of the thyroid bed demonstrates an enhancing PTA posterior to the left lobe of the thyroid in the left tracheoesophageal groove.

Thyroid and Parathyroid Anatomy

GRAPHICS OF PARATHYROID AND GLAND EMBRYOLOGY

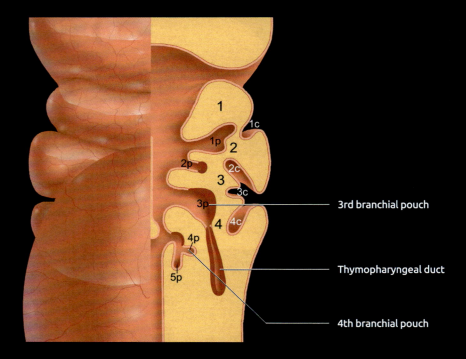

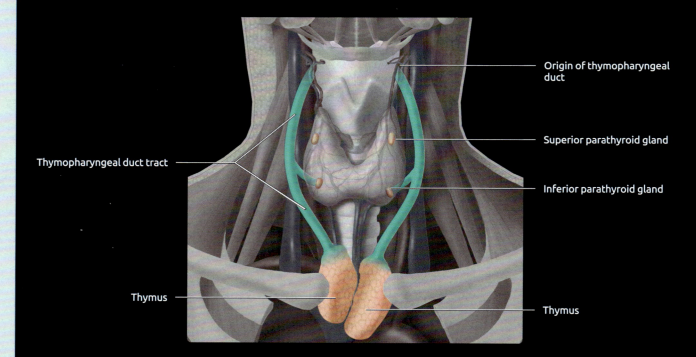

(Top) AP graphic of a 6-week-old fetus shows embryologic anatomy of branchial apparatus. Branchial apparatus includes 6 arches (mesoderm) interfaced by 4 clefts (ectoderm) & pouches (endoderm) on each side at end of 4th week of embryonic life. The 5th arch is rudimentary & does not contribute to formation of any adult structure. Superior PTGs develop from 4th branchial pouches, along with primordial thyroid. Superior PTGs & thyroid gland migrate caudally along thyroglossal duct. Less than 2% of superior PTGs are ectopic. Inferior PTGs develop from 3rd branchial pouches along with anlage of thymus. Inferior PTGs & primordial thymus migrate caudally along thymopharyngeal duct & may descend into anterior mediastinum. Up to 35% of inferior PTGs can be in ectopic locations.
(Bottom) AP graphic of neck shows course of inferomedial migration of thymic primordia & inferior PTGs along paired thymopharyngeal duct tracts. Note tracts extend from lateral hypopharyngeal area to anterior mediastinum. The most frequent ectopic inferior PTG site is just below inferior thyroid pole & less commonly in superior & anterior mediastinum.

Thyroid and Parathyroid Anatomy

ECTOPIC PARATHYROID ADENOMA

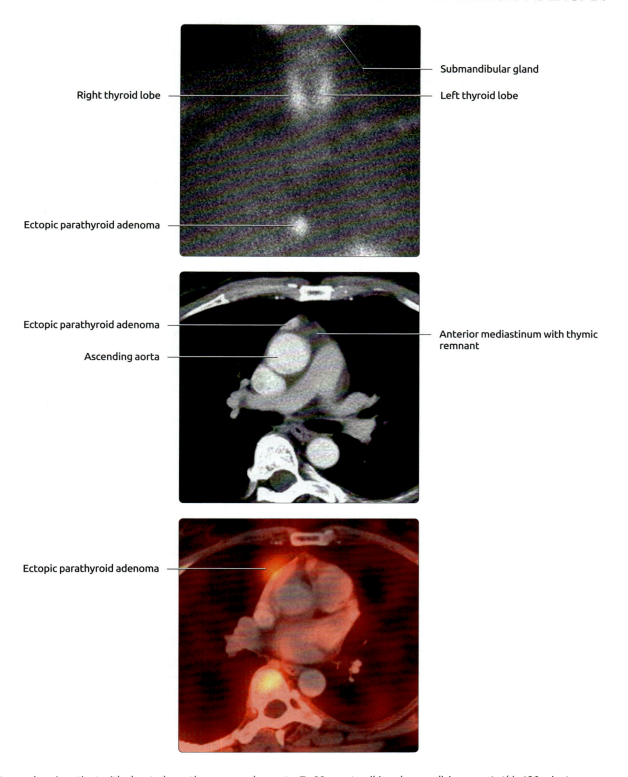

(Top) Hypercalcemic patient with elevated parathormone underwent a Tc-99m sestamibi nuclear medicine scan. In this 120-minute delayed scan, an area of persistent concentration of isotope is visible in the mediastinum. In this clinical setting, an ectopic PTA can be diagnosed. Persistent activity is also visualized in the thyroid and submandibular salivary glands. CECT is ordered for presurgical localization. (Middle) Axial CECT at the level of the main pulmonary artery demonstrates an enhancing PTA in the anterior mediastinum, anterior to ascending aorta. (Bottom) Axial fusion image of a CECT and Tc-99m sestamibi nuclear medicine scan at the level of the left atrium shows ectopic radiotracer activity in an anterior mediastinal PTA.

Thyroid and Parathyroid Anatomy

CLINICAL CORRELATES: PARATHYROID ADENOMA

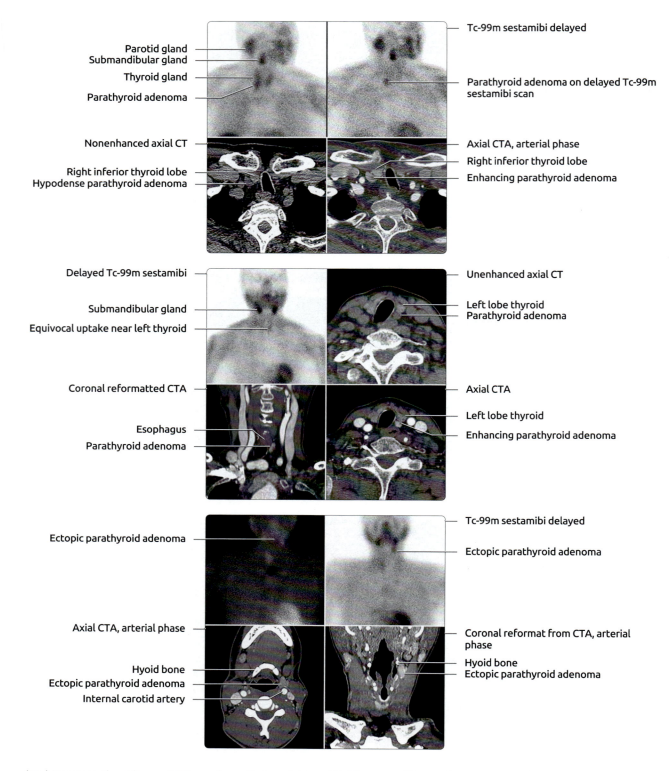

(Top) Hyperparathyroidism and PTA are shown. Early and delayed Tc-99m sestamibi scans demonstrate uptake in PTA just adjacent to the inferior margin right lobe thyroid gland. Thyroid uptake disappears on delayed images, allowing greater conspicuity of PTA. Nonenhanced CT scan through this region demonstrates slightly hyperdense thyroid tissue medially and hypodense PTA posterolaterally. During the early arterial phase, PTA enhances and is now isodense to the thyroid gland. (Middle) Hyperparathyroidism and PTA are shown. Sestamibi scan is equivocal in demonstrating left PTA. Unenhanced CT demonstrates small soft tissue nodule in the left tracheoesophageal groove. CTA, arterial phase, demonstrates brisk enhancement of nodule, helping localize the PTA. (Bottom) Hyperparathyroidism and PTA are shown. Patient underwent exploration for PTA, but no PTA was found. Sestamibi revealed small focus of abnormal uptake in the left suprahyoid neck, just below the submandibular gland; CTA shows enhancing PTA just anterior to the internal carotid artery and just below the submandibular gland.

Thyroid and Parathyroid Anatomy

PARATHYROID ULTRASOUND

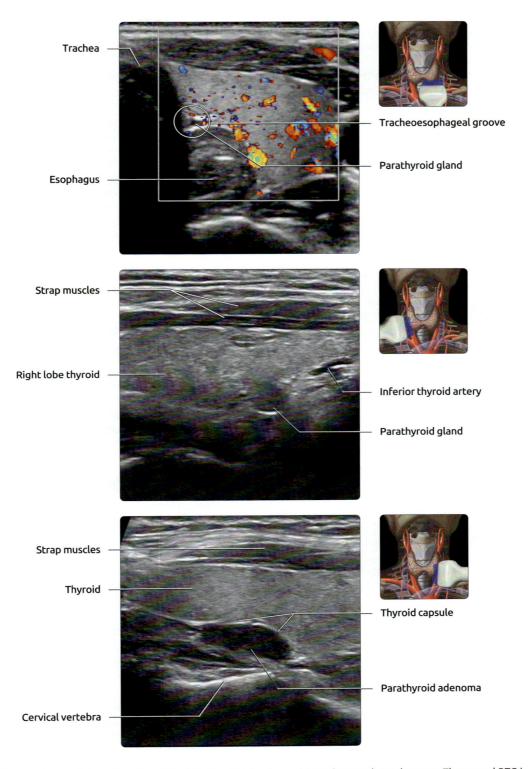

(Top) Transverse color Doppler US of the midportion of the left thyroid lobe shows the tracheoesophageal groove. The normal PTG is located in this area and is small, round to elliptical, and hypoechoic but is often difficult to identify with certainty. (Middle) Longitudinal scan of the right thyroid shows a larger, hypoechoic nodule in the expected location of the PTG, posterior middle 1/3 of the thyroid gland. This is the typical location of the superior PTGs. Careful analysis during a real-time scan should be done to prove they are outside the thyroid capsule and not a thyroid nodule. A PTG may also sometimes be confused with a small lymph node, but a normal lymph node should have an echogenic hilum. (Bottom) Longitudinal ultrasound of the left lobe of the thyroid in a patient with hypercalcemia shows a well-defined, ovoid, hypoechoic mass. Note the distinct thyroid capsule, confirming this is posterior to the thyroid and therefore likely a PTG rather than a thyroid nodule.

Cervical Trachea and Esophagus

TERMINOLOGY

Definitions

- Cervical trachea: Air-conveying flexible tube made of cartilage and fibromuscular membrane connecting larynx to lungs
- Cervical esophagus: Muscular food and fluid-conveying tube connecting pharynx to stomach

IMAGING ANATOMY

Overview

- Trachea
  - 10- to 13-cm tube extending in midline from inferior larynx at ~ 6th cervical vertebral body to carina at upper margin of 5th thoracic vertebral body (carina)
- Esophagus
  - 25-cm tube extending in midline from inferior hypopharynx at ~ 6th cervical vertebral body to 11th thoracic vertebral body
  - Descends behind trachea and thyroid, lying in front of lower cervical vertebrae
    - Inclines slightly to left in lower cervical neck and upper mediastinum, returning to midline at T5 vertebral body level

Anatomy Relationships

- Cervical trachea
  - Anterior structures: Infrahyoid strap muscles; isthmus of thyroid gland (2nd-4th tracheal cartilages)
  - Lateral structures: Lobes of thyroid gland
    - Tracheoesophageal groove structures: Recurrent laryngeal nerve, paratracheal nodes, parathyroid glands
  - Posterior structure: Cervical esophagus
- Cervical esophagus
  - Anterior structure: Cervical trachea
  - Anterolateral structures: Tracheoesophageal groove structures
  - Lateral structures: Carotid spaces on both sides, thoracic duct on left side at C6 level
  - Posterior structures: Retropharyngeal/danger spaces

Internal Contents

- Cervical trachea
  - **Cartilage anatomy**
    - Total 15-20 cartilages; each cartilage is "incomplete ring" of cartilage surrounding anterior 2/3 of trachea
    - Flat cartilage-deficient posterior portion is formed by fibromuscular tissue
    - Cross-sectional shape of trachea is that of letter D with flat side posterior
    - Smooth muscle fibers in posterior membrane (trachealis muscle) attach to free ends of tracheal cartilages and provide alteration in tracheal cross-sectional area
  - **Cervical tracheal mucosa**
    - Continuous sheet from larynx above
    - Layer of pseudostratified ciliated columnar epithelium interspersed with goblet cells with both lying on basal lamina
    - Minor salivary glands sporadically distributed in tracheal mucosa
    - Trachea has 3 layers: Mucosa, cartilage, and adventitia
  - **Blood supply**: Inferior thyroid arteries and veins
  - **Lymphatic drainage**: Level VI, pretracheal and paratracheal nodes
- Cervical esophagus
  - Begins at lower border of cricoid cartilage as continuation of hypopharynx
    - Cricopharyngeus muscle arises from either side of cricoid cartilage and creates muscular sling that encircles proximal esophagus, helping to form upper esophageal sphincter complex
    - Innervated by pharyngeal plexus
  - **Cervical esophageal mucosa**
    - Nonkeratinized stratified squamous epithelium
  - **Blood supply**: Inferior thyroid arteries and veins
  - **Lymphatic drainage**: Level IV, level VI, and paratracheal nodes

Fascia

- Middle layer, deep cervical fascia surrounds visceral space with trachea and esophagus inside

ANATOMY IMAGING ISSUES

Imaging Approaches

- Cervical trachea
  - **Multislice CT** with sagittal and coronal reformations exam of choice for trachea
- Cervical esophagus
  - **Air-contrast barium swallow** is **primary diagnostic tool** in esophageal evaluation
  - Multislice CECT for esophageal tumor staging

CLINICAL IMPLICATIONS

Clinical Importance

- Cervical tracheal lesions present with shortness of breath and stridor
  - May be treated for asthma prior to diagnosis
- Cervical esophageal lesions present with dysphagia
  - Aspiration pneumonia may occur prior to diagnosis

EMBRYOLOGY

Embryologic Events

- During 4th gestational week, respiratory primordium begins with formation of laryngotracheal groove that extends lengthwise in floor of gut just caudal to pharyngeal pouches
- Groove then deepens into laryngotracheal diverticulum whose ventral ectoderm become larynx and trachea
- Lateral furrows develop on either side of laryngotracheal diverticulum, then deepen to form laryngotracheal tube
- Tracheoesophageal septum then develops caudally to cranially, separating respiratory system from esophagus

Cervical Trachea and Esophagus

BARIUM SWALLOW

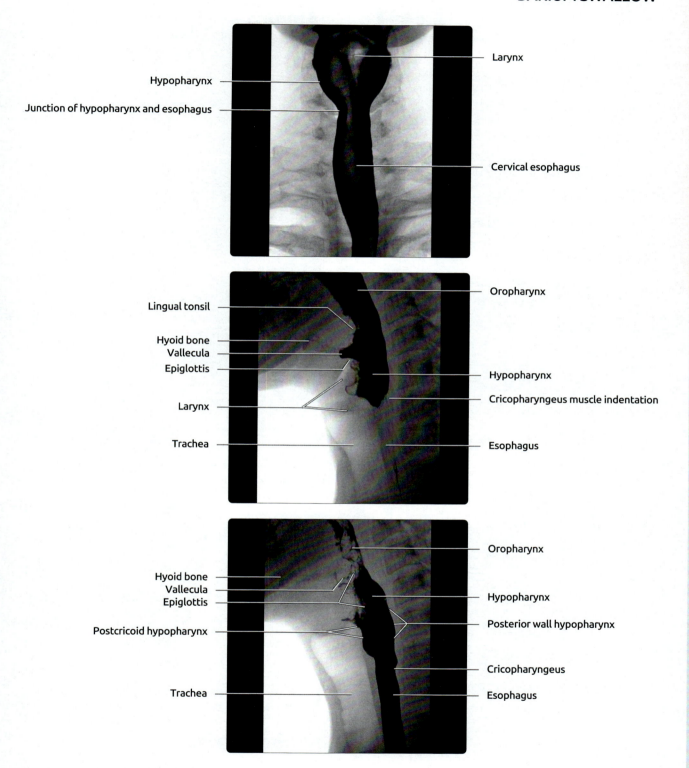

(Top) *Frontal view of a normal barium swallow shows barium deflected around the larynx that appears as a filling defect. Inferior cricoid cartilage delineates the inferior larynx and hypopharynx on CT studies as well as the junction of the hypopharynx with the cervical esophagus.* (Middle) *Lateral view of a barium swallow of the upper pharynx shows the junction of the oropharynx and hypopharynx at the hyoid bone. The lingual tonsil (base of tongue) causes a lobulated impression upon the anterior oropharynx. Epiglottis closes during swallowing to protect the larynx from aspiration. Valleculae are recesses between the tongue and epiglottis.* (Bottom) *Lateral view of a barium swallow shows the hypopharynx and cervical esophagus posterior to the larynx and trachea. The hypopharynx extends from the hyoid bone to the cricopharyngeus muscle. The cricopharyngeus muscle demarcates the hypopharynx from the cervical esophagus on barium studies and is typically located at C5/6 level.*

Cervical Trachea and Esophagus

GRAPHICS: MUSCLES AND SPACES

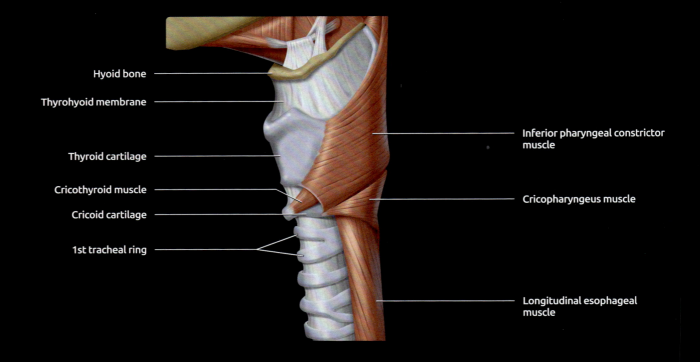

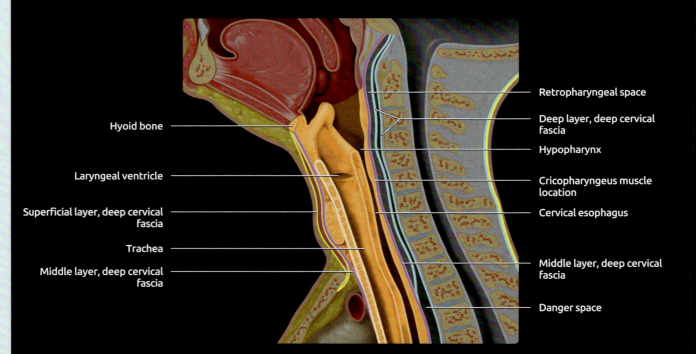

(Top) Lateral graphic shows the junction of the larynx and hypopharynx with the trachea and esophagus. The cricopharyngeus muscle, which separates the hypopharynx from the cervical esophagus, is part of the inferior constrictor muscle. The esophagus is composed of outer longitudinal muscles and an inner circular muscle layer (not shown). The 1st tracheal ring is the broadest of all tracheal cartilages and is often merged to cricoid cartilage or the 2nd tracheal ring. Mucosal portions of the posterior trachea are separated from the esophagus by a thin layer of connective tissue, often called the "party wall," as it separates the trachea anteriorly from the esophagus posteriorly. (Bottom) Sagittal graphic shows the longitudinal relationships of the infrahyoid neck. Note the middle layer of the deep cervical fascia (pink) encircles the trachea and esophagus as part of the visceral space. The trachea and esophagus are an inferior continuation of the airway and pharynx.

Cervical Trachea and Esophagus

GRAPHICS

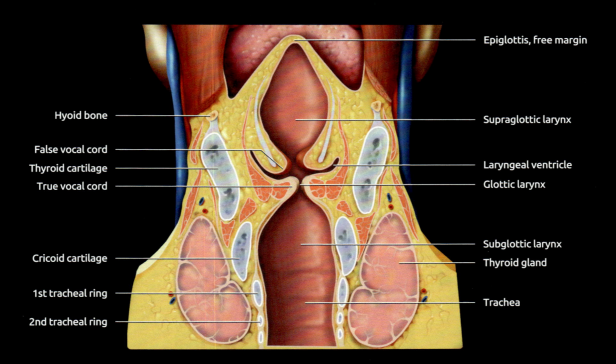

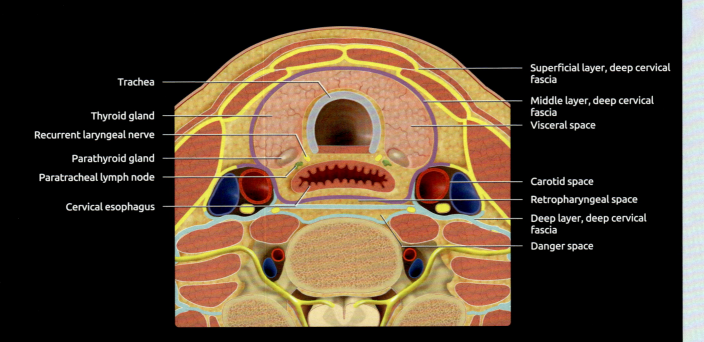

(Top) Coronal graphic shows the larynx and trachea. The supraglottic larynx includes the epiglottis, aryepiglottic folds, false vocal cords, and preepiglottic and paraglottic spaces. The glottic larynx includes true vocal cords. The subglottic larynx is separated from the trachea at the inferior cricoid cartilage. The 1st tracheal ring is located 1.5-2 cm below true vocal cords and is broadest of all the cartilage rings. The 2nd, 3rd, and 4th tracheal rings are surrounded by the thyroid gland, anteriorly and laterally. Coronal and sagittal reformatted images are particularly helpful in evaluation of tracheal stenosis and other disorders. (Bottom) Axial graphic shows layers of deep cervical fascia in the infrahyoid neck. Note the middle layer of deep cervical fascia as it surrounds the visceral space. Important components of the tracheoesophageal groove include the recurrent laryngeal nerve, paratracheal nodes, and parathyroid glands.

Cervical Trachea and Esophagus

AXIAL CECT

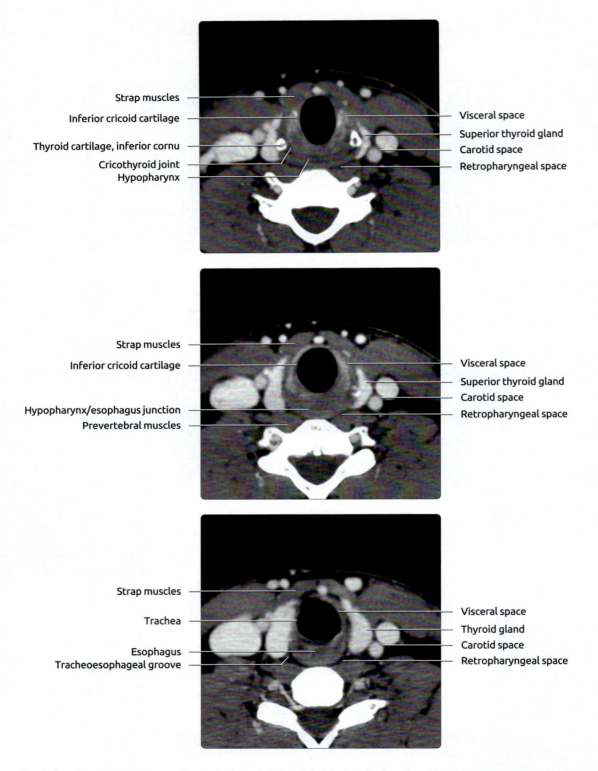

(Top) *First of 6 axial CECT images from superior to inferior shows the inferior larynx and hypopharynx and transition to the cervical trachea and esophagus. The inferior larynx and hypopharynx are defined by the inferior cricoid cartilage on cross-sectional imaging. This image shows the subglottic larynx, an area from the undersurface of true vocal cords to the inferior surface of cricoid cartilage. The cricothyroid joint lies adjacent to the recurrent laryngeal nerve, and dislocation of this joint may result in vocal cord paralysis.* (Middle) *This image shows the junction of the hypopharynx and larynx, which is defined by the cricopharyngeus muscle on barium swallow studies. This muscle is an inferior portion of the inferior pharyngeal constrictor muscle and is typically present at C5/6.* (Bottom) *Image more inferior shows the cervical trachea and esophagus. The upper 2nd through 4th tracheal rings are surrounded by the thyroid gland.*

Cervical Trachea and Esophagus

AXIAL CECT

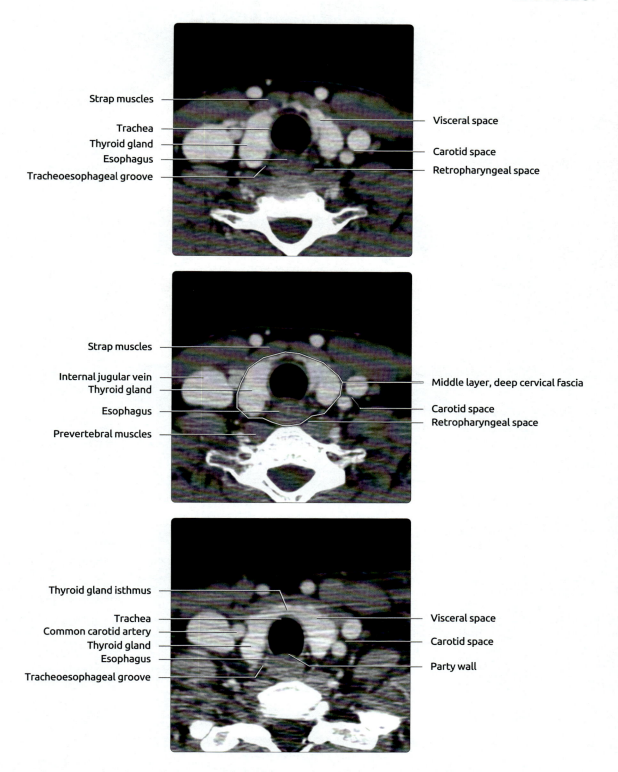

(Top) Image more inferior shows the cervical trachea and esophagus within the inferior visceral space. The cervical trachea is bordered anteriorly by the infrahyoid strap muscles, anteriorly and laterally by the thyroid gland and tracheoesophageal groove structures, and posteriorly by the esophagus. The esophagus is bordered anteriorly by the cervical trachea, anterolaterally by the tracheoesophageal groove structures, laterally by the carotid spaces, and posteriorly by the retropharyngeal space. (Middle) This image shows the middle layer of the deep cervical fascia encircling the visceral space. (Bottom) This image shows the "party wall," the thin layer of connective tissue that separates mucosal portions of the posterior trachea from the anterior esophagus. Tracheoesophageal groove structures include the recurrent laryngeal nerve, paratracheal lymph nodes, and parathyroid glands.

Cervical Trachea and Esophagus

GENERIC TRACHEAL MASS GRAPHIC AND CECT

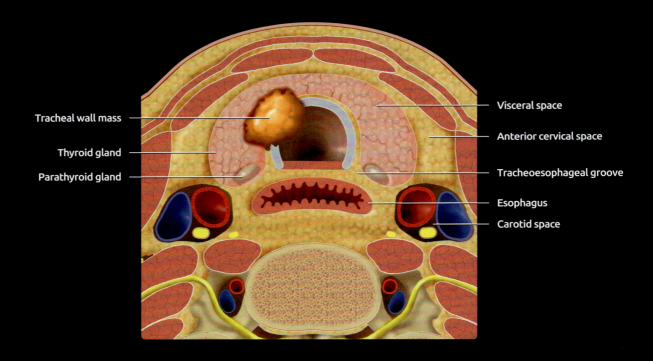

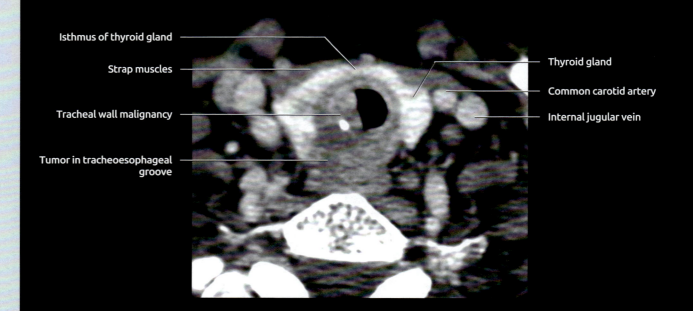

(Top) Axial graphic shows a generic tracheal wall mass. A mass within the tracheal wall typically displaces the thyroid gland laterally and esophagus posteriorly. Primary tumors of the trachea are rare, representing 2% of upper airway tumors. The most common primary malignant tumors include squamous cell carcinoma (SCCa) and adenoid cystic carcinoma. SCCa usually arise in the lower trachea and carina. Adenoid cystic carcinomas are usually located on the posterolateral tracheal wall. (Bottom) Axial CECT demonstrates a right tracheal wall adenoid cystic carcinoma that has spread posteriorly to involve the right tracheoesophageal groove and anterior wall of the cervical esophagus. Such lesions can be relatively asymptomatic until stridor supervenes.

Cervical Trachea and Esophagus

GENERIC ESOPHAGEAL MASS GRAPHIC AND CECT

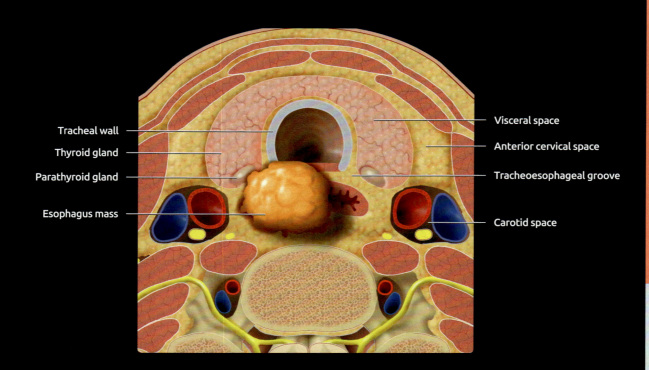

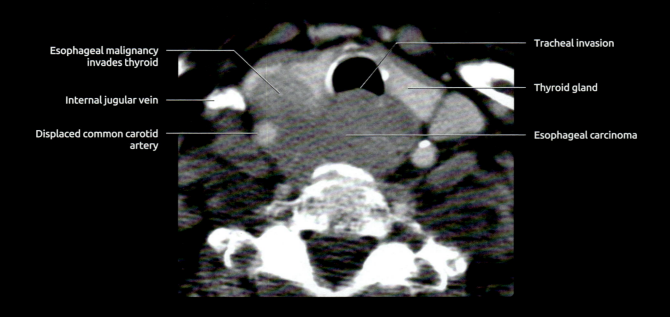

(Top) Axial graphic of a generic esophageal mass, which is typically midline and displaces the trachea and thyroid gland anteriorly, is shown. Ninety percent of esophageal carcinomas are SCCa, while the remainder is adenocarcinomas related to Barrett esophagus. CT is particularly useful to define the extent of disease and associated metastases, typically to periesophageal, paratracheal, supraclavicular, and mediastinal lymph nodes and the liver. Leiomyoma is the most common benign tumor of the esophagus and is usually incidentally discovered. (Bottom) Axial CECT through the lower thyroid bed in the cervical neck reveals a large retrotracheal invasive mass (esophageal carcinoma) that has lifted the trachea and left thyroid lobe anteriorly. The right common carotid artery is displaced laterally. The tumor has invaded the right thyroid lobe and the posterior trachea.

Cervical Trachea and Esophagus

TRANSVERSE ULTRASOUND

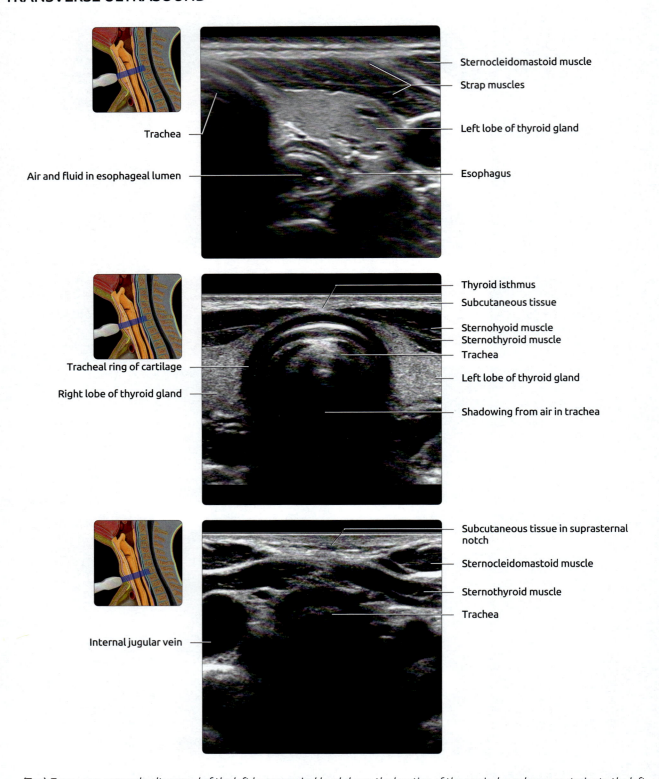

(Top) Transverse grayscale ultrasound of the left lower cervical level shows the location of the cervical esophagus posterior to the left lobe of the thyroid gland and posterolateral to the trachea. It is easily recognized by the alternating hypo-/hyperechoic rings (gut signature). If there is any question, have the patient swallow. The recurrent laryngeal nerve is located in the tracheoesophageal groove. The nerve is not visualized on ultrasound. (Middle) Transverse grayscale ultrasound of the midline anterior neck at the level of thyroid gland shows the trachea as a midline structure underneath the isthmus of the thyroid gland and related laterally to the thyroid lobes. Note the hypoechoic tracheal ring composed of hyaline cartilage that is incomplete posteriorly. (Bottom) Transverse grayscale ultrasound of the suprasternal region shows the lower cervical trachea underneath the insertion sites of the strap muscles.

Cervical Trachea and Esophagus

LONGITUDINAL ULTRASOUND AND CT

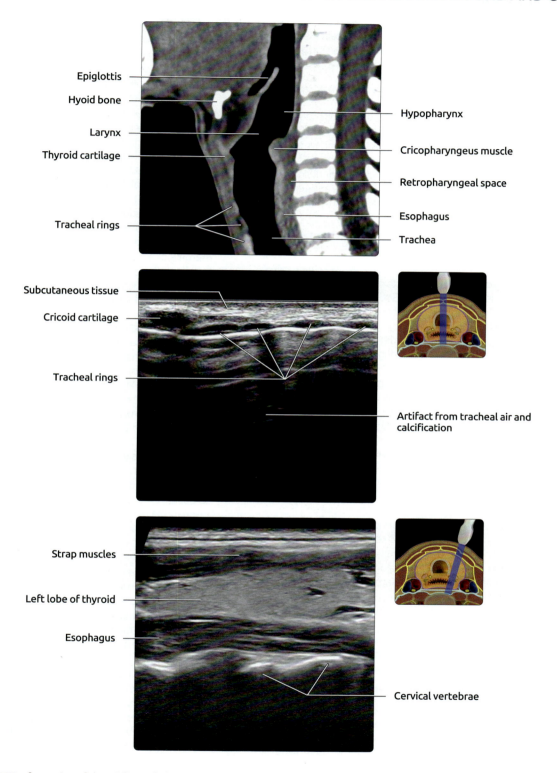

(Top) Sagittal NECT reformation of the midline infrahyoid neck shows noncalcified tracheal rings anteriorly. These rings form an arch around the trachea and are incomplete posteriorly. The posterior wall is composed of a thick fibromuscular membrane and is immediately adjacent to the esophagus. (Middle) Longitudinal grayscale US of the midline anterior neck shows the presence of hypoechoic tracheal rings along the cervical portion of the trachea. Note the hypoechoic, noncalcified, cricoid cartilage above the tracheal rings. (Bottom) Longitudinal grayscale ultrasound of the lower left neck at the thyroid gland level shows the cervical esophagus posterior to the left lobe of the thyroid gland. It is a long tubular structure with alternating echogenic/hypoechoic layers representing the mucosal, submucosal, muscular, and serosal layers.

Cervical Lymph Nodes

TERMINOLOGY

Abbreviations

- Internal jugular chain (IJC); spinal accessory chain (SAC); sternocleidomastoid muscle (SCM); internal carotid artery (ICA); common carotid artery (CCA); retropharyngeal (RP); retropharyngeal space (RPS)

Definitions

- **Lymph nodes** are small, bean-shaped organs distributed throughout body that function as part of lymphatic system
  - Mechanical filtration of lymph collected along lymphatic vessels
  - Provides environment in which cellular elements of immune system can interact with & identify antigens within lymph fluid & mount appropriate immune response

IMAGING ANATOMY

Overview

- **Lymphatic system** in neck consists of extensive lymphatic capillary & vessel network, up to 300 individual lymph nodes, & Waldeyer ring: Palatine tonsils, nasopharyngeal tonsil (adenoid), & lingual tonsil
- Lymph node is bean-shaped gland that receives 1 or more afferent lymphatic vessels that bring lymph from peripheral tissue (or from upstream lymph node)
- Focal concavity along margin of lymph node is its hilum & contains small arterioles, venules, & efferent lymphatic vessels
- Supporting architecture of lymph node includes **peripheral capsule** of thin fibrous connective tissue, internal fibrous trabeculae that penetrate gland from capsule, & fine network of reticular cells
- Lymph node contains variety of immune cells specifically organized into functional regions to maximize cellular exposure to antigens & provoke immune response
  - **Cortex**: Located in periphery of node, contains **lymphoid follicles** composed mostly of B-cell lymphocytes & responsible for humoral immunity
  - **Paracortex**: Main site of cellular immunity; T cells reside here & proliferate when stimulated
  - **Medulla**: Contains lymphocytes, plasmacytoid lymphocytes, & plasma cells; main site of antibody production
- Cervical nodes drain into thoracic duct on left & right lymphatic duct on right side; both open into their respective angle of internal jugular & subclavian veins

Nodal Nomenclature & Classifications

- Earliest classifications of cervical lymph nodes (Rouvière, Trotter, & Poirier & Charpy) were largely based on palpable landmarks of neck
- Shah suggested level-based system of nomenclature in 1981
- Since 1981, several level-based systems have been developed in attempt to standardize head & neck cancer staging & surgical approaches based on predictable patterns of tumor spread
- 1997: American Joint Committee on Cancer classification
- 1998: American Academy of Otolaryngology-Head & Neck Surgery classification
- 1999: Imaging-based classification based on cross-sectional CT or MR images (Som, Curtin, & Mancuso)

Image-Based Classification Method

- Relies on identification of anatomic landmarks easily determined on cross-sectional CT or MR images
- Requires placement of lines along margins of specific anatomic structures in axial plane to determine boundaries of lymph node levels
- Lines defining boundaries of lymph node levels must be **drawn separately** for each side of neck
- If lymph node lies in both adjacent levels on either side of line, it should be assigned to level that has most cross-sectional area of node
- **Level I: Submental & submandibular nodes**
  - Nodes below mylohyoid muscle, above inferior margin of hyoid bone, & anterior to transverse lines drawn along posterior margins of each submandibular gland
  - Level IA (submental nodes): Found between **medial margins** of anterior bellies of digastric muscles
  - Level IB (submandibular nodes): Nodes posterior & lateral to medial margin of anterior belly of digastric muscle, around submandibular gland in submandibular space
- **Level II: Upper IJC nodes (suprahyoid)** from skull base at lower jugular fossa to **lower margin** of hyoid bone body
  - Anterior to **transverse line** along posterior border of SCM, & posterior to transverse line along posterior edge of submandibular gland on either side
  - If node within 2 cm of skull base lies lateral, anterior, or posterior to carotid sheath, it is level II node, whereas if node lies within 2 cm of skull base & medial to ICA, it is RP node
  - Below 2 cm of skull base, level II node can lie medial, lateral, anterior, or posterior to internal jugular vein (IJV)
  - Level IIA: Level II node anterior, medial, lateral, anterior, or posterior to IJV; if posterior to IJV, node must be inseparable from IJV
  - Level IIB: Level II node posterior to IJV with fat plane visible between node & IJV; lies above & behind spinal accessory nerve
    - Previously classified as upper spinal accessory nodes
- **Level III: Mid-IJC nodes** from lower margin of hyoid bone to **lower margin** of cricoid cartilage arch
  - Anterior to **transverse line** along posterior border of SCM; lateral to **medial margin** of CCA/ICA here (level VI nodes are seen medial to medial margin of CCA/ICA)
  - Anterior boundary of levels III & IV is sternohyoid muscle
- **Level IV: Low IJC nodes (infracricoid)** from **lower margin** of cricoid arch to clavicle
  - Anterior & medial to **oblique line** along posterior border of SCM & posterolateral border of anterior scalene muscle; lateral to **medial margin** of CCA (level VI nodes are seen medial to medial margin of CCA)
- **Level V: Nodes of posterior cervical space (SAC)**
  - Anterior to transverse line along anterior border of trapezius muscle
  - Level VA: Upper SAC nodes from skull base to lower margin of cricoid cartilage arch; posterior to **transverse line** along posterior border of SCM

Cervical Lymph Nodes

- Level VB: Lower SAC (transverse cervical) nodes from lower margin of cricoid cartilage arch to clavicle; posterior to **oblique line** along posterior border of SCM & posterolateral border of anterior scalene muscle
- **Level VI: Visceral nodes** found from lower margin of hyoid bone above to top of manubrium below; includes prelaryngeal, pretracheal, & paratracheal subgroups
  - Medial to **medial margin** of CCA/ICA
- **Level VII: Superior mediastinal nodes** found between carotid arteries from top of manubrium above to innominate vein below
  - Medial to **medial margin** of CCA
- **Supraclavicular nodes**: Lymph nodes lateral to medial margin of common carotid artery in lower neck if any portion of clavicle is seen on that side in axial image
  - If level of axial image is cranial & does not show any portion of clavicle on that side, then lower lateral neck node is classified as either level IV (anteriorly) or VB (posteriorly)
- **Axillary nodes**: Nodes below clavicle level & lateral to ribs
- **Parotid nodal group**: Intraglandular or extraglandular
  - Both intraglandular & extraglandular nodes are within fascia circumscribing parotid space
  - Drains into upper IJC nodes (level II)
  - Most common tumors to involve this group are skin squamous cell carcinoma (SCCa), melanoma, & parotid malignancy
- **RP nodal group**: 2 subgroups
  - Nodes within 2 cm of skull base & medial to ICA
  - Medial RPS nodes: Found in paramedian RPS in suprahyoid neck (SHN)
  - Lateral RPS nodes: Found in lateral RPS in SHN, lateral to prevertebral muscles, medial to ICA
  - Drainage pattern: Drains posterior pharynx into high IJC
- **Facial nodal groups**
  - Mandibular nodes: Along external mandibular surface
  - Buccinator nodes: In buccal space
  - Infraorbital nodes: In nasolabial fold
  - Malar nodes: On malar eminence
  - Retrozygomatic nodes: Deep to zygomatic arch

ANATOMY IMAGING ISSUES

Imaging Approaches

- **SCCa nodal staging**: CECT or T1 C+ MR; scan extent: Skull base to clavicles
- PET/CT utility in head & neck SCCa nodal work-up: Small active malignant node identification & treatment planning
- **Thyroid or cervical esophageal cancer**
  - Scan extent: Skull base to **carina to include superior mediastinum**
  - MR preferred for thyroid cancer as iodinated contrast for CECT may interfere with decision for I-131 radioiodine thyroid ablation treatment

CLINICAL IMPLICATIONS

Clinical Importance

- Recognizing enlarged or pathologic-appearing nodes important in infectious, inflammatory, & neoplastic processes
- Differentiation between **benign vs. malignant nodes**

- Most normal lymph nodes in neck not visualized by routine imaging
- Normal nodes are smoothly marginated
- Identifying metastatic nodes critical for cancer staging & treatment
- Normal size criteria: < 1.5-cm IJC nodes near angle of mandible; < 8-mm RP nodes; < 1-cm all other nodal groups
- 1-cm cutoff in largest axial diameter shows 88% sensitivity & 39% specificity, whereas 1.5-cm cutoff shows 56% sensitivity & 84% specificity for metastatic head & neck cancer
- Nodes smaller than cutoff size criteria can also be malignant, especially if in drainage areas of primary tumor, & should be evaluated carefully for abnormal morphology
- Morphology: Oval nodes with central fatty hila normally; metastatic disease may be round, replace normal fatty hila, & show necrosis, cystic change, hyperenhancement, or calcification
- IJC is final common pathway for all lymphatics of upper aerodigestive tract & neck
  - Since IJC empties into thoracic duct on left & right lymphatic duct on right (both opening into angle of internal jugular & subclavian veins on their respective sides), SCCa does not normally drain directly into mediastinum
  - Neck imaging to stage SCCa: Skull base to clavicles
  - Distal thoracic duct or right lymphatic duct could be mistaken for supraclavicular lymphadenopathy; for pseudoaneurysm on NECT, for neurogenic tumor similar to schwannoma due to their location near carotid sheath, & in younger patients for congenital cystic mass similar to branchial anomaly or lymphatic malformation
- **RP space nodal group**
  - Reactive-appearing RPS nodes commonly seen in younger patients on brain MR exam
  - Important when identified on imaging in SCCa setting, as often clinically silent
- **Parotid nodal group**
  - Receives lymph drainage from external auditory canal, eustachian tube, skin of lateral forehead & temporal region, posterior cheek, gums, & buccal mucous membrane (especially due to skin SCCa & melanoma)
- **Notable named nodes**
  - **Signal (Virchow) node**: Lowest node in IJC; if no primary tumor evident in neck, consider chest or abdomen primary, with metastasis carried via thoracic duct; left > right
  - **Rouvière node**: Highest node in RP group; lies within 2 cm of skull base; site of spread for nasopharyngeal carcinoma, esthesioneuroblastoma
  - **Jugulodigastric (sentinel) node**: Lies within IJC just above hyoid bone; larger than surrounding nodes
  - **Delphian (prelaryngeal/precricoid) node**: Not normally identified on imaging; pathologically enlarged in cases of advanced thyroid cancer & head & neck SCCa
  - **Jugulo-omohyoid node**: "Lymph node of tongue," found near intermediate tendon of omohyoid muscle (in level III)

Cervical Lymph Nodes

GRAPHIC LYMPH NODE ANATOMY AND HISTOLOGY

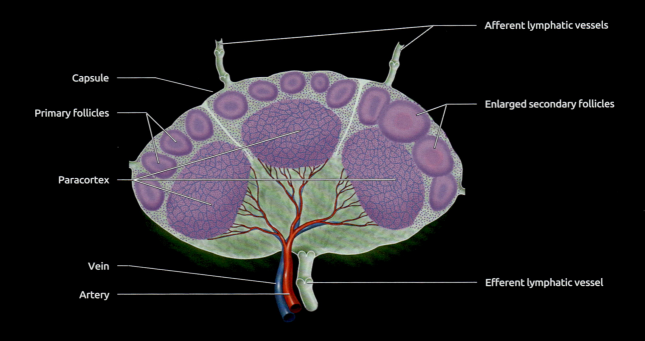

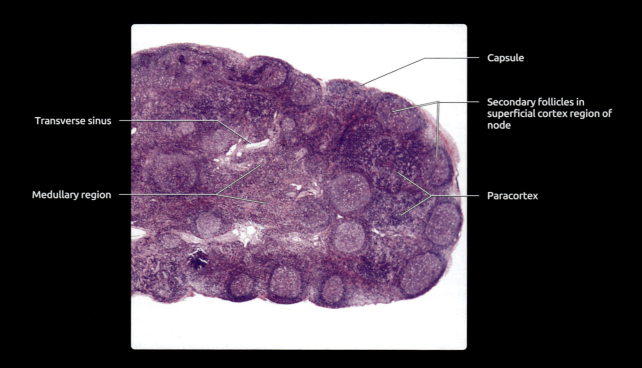

(Top) Several afferent lymphatic vessels enter the broad convex side of the lymph node. Lymph flows through a series of sinuses from the periphery toward the hilum. Peripherally, the lymphatic tissue is organized into the superficial cortex that contains the primary follicles. When the primary follicles are stimulated, secondary follicles with germinal centers are formed. The follicles preferentially contain B cells. The paracortex contain the so-called deep cortical units where T cells congregate and proliferate when stimulated. Plasma cell precursors produced by B-cell proliferation migrate to the medulla where they ultimately secrete antibodies. (Bottom) Histologic slide of a reactive lymph node demonstrates the principle regions of the node from the superficial cortex that contains the follicles (B cells), the paracortex that contains the deep cortical units (T cells), and the medullary region where B cells mature and produce antibodies.

Cervical Lymph Nodes

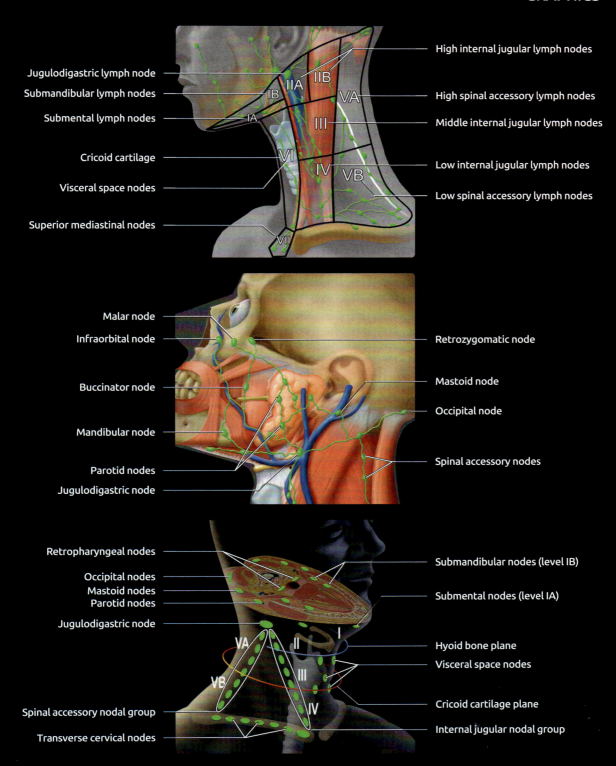

(Top) Lateral oblique graphic of the neck shows anatomic locations of major nodal groups of the neck. Division of the internal jugular nodal chain into high, middle, and low regions is defined by the level of the lower borders of the hyoid bone and cricoid cartilage. Similarly, the spinal accessory nodal chain is divided into high and low regions by lower cricoid cartilage level. (Middle) Lateral view of facial nodes and parotid nodes is shown. None of these nodes bear level numbers and must be described by their anatomic location. (Bottom) Lateral oblique graphic of the cervical nodes depicts an axial slice through the suprahyoid neck. Note retropharyngeal nodes behind the pharynx, which are often clinically occult. The hyoid bone (blue arc) and cricoid cartilage (orange circle) planes are highlighted as they serve to subdivide the internal jugular and spinal accessory nodal group levels. Neck lymph nodes empty into the thoracic duct on the left and right lymphatic duct on the right, both opening into angle of internal jugular and subclavian veins on their respective sides.

Cervical Lymph Nodes

IMAGING CLASSIFICATION: AXIAL CT

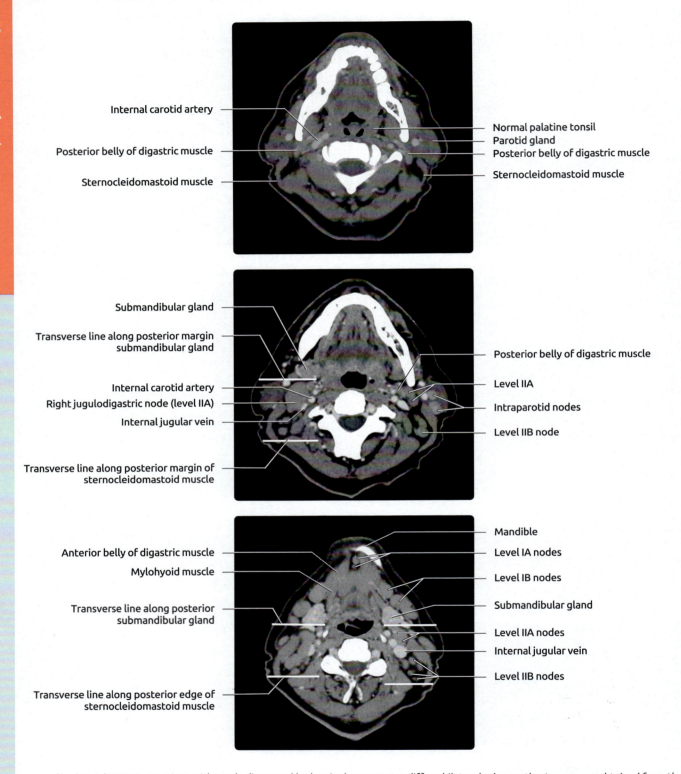

(Top) Axial CECT in a patient with newly diagnosed leukemia demonstrates diffuse bilateral adenopathy. Images are obtained from the skull base through clavicles inferiorly. The posterior belly of the digastric muscle arises from the mastoid tip and passes between the parotid gland and the carotid sheath. It is a good landmark on axial CT images. Immediately below the posterior belly, the jugulodigastric node is found, often the largest lymph node in normal neck with upper limits of normal 1.5 cm. (Middle) In this section, multiple enlarged nodes are present, including a significantly enlarged right level II node, the jugulodigastric node. Transverse lines are drawn along the posterior margin of the submandibular gland (to demarcate level IB from level IIA nodes) and along the posterior margin of the sternocleidomastoid muscle (SCM) (to distinguish level II from level V nodes). (Bottom) Axial CECT of the submandibular region above the hyoid bone is shown. Tranverse lines are drawn along the posterior margins of submandibular glands and SCMs. Diffusely enlarged lymph nodes are identified. In a normal subject, a small number of these nodes would be identifiable on CT.

Cervical Lymph Nodes

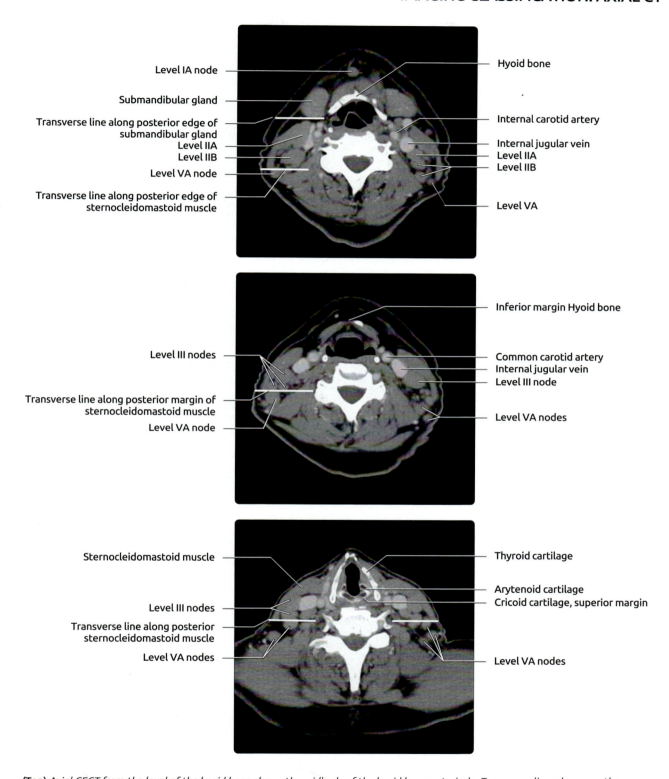

(Top) Axial CECT from the level of the hyoid bone shows the midbody of the hyoid bone anteriorly. Transverse lines drawn on the patient's right again separate level I from level II and level II from level V. Level IIB nodes lie posterior to internal jugular vein (IJV) with fat plane visible between the node and IJV. Note that 1 of the nodes posterior to left IJV contacts the vein and is denoted as level IIA. **(Middle)** Axial CECT just below the level of the hyoid bone is shown. The inferior margin of the hyoid bone is an important landmark, marking the transition from level II IJC nodes above to level III IJC nodes below. Level III extends from the inferior margin of the hyoid bone to the inferior margin of the cricoid cartilage. A transverse line is drawn on the patient's right, along the posterior margin of the SCM, separating the level II nodes from more posterior level VA nodes. **(Bottom)** Axial CECT below the hyoid and above the inferior margin of cricoid cartilage is shown. A transverse line is drawn bilaterally along the posterior margins of SCMs. This separates the level III nodal group from level VA.

Cervical Lymph Nodes

IMAGING CLASSIFICATION: AXIAL CT

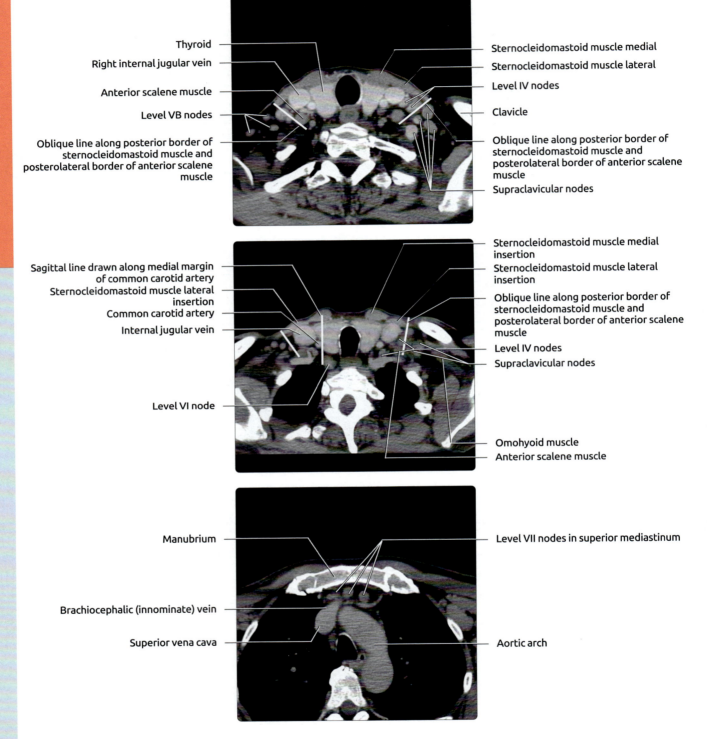

(Top) Axial CECT just below the inferior margin of the cricoid cartilage is shown. The inferior margin of the cricoid is important because it separates level III internal jugular chain (IJC) nodes above from level IV IJC nodes below and also marks the inferior extent of level VA. Notice on the patient's right, the clavicle is not in view, and the nodes lateral to the oblique line is designated as level VB. On the patient's left, the clavicle is in view and by convention, the nodes lateral to the oblique line is designated as supraclavicular nodes. (Middle) Axial CECT at the thyroid level is shown. Oblique lines separate the level IV nodes from more lateral supraclavicular nodes bilaterally as clavicles are visualized in the image on both sides. An anteroposterior line is drawn in the sagittal plane along the medial margin of the right common carotid artery to separate level IV nodes lateral to it from the more medially located level VI nodes. A single level VI node is identified in the right tracheoesophageal groove. (Bottom) Axial CECT below the upper margin of the manubrium shows the top of the manubrium marks the separation between level VI nodes above and level VII superior mediastinal nodes below.

Cervical Lymph Nodes

AXIAL CECT

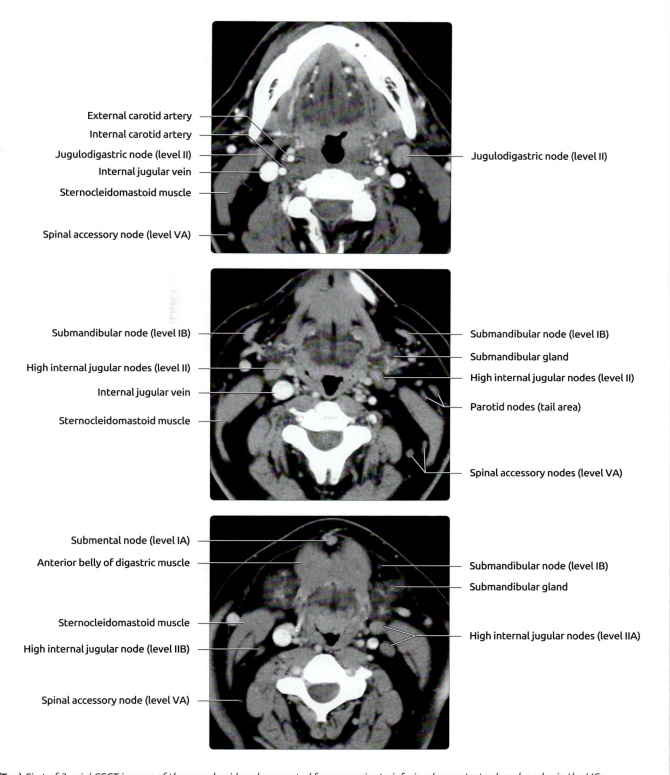

(Top) First of 3 axial CECT images of the suprahyoid neck presented from superior to inferior demonstrates lymph nodes in the IJCs (level II) and spinal accessory chains (level V). The jugulodigastric node is the highest or "sentinel" node of the IJC. (Middle) In this image, the internal jugular and spinal accessory lymph nodes are seen along with submandibular nodes (level IB) anterolateral to the submandibular glands in the submandibular space. Note the internal jugular nodes are closely applied to the carotid space while the spinal accessory nodes are in the posterior cervical space. (Bottom) In this image just above the hyoid bone, a submental (level IA) node is seen between the anterior bellies of digastric muscles. Note also the submandibular (level IB), high internal jugular nodes (level IIA and IIB), and spinal accessory (level VA) nodes.

Cervical Lymph Nodes

AXIAL T1 & T2 MR

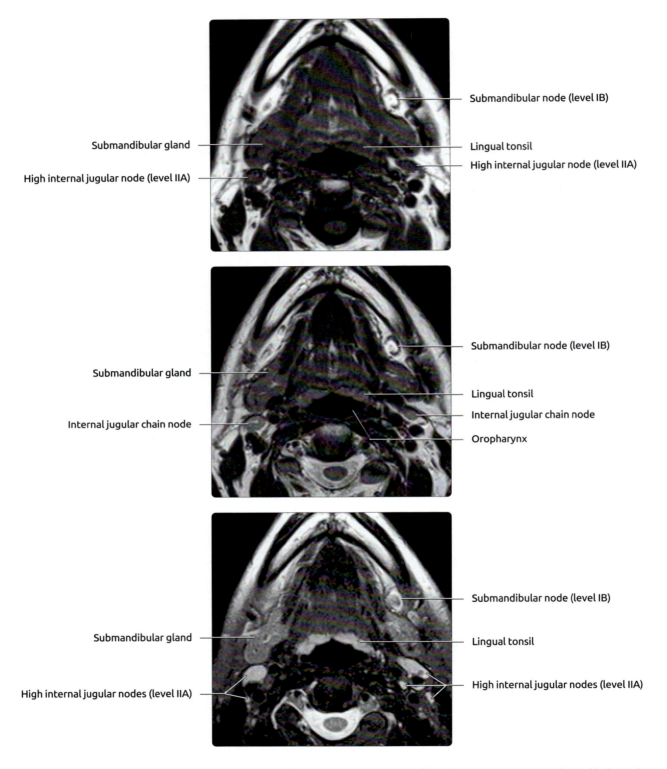

(Top) Axial T1 MR through the low oropharynx shows characteristic low T1 signal of lymph nodes. A prominent submandibular node with a fatty hilum is seen on the left. Level IIA internal jugular nodes are observed bilaterally. (Middle) Axial T2 MR at the bilateral level of the low oropharynx shows high internal jugular nodes as intermediate signal intensity. (Bottom) Axial T2 MR with fat saturation creates increased conspicuity of lymph nodes. The smaller high internal jugular nodes surrounding the carotid space are easily identified on this fat-saturated T2 image. STIR MR sequences create the same level of nodal conspicuity. Lingual tonsil tissue is also made more conspicuous with the fat-saturation T2 sequence.

Cervical Lymph Nodes

RETROPHARYNGEAL NODES

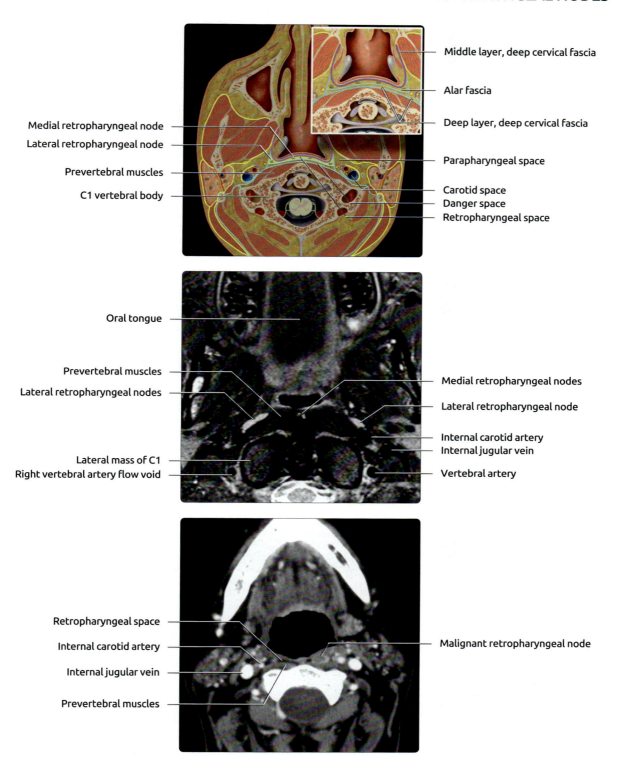

(Top) Axial graphic at the base of the skull demonstrates medial retropharyngeal nodes in the paramedian retropharyngeal space; the lateral retropharyngeal nodes are lateral to the prevertebral muscles and medial to the internal carotid artery (ICA). If a node lies within 2 cm of the skull base and medial to ICA, it is classified as retropharyngeal node, whereas if a node within 2 cm of skull base lies lateral, anterior, or posterior to the carotid sheath, it is a level II node. Note that below 2 cm of skull base, a level II node can lie medial, lateral, anterior, or posterior to the IJV. (Middle) Axial T2 MR with fat saturation shows the location of both medial and lateral retropharyngeal lymph nodes. Note the lateral group is located on the anterolateral surface of prevertebral muscles, just medial to the carotid space. (Bottom) Axial CECT at the level of the low oropharynx shows a small medial retropharyngeal node in a patient with posterior wall hypopharynx squamous cell carcinoma (not shown). Central low density suggests a malignant node despite the small size.

Cervical Lymph Nodes

NORMAL AND REACTIVE NODES: GRAYSCALE ULTRASOUND

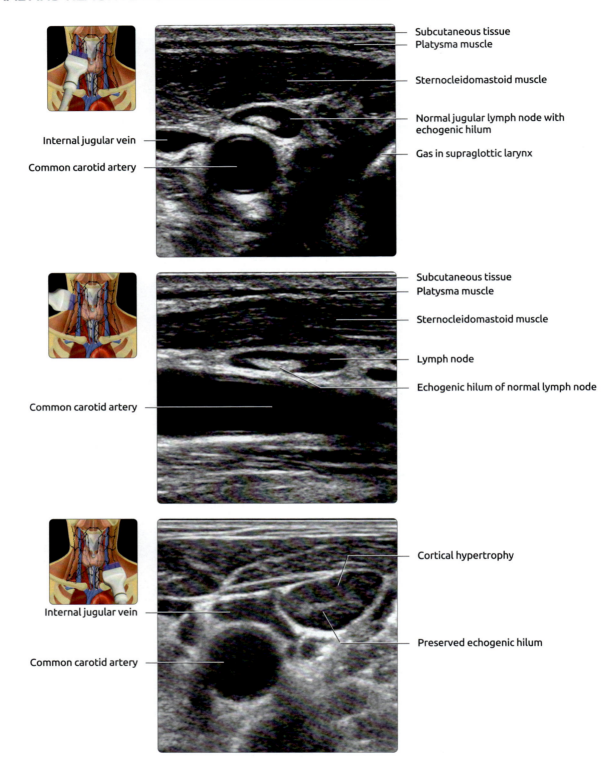

(Top) Transverse grayscale ultrasound of the midcervical level shows the normal appearance of a cervical lymph node (i.e., ovoid shape with echogenic hilum). It is commonly found anterior to the carotid artery/internal jugular vein. (Middle) Longitudinal grayscale ultrasound of the midcervical level shows a normal elliptical hypoechoic lymph node with echogenic hilum anterior to the common carotid artery. (Bottom) Transverse grayscale ultrasound shows a hypoechoic node with cortical hypertrophy and preserved echogenic hilum along the deep cervical/jugular chain. This is the classic appearance of a reactive node. Note its relation to internal jugular vein & common carotid artery. This is a common site of reactive nodes, which are often bilateral & symmetric.

Cervical Lymph Nodes

NORMAL AND REACTIVE NODES: POWER DOPPLER ULTRASOUND

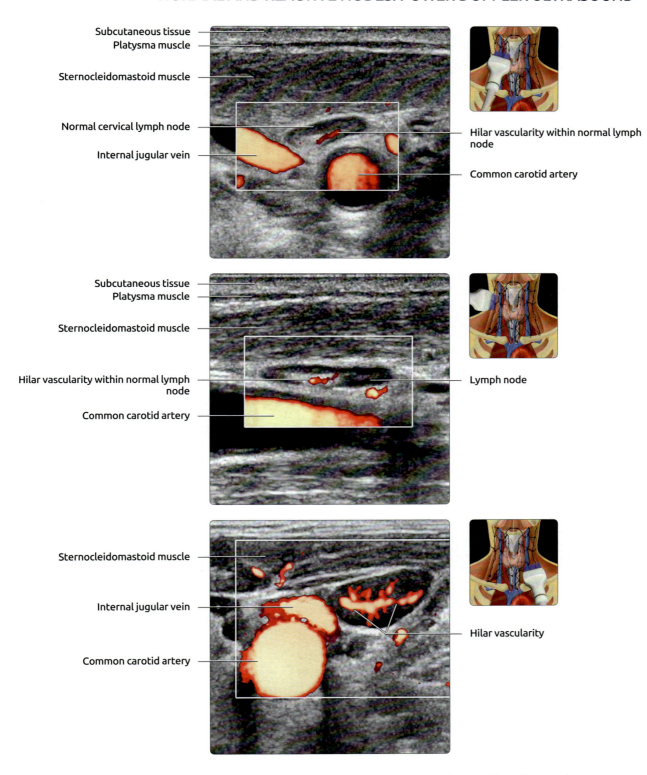

(Top) Transverse power Doppler ultrasound shows the presence of hilar vascularity within the echogenic hilum of a normal cervical lymph node. (Middle) Longitudinal power Doppler ultrasound shows hilar vascularity within the echogenic hilum of a normal cervical lymph node. The presence of echogenic hilum and hilar vascularity are good signs of cervical lymph node benignity. (Bottom) Power Doppler ultrasound of a reactive node clearly defines radiating hilar vascularity and relation to IJV and CCA.

Cervical Lymph Nodes

PATHOLOGY: GRAYSCALE ULTRASOUND

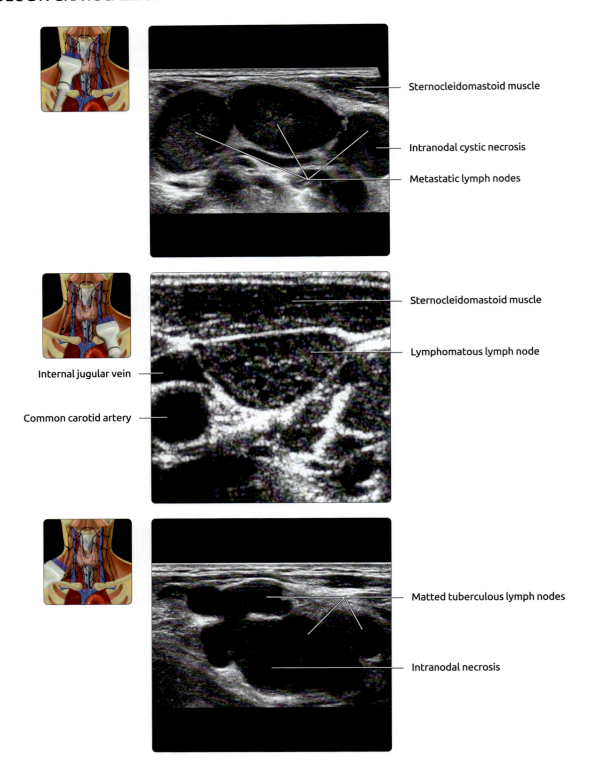

(Top) Transverse grayscale ultrasound of the upper neck shows multiple enlarged, round, predominantly solid, hypoechoic lymph nodes. Patient has a known history of H&N cancer. Presence of intranodal cystic necrosis in a patient with known primary malignancy is indicative of the metastatic nature of lymph nodes. (Middle) Transverse grayscale ultrasound of a lymphomatous lymph node in midjugular chain demonstrates the typical reticulated echo pattern without central necrosis. (Bottom) Transverse grayscale ultrasound shows multiple matted, enlarged, heterogeneous, hypoechoic lymph nodes in the posterior triangle of a patient with tuberculosis. Some of them demonstrate intranodal necrosis. A mild degree of edema is noted in the adjacent soft tissue. Features are compatible with tuberculous lymphadenitis.

Cervical Lymph Nodes

PATHOLOGY: POWER DOPPLER ULTRASOUND

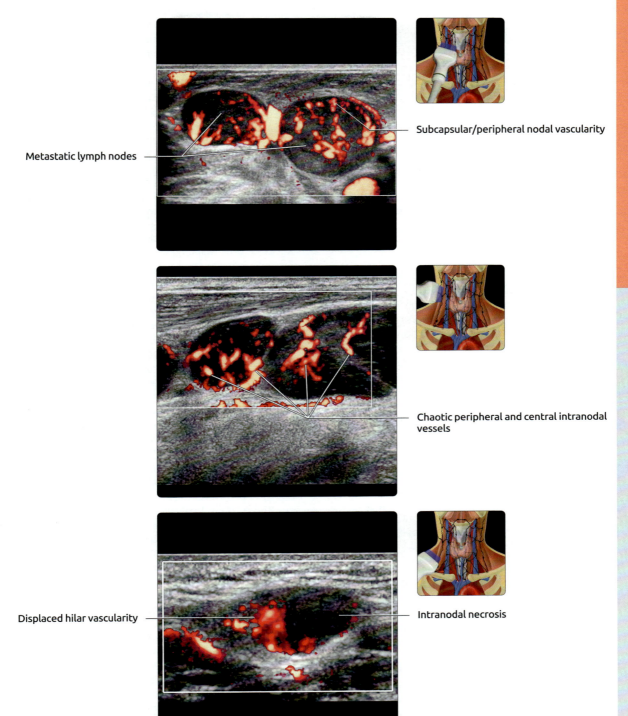

(Top) Transverse power Doppler ultrasound shows multiple subcapsular/peripheral intranodal vessels in multiple round, hypoechoic, solid lymph nodes at the upper cervical level. Pathology confirmed metastatic squamous cell carcinoma. (Middle) Longitudinal power Doppler ultrasound of multiple lymphomatous lymph nodes shows chaotic peripheral and central intranodal vessels. Note that hilar vascularity is more prominent than peripheral vascularity. (Bottom) Transverse power Doppler ultrasound shows a tuberculous lymph node in posterior triangle that is predominantly hypovascular with displaced hilar vascularity. The hypovascular portion corresponds to intranodal caseating necrosis.

Facial Muscles and Superficial Musculoaponeurotic System

TERMINOLOGY

Abbreviations

- Superficial musculoaponeurotic system (SMAS)

Definitions

- Termed "mimetic muscles/mimic muscles/muscles of facial mimicry" as primary function of facial muscles is facial expression
  - In face, muscles insert directly into dermis via SMAS allowing for facial expression (whereas in remainder of body, subcutaneous tissue is separated from muscle by investing layer of fascia)
- SMAS: Continuous organized fibrous network connecting facial muscles to dermis
- Modiolus: Dense fibromuscular structure at lateral border of corner of mouth formed by convergence of muscles attaching here

IMAGING ANATOMY

Overview

- Muscles of facial mimicry have their origin on bone but insert directly into dermis (through SMAS)
- Exceptions are inconsistently found risorius & malaris muscles, with both origin & insertion in soft tissue
- Other exceptions are tiny nasal muscles, namely compressor narium minor, dilator naris anterior (DNA) (both have origin from nasal cartilages & insert into skin), & dilator naris vestibularis (DNV) (origin & insertion in skin)
- Mimetic muscles act as sphincters & dilators of facial orifices & elevators & depressors of facial structures
- Adjacent muscles closely intertwined due to their common origin from mesoderm of 2nd branchial arch; large muscular sheets later differentiate into individual muscles
- Groups of facial muscles share common insertion sites; therefore identification is often easiest tracing them back from their insertion to less crowded origins
- 6 groups for purpose of easy identification, namely muscles inserting at 1) scalp, 2) orbit, 3) nose, 4) upper lip, 5) modiolus/angle of mouth, & 6) lower lip

Anatomy Relationships

- Layers of face, from superficial to deep
  - **Skin**
  - **Subcutaneous fat**: Deficient in eyelid, lips, & nose; extensive in cheek region called **malar fat pad** (fat pad beneath orbicularis oculi (OOc) muscle called **suborbicularis oculi fat pad**)
    - Malar fat pad is firmly fixed to dermis & also to thicker superior part of SMAS but loosely attached to thinner inferior SMAS; zygomatic ligament, which is osteocutaneous ligament on zygoma lateral to zygomaticus minor (Zmi) muscle origin, anchors malar fat to deeper tissue layers
    - Malar fat pad slides downward & inward over SMAS with aging, deepening nasolabial crease

- **SMAS** (superficial fascia): Connects muscles to overlying dermis of skin; SMAS continuous above with **temporoparietal fascia** (a.k.a. superficial temporal fascia or epicranial aponeurosis as it passes over zygomatic arch, which in turn is continuous with galea aponeurotica in scalp superiorly, frontalis muscle anteriorly, & occipitalis muscle posteriorly)
  - Temporoparietal fascia usually fibrous, sometimes contains vestigial muscles, namely **temporoparietal muscle** & **superior auricular muscle**
  - SMAS extremely thin beyond anterior border of masseter as it enters cheek area, barely traceable by position of split peripheral part of platysma
  - SMAS blends with platysma inferiorly & begins fading medially as it reaches lateral nasal margin
  - Lower 1/2 of SMAS is extremely thin & somewhat discontinuous with no mechanical bearing capacity
  - SMAS invests in & extends into external aspects of facial muscles, mainly frontalis, OOc, Zmi, zygomaticus major (Zmj), risorius, orbicularis oris (OOr), & platysma
  - SMAS composed of 3D scaffold of collagen & elastic fibers with interspersed fat cells
  - 2 distinct histological subtypes of SMAS described
    - **Type 1** comprises all of SMAS lateral to nasolabial fold, has meshwork of fibrous septa that envelop large lobules of fat cells & allow for connections with both facial muscles as well as periosteum; more susceptible to aging process than type 2
    - **Type 2** comprises SMAS medial to nasolabial fold in upper & lower lip, has meshwork of intermingled collagen, elastic & muscle fibers that reach up into dermis, much firmer connection to skin than type 1, dispersed fat cells seen as opposed to distinct fat lobules in type 1
    - Transition between type 1 & 2 SMAS at nasolabial fold is challenge for facial rejuvenation surgeries
    - CT: Hyperdense line between superficial & deep fibroadipose tissue; MR: T1/T2 hypointense line
  - **Facial nerve** (CNVII) dividing into branches inside parotid gland lies underneath investing fascia of parotid/parotideomasseteric fascia (deep fascia) in cheek that is deep to SMAS; making sub-SMAS dissection safe during facelift surgery
  - Facial nerve branches eventually traverse deep fascia in their anteromedial superficial course to innervate muscles of SMAS, most of which receive innervation from their deep surfaces
  - Facial nerve fibers become more superficial medially beyond facial artery & vein; knowledge of this anatomy is very important during face lift surgery to avoid nerve injury
  - Facial nerve branches lie in loose areolar plane between periosteum & temporoparietal fascia at zygomatic arch level, between temporalis fascia & temporoparietal fascia at 1 cm above zygomatic arch & then penetrates loose areolar plane & more superficial temporoparietal fascia at ~ 2 cm above arch to travel along with anterior branch of superficial temporal artery

Facial Muscles and Superficial Musculoaponeurotic System

- **Facial artery** curves upward over body of mandible at anteroinferior angle of masseter muscle → pass anterosuperiorly across cheek to location 8-23 mm lateral to labial commissure → ascends along side of nose to end at medial commissure of eye as **angular artery**; accompanied by **facial & angular veins**
- Internal maxillary artery, including its infraorbital artery branch lying in between levator labii superioris (LLS) & levator anguli oris (LAO) muscles, superficial temporal artery also supplies face
- **Superficial facial muscles** ("**mimic**" muscles")
- **Deep fascia**: **Parotideomasseteric fascia** enveloping parotid gland, duct, & masseter muscle; also envelops facial nerve peripheral branches, part of **buccal fat pad**; continues to superficial layer of deep cervical fascia inferiorly & superiorly to **temporalis fascia** (a.k.a. deep temporal fascia, which in turn covers temporalis muscle & splits inferiorly attaching around zygomatic arch & attaches superiorly to pericranium at & above superior temporal line on skull)
- **Retaining ligaments**: Connects overlying structures to underlying periosteum of facial bones

Internal Contents

- 6 groups of facial muscles based on insertion site

I: Muscles Inserting at Scalp

- **Frontal belly of occipitofrontalis (frontalis muscle)**: Origin from epicranial aponeurosis near coronal suture & insertion at skin of frontal region & galea aponeurotica
  - Partially intertwined with muscle fibers of adjacent corrugator supercilii (CS), procerus, & OOc
  - Furrows forehead, raises eyebrows, & widens eyes
  - Can cause horizontal hyperfunctional facial lines on forehead; botulinum toxin is commonly injected in this muscle to decrease these lines

II: Muscles Inserting at Orbit

- **OOc**: Origins: **Palpebral** portion from medial palpebral ligament, a.k.a. medial canthal tendon (inserts on lateral palpebral raphe), **orbital** portion from medial orbital rim (inserts laterally to palpebral portion), & **lacrimal** portion from lacrimal bone (insertion at upper & lower eyelids)
  - Medially, muscle is deep to medial canthal tendon
  - Palpebral part helps in light closure of eyelids whereas orbital part is used more forceful closure along with medial displacement of eyelids; thereby compressing eye globe & lacrimal sac, which in turn initiate flow of tears into nasolacrimal duct
  - Hyperactivity of lateral OOc can produce radial lines stemming from lateral canthus ("crow's feet")
  - **Malaris** muscle is inconsistent lateral muscular band of OOc that originates from superficial temporal fascia & terminates at either zygomatic arch or cheek region or angle of mouth; plays role in facial animation
  - Inconsistent medial muscular bands preventing drooping of OOc
  - Many muscular connections between OOc & ZMi may play role in facial expression
- **CS**: Origin on frontal bone at medial supraorbital margin & inserts into frontalis; 2 bellies, deep transverse belly & superficial oblique belly
  - Deep to frontalis

- Depresses brow, pulls it medially, & creates vertical skin creases as in frowning
- **Depressor supercilii (DS)**: Origin in region of medial orbital rim on frontal process of maxilla 2-5 mm below frontomaxillary suture; some fibers from lacrimal sac
  - Inserts into dermis 14-15 mm superior to medial canthal tendon (medial palpebral ligament)
  - DS interdigitates with adjacent OOc & CS
  - Depresses medial aspect of brow during frowning
- **Procerus**: Origin on lower end of nasal bone & upper part of upper lateral nasal cartilage
  - Inserts on forehead skin medial to eye & interdigitates with frontalis muscle
  - Displaces medial angle of eyebrow inferiorly, which also causes horizontal facial skin creases, frowning
  - Elevator of nose

III: Muscles Inserting at Nose

- Consists of nasal elevators (anomalous nasi, & 2 extrinsic muscles, namely procerus, which is described under muscles inserting at orbit & levator labii superioris alaeque nasir (LLSAN), which inserts at upper lip with medial slip inserting into alar cartilage); compressors (transverse nasalis & compressor narium minor), depressors (alar nasalis & depressor septi nasi), & dilators (DNA, DNV, & contribution from alar nasalis)
- **Anomalous nasi**: Origin on frontal process of maxilla & inserts into nasal bone, upper lateral nasal cartilage, procerus, & transverse nasalis; nasal elevator
- **Transverse nasalis**: Nasalis muscle has 2 parts, namely transverse nasalis & alar nasalis
  - Origin of transverse nasalis on canine eminence of maxilla superolateral to incisive fossa & inserts expanding into thin aponeurosis continuous on bridge of nose with contralateral transverse nasalis & aponeurosis of procerus; main nasal compressor
  - Hyperactivity can cause radial lines along dorsum of nose as far down to lower border of lower lateral cartilage (greater alar cartilage), so called "bunny lines"
- **Alar nasalis**: Origin on maxilla just medial to transverse nasalis above lateral incisor tooth; is located anterior to transverse nasalis & ascends anterolaterally to insert on alar-facial crease & adjacent deep surface of external skin of alar lobule; nasal depressor & also helps to dilate nares (hence it is also sometimes called dilator naris posterior) & prevent collapse during breathing
- **Depressor septi nasi**: Origin in incisive fossa of maxilla located further medial to origin of alar nasalis & inserts on base & lateral surface of medial crus of greater alar cartilage; nasal depressor
  - Medially, attaches to dermocartilagenous ligament, which is sandwiched by medial crus of greater alar cartilage
- **DNA**: Origin on frontal surface of lateral 1/2 of lateral crus of greater alar cartilage & adjacent accessory alar cartilage & inserts on skin of nose superior to alar groove (supraalar crease); dilator of nasal vestibule (nasal vestibule is most anterior nasal cavity)
- **DNV**: Origin on external skin of alar lobule, radiates along dome of nasal vestibule & inserts on vestibular skin of alar lobule; dilator of nasal vestibule

Suprahyoid and Infrahyoid Neck

441

Facial Muscles and Superficial Musculoaponeurotic System

- **Compressor narium minor**: Origin on anterior part of greater alar cartilage & inserts into skin near margin of nostril; nasal compressor

IV: Muscles Inserting at Upper Lip

- **LLS**: Origin on inferior margin of orbit just above infraorbital foramen deep to OOc & inserts on upper lip; raises upper lip
- **LLSAN**: Origin on frontal process of maxilla & inserts in 2 places, one at greater alar cartilage & skin of nose & another at muscles of upper lip; elevates nose & dilates nares & displaces upper lip superomedially
  - LLSAN & LLS can be injected with botulinum toxin to decrease gingival show or "gummy smile" whereby they are prevented from contracting, which in turn decreases superior displacement of upper lip
- **ZMi**: Origin on zygoma posterior to zygomaticomaxillary suture & inserts on upper lip; displaces upper lip superiorly resulting in deepening of nasolabial furrow during expression of contempt
  - Attaches to both upper lip & ala of nose in ~ 1/4 of cases
  - LLS, LLSAN, & ZMi pass through OOr at upper lip insertion contributing to nasolabial fold

V: Muscles Inserting at Modiolus/Angle of Mouth

- Tendinous tissue nodule in modiolus seen in 20%; facial artery passes 1 mm lateral to lateral border of modiolus
- **ZMj**: Origin on zygoma (behind ZMi origin) anterior to zygomaticotemporal suture & inserts at modiolus; raises angle of mouth superiorly & posteriorly & helps to smile or laugh; bifid ZMj can cause cheek "dimple" due to fascial strands inserting into dermis & causing dermal tethering effect
  - At modiolar insertion, deep to LAO, or if ZMj is bifid, then LAO passes between its 2 heads
  - Main insertion of deep muscle band of ZMj is at anterior margin of buccinator muscle & its fascia; key relationship in facial animation (even though buccinator is not classified as muscle of facial mimicry)
- **OOr**: Origin from other facial muscles converging to mouth; bony origin of upper portion on alveolar border of maxilla & lower portion on mandible lateral to mentalis; insert at angle of mouth
  - Sphincter of mouth, which brings lips close to teeth & alveoli, brings lips together & protrudes lips forward
  - Hyperactivity can result in radial lines around mouth, also known as "lipstick lines" or "smoker's lines"; treated with botulinum toxin in combination with lip fillers
- **LAO**: Origin in canine fossa of maxilla well below infraorbital foramen & inserts at modiolus just superficial to ZMj insertion; displaces lip angle superiorly & results in deepening of nasolabial furrow
  - In its superior aspect, LAO is deep to LLS; **infraorbital vessels & nervous plexus** lie between them
- **Depressor anguli oris (DAO)**: Origin on oblique line of mandible lateral & inferior to depressor labii inferioris (DLI), also interdigitates with platysma & inserts at corner of mouth as narrow fasciculus; depresses angle of mouth during expression of grief & displaces angle medially when contracted simultaneously with LAO
  - Some fibers may continue below mental tubercle joining contralateral DAO & creating **transversus menti** muscle

- **Risorius**: Inconsistent muscle, most fibers originating from SMAS (superficial fascia), some fibers from parotidomasseteric fascia (deep fascia); in some cases receives platysma fibers & inserts at modiolus in 3 distinct superficial, flush, & deep layers in relation to DAO; displaces skin of cheek posteriorly, stretches lower lip & displaces corner of mouth inferolaterally during grinning

VI: Muscles Inserting at Lower Lip

- **DLI**: Origin on oblique line of mandible between mental foramen & symphysis (superomedial to DAO origin), also interdigitates with platysma & inserts on skin of lower lip & OOr; displaces lower lip inferiorly & slightly laterally
- **Mentalis**: Origin in incisive fossa of mandible & inserts on skin of chin; only elevator of lower lip; elevates & protrudes lower lip & can wrinkle chin, which if deep may be treated with botulinum toxin
- **Platysma**: Origin on superficial pectoral & deltoid fascia & inserts on inferior body of mandible & into skin & hypodermis; depresses lower mandible & lower lip

ANATOMY IMAGING ISSUES

Imaging Recommendations

- Most of "mimic muscles" identified in thin-section CT & 3-mm T1 & T2W MR with accurate knowledge of anatomy

CLINICAL IMPLICATIONS

Clinical Importance

- Important landmarks for surgical procedures: Facial rejuvenation, rhytidectomy (face lift), cleft lip/palate repair
- Wrinkles on face are actually perpendicular to action of muscles there, very important point when considering injection treatment like botulinum toxin to get rid of them
- Atrophy of facial fat pads plays significant role in aging process, & its anatomy is important in cosmetic surgery
- "Marionette lines" or "melomental folds" are long vertical lines laterally circumscribing chin, extending downward from oral commissures, appear with aging when ligaments, skin & fat around mouth & chin sag; treated with injectable fillers & surgeries, including face lift
- Imaging identification of denervation changes in facial muscles: Numerous etiologies, including neoplasms (CNVII & CNVIII schwannoma), Bell palsy, myotonic dystrophy, myasthenia gravis, iatrogenic (parotidectomy)
- Involved in tumors, including lesions along SMAS & facial muscles & perineural spread along CNV & CNVII in relation to SMAS: Lymphoma, squamous cell cancer

Major Contributor Muscles to Common Facial Expressions

- **Surprise**: Frontalis
- **Frowning**: CS, DS, & procerus
- **Anger**: DNA, DNV, depressor septi nasi
- **Contempt**: ZMi
- **Smiling & laughing**: ZMj
- **Grinning**: Risorius
- **Sadness**: LLS, LAO; **grief**: DAO
- **Doubt**: Mentalis
- **Whistling**: Buccinator, OOr
- **Horror, terror, & fright**: Platysma

Facial Muscles and Superficial Musculoaponeurotic System

GRAPHIC: FACIAL MIMIC MUSCLES

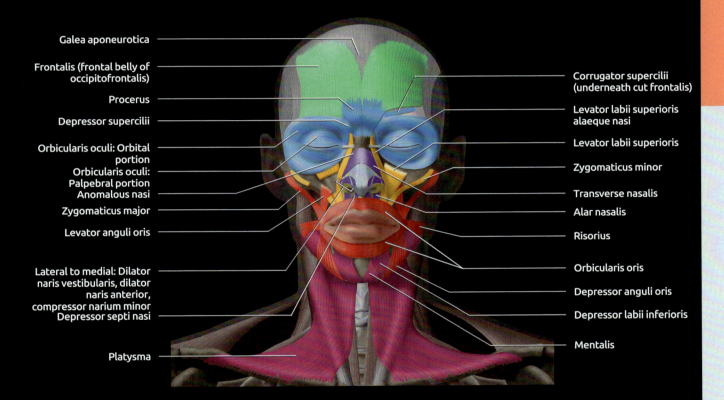

Frontal graphic shows facial mimic muscles color coded into 6 groups according to common insertion sites: Scalp is green, orbit is blue, nose is purple, upper lip is yellow, modiolus/angle of mouth is red, and lower lip is magenta.

Facial Muscles and Superficial Musculoaponeurotic System

GRAPHIC: ORIGIN OF FACIAL MUSCLES

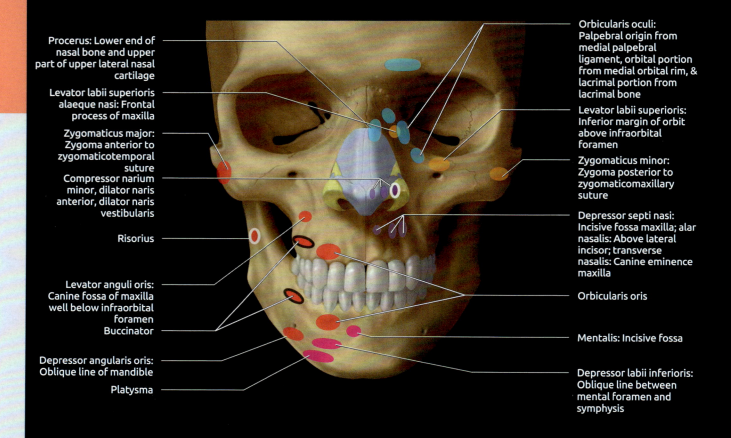

Muscle groups follow color coding similar to the graphic above. Muscles of facial mimicry originate on bone and insert into the dermis through the superficial musculoaponeurotic system (SMAS); exceptions are inconsistently found risorius and malaris muscles that originate and insert in soft tissue and also tiny nasal muscles, namely compressor narium minor and dilator naris anterior (both originate from nasal cartilages and insert into skin) and dilator naris vestibularis (originate and insert into skin). Note that the buccinator muscle making up the bulk of the cheek and forming the lateral wall of oral cavity is not classified as a muscle of facial mimicry, it originates on the alveolar processes of the mandible and maxilla near molar teeth and the pterygomandibular raphe and inserts around the mouth; medial fibers decussate and merge with the upper and lower lip muscles.

Facial Muscles and Superficial Musculoaponeurotic System

CORONAL T2 MR

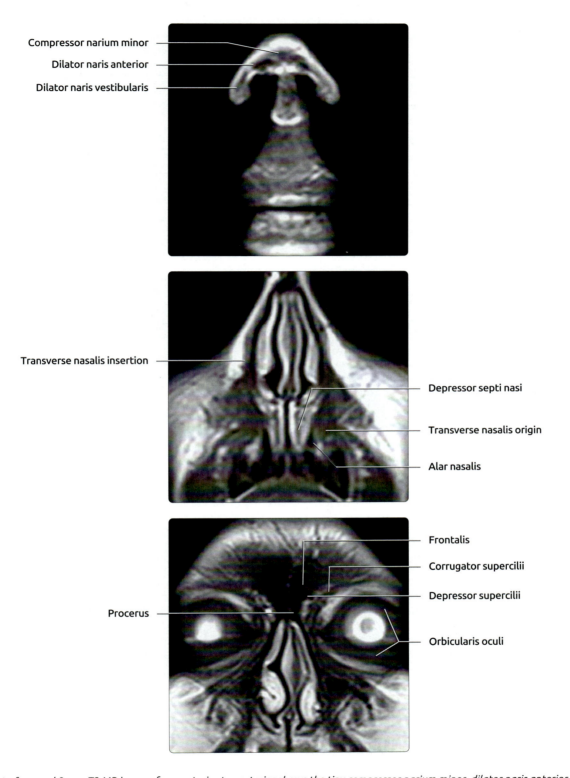

(Top) First of coronal 3-mm T2 MR images from anterior to posterior shows the tiny compressor narium minor, dilator naris anterior, and dilator naris vestibularis, which do not have bony origins. **(Middle)** Coronal T2 MR though the soft tissues of the nose shows the depressor septi nasi originating in the maxillary incisive fossa, just laterally is the alar nasalis originating above the maxillary lateral incisor, and further laterally is the transverse nasalis originating from the maxillary canine eminence. The depressor septi nasi inserts near the nasal septum into the medial crus of the greater alar cartilage, the alar nasalis lies anterior to the transverse nasalis and inserts into the nasal alar lobule skin and alar-facial crease, and the transverse nasalis continues up across the nasal bridge. **(Bottom)** Coronal T2 MR though the ventral aspects of the orbits shows the frontalis inserting at the scalp, corrugator and depressor supercilii, and procerus, and the orbicularis oculi inserting around the eye region.

Facial Muscles and Superficial Musculoaponeurotic System

AXIAL T1 MR

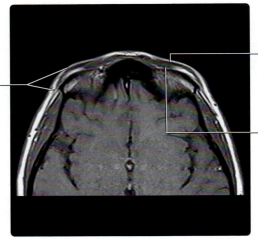

- Temporoparietal fascia merging with frontalis muscle
- Frontalis (frontal belly of occipitofrontalis)
- Corrugator supercilii

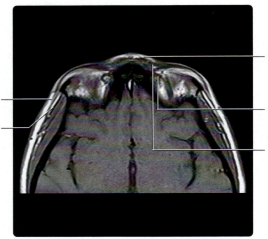

- Temporoparietal fascia (superficial fascia)
- Temporalis fascia (deep fascia)
- Procerus: Insertion into skin and frontalis
- Trochlea of superior oblique muscle near its attachment on superior nasal aspect of frontal bone
- Depressor supercilii: Insertion into dermis

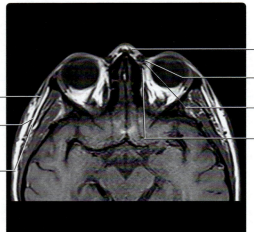

- Temporoparietal fascia (superficial fascia)
- Loose areolar plane in between superficial and deep fascia (facial nerve branches location)
- Temporalis fascia (deep fascia)
- Procerus: Origin on nasal bone
- Depressor supercilii: Origin on frontal process of maxilla
- Medial canthal tendon
- Anomalous nasi: Origin on frontal process of maxilla

(Top) Axial 3-mm T1 MR image series from superior to inferior is shown. MR at the forehead shows the corrugator supercilii originating from the frontal bone at the medial supraorbital rim and lying deep to the frontalis to which it attaches. Note the temporoparietal fascia (superficial fascia) merging with the frontalis muscle. (Middle) Axial T1 MR at the uppermost orbital level shows the insertion of the procerus and depressor supercilii. (Bottom) Axial T1 MR at eye lens level shows the origin of the procerus muscle on the nasal bone (inserts around the orbit and acts as a nasal elevator also) and depressor supercilii (inserts around orbit) and anomalous nasi (inserts at nose) on frontal process of the maxilla. Note that facial nerve branches at the temple lie in the fat of the loose areolar plane between the temporoparietal fascia and temporalis fascia until 2 cm above the zygomatic arch and then pierce the temporoparietal fascia.

Facial Muscles and Superficial Musculoaponeurotic System

AXIAL T1 MR

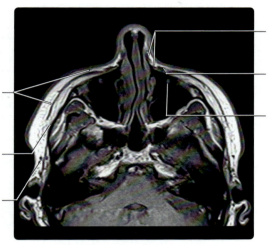

- Superficial musculoaponeurotic system merging with orbicularis oculi anteriorly and temporoparietal fascia (superficial fascia) superiorly
- Zygomatic arch
- Parotideomasseteric fascia (deep fascia) merging with temporalis fascia (deep fascia) superiorly
- Levator labii superioris alaeque nasi: Fibers to nose anteriorly and upper lip posteriorly
- Levator labii superioris just below its origin on inferior margin of orbit
- Infraorbital vessels and nerve partial volume in upper maxillary sinus

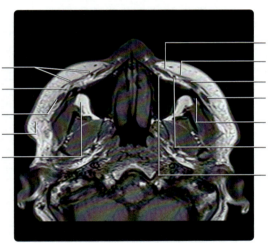

- Superficial musculoaponeurotic system
- Zygomaticus minor extremely thin on right
- Zygomaticus major
- Malar fat pad
- Retromaxillary fat pad (part of buccal space)
- Levator labii superioris
- Superficial musculoaponeurotic system
- Zygomaticus minor
- Zygomaticus major
- Zygoma
- Facial vessels
- Infraorbital vessels/nerve

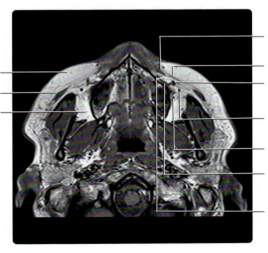

- Malar fat pad
- Zygomaticus major
- Buccal pat pad
- Levator labii superioris near upper lip insertion
- Superficial musculoaponeurotic system
- Facial vein (predictable course; larger than artery)
- Facial artery (variable tortuous course)
- Buccal artery
- Levator anguli oris: Origin from canine fossa of maxilla (deepest muscle anterior to maxilla)
- Infraorbital vessels and nerve in between levator labii superioris and levator anguli oris

(Top) Axial T1 MR just below inferior orbit at upper maxillary sinus level shows 2 main muscles inserting at upper lip: Levator labii superioris alaeque nasi (LLSAN) (also nasal elevator) & levator labii superioris (LLS). Third upper lip muscle is zygomaticus minor (ZMi) shown in next image. LLSAN can be easily tracked down from its origin on frontal process of maxilla. LLS originates on infraorbital margin above infraorbital foramen, so infraorbital vessels & nerve run down deep to it over maxilla. **(Middle)** Axial T1 MR at lower zygomatic arch level shows that ZMi (attaching at upper lip) origin on zygoma is anterior to that of zygomaticus major (attaching at modiolus/angle of mouth). ZMi can be extremely thin uni/bilaterally. **(Bottom)** Axial T1 MR just above maxillary alveolus shows levator anguli oris (LAO) origin at maxillary canine fossa. LAO is deepest muscle anterior to maxilla; this is a key feature to separate this muscle (inserting into modiolus/angle of mouth region) from more superficial LLS & LLSAN (which can be traced towards upper lip). Infraorbital vessels & nerve running down deep to LLS now lies between LLS & LAO, whereas facial vessels run more laterally.

Facial Muscles and Superficial Musculoaponeurotic System

AXIAL T1 MR

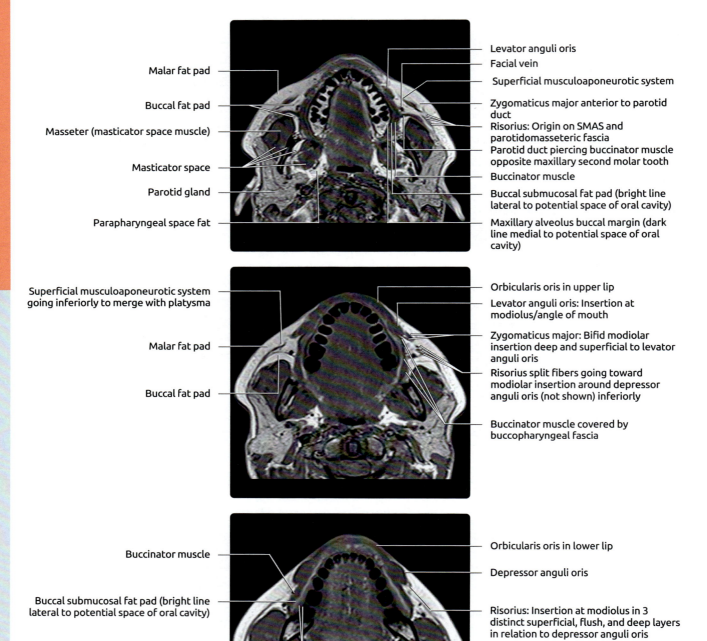

(Top) *Axial T1 MR at maxillary alveolus shows that the parotid duct divides the fat-filled buccal space into 2 compartments, with the anterior compartment fat pad extending anterior to the parotid duct and facial vein. Malar fat pad is subcutaneous, whereas buccal fat pad is deeper. Note that ZMj or risorius could be confused for parotid duct.* (Middle) *Axial T1 MR through the upper lip shows the orbicularis oris muscle makes up the bulk of the lip. ZMj insertion is bifid and LAO passes between its 2 heads at modiolar insertion (if not bifid, ZMj insertion is deep to LAO). The main insertion of the deep band of the ZMj is at the anterior margin of the buccinator muscle/fascia, key for facial animation.* (Bottom) *Axial T1 MR through the lower lip shows the orbicularis oris makes up the bulk of the lip, depressor anguli oris (DAO) and trilaminar insertion of risorius. DAO stands out at the lower lip and mandibular levels, but is not a muscle inserting at the lower lip. DAO can be traced superiorly to its modiolar insertion.*

Facial Muscles and Superficial Musculoaponeurotic System

AXIAL AND CORONAL T1 MR

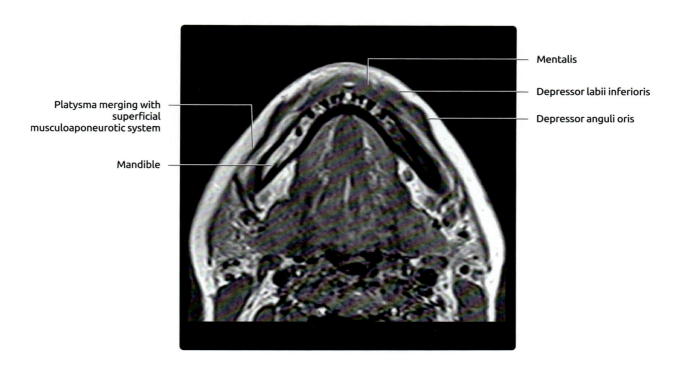

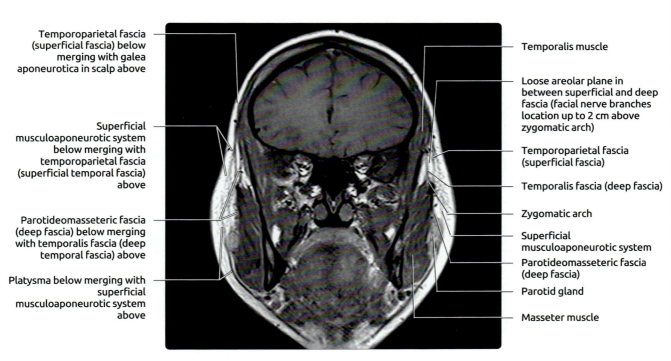

(Top) Axial T1 MR at lower mandible shows muscles inserting at the lower lip: Depressor labii inferioris, mentalis, and platysma. (Bottom) Coronal T1 MR shows fascial reflections. Parotidomasseteric fascia is continuous above with temporalis fascia (a.k.a. deep temporal fascia), which in turn covers the temporalis muscle and attaches inferiorly to zygomatic arch splitting over its superficial and deep surfaces, and superiorly to pericranium at and above the superior temporal line on skull. SMAS is continuous above with temporoparietal fascia (a.k.a. superficial temporal fascia) as it passes over the zygomatic arch, which in turn is continuous with galea aponeurotica in scalp superiorly, frontalis muscle anteriorly, and occipitalis muscle posteriorly. Facial nerve branches lie in the loose areolar plane between the periosteum and temporoparietal fascia at zygomatic arch level, between temporalis fascia and temporoparietal fascia at 1 cm above zygomatic arch, and then penetrate the loose areolar plane and more superficial temporoparietal fascia at about 2 cm above arch.

SECTION 6
Oral Cavity

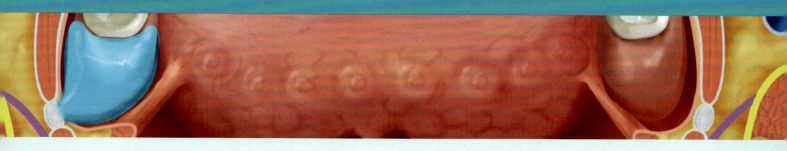

Oral Cavity Overview	**452**
Oral Mucosal Space	**460**
Sublingual Space	**462**
Submandibular Space	**468**
Buccal Space	**474**
Tongue	**480**
Retromolar Trigone	**486**
Mandible and Maxilla	**490**

Oral Cavity Overview

TERMINOLOGY

Definitions

- Oral cavity (OC): Area of suprahyoid neck below sinonasal region and anterior to oropharynx

IMAGING ANATOMY

Overview

- OC is separated from oropharynx by soft palate, anterior tonsillar pillars, and circumvallate papillae
- Suggested approach to OC imaging anatomy is to consider 4 distinct regions
  - **Oral mucosal space/surface (OMS)**
  - **Sublingual space (SLS)**: Nonfascial-lined area superomedial to mylohyoid muscle
  - **Submandibular space (SMS):** Located inferolateral to mylohyoid muscle
  - **Root of tongue (ROT)**: Made up of genioglossus-geniohyoid complex and lingual septum

Anatomy Relationships

- OC regional relationships
  - Superior: Hard palate, maxillary alveolar ridge
  - Lateral: Cheek-buccal space
  - Inferior: Mylohyoid muscle, mandibular alveolar ridge, and teeth
  - Posterior: Soft palate, anterior tonsillar pillars, and lingual tonsil (tongue base)
  - Anterior: Orbicularis oris sphincter with mucocutaneous junctions of upper and lower lips
- SLS relationships
  - Situated below floor of mouth mucosa and superomedial to mylohyoid muscle; lateral to extrinsic tongue muscles (genioglossus-geniohyoid)
  - Both SLSs communicate anteriorly beneath frenulum
    - Form "**horizontal horseshoe**" below oral tongue
  - Posteriorly SLS empties into posterosuperior aspect of SMS and inferior parapharyngeal space (PPS)
  - No fascia separates posterior SLS from SMS and inferior PPS
- SMS relationships
  - SMS is "**vertical horseshoe**" space between hyoid bone below and mylohyoid muscle sling above
  - SMS communicates posteriorly with inferior PPS and posterior SLS
  - SMS continues inferiorly as anterior cervical space
- ROT relationships
  - Inferiorly, ROT ends at hyoid and mylohyoid sling
  - Anteriorly, ends at mandibular symphysis (genioglossus/geniohyoid muscles insert on genial tubercles)

Internal Contents

- **Oral tongue**
  - Oral tongue: Anterior 2/3 of tongue
    - Base of tongue: Posterior 1/3 of tongue, including lingual tonsil of oropharynx considered part of oropharynx
  - **Intrinsic tongue muscles:** Represents major tissue of oral tongue
  - **Extrinsic tongue muscles**

- Genioglossus, hyoglossus, styloglossus, and palatoglossus serve to anchor main body of oral tongue to osseous structures and fibrous connective tissue to affect tongue movement and alter shape of tongue
- **Mylohyoid muscle**
  - Separates lower OC into SMS and SLS, except along free posterior margin
  - Arises from **mylohyoid line** of mandible
  - **Mylohyoid cleft** at junction of anterior 1/3 and posterior 2/3 of mylohyoid muscle
    - May be prominent with fat ± vessels ± accessory salivary tissue
- **OMS**
  - Squamous epithelial lining of OC, including tongue, buccal, gingival, palatal, and lingual surfaces
  - Submucosal **minor salivary glands** throughout OC
    - Most common locations are inner surface of lip, buccal mucosa, and palate
  - **Retromolar trigone**: Small, triangular-shaped region of mucosa behind last molar on mandibular ramus
    - Anatomical crossroads of OC, oropharynx, soft palate, buccal space, floor of mouth, masticator space, and PPS
- **SLS**
  - Lingual nerve: V3 sensory combined with CNVII chorda tympani nerve (anterior 2/3 of tongue taste) via submandibular ganglion
  - Distal CNIX (motor to stylopharyngeus muscle) and CNXII (motor to tongue)
  - Deep lingual artery and veins
  - Sublingual glands and Wharton ducts
  - Hyoglossus muscle anterior margin projects into posterior SLS
  - Deep portion of submandibular gland and submandibular gland duct
  - Deep lingual lymph nodes
- **SMS**
  - Large superficial portion of submandibular gland
  - Submental (level IA) and submandibular (level IB) lymph node groups
  - Facial vein and artery
  - Inferior loop of CNXII
  - Anterior belly of digastric muscles
- **Pterygomandibular raphe**
  - Fibrous band extending from posterior mandibular mylohyoid line to medial pterygoid plate hamulus
  - Buccinator and superior pharyngeal constrictor meet at pterygomandibular raphe
  - Lies beneath mucosa of retromolar trigone
  - Perifascial route of spread for squamous cell carcinoma

Fascia

- SLS is **not** lined by fascia
- SMS is lined by superficial layer of deep cervical fascia
  - Deeper slip of fascia runs along external surface of mylohyoid muscle, and more shallow slip parallels deep margin of platysma
  - No fascia separates posterior SMS and SLS from inferior PPS

Oral Cavity Overview

GRAPHICS

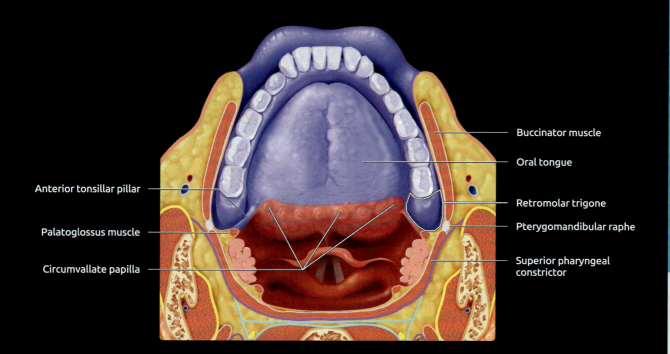

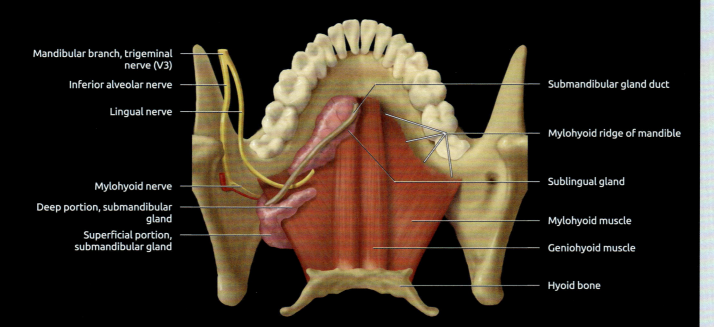

(Top) *Graphic from above shows the oral mucosal space/surface shaded in blue. Notice the circumvallate papilla, a superficial line of taste buds, divides the anterior oral cavity from the posterior oropharynx. The lingual tonsil is part of the oropharynx, not the oral cavity. The pterygomandibular raphe connects the posterior margin of the buccinator muscle to the anterior margin of the superior pharyngeal constrictor muscle. It also represents a key route of perifascial spread of squamous cell carcinoma of the retromolar trigone.*
(Bottom) *Graphic shows the floor of the mouth from above. The mylohyoid muscle sling is the principal structure of the floor of the mouth. This muscle attaches to the hyoid bone inferiorly and the mylohyoid ridge of the medial mandibular cortex. Superomedial to the mylohyoid muscle is the sublingual space, while the submandibular space is inferolateral to this muscle.*

Oral Cavity Overview

GRAPHICS

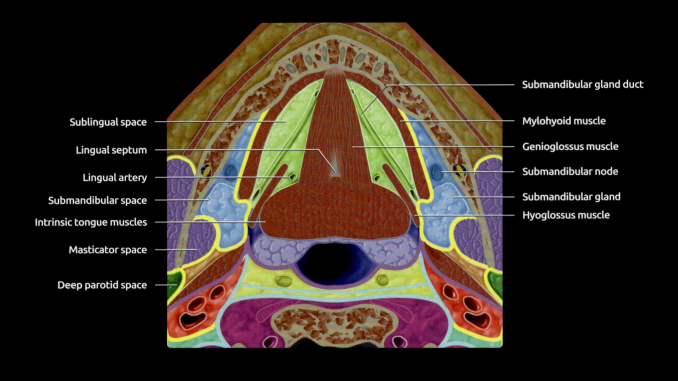

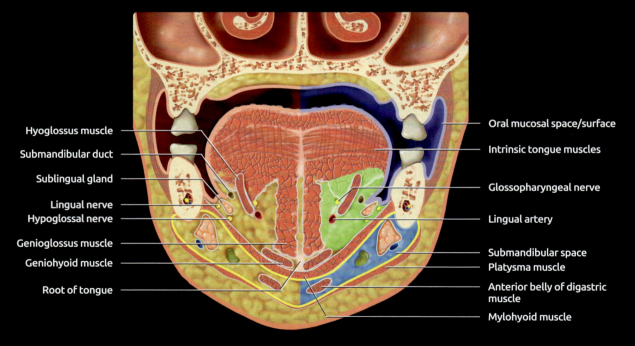

(Top) Axial graphic through the oral cavity shows the superficial layer of the deep cervical fascia (yellow line) circumscribing masticator and parotid spaces posteriorly and defining the deep margin of the submandibular space anteriorly, colored in blue. Note the principal occupants of the submandibular space are the submandibular gland and nodes. The green sublingual space has many structures within it, including the sublingual gland, submandibular duct, and anterior margin of the hyoglossus, to name a few. **(Bottom)** In this coronal graphic through the oral cavity, the mylohyoid muscle is seen stretched from side to side from the mylohyoid ridges. The mylohyoid muscle separates the sublingual space (green) from the submandibular space (blue). The sublingual space contains the lingual nerve and artery, submandibular duct, CNIX and CNXII, and sublingual gland. Genioglossus and geniohyoid complex with the lower lingual septum forms the root of the tongue.

Oral Cavity Overview

AXIAL CECT

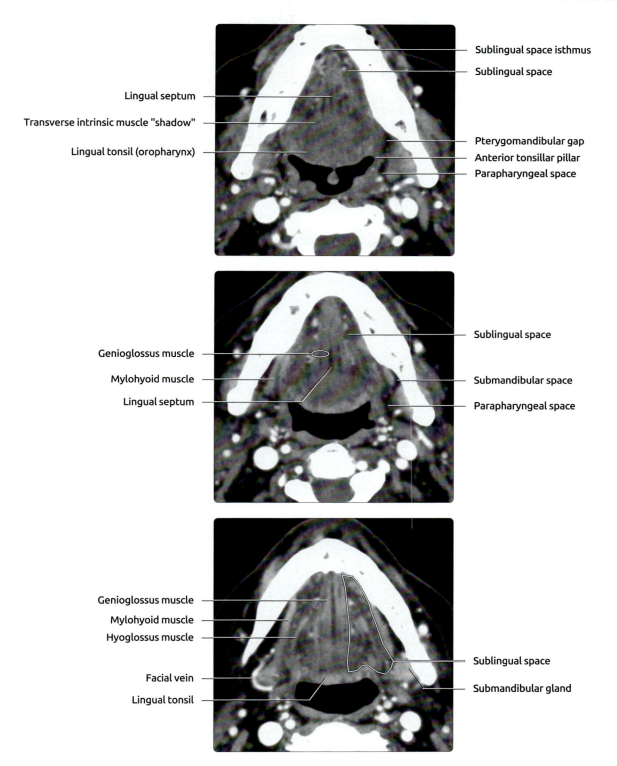

(Top) First of 6 axial CECT images of the oral cavity presented from superior to inferior is shown. On the most cephalad image, the parapharyngeal space can be seen emptying anteriorly into the submandibular space via the pterygomandibular gap. (Middle) The large paired genioglossus muscles are seen on either side of the lingual septum. The cephalad submandibular space fat is just coming into view. (Bottom) The sublingual space is lateral to the genioglossus muscle, superomedial to the mylohyoid muscle, and anterior to the lingual tonsil. On the patient's right, the facial vein curves around the lateral margin of the submandibular gland.

Oral Cavity Overview

AXIAL CECT

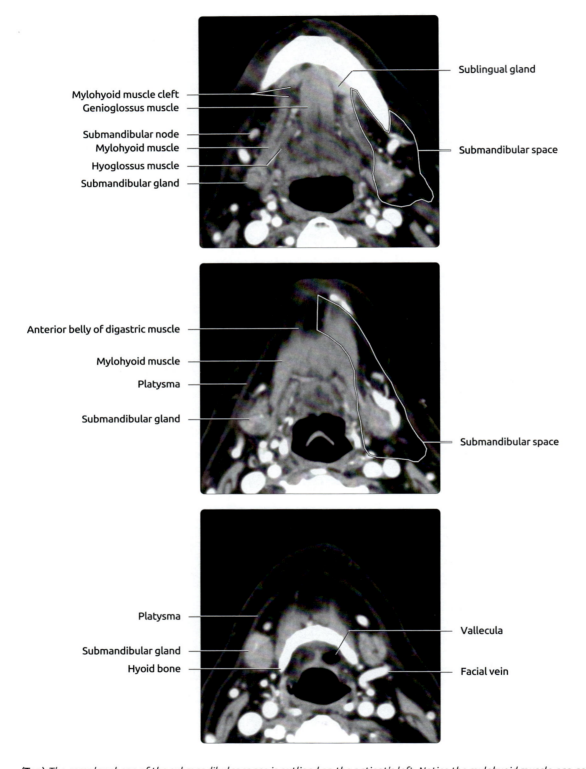

(Top) The complex shape of the submandibular space is outlined on the patient's left. Notice the mylohyoid muscle gap anteriorly on the right. This is a normal variant and can be large and fat-filled, as in this image. (Middle) The left 1/2 of the more inferior submandibular space is outlined. The submandibular gland and anterior belly of the digastric muscles are seen as normal occupants of this space. Remember, there is no vertical fascia dividing the 2 sides of the submandibular space. (Bottom) The platysma muscle represents the superficial border of the submandibular space. The anterior cervical space connects to the submandibular space in the infrahyoid neck.

Oral Cavity Overview

AXIAL T2 MR

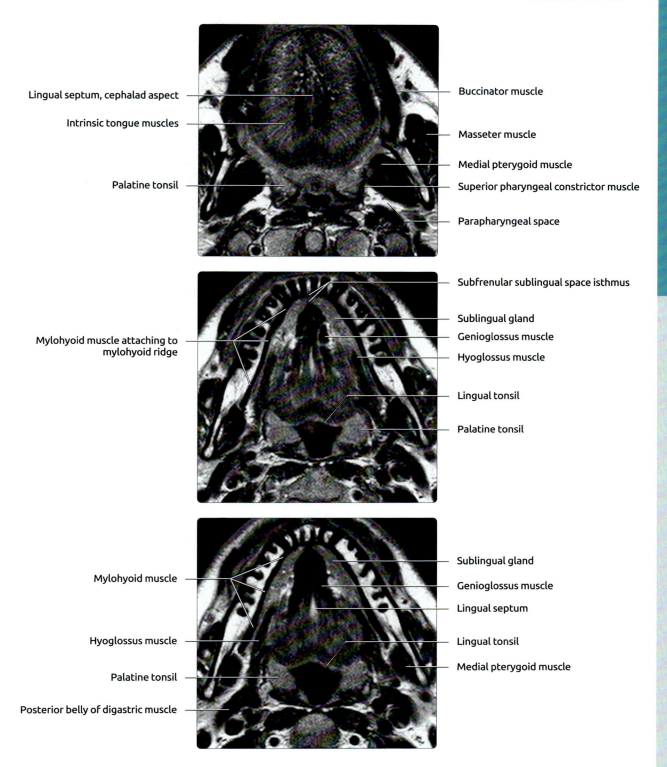

(Top) First of 6 axial T2 MR images through the oral cavity presented from superior to inferior is shown. This 1st image reveals the cephalad surface of the oral tongue. (Middle) In this image, the mylohyoid muscle can be seen attaching to the mylohyoid ridge bilaterally. The sublingual space communicates anteriorly in the subfrenular isthmus. (Bottom) In this image, the hyoglossus muscle is seen projecting into the posterior aspect of the sublingual space.

Oral Cavity Overview

AXIAL T2 MR

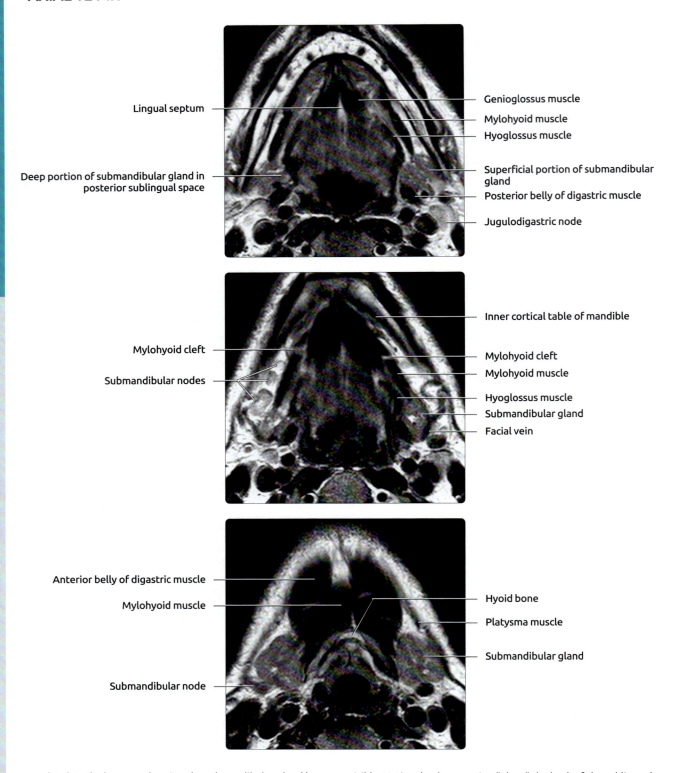

(**Top**) *In the lower oral cavity, the submandibular gland becomes visible. Notice the deep portion "plugs" the back of the sublingual space (visible on the left). The larger, superficial submandibular gland is in the submandibular space proper.* (**Middle**) *At the level of the inferior body of the mandible, the fatty gap in the mylohyoid muscle is visible. Also notice the multiple reactive submandibular nodes on the left.* (**Bottom**) *At the level of the hyoid bone, the bulk of the anterior bellies of the digastric muscles are visible. The platysma is seen as the superficial margin of the submandibular space.*

Oral Cavity Overview

CORONAL T1 MR

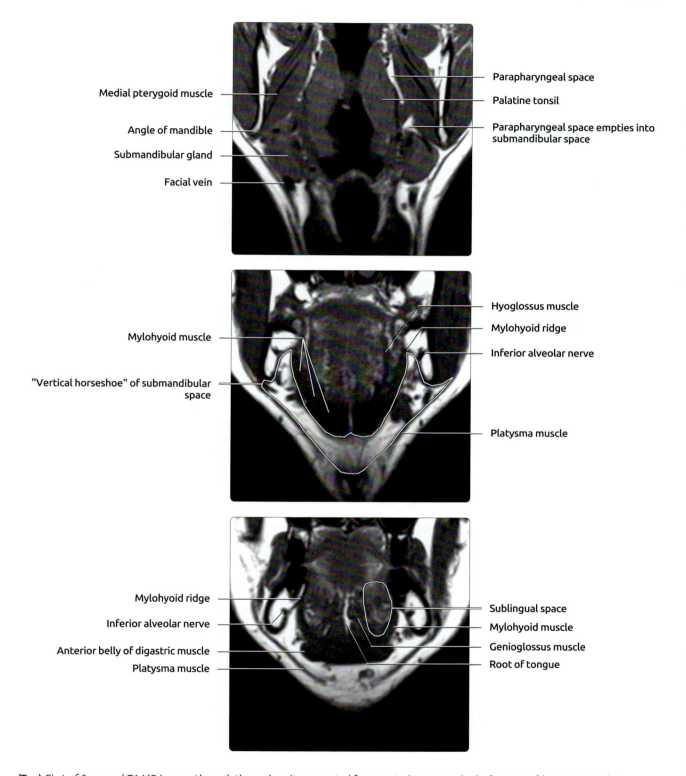

(Top) First of 3 coronal T1 MR images through the oral cavity presented from posterior to anterior is shown. In this most posterior image, the parapharyngeal space can be seen "emptying" inferiorly into the posterior submandibular space on the right. (Middle) This more anterior view delineates the "vertical horseshoe" of the submandibular space bounded superficially by the platysma and superomedially by the mylohyoid muscle. (Bottom) The sublingual space becomes more obvious in the anterior oral cavity. Notice it is a potential space drawn in on the right, lateral to the genioglossus muscle and superomedial to the mylohyoid muscle.

Oral Mucosal Space

TERMINOLOGY

Abbreviations
- Oral mucosal space/surface (OMS)

Definitions
- Mucosal surface of oral cavity extending from skin-vermilion junction of lips to junction of hard and soft palate above and to line of circumvallate papillae below

IMAGING ANATOMY

Overview
- OMS is constructed to complete radiologist's thinking regarding oral cavity (OC) locations where specific lesions primarily occur
- Since OMS describes mucosal surface of entire oral cavity, it represents continuous sheet of mucosa where squamous cell carcinoma (SCCa) may originate

Extent
- Anterior extent of OMS: Skin-vermilion junction of upper and lower lips
- Posterior extent of OMS
  - Posterosuperior extent: Junction of hard and soft palate
  - Posteroinferior extent: Junction of anterior 2/3 of tongue and posterior 1/3 of tongue at circumvallate papillae
    - Anterior 2/3 of tongue is **oral tongue**
    - Posterior 1/3 of tongue is **lingual tonsil**; part of **oropharynx**

Anatomy Relationships
- OMS represents continuous mucosal surface of OC, which sits anterior to mucosal surface of oropharynx
- Superior OMS overlies hard palate
  - Floor of nose and maxillary sinuses (palatine process of maxillary palatine bones) lie deep to this mucosa
- Inferior OMS overlies sublingual spaces and mylohyoid muscles

Internal Contents
- OMS is divided into 8 specific areas
  - **Mucosal lip**
    - Lip begins at vermilion border junction with skin
    - Includes only vermilion surface or portion of lip that makes contact with opposing lip
  - **Upper alveolar ridge mucosal surface**
    - Refers to mucosa overlying alveolar process of maxilla
    - Extends from line of attachment of mucosa in upper gingival buccal gutter to junction of hard palate
    - Posterior margin is upper end of pterygopalatine arch
  - **Lower alveolar ridge mucosal surface**
    - Refers to mucosa overlying alveolar process of mandible
    - Extends from line of attachment of mucosa in buccal gutter to line of free mucosa of floor of mouth
    - Posteriorly extends to ascending ramus of mandible
  - **Retromolar trigone** mucosal surface
    - Attached mucosa overlying ascending ramus of mandible
    - Extends from level of posterior surface of last molar tooth to apex superiorly, adjacent to tuberosity of maxilla
  - **Buccal mucosa**
    - Includes all membranes that line inner surface of cheeks and lips
    - Extends from line of contact of opposing lips to line of attachment of mucosa of alveolar ridge (upper and lower) and pterygomandibular raphe
  - **Floor of mouth mucosal surface**
    - Semilunar mucosal surface overlying mylohyoid and hyoglossus muscles
    - Extends from inner surface of lower alveolar ridge to undersurface of tongue
    - Posterior boundary is base of anterior pillar of tonsil
    - Divided into 2 sides by tongue **frenulum**
    - Contains ostia of submandibular and sublingual salivary glands
  - **Hard palate mucosal surface**
    - Semilunar mucosal area between upper alveolar ridge and mucous membrane covering palatine process of maxillary palatine bones
    - Extends from inner surface of superior alveolar ridge to posterior edge of palatine bone
  - **Anterior 2/3 of tongue (oral tongue) mucosal surface**
    - Mucosal surface overlying oral tongue
    - Extends anteriorly from line of circumvallate papillae (anterior edge of lingual tonsil) to undersurface of tongue at junction of mucosal surface of floor of mouth
    - Composed of 4 areas, including tongue tip, lateral borders, dorsum, and undersurface (nonvillous oral tongue ventral surface)
- Contents of OMS
  - Mucosal surface of OC
  - **Minor salivary glands** (MSG)
    - Lie within submucosa of OC, paranasal sinuses, pharynx, larynx, trachea, and bronchi
    - Particularly concentrated in buccal, palatal, and lingual submucosal regions
    - Mucinous or seromucinous in nature

Fascia
- **No** fascia exists to define OMS

CLINICAL IMPLICATIONS

Clinical Importance
- Primary malignancies arising from OMS include SCCa and MSG malignancy
- Vast majority of malignancies of OMS are SCCa whereas MSG malignancy is relatively rare
- Histologic transition from keratinized oral mucosa to nonkeratinized lining mucosa of oropharynx provides important route for viral invasion in human papillomavirus-related SCCa

Oral Mucosal Space

GRAPHICS

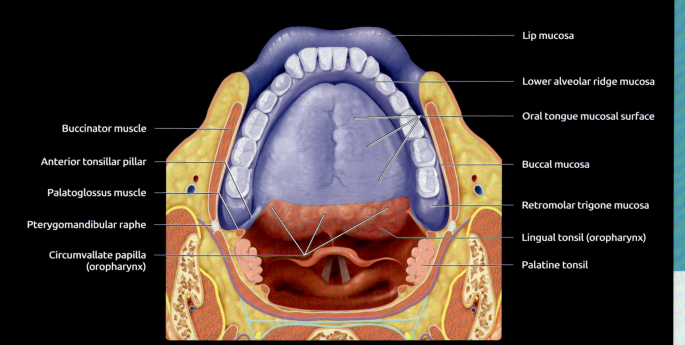

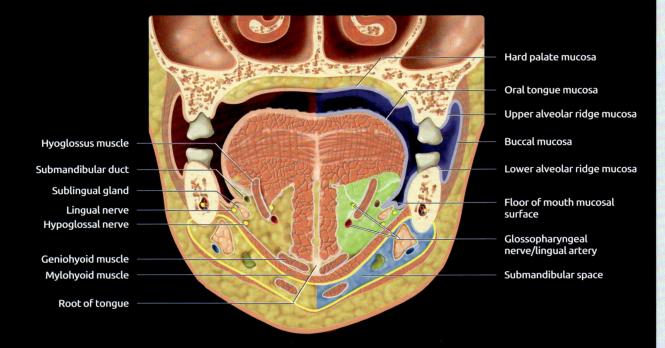

(Top) Axial graphic through the oral cavity and oropharynx is shown. The area in blue delineates the oral mucosal space/surface. Notice the posterior oropharynx contains the lingual and palatine tonsils. The circumvallate papilla are a superficial line of taste buds that separate the anterior oral cavity from the posterior oropharynx. (Bottom) In this coronal graphic through the oral cavity, the oral mucosal space/surface is again highlighted in blue. In this image, the hard palate, oral tongue, upper and lower alveolar ridge, buccal and floor of mouth mucosal surfaces are seen. Also notice that the 4 main areas of the oral cavity are all present: (1) Oral mucosal space/surface (blue), (2) sublingual space (green), (3) submandibular space (light blue), and (4) root of tongue.

Sublingual Space

TERMINOLOGY

Abbreviations

- Sublingual space (SLS)

Definitions

- SLS: Paired submucosal, nonfascial-lined spaces of oral cavity between floor of mouth (FOM) mucosa and mylohyoid muscular sling; separated by extrinsic tongue muscles in midline

IMAGING ANATOMY

Overview

- SLS contains sublingual gland, submandibular duct, and key neurovascular structures, including hypoglossal nerve (CNXII), lingual nerve (branch of V3), glossopharyngeal nerve (CNIX), lingual artery and vein

Anatomy Relationships

- SLS situated below FOM mucosa and **superomedial to mylohyoid muscle**; lateral to extrinsic tongue muscles (genioglossus-geniohyoid)
- Communication between SLSs occurs in midline anteriorly as narrow **isthmus** beneath frenulum; when lesion involves both SLSs and crosses isthmus anteriorly, it assumes the shape of **horizontal horseshoe** paralleling internal surface of mandible
- SLS communicates with submandibular space (SMS) at posterior margin of mylohyoid muscle
- **Mylohyoid** muscle may contain variable-sized **cleft** in its midportion that may allow communication between SLS and SMS

Internal Contents

- SLS is partially divided posteriorly into medial and lateral compartments by hyoglossus muscle
- **Lateral compartment contents**
  - **Sublingual gland and ducts**
    - Sublingual gland is smallest major salivary gland, measuring ~ 3 cm x 1 cm
    - Lies in anterior and lateral SLS; can extend into SMS through mylohyoid defect
    - ~ 5-15 small ducts (of Rivinus) open under oral tongue on summit of sublingual fold and drain into oral cavity; occasionally, few ducts unite to form Bartholin duct that joins submandibular duct
  - **Submandibular gland deep portion and submandibular (Wharton) duct**
    - Submandibular gland deep margin extends into posterior opening of SLS
    - Enlarging lesions of SLS in effect push this deep margin of submandibular gland out of way as they emerge from SLS into SMS
    - Submandibular duct runs anteriorly to sublingual papillae in anteromedial subfrenular mucosa
  - **Hypoglossal nerve**: Motor to tongue muscles
    - Intrinsic muscles of tongue include inferior lingual, vertical, and transverse muscles
    - Extrinsic muscles of tongue include genioglossus, hyoglossus, styloglossus, and palatoglossus muscles
  - **Lingual nerve**: Combined with chorda tympani nerve

- Lingual nerve branch of CNV3 (mandibular division of trigeminal): Sensation to anterior 2/3 of oral tongue
- Chorda tympani branch of facial nerve: Taste to anterior 2/3 of tongue; and parasympathetic secretomotor fibers to submandibular and sublingual salivary glands via its preganglionic parasympathetic supply from pontine superior salivatory nucleus to submandibular ganglion
- Chorda tympani nerve exits middle ear through petrotympanic fissure into masticator space and joins lingual nerve 2 cm below skull base
  - **Submandibular ganglion**
    - Fusiform ganglion, lies on hyoglossus muscle just above deep part of submandibular salivary gland
    - Suspended from lingual nerve by 2 roots; posterior root carries parasympathetic fibers to ganglion
    - Anterior root has postganglionic parasympathetic fibers reentering lingual nerve to supply sublingual salivary gland; those for submandibular salivary gland reach it through 5-6 direct branches from ganglion
    - Sympathetic fibers from plexus around facial artery contain postganglionic fibers arising from superior cervical ganglion and pass through submandibular ganglion without relay
- **Medial compartment contents**: Glossopharyngeal nerve above and lingual artery and vein below
  - **Glossopharyngeal nerve** (CNIX)
    - Provides sensation to posterior 1/3 of tongue
    - Carries taste input from posterior 1/3 of tongue
  - **Lingual artery and vein**: Supply oral tongue
    - Seen running just lateral to genioglossus muscle

ANATOMY IMAGING ISSUES

Imaging Recommendations

- CECT or T1 C+ MR with fat saturation are both excellent to evaluate SLS lesions
- MR better in cooperative patient, permits direct coronal imaging to assess relationship of lesion to mylohyoid muscle, and is less affected by dental amalgam artifact
- Bone windows on CT critical to evaluate
  - Glandular or ductal calculi in setting of sialolithiasis
  - Mandibular bony invasion by tumor in FOM
  - Odontogenic source of infection in SLS

Imaging Pitfalls

- Dental amalgam artifact obscures anatomy and pathology of FOM and SLS
- On MR or CT, difficult to differentiate enhancing tumor from normal enhancement of sublingual gland and adjacent oral mucosa

Imaging Issues Related to Malignancy

- While primary tumors of sublingual glands are uncommon, percentage of malignant tumors is high (70-85%)
- For squamous cell carcinoma (SCCa) of FOM, it is critical to evaluate for deep extension to tongue musculature and bony invasion of mandible
- Since neurovascular bundle to tongue travels in SLS, oral cavity SCCa involving posterior SLS is challenging to treat

Sublingual Space

GRAPHIC & AXIAL CECT

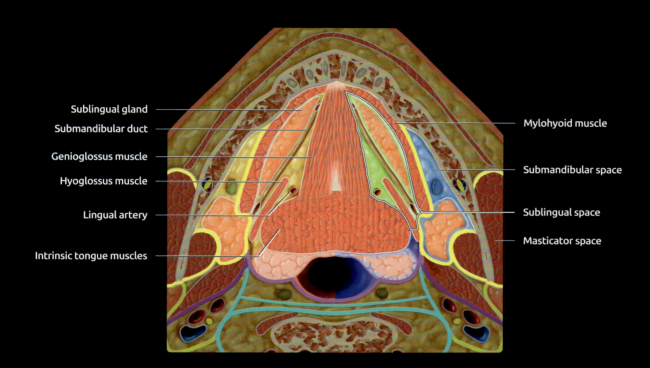

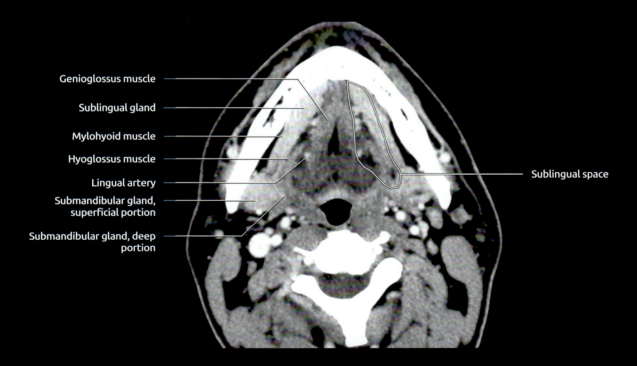

(Top) Axial graphic through the body of the mandible shows the sublingual space (on patient's left, shaded in green) situated superomedial to the mylohyoid muscle and lateral to the genioglossus muscle. Notice the absence of fascia surrounding the sublingual space. The yellow line represents the superficial layer of deep cervical fascia. (Bottom) Axial CECT shows the sublingual space outlined on the patient's left. Notice the difficulty on enhanced CT in separating the mylohyoid muscle from the sublingual gland. The deep portion of the submandibular gland projects into the posterior margin of the sublingual space.

Sublingual Space

GRAPHIC & CORONAL T1 MR

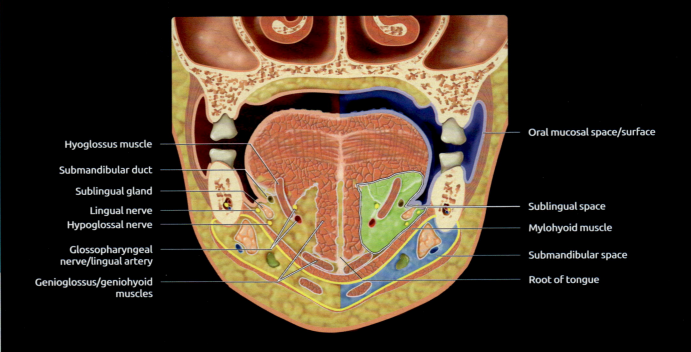

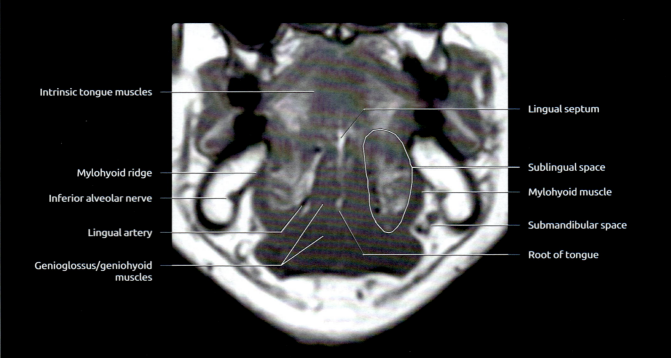

(Top) In this coronal graphic through the oral cavity, the sublingual space is shaded in green. The sublingual space medial compartment contents include the glossopharyngeal nerve (CNIX) superiorly and the lingual artery and vein inferiorly. Lateral sublingual space compartment contents include the lingual nerve superolaterally and submandibular (Wharton) duct and sublingual salivary gland and deep part of submandibular salivary gland in the middle and hypoglossal nerve (CNXII) inferomedially. Submandibular duct and lingual nerve cross each other at anterior border of hyoglossus. The fascia-lined (yellow line) submandibular space is inferolateral to the mylohyoid muscle. **(Bottom)** In this coronal T1 MR image, the sublingual space (a potential space not lined by fascia) is superomedial to the mylohyoid muscle and lateral to the genioglossus muscle. It is difficult to identify the margins of the genioglossus muscles.

Sublingual Space

AXIAL CECT

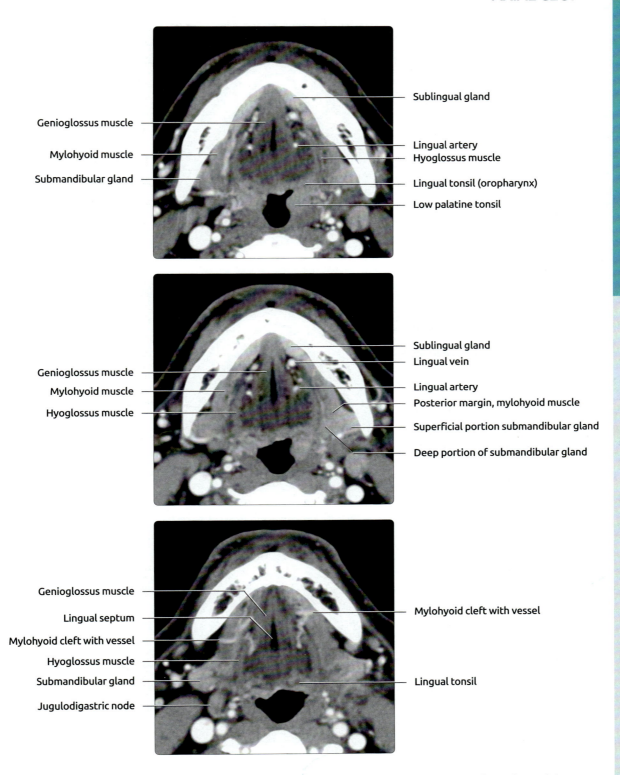

(Top) First of 3 axial CECT images of the sublingual space within the oral cavity is shown. This most superior image shows the medial border of the sublingual space is the genioglossus muscle. The hyoglossus muscles are seen projecting into the posterior sublingual spaces. (Middle) More inferiorly, a larger portion of the mylohyoid muscle can be seen forming the inferolateral border of the sublingual space. Notice the submandibular gland wrapping around the posterior margin of this muscle on the patient's left. The deep portion of the submandibular gland is found in the posterior sublingual space. (Bottom) Inferiorly, the sublingual spaces become smaller with the hyoglossus muscle filling most of this space. Both mylohyoid muscles demonstrate small clefts with a vessel present bilaterally.

Sublingual Space

AXIAL T2 FS MR

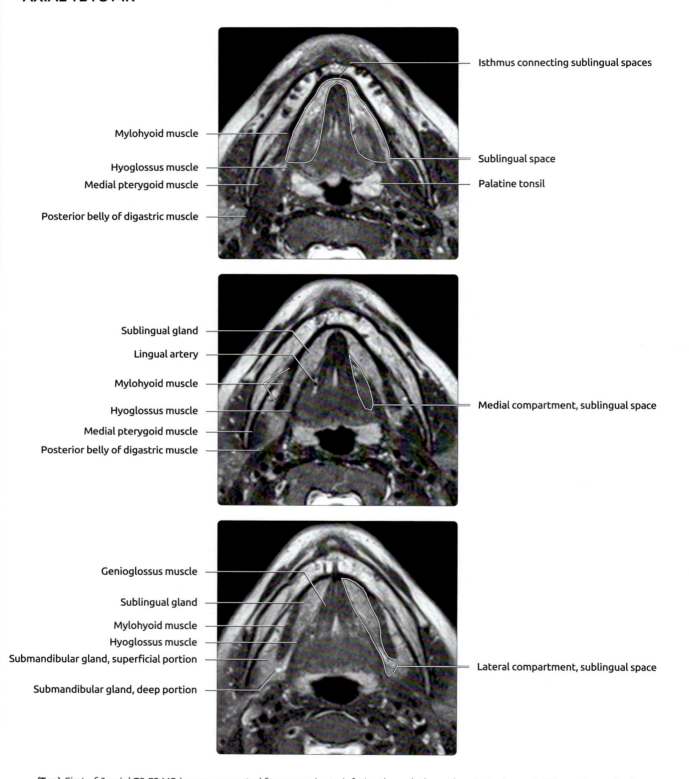

(Top) First of 3 axial T2 FS MR images presented from superior to inferior through the oral cavity is shown. In this most superior image, the 2 sublingual spaces are outlined to highlight the anterior connecting isthmus that is present under the frenulum of the oral tongue. (Middle) Slightly inferior, the medial compartment of the sublingual space is outlined on the patient's left. The medial compartment is defined as the sublingual space area medial to the hyoglossus muscle containing the lingual artery and vein as well as the glossopharyngeal nerve (CNIX). (Bottom) Continuing inferiorly, the submandibular gland deep portion is seen projecting into the posterior margin of the sublingual space. The lateral compartment of the sublingual space is outlined. It is defined as the sublingual space component lateral to hyoglossus muscle. It contains the sublingual gland, lingual nerve, hypoglossal nerve, and submandibular gland duct.

Sublingual Space

CORONAL T1 MR

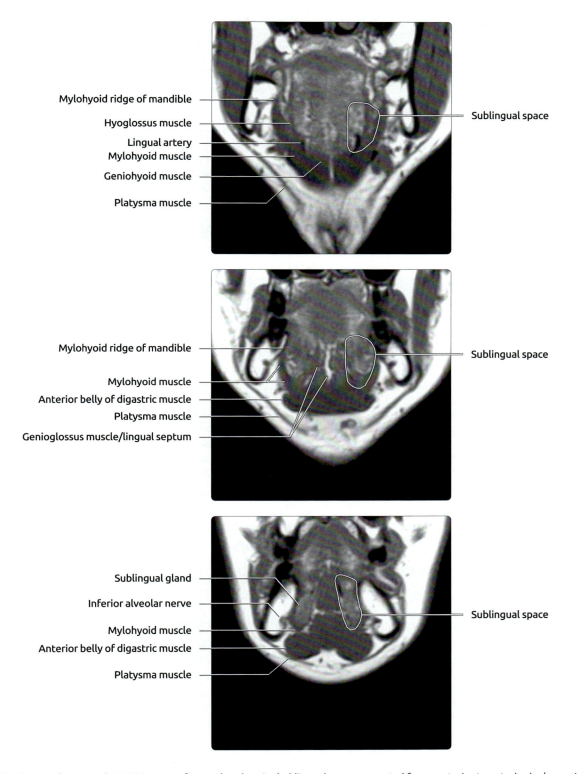

(Top) First of 3 coronal T1 MR images of normal oral cavity/sublingual space presented from posterior to anterior is shown. In this most posterior image, the mylohyoid sling is slung from side to side between mylohyoid ridges of inner mandibular cortex. The sublingual space is superomedial to the mylohyoid muscle and lateral to the genioglossus and geniohyoid muscles. (Middle) Anteriorly, in the oral cavity, the true size of sublingual space is visible as delineated on the patient's left. Although it is possible to see the low-signal lingual artery, the remaining normal sublingual space structures are blended into the fibrofatty space itself. (Bottom) In the very anterior floor of the mouth, the anterior belly of digastric muscles are the most prominent occupants of the submandibular space. The sublingual gland is mostly found within the anterior sublingual space where it takes up much of the space's volume.

Submandibular Space

TERMINOLOGY

Abbreviations

- Submandibular space (SMS)

Synonyms

- Term "submaxillary space" used by surgeons

Definitions

- Fascial-lined space inferolateral to mylohyoid muscle containing submandibular gland (SMG), nodes, and anterior belly of digastric muscles

IMAGING ANATOMY

Overview

- SMS is 1 of 4 distinct locations within oral cavity used to develop location-specific differential diagnoses
  - Other 3 locations include oral mucosal space/surface, sublingual space, and root of tongue

Extent

- SMS is defined as superficial space above hyoid bone deep to platysma and superficial to mylohyoid sling

Anatomy Relationships

- **Inferolateral to mylohyoid muscle**
- Deep to platysma muscle
- Cephalad to hyoid bone
- **Vertical horseshoe-shaped** space between hyoid bone below and mylohyoid sling above
- Communicates posteriorly with sublingual space and inferior parapharyngeal space at posterior margin of mylohyoid muscle
- Continues inferiorly into infrahyoid neck as anterior cervical space

Internal Contents

- **SMG**
  - Superficial portion is larger and in SMS itself
    - Superficial layer, deep cervical fascia (SL-DCF) forms SMG capsule
    - Crossed by facial vein and cervical branches of facial nerve (marginal mandibular branch)
  - Smaller deep portion often called deep "process"
    - Deep process is tongue-like extension of gland
    - Wraps around posterior margin of mylohyoid muscle
    - Projects into posterior aspect of sublingual space
    - Submandibular (Wharton) duct projects off deep process into sublingual space
  - SMG innervation: Branches from submandibular ganglion located in sublingual space
    - Parasympathetic secretomotor supply from chorda tympani (CNVII branch)
      - □ Via lingual nerve (CNV3)
- **Submental (level IA) and submandibular (level IB) nodal groups**
  - Receive lymph drainage from anterior facial region, including oral cavity and anterior sinonasal and orbital areas
- Facial vein and artery pass through SMS

- Facial vein in SMS courses just lateral to SMG and joins anterior branch of retromandibular vein (coursing along posterior aspect of SMG) to form common facial vein that in turn enters internal jugular vein slightly below this level
- **Caudal loop of CNXII** passes through SMS on way before looping anteriorly and cephalad into tongue muscles
- **Anterior belly of digastric muscles**
- Tail of parotid may "hang down" into posterior SMS

Fascia

- **SMS is lined by SL-DCF**
  - Superficial surface of mylohyoid covered by SL-DCF
  - Deep surface of platysma covered by SL-DCF
- There is **no midline fascia** separating 2 sides of SMS
  - Consequently, lesion growth from side to side in SMS is unobstructed

ANATOMY IMAGING ISSUES

Questions

- Major clinical/imaging question when mass present in SMS: Is lesion nodal or SMG in origin?
  - Fatty cleavage plane between mass and SMG identifies lesion as nodal in origin
    - If facial vein separates lesion from SMG, then lesion is from node
  - "Beaking" of SMG tissue around lesion margin identifies lesion as SMG in origin
- What are major diagnoses in SMS differential diagnoses list?
  - Congenital: Epidermoid, cystic hygroma
  - Inflammatory: SMG sialoadenitis with ductal calculus; diving ranula; reactive or suppurative adenopathy
  - Benign tumor: Benign mixed tumor of SMG, lipoma
  - Malignant tumor: Salivary gland carcinomas; nodal squamous cell carcinoma and non-Hodgkin lymphoma

Imaging Recommendations

- CECT or T1 C+ fat-saturated MR both effective
- Ultrasound with needle aspiration of lesion also used

Imaging Pitfalls

- Do not mistake obstructed, enlarged SMG for malignant node in setting of anterior floor of mouth primary squamous cell carcinoma

CLINICAL IMPLICATIONS

Clinical Importance

- Majority of lesion of SMS are either from SMG or nodes
  - Sorting lesions into these 2 categories helps work through imaging differential diagnosis
  - SMGs are frequently excised during neck dissection due to their proximity to primary lesion and afferent lymph nodes
- Remember, clinicians can see and feel area of SMS
  - Fine-needle cytopathology may have already been done at time of imaging
- Incision to perform SMG excision for calculus or tumor must be placed ≥ 4 cm below angle of mandible to preserve marginal mandibular branch of facial nerve, which passes posteroinferior to angle
- Lesions of parotid tail may appear in posterior SMS clinically

Submandibular Space

GRAPHIC AND AXIAL T2 MR

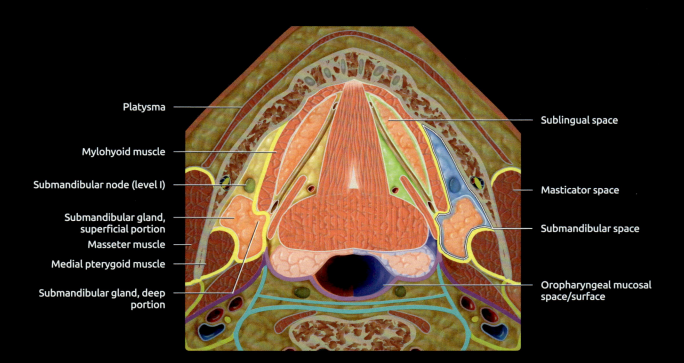

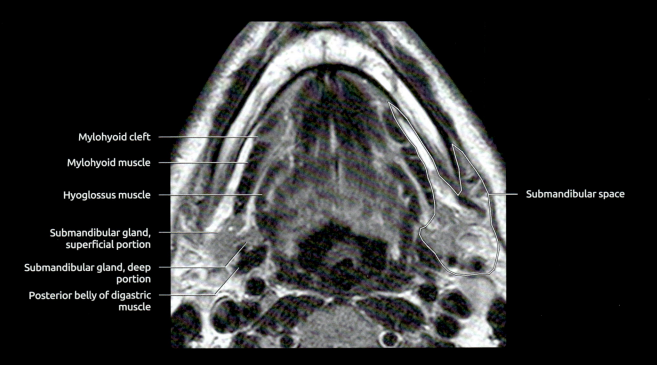

(Top) Axial graphic shows oral cavity with emphasis on the submandibular space (SMS) shaded in light blue on the patient's left. The SMS is inferolateral to the mylohyoid muscle. Note the principal occupants of the SMS are the submandibular gland and nodes.
(Bottom) Axial T2 MR demonstrates the axial appearance of the SMS outlined on the patient's left. The principal occupants of the SMS are the submandibular gland and nodes. Consequently, the differential diagnosis of lesions of this space includes gland tumors and lymph node diseases.

Submandibular Space

GRAPHIC & CORONAL T1 MR

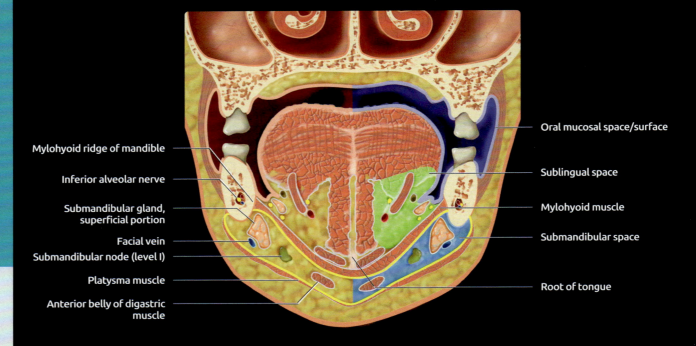

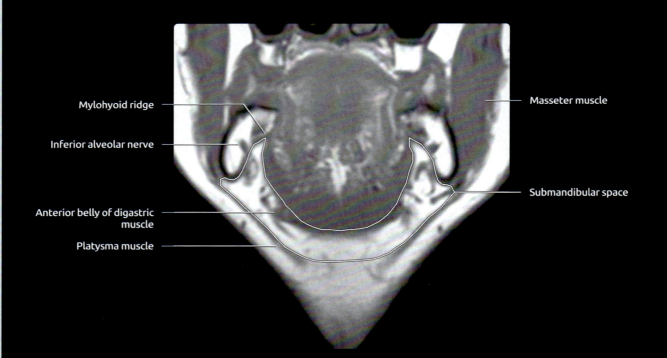

(Top) In this coronal graphic through the oral cavity, the SMS is shaded in light blue. The superficial layer of deep cervical fascia (yellow line) is seen lining the vertical horseshoe-shaped SMS inferolateral to the mylohyoid muscle. Contents of the SMS are the anterior belly of the digastric muscle, submandibular nodes, submandibular gland, and facial vein. Notice the platysma forms the superficial margin of the SMS. *(Bottom)* Coronal T1 MR shows the horseshoe-shaped SMS extending from side to side inferior and inferolateral to the mylohyoid muscle and deep to the platysma muscle. Notice the lack of vertical fascia or septation. Consequently, lesions of the SMS spread readily across the midline.

Submandibular Space

AXIAL CECT

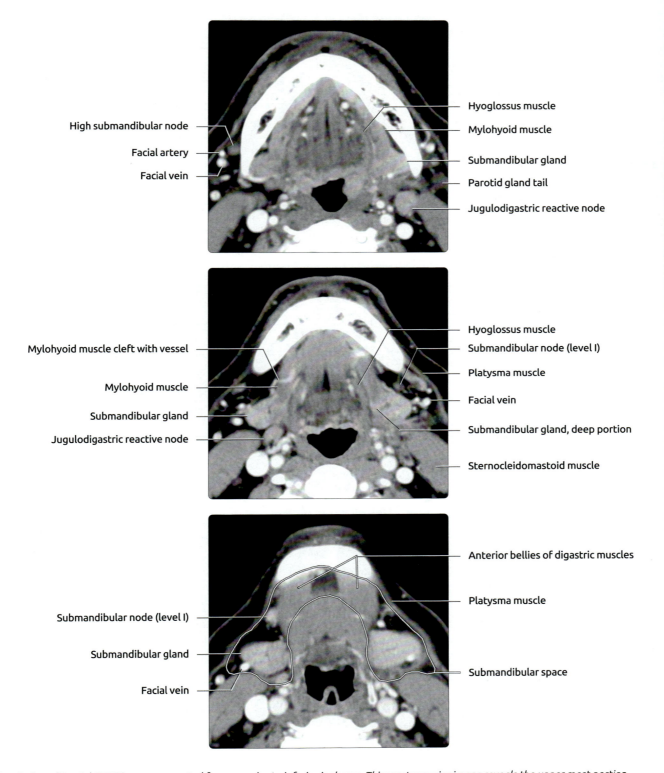

(Top) First of 3 axial CECT images presented from superior to inferior is shown. This most superior image reveals the upper most portion of the SMS. Notice the parotid gland tail projecting into the posterior SMS on the patient's left. (Middle) More inferiorly, this image shows the enlarging SMS filled with the submandibular gland, nodes, and facial vein. The submandibular gland deep portion extends to fill the posterior margin of the sublingual space on the patient's left. (Bottom) Low SMS axial CECT image highlights the full extent of these spaces. Notice how large the submandibular glands become inferiorly. Also note that the anterior bellies of the digastric muscles fill the anteromedial SMS.

471

Submandibular Space

AXIAL T2 MR

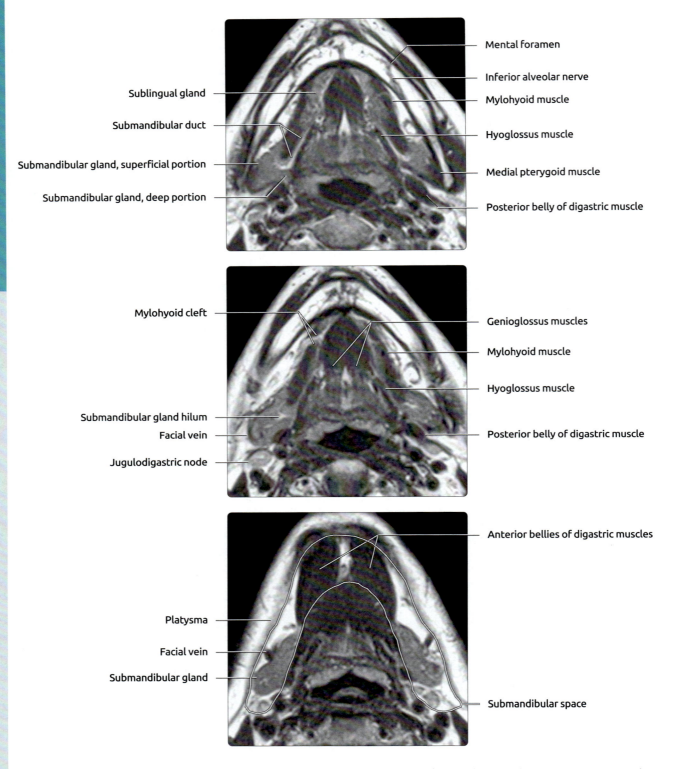

(Top) First of 3 axial T2 MR images of the oral cavity presented from superior to inferior is shown. In this most superior image, the upper SMS is evident, filled with fat and the upper submandibular glands. Notice the high-signal submandibular ducts entering the posterior sublingual spaces bilaterally. (Middle) Moving inferiorly, more fat is seen in the SMS bilaterally surrounding the submandibular glands. Both submandibular glands can be seen wrapping around the posterior margins of the mylohyoid muscles. Remember that the neurovascular pedicle to each side of the tongue enters closely approximated to the hyoglossus muscles. (Bottom) Low in the SMS, the full extent of both SMSs is visible. Notice that the anterior bellies of the digastric muscles fill the anteromedial SMS. Remember, there is no midline fascia, so diseases can move across midline from side to side.

Submandibular Space

CORONAL T1 MR

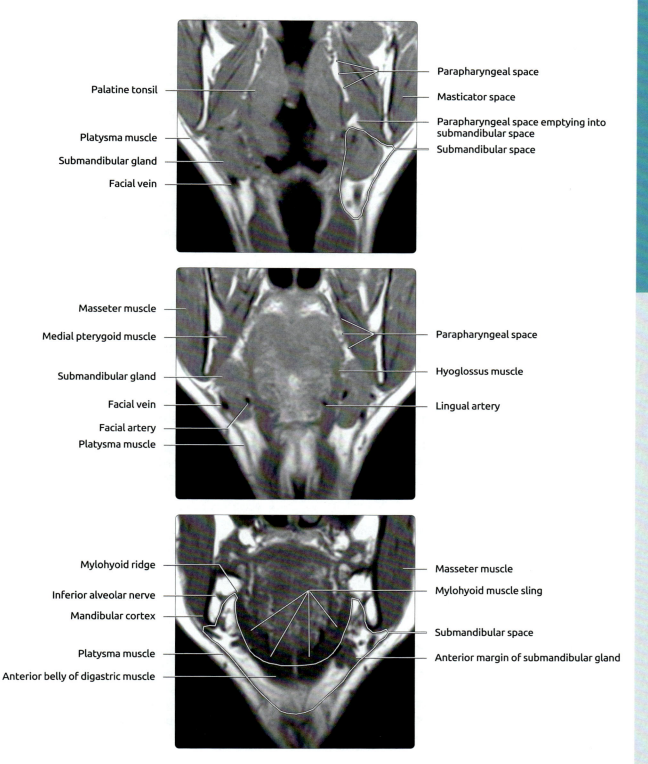

(Top) First of 3 coronal T1 MR images presented from posterior to anterior is shown. This most posterior image shows the area of the SMS outlined on the patient's left. Notice the parapharyngeal space empties inferiorly into the posterior SMS. (Middle) More anteriorly, the connection between the parapharyngeal space and the SMS is still visible. The facial vein is visible snaking along the inferolateral margin of the submandibular gland. Remember that if the facial vein is seen between a mass and the gland, it is most likely nodal in origin. (Bottom) In this image through the midoral cavity, the full extent of the SMS is clearly visible from side to side. The location of the superficial layer of deep cervical fascia is outlined. The mylohyoid sling forms the superomedial border of the SMS. The superficial margin of the SMS is the platysma muscle.

Buccal Space

Oral Cavity

TERMINOLOGY

Abbreviations

- Buccal space (BS)

Definitions

- Small anatomic space or compartment in deep face situated between buccinator muscle medially, greater and lesser zygomatic muscles laterally, and masticator space posteriorly; contains buccal fat pad, distal parotid duct, and facial artery and vein

IMAGING ANATOMY

Overview

- BS has received less attention in anatomic and radiologic literature than other spaces in neck
- BS interdigitates between oral cavity, superficial muscular aponeurotic system (SMAS), and masticator space
- Contains adipose tissue with conspicuous **buccal fat pad** that is easily identified with CT and MR

Extent

- Bounded by, but does not include, **buccinator muscle** medially
  - **BS does not include buccal mucosa** (part of oral cavity mucosal space) or minor salivary glands
  - BS is separated from buccal mucosa by buccinator muscle and thin layer of submucosal fat
  - Buccinator attachments: Alveolar ridge of maxilla superiorly, alveolar ridge of mandible inferiorly, pterygomandibular raphe posteriorly, and orbicularis oris anteriorly
- Lateral border is defined by several muscles of facial expression in cheek and their associated investing fascia (SMAS), including greater and lesser zygomatic muscles and risorius muscle
- Anterior border formed by orbicularis oris and ventral attachments of zygomatic muscles
- Posterior border defined by parotid gland laterally and anterior border of masticator space medially

Internal Contents

- **Buccal fat pad**
  - Represents distinct adipose tissue, composed of specialized type of fat termed syssarcosis, fat that facilitates adjacent muscular motion
  - **4 projections** of adipose tissue extend from main buccal fat pad
    - **Posterolateral**: Extends along parotid duct to parotid gland
      - Bounded by superficial layer of deep cervical fascia and facial muscles laterally and parotidomasseteric fascia medially
    - **Posteromedial**: Interposed between mandible laterally and maxilla medially
      - Contiguous with retromaxillary fat
      - Communication is often observed between posteromedial projection and masticator space itself
    - **Anterior**: Lies ventral to distal parotid duct and insinuates between buccinator muscle medially and adjacent muscles of facial expression laterally

    - **Temporal**: Extends superiorly and divides into superficial and deep portion, relative to temporalis muscle
      - Thin superficial portion lies between temporalis muscle and overlying superficial fascia
      - Deep portion passes behind lateral orbital wall and extends to greater wing of sphenoid
- **Distal parotid duct**
  - Duct can be used to divide BS into **anterior and posterior divisions**
  - As duct passes medially, it crosses through buccal fat pad on its way to its termination in oral cavity
  - Parotid duct passes anteriorly from parotid gland, lateral to masseter muscle, and then turns medially along ventral aspect of masseter muscle
- **Minor salivary gland tissue**
  - Microscopic submucosal structures found throughout upper aerodigestive tract
  - Most concentrated in tongue base and hard palate
  - Occasionally, present in BS; can give rise to minor salivary gland tumors, most common of primary BS tumors
- **Vessels**
  - **Facial vein** is typically located just anterior to parotid duct on axial images; ultimately drains into external jugular system
  - **Facial artery** is branch of external carotid artery that extends through BS to nasolabial fold region
  - **Buccal artery** arises from internal maxillary artery in masticator space and extends to BS, passing between medial margin of masseter muscle and lateral margin of buccinator muscle; anastomoses with facial artery
- **Nerves**
  - **Buccal branch of facial nerve (VII)** innervates buccinator muscles and nearby muscles of facial expression
  - **Buccal branch of mandibular nerve (V3)** provides sensory innervation to BS as well as buccal mucosa
- **Accessory parotid tissue**
  - Present in 20%; usually anterior to parotid gland and superficial to masseter muscle
  - Can give rise to common parotid gland pathology, including inflammation and neoplasm
- **Lymph nodes**
  - 1-3 buccal lymph nodes are present along lateral edge of buccinator muscle
  - Buccal nodes ultimately drain into submandibular nodes

ANATOMY IMAGING ISSUES

Imaging Recommendations

- CECT of neck/face is generally 1st-line imaging tool
- Multiplanar MR, including T1 without fat saturation and T1 C+ with fat saturation in axial and coronal planes

Buccal Space

GRAPHICS

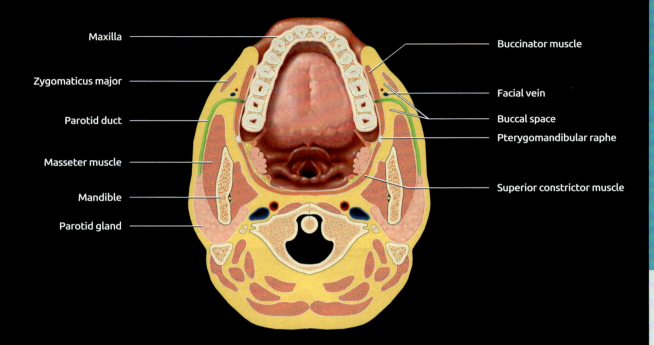

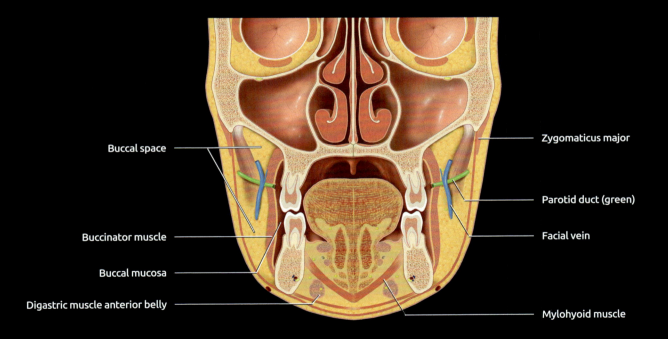

(Top) Axial graphic through the maxillary ridge demonstrates the course of the parotid duct as it passes around the ventral aspect of the masseter muscle and through the buccal space (BS) fat. The buccinator muscle represents the medial margin of the BS. Notice the BS fat extends posteriorly and medially. The facial vein passes in front of the parotid duct. (Bottom) Graphic through the posterior oral cavity demonstrates the anterior margins of the parotid ducts as they pass through the BSs that consist mostly of fat. The facial vein passes in front of the duct. The parotid ducts pass along the ventral margins of the masseter muscles. There is localized tenting of the buccinator muscle and buccal mucosa at the point where the duct penetrates these structures.

Buccal Space

BUCCAL SPACE ANATOMY: AXIAL CT

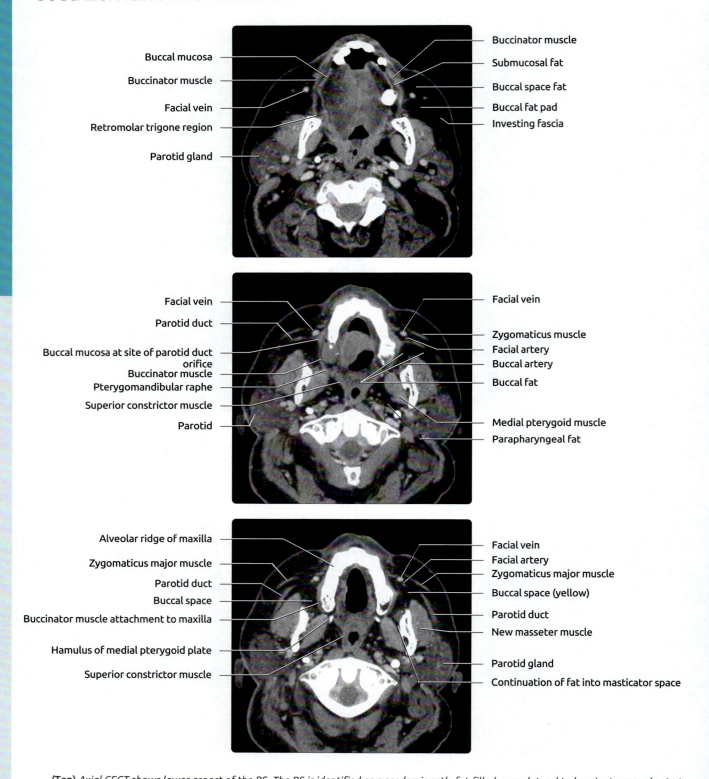

(Top) Axial CECT shows lower aspect of the BS. The BS is identified as a predominantly fat-filled space lateral to buccinator muscle. Just medial to buccinator muscle is a thin band of submucosal fat separating buccinator muscle from oral mucosa. Facial vein & artery enter BS from below. BS fat is separated from subcutaneous fat by a thin band of investing fascia that is part of superficial muscular aponeurotic system. (Middle) Axial CECT through midportion of BS demonstrates anterior portion of parotid duct crossing the space, piercing buccinator muscle. Parotid duct divides BS into anterior & posterior regions. The space is bounded anteriorly by thin zygomaticus major at this level. The angular portion of facial vein & facial artery are identified ventral to parotid duct. Fascial boundary that separates buccal fat from subcutaneous fat is less conspicuous. Fat projects medially between mandible & maxilla as well as posterolaterally along masseter muscle. (Bottom) Axial CECT shows upper BS. Proximal parotid duct is visualized as a linear soft tissue density surrounded by fat within posterolateral projection. Posterolateral component extends to hilum of parotid gland. Note a thin band of fat passes from BS medially into masticator space proper where fascia is deficient.

Buccal Space

BUCCAL SPACE ANATOMY: CORONAL CT

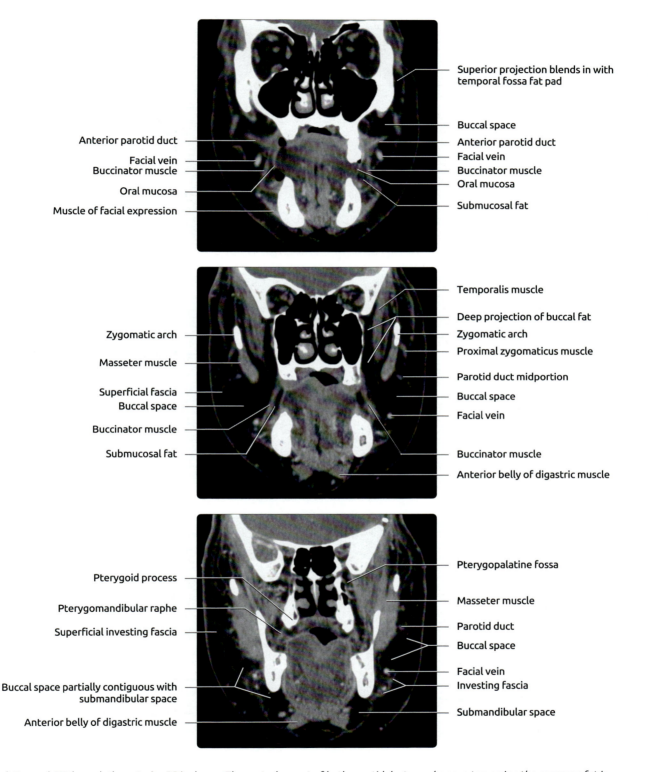

(Top) Coronal CT through the anterior BS is shown. The ventral aspect of both parotid ducts can be seen traversing the generous fat in BSs bilaterally. The buccinator muscle and adjacent buccal mucosa is "tented" where the duct empties into the oral cavity. The buccinator muscle is separated from the buccal mucosa by a thin rim of submucosal fat. Superior projection of fat extends to the region of the temporal fossa fat and merges with it. Facial vein is traversing obliquely from inferior to superior through the fat. (Middle) Coronal CECT through the midportion of oral cavity is shown. There is generous buccal fat identified bilaterally. The parotid duct is visualized in cross section just lateral to the masseter muscle. A deep portion of the buccal fat extends posteriorly and superiorly, extending between the temporalis muscle and the maxillary sinus. (Bottom) Coronal CT through posterior margin of the oral cavity is shown. The buccinator muscle fuses posteriorly with the pterygomandibular raphe, a band of firm fibrous tissue between the superior constrictor muscle and the buccinator. Buccal fat extends superiorly along the lateral margin of the masseter muscle.

Buccal Space

BUCCAL SPACE ANATOMY: AXIAL MR

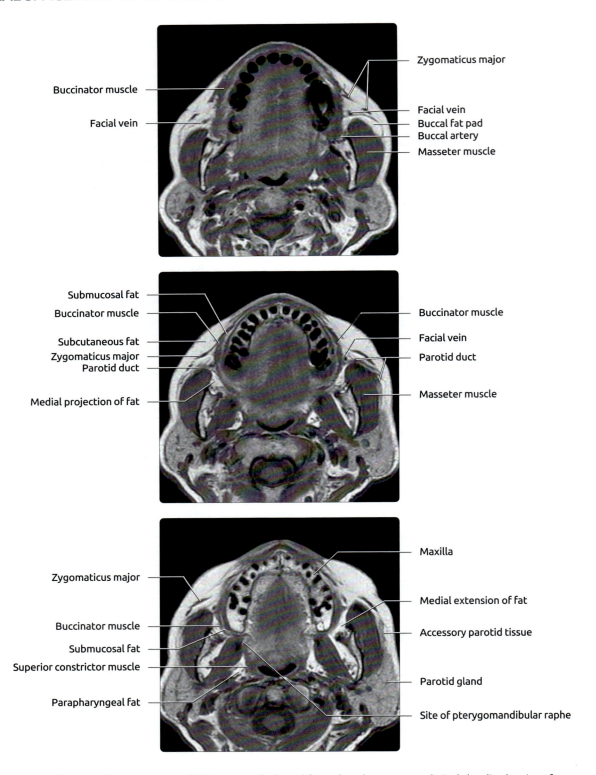

(Top) Axial T1 MR though the lower aspect of BS is shown. The buccal fat pad can be seen as a relatively localized region of homogeneous fat. In this image, the BS is triangular in shape and includes fat anterior and posterior to the facial vein. It is interposed between the buccinator muscle medially and the more superficial muscles of facial expression. (Middle) Axial T1 MR through the midportion of the BS is shown. The parotid duct passes anteriorly from the parotid gland, just lateral to the masseter muscle, and passes along the anterior margin of the masseter muscle, through the buccal fat, ultimately passing though the buccinator muscle and opening along the buccal mucosa at the parotid ampulla near the 2nd maxillary molar. The facial vein passes just anterior to the parotid duct. (Bottom) Axial T1 MR through upper BS is shown. Fat projects medially between the mandible and maxilla. Notice a thin band of fat passes from the BS medially into the masticator space proper where the fascia is deficient.

Buccal Space

ANATOMIC-PATHOLOGIC CORRELATION SQUAMOUS CELL CARCINOMA

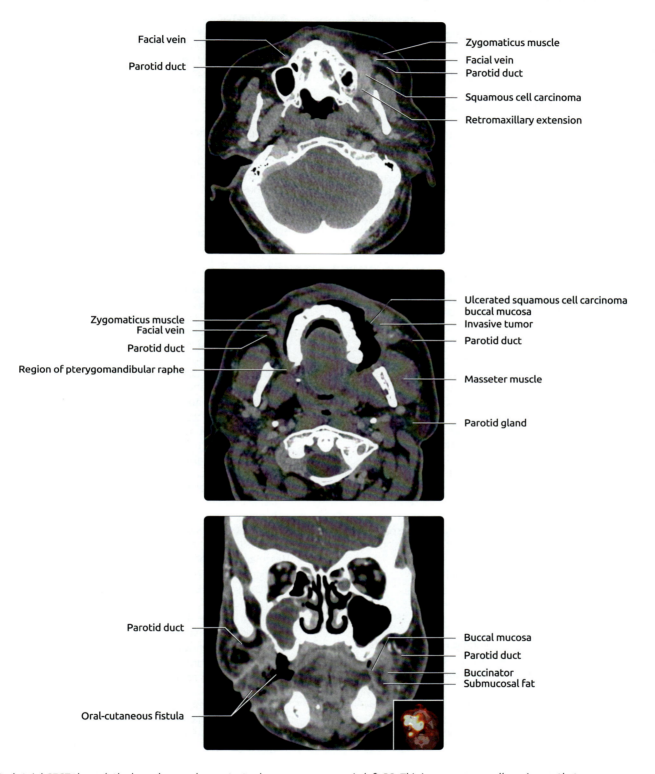

(Top) Axial CECT through the buccal space demonstrates homogeneous mass in left BS. This is a squamous cell carcinoma that originated on the buccal mucosa and buccal gingival sulcus, then eroded through the mucosa and buccinator space into the BS. The mass causes displacement of the parotid duct but no definite parotid duct enlargement. (Middle) Axial CECT through the BS is shown. This CT was performed using "puffed cheek" technique, allowing increased air in the lateral oral cavity recesses. There is an ulcerated lesion arising from the buccal mucosa (part of oral cavity mucosa) and invading laterally into the buccinator muscle and BS. There is nodular tissue near the junction of the facial vein and parotid duct. The parotid duct is normal in size despite the potential obstruction. (Bottom) Coronal CECT is performed after chemoradiation in patient with large unresectable squamous cell carcinoma that extended from the right tonsil to the BS. The pretreatment PET scan is seen in the inset. Posttreatment coronal image shows that the tumor has undergone significant necrosis, leaving a large oral cutaneous fistula through the BS.

Tongue

TERMINOLOGY

Definitions

- **Oral tongue**: Anterior 2/3 of tongue not including tongue base; mucosal covering of oral tongue **part of oral mucosal space/surface (OMS)**
  - By imaging, includes freely mobile portion of tongue that is anterior to lingual tonsil
- **Root of tongue (ROT)**: Undersurface of oral tongue at its junction with anterior FOM and mandible
  - By imaging, includes lingual septum, inferior portion of genioglossus muscles, and geniohyoid muscles
- **Floor of mouth (FOM)**: Crescent-shaped region of mucosa overlying mylohyoid and hyoglossus muscles, extending from inner aspect of lower alveolar ridge to undersurface of anterior oral tongue
  - Be aware, some authors have historically used term "floor of mouth" to refer to mylohyoid muscle sling
- **Base of tongue**: Posterior 1/3 of tongue (**part of oropharynx**)
  - By imaging, includes lingual tonsil

IMAGING ANATOMY

Anatomy Relationships

- **Sublingual space (SLS)**
  - Nonfascia-lined potential space containing lingual nerve, CNIX, CNXII, lingual artery and vein, sublingual glands and ducts, submandibular gland deep portion, submandibular duct, and anterior part of hyoglossus muscle
  - SLS situated below FOM mucosa and superomedial to mylohyoid muscle; lateral to extrinsic tongue muscles (genioglossus-geniohyoid)
  - Communicates with contralateral SLS beneath **frenulum** anteriorly
  - Posterior boundary partly formed by insertion of anterior tonsillar pillar into tongue
  - Empties posteriorly into posterosuperior aspect of submandibular space and inferior parapharyngeal space
- **ROT**
  - Inferiorly, ROT ends at mylohyoid sling
  - Superiorly ends at intrinsic tongue muscles
  - Anteriorly ends at mandibular symphysis

Internal Contents

- Oral tongue consists of 4 anatomic regions: Tip, lateral borders, dorsum, and undersurface (nonvillous surface)
- **Extrinsic tongue muscles**: Move tongue body and alter shape
  - **Genioglossus**: Large, fan-shaped muscle lying parallel to median plane in sagittal plane
  - Origin from upper genial tubercle and internal surface of symphysis menti of mandible; inserts along entire length of under surface of tongue
  - Protrudes tongue (safety muscle; if paralyzed tongue falls back into airway of oropharynx); nerve: CNXII
  - **Hyoglossus**: Thin and quadrilateral-shaped muscle; "arms reaching up from posteroinferior FOM into posterior SLS"
  - Origin from body and greater cornu of hyoid bone; passes vertically upward to insert into side of tongue

- Depresses tongue; nerve: CNXII
- **Styloglossus**: Origin from styloid process and stylomandibular ligament; passes anteroinferiorly between internal and external carotid arteries to insert into side of tongue, merging with hyoglossus muscle
- Retracts tongue upward and backward; nerve: CNXII
- **Palatoglossus**: Origin from undersurface of palatine aponeurosis; inserts into side and dorsum of tongue
- Forms palatoglossal arch (anterior tonsillar pillar); nerve: CNX, pharyngeal plexus branch
- **Intrinsic tongue muscles**: Alters shape of tongue during deglutition and speech; complicated bundles of interlacing fibers innervated by CNXII
  - **Superior longitudinal muscle**: Origin from median fibrous septum close to epiglottis; inserts into edges of tongue; elevates apex and sides of tongue, shortening and making its dorsum concave
  - **Inferior longitudinal muscle**: Origin from ROT and inserts into its apex, seen between genioglossus and hyoglossus; depresses apex and sides of tongue, shortening and making its dorsum convex
  - **Transverse muscle**: Origin from fibrous lingual septum; runs transversely to insert into submucosal fibrous tissue at lateral tongue margins; makes tongue narrow and elongated (sticks out tongue)
  - **Vertical muscle**: Origin from submucosal fibrous layer of dorsum of tongue; inserts into its inferior surface borders, found at borders of anterior tongue; makes tongue broad and flattened
- **Innervation of tongue**
  - Sensory supply (touch, pain, temperature, and **taste**): Anterior 2/3: Lingual nerve (taste fibers are from chorda tympani branch of CNVII); posterior 1/3: CNIX
  - **Hypoglossal nerve** (CNXII): Emerges from nasopharyngeal carotid space; receives fibers from 1st and 2nd cervical nerves; loops inferiorly to level of hyoid bone; rises anteriorly to enter posterior SLS just lateral to hyoglossus muscle; runs in SLS on lateral surface of genioglossus muscle; and innervates extrinsic and intrinsic tongue muscles
- **Vasculature of tongue**
  - Lingual artery: 2nd branch of external carotid artery
    - Divides in SLS into sublingual and deep lingual branches
  - Lingual vein: Parallels lingual artery; drains into internal jugular or facial veins
- **Lymphatics of tongue**
  - **Tip of tongue** drains bilaterally to submental nodes; **anterior 2/3 of remaining lateral tongue** drains unilaterally to submandibular nodes of either side and central lymphatics here drain bilaterally to deep cervical or submandibular nodes; **posterior tongue** drains to upper deep cervical nodes, including jugulodigastric nodes (level II), and finally all drain into **jugulo-omohyoid** nodes (level III) known as lymph nodes of tongue

Tongue

GRAPHICS

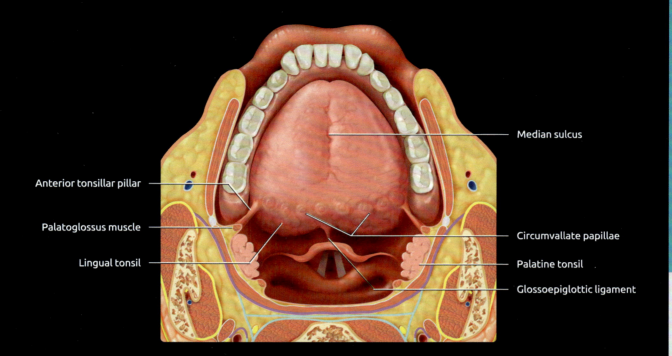

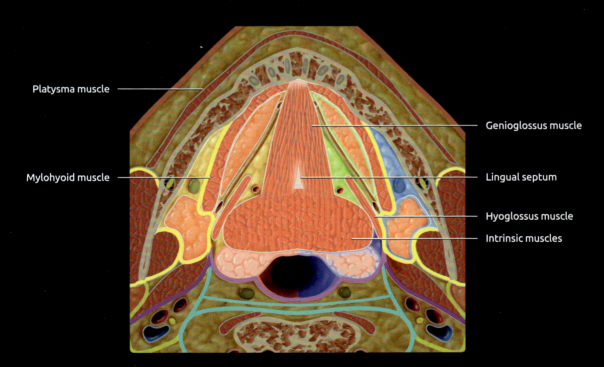

(Top) Axial graphic of the surface of the oral tongue is shown. The oral tongue sits anterior to the oropharyngeal lingual tonsil. The line of the circumvallate papillae delineates the mucosal surface transition to the more anterior oral cavity. (Bottom) In this axial graphic through the deep portion of the oral tongue, it is possible to see the large, bilateral paramedian genioglossus muscles bordering the midline lingual septum. The genioglossus muscles rise to mingle with the complex tangle of intrinsic tongue muscles. The hyoglossus muscles are also seen rising from the hyoid bone below into the posterior sublingual space.

Tongue

GRAPHICS

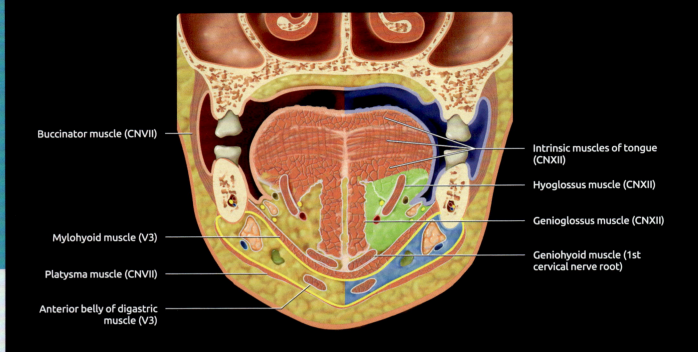

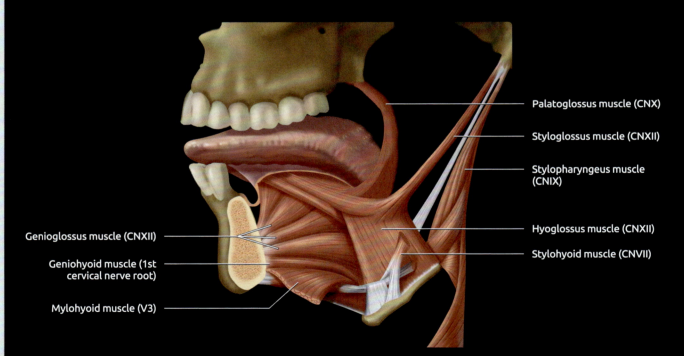

(Top) Coronal graphic through oral cavity highlights all major muscles with their innervations indicated in parentheses. Note all intrinsic and extrinsic (genioglossus, hyoglossus, styloglossus, palatoglossus) tongue muscles are innervated by CNXII except palatoglossus. The buccinator and platysma, both muscles of facial expression, are innervated by CNVII. (Bottom) Sagittal graphic shows muscles of the tongue area. Each muscle is labeled with its innervating nerve in parentheses. Pay attention to fan-shaped genioglossus, which represents much of the oral tongue extrinsic musculature. Note the hyoglossus muscle projecting upward from the hyoid bone like 2 big arms into the oral tongue's posterior sublingual space. Geniohyoid muscle is not considered part of the extrinsic muscles of the tongue but instead is the suprahyoid neck muscle innervated by the CNXII branch with the 1st cervical nerve root in it.

Tongue

SAGITTAL AND CORONAL T1 MR

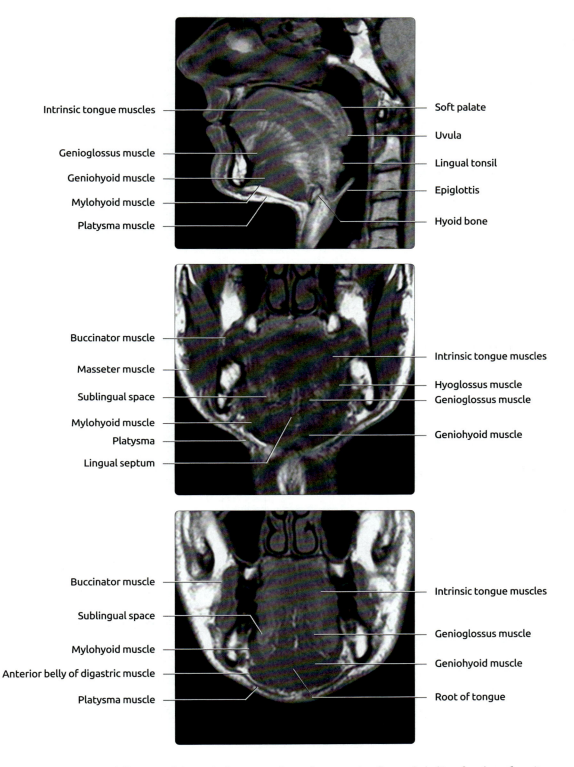

(Top) In this sagittal T1 MR, the full extent of the genioglossus muscle can be seen extending cephalad in a fan shape from its attachment to the posteroinferior mandible. Notice that it is difficult to distinguish the mylohyoid, geniohyoid, and inferior genioglossus muscles. (Middle) More posterior coronal T1 MR reveals the oral tongue superomedial to the mylohyoid muscle. Again, the 3 stacked muscles (mylohyoid, geniohyoid, and genioglossus) are difficult to distinguish. Remember that the sublingual spaces lie lateral to the genioglossus muscles and superolateral to the mylohyoid muscle. (Bottom) In this more anterior coronal T1 MR, 4 muscles can be identified from inferior to superior, namely the anterior belly of the digastric, mylohyoid, geniohyoid, and genioglossus muscles. Notice also the root of tongue area.

Tongue

AXIAL T2 MR

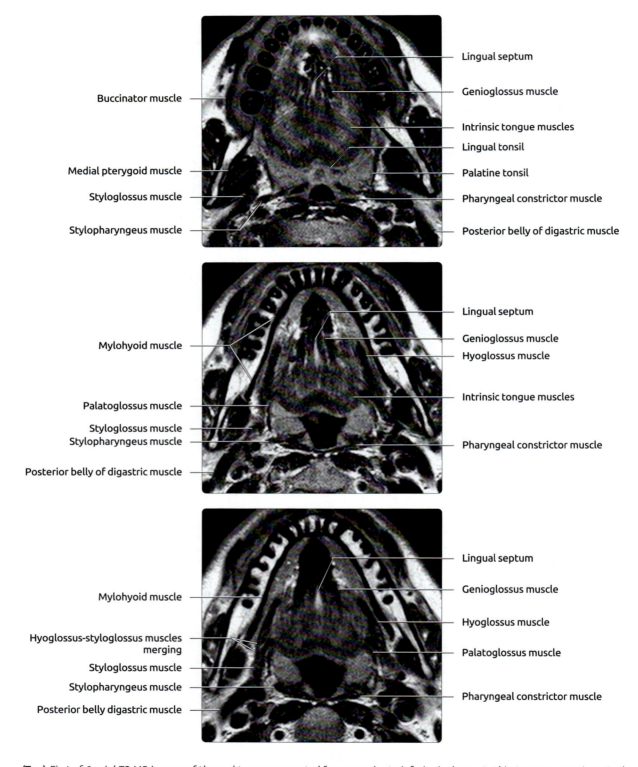

(Top) First of 6 axial T2 MR images of the oral tongue presented from superior to inferior is shown. In this 1st most superior MR, the superior aspect of the oral tongue is seen. The intrinsic muscles, especially the transverse group, are well seen with just the top of the genioglossus muscle visible. The styloglossus muscle is seen in its expected location just medial to the medial pterygoid muscle. The stylopharyngeus is identified melding with the pharyngeal constrictor muscle. (Middle) In this inferior MR, the hyoglossus upper margin is seen rising into the posterior sublingual space. The genioglossus is now readily apparent on either side of the fibrofatty lingual septum. (Bottom) In this MR, the styloglossus can be seen merging with the hyoglossus (labeled on the patient's right). The palatoglossus is now visible along the anterior margin of the palatine tonsil.

Tongue

AXIAL T2 MR

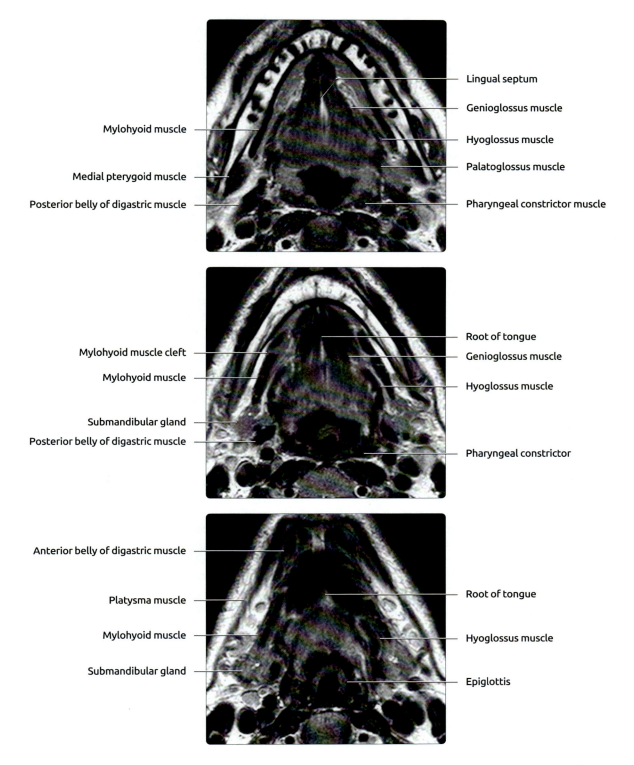

(Top) At the level of the mandibular teeth roots, the posterior belly of the digastric muscle is seen passing deep to the most inferior aspect of the medial pterygoid muscle on the patient's right. The posterior belly of the digastric muscle is larger and more inferior than the styloglossus muscle. **(Middle)** In this MR, the mylohyoid muscle has left the mylohyoid ridge of the mandible. A prominent mylohyoid muscle cleft is present on the patient's right. The area of the root of tongue is labeled. **(Bottom)** This most inferior MR shows the convergence of the anteroinferior genioglossus muscle with the geniohyoid muscle to form the area of the root of the tongue. The origins of the hyoglossus muscles are also seen rising off the hyoid bone. The free margin of the epiglottis is visible within the pharyngeal airway.

Retromolar Trigone

TERMINOLOGY

Abbreviations
- Retromolar trigone (RMT)

Definitions
- RMT: Small triangular subsite of oral cavity composed of mucosa posterior to last mandibular molar that covers anterior surface of lower ascending ramus of mandible and extends superiorly up to maxillary tuberosity
- Pterygomandibular raphe (PMR): Thick fascial band that extends between posterior border of mandibular mylohyoid ridge and hamulus of medial pterygoid plate
  - Fascial band represents thickening of middle layer of deep cervical fascia condensed between posterior margin of buccinator muscle and anterior margin of superior constrictor muscle

IMAGING ANATOMY

Overview
- PMR lies posteriorly beneath mucosa of RMT
- If RMT is affected by squamous cell carcinoma (SCCa), PMR is involved early
- PMR provides both inferior and superior routes of spread for SCCa

Extent
- RMT extent
  - Cephalad tip (apex of trigone) is in continuity with maxillary tuberosity behind last upper molar tooth
  - Base of mucosal triangle is posterior margin of last mandibular molar tooth
  - Bounded laterally by gingivobuccal sulcus and medially by anterior tonsillar pillar

Anatomy Relationships
- RMT is seen on few contiguous axial CT scan sections, its superior limit being maxillary tuberosity/3rd molar and inferior limit being mandibular 3rd molar
  - Oblique CT reformats help to evaluate entire superoinferior extent of RMT
- PMR can be located at line of junction between buccinator (posterior margin) muscle and superior constrictor muscle (anterior margin)
  - PMR represents junction of oropharynx posteriorly and oral cavity anteriorly

Internal Contents
- PMR: Fascia made up of focally thickened middle layer of deep cervical fascia
  - Middle layer of deep cervical fascia runs along superficial margin of buccinator muscle and along deep and lateral margins of superior constrictor muscle

ANATOMY IMAGING ISSUES

Questions
- RMT SCCa can spread in multiple directions
  - Posterior spread of SCCa
    - Posterolaterally to buccal fat and masticator space and rarely perineural CNV3
    - Posteromedially to tongue
    - Posteriorly to anterior tonsillar pillar/oropharynx
  - Anterior spread of SCCa
    - Along alveolar ridge and anterolaterally to buccinator muscle and cheek
  - Inferior spread of SCCa
    - If directly into mandible, may extend anteriorly via perineural spread along inferior alveolar nerve
    - If along caudal spread along PMR, reaches posterior mylohyoid line of mandible and thereby posterior margin of mylohyoid muscle
  - Superior spread of SCCa
    - Cephalad spread along PMR to inferior margin of medial pterygoid plate at hamulus; maxillary tuberosity may be involved at apex of RMT

Imaging Recommendations
- Tiny RMT lesions may be missed due to opposition of mucosal surfaces
  - Loss of adjacent fat planes act as diagnostic clue in CT and MR
- Puffed-cheek technique may help to detect small, obscure lesions in CT scan
- CECT provides both soft tissue and bone information
  - May be severely degraded by dental amalgam artifact
  - Bone window critical for bony invasion of mandible or secondary involvement of pterygoid plates
- MR less affected by dental amalgam artifact in most cases
  - Reserve for invasive RMT SCCa
  - Axial T2 and T1 fat-saturated enhanced MR sequences best for evaluation of cephalad PMR

Imaging Pitfalls
- Dental amalgam artifact on CECT may obscure RMT SCCa primary site ± spread along PMR in cephalad direction
  - Key CT observation
    - Always check **above CT artifact** in oral cavity in area of cephalad PMR (inferior margin of pterygoid plate) for evidence of tumor spread if primary RMT SCCa is known to be present

CLINICAL IMPLICATIONS

Clinical Importance
- Most RMT tumors are SCCas; minor salivary gland tumors are sometimes diagnosed
- SCCa of RMT may spread along PMR
  - Cephalad spread along PMR takes tumor up to inferolateral pterygoid plate-anteromedial masticator space (especially medial pterygoid producing trismus)
    - Tumor is seen at level of inferior pterygoid plate involving posterior buccinator muscle and anterior superior constrictor muscle
    - Enlarging tumor involves maxillary sinus, buccal and masticator spaces
  - Caudal spread along PMR takes tumor inferiorly to posterior margin of mylohyoid muscle
    - Enlarging tumor in this location involves floor of mouth of oral cavity

Retromolar Trigone

GRAPHICS

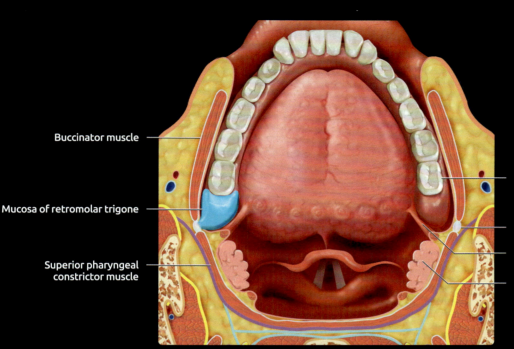

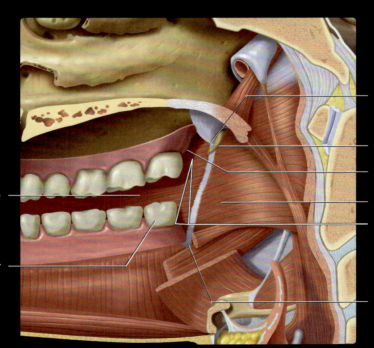

(Top) Axial graphic highlights the retromolar trigone (RMT) (shaded in blue on the left) and the pterygomandibular raphe (PMR). Notice that the mucosal surface of the RMT is found directly behind the mandibular 3rd molar. Its proximity to the PMR (fascial band connecting the buccinator and superior pharyngeal constrictor muscles) is important when squamous cell carcinoma occurs here because of this tumor's propensity for spreading cephalad on this fascia. (Bottom) Sagittal graphic viewed from inside the mouth delineates the full extent of the PMR. Note the cephalad PMR attachment to the hamulus of the medial pterygoid plate and its inferior attachment to the posterior aspect of the mylohyoid ridge on the inner mandibular cortex. The PMR "connects" the buccinator muscle to the superior pharyngeal constrictor muscle. Note that the cephalad apex of the RMT reaches up to the maxillary tuberosity. Maxillary tuberosity is the most posterior aspect of maxilla with its posterior border curving upward. The 3rd maxillary molar tooth lies just in front and within the maxillary tuberosity.

Retromolar Trigone

AXIAL T2 MR

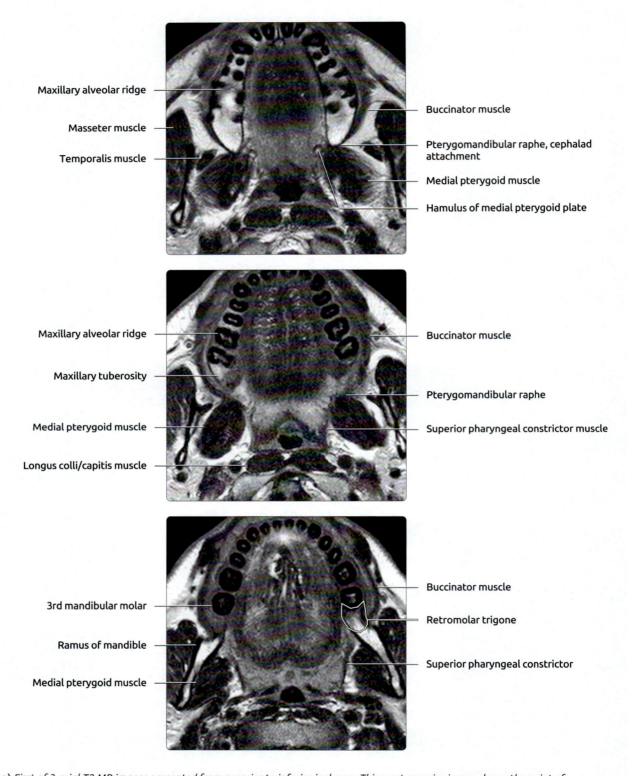

(Top) First of 3 axial T2 MR images presented from superior to inferior is shown. This most superior image shows the point of attachment of the PMR to the hamulus of the medial pterygoid plate. (Middle) On this more inferior image, the buccinator can be seen meeting the superior pharyngeal constrictor muscle at the PMR. The raphe itself is difficult to visualize. Note that the superior apex of the triangular RMT extends up to the maxillary tuberosity. (Bottom) At the level of the mandibular alveolar ridge, the area of the RMT can be outlined. Notice it is found directly behind the mandibular 3rd molar tooth. The buccinator is seen along its lateral margin while the superior pharyngeal constrictor can be seen approaching its medial margin. Just above this slice, these 2 muscles meet at the PMR. Squamous cell carcinoma of the RMT often spreads cephalad along this raphe.

Retromolar Trigone

AXIAL T1 MR

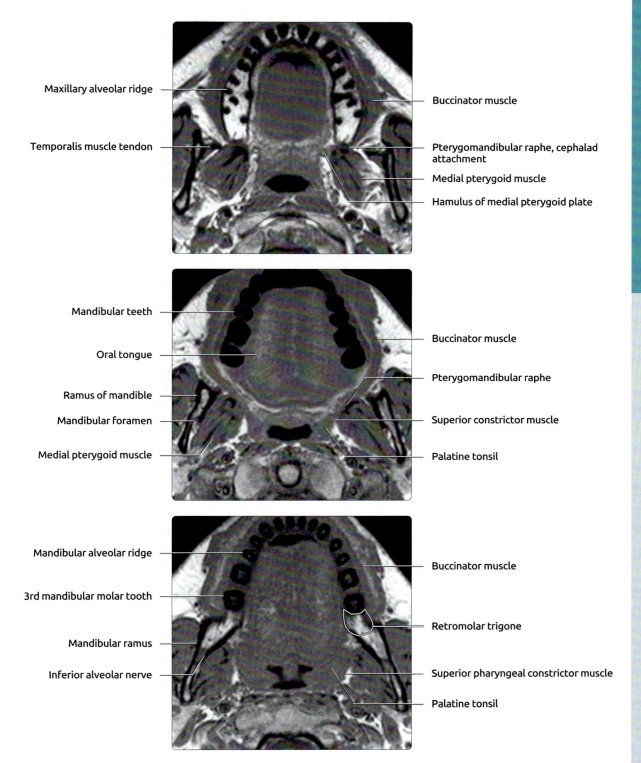

(Top) First of 3 axial T1 MR images through oropharynx-oral cavity presented from superior to inferior is shown. On this most superior image, the buccinator can be seen inserting at the inferolateral margin of the pterygoid plate with the most superior aspect of the PMR. (Middle) Inferiorly at the level of the mandibular teeth, the buccinator and the superior constrictor muscle meet at the PMR. The superior constrictor muscle cannot be differentiated from the palatine tonsil on T1 images. (Bottom) On this most inferior image at the level of the mandibular alveolar ridge, the area of the RMT is outlined on the patient's left. Note that the RMT is found directly behind the 3rd mandibular molar tooth. Squamous cell carcinoma can spread up the PMR from this location.

Mandible and Maxilla

TERMINOLOGY

Abbreviations
- Mandible
- Maxilla

Definitions
- Angle of mandible: Obtuse angle of mandible where inferior segment of ramus meets posterior mandible body

IMAGING ANATOMY

Internal Contents
- Mandible anatomy: Bony
  - 2 vertical rami attached to horizontal, horseshoe-shaped body
  - Each ramus has 2 upwardly directed processes
    - **Condylar process**: Condylar head & neck contains articular surface of temporomandibular joint
    - **Coronoid process**: Temporalis muscle inserts here
    - Mandibular notch separates these 2 processes
    - Mandibular ramus divides masticator space into lateral & medial compartments
  - **Mandibular foramen**
    - Location: Center, medial surface of mandible ramus
    - Nerve transmitted: Inferior alveolar nerve
    - Lingula: Small, osseous lip extending from anterior aspect of mandibular foramen
  - Mandibular body
    - U-shaped, horizontal body composed of 2 halves; fuses in anterior midline at **symphysis menti**
    - Alveolar process consists of external buccal & internal lingual plates, covered by periosteum
    - **Mental foramen**: Paired external openings of mandibular canal that transmits mental nerve
    - **Mylohyoid ridge**: Bony ridge on lingual mandible body; site of attachment of mylohyoid muscle
  - Mandibular canal
    - Lies within distal ramus & proximal body of mandible
    - Extends from mandibular to mental foramen
    - Contains inferior alveolar nerve & vessels
- Mandible anatomy: Nerves
  - **Inferior alveolar nerve**
    - Extends from mandibular foramen, through mandibular canal to mental foramen
    - Innervates ipsilateral premolars & molars
    - Divides into mental & incisive branches
  - **Mental nerve**
    - Exits mental foramen
    - Provides sensory innervation to skin & mucosa of lower lip & labial gingiva
  - **Incisive nerve**
    - Innervates ipsilateral canine & incisors
- Maxillary alveolar & palatine processes: Bony
  - Represents inferior aspect of maxillary bone
  - Maxillary alveolar ridge (arch)
    - Adult version contains 16 teeth
  - **Premaxilla**: Anterior hard palate & alveolar ridge
    - Contains **incisive foramen** (nasopalatine nerve)
    - Paired nasopalatine canals terminate as single incisive foramen
  - Palatine process of maxillary bone
    - Forms anterior 2/3 of hard palate
  - Posterior 1/3 of hard palate formed by horizontal plate of palatine bone
- Maxillary alveolar & palatine processes: Nerves
  - **Nasopalatine nerve** (V2 sensory branch) travels through incisive foramen
    - Supplies sensory fibers to anterior hard palate
  - **Greater palatine nerve** comes down greater palatine canal in palatine bone
    - Supplies sensation to posterior 2/3 of hard palate
    - Exits greater palatine foramen anteriorly to hard palate mucosa
  - **Lesser palatine nerve** comes down lesser palatine canal in palatine bone
    - Exits lesser palatine foramen posterior to greater palatine foramen
    - Supplies sensory fibers to palatine tonsil
- Dental anatomy, mandible & maxilla
  - 32 total permanent teeth in mandible (16) & maxilla (16)
    - Each tooth has crown, root, & pulp
  - 16 adult teeth in each "dental arch"
    - Each arch consists of 2 quadrants
    - Each quadrant contains 3 molars, 2 premolars, 1 canine, 1 lateral incisor, & 1 medial incisor
  - **Teeth numbering convention**
    - Maxillary alveolar ridge: Begin with right 3rd molar, 1-16 across to left 3rd molar
    - Mandibular alveolar ridge: Begin with left 3rd molar, 17-32 across to right 3rd molar
  - Each crown: Outer enamel surrounding dentin; pulp in center
    - **Enamel**: Densest material in body
    - **Dentin**: Encases pulp
    - **Pulp**: Nourishes dentin
  - Tooth root covered by cementum
    - Cementum acts as medium for attaching fibers of periodontal ligament to tooth
    - Periodontal ligament located in periodontal space
    - Periodontal space is radiolucency surrounding root

ANATOMY IMAGING ISSUES

Questions
- **V2** perineural malignant tumor?
  - If malignancy affects skin of upper lip, **hard palate**, soft palate, check for V2 perineural tumor (PNT)
  - Major locations to identify V2 PNT extend from incisive canal-greater palatine foramen to root entry zone of V in lateral pons
  - If imaging for V2 PNT, check incisive canal, greater & lesser palatine foramen, pterygopalatine canal & fossa, foramen rotundum, Meckel cave, preganglionic segment of CNV, & root entry zone
- **V3** perineural malignant tumor?
  - If malignant tumor of skin of chin, mandibular alveolar ridge, or masticator space, check for V3 PNT
  - If imaging for V3 PNT, check entire length of V3 to root entry zone
    - Pay special attention to inferior alveolar canal, mandibular foramen, masticator space

Mandible and Maxilla

GRAPHICS

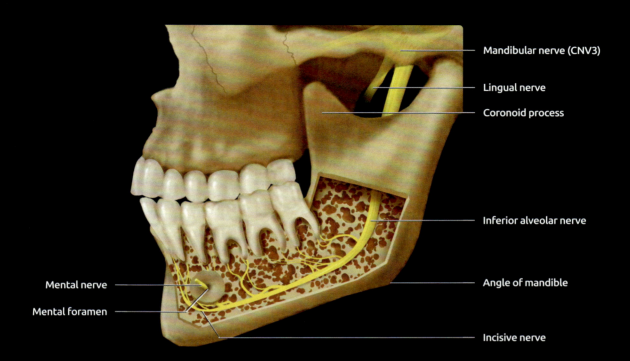

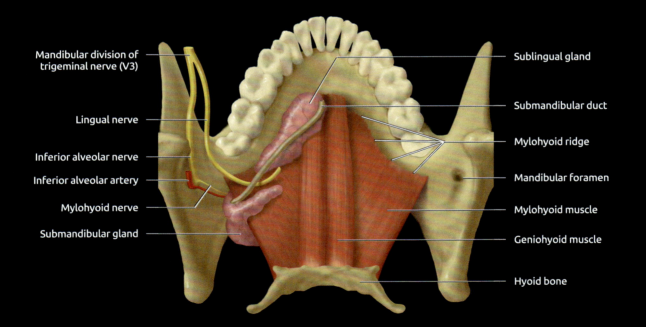

(Top) Lateral graphic of mandible with its lateral cortex removed reveals the mandibular nerve divides into lingual and inferior alveolar nerves. The inferior alveolar nerve divides distally into mental and incisive branches. The mental nerve branch reaches the superficial chin through the mental foramen. (Bottom) Graphic of the posterior view of the floor of mouth and mandible shows the S-shaped mylohyoid ridge where the mylohyoid muscle attaches to the mandible. Also note the mandibular division of the trigeminal nerve bifurcates into the lingual nerve and the inferior alveolar nerve. Just prior to entering the mandibular foramen, the inferior alveolar nerve gives off the mylohyoid motor branch that innervates the mylohyoid and anterior belly of the digastric muscles.

Mandible and Maxilla

GRAPHICS

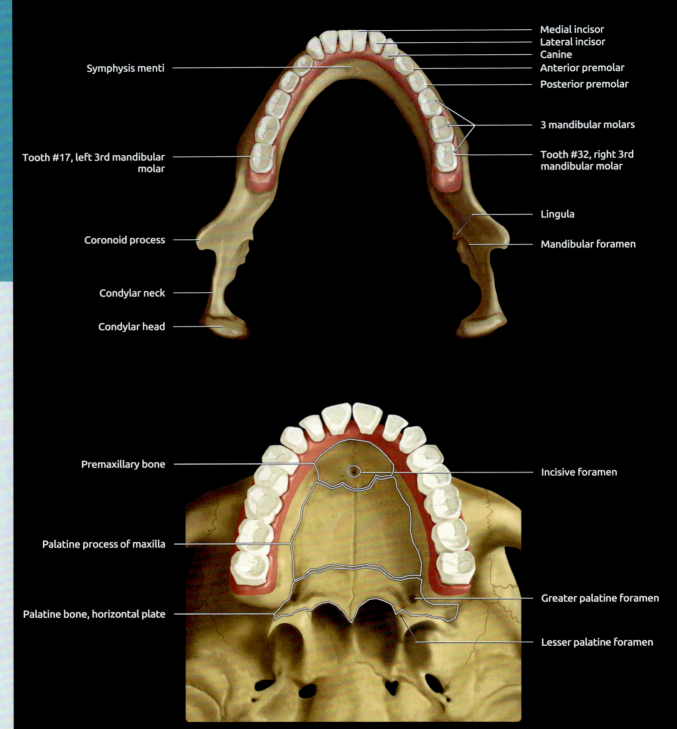

(Top) Axial graphic of the mandible seen from above demonstrates the cephalad condylar head and neck leading to the more inferior ramus. The mandibular foramen is seen on the inner surface of the mandibular ramus. The cephalad projecting coronoid processes attach to the temporalis muscle tendons. The U-shaped mandibular bodies fuse in the midline at the symphysis menti. Notice there are 16 adult teeth, numbered beginning at the left 3rd molar from 17-32 (right 3rd molar tooth). (Bottom) Axial graphic of the hard palate and maxillary alveolar ridge viewed from below shows the anterior premaxillary bone and the larger, more posterior palatine process of the maxillary bone. The horizontal plate of the palatine bone completes the hard palate picture. Notice the anterior midline incisive canal and the posterolateral greater and lesser palatine foramina.

Mandible and Maxilla

GRAPHIC & BONE CT

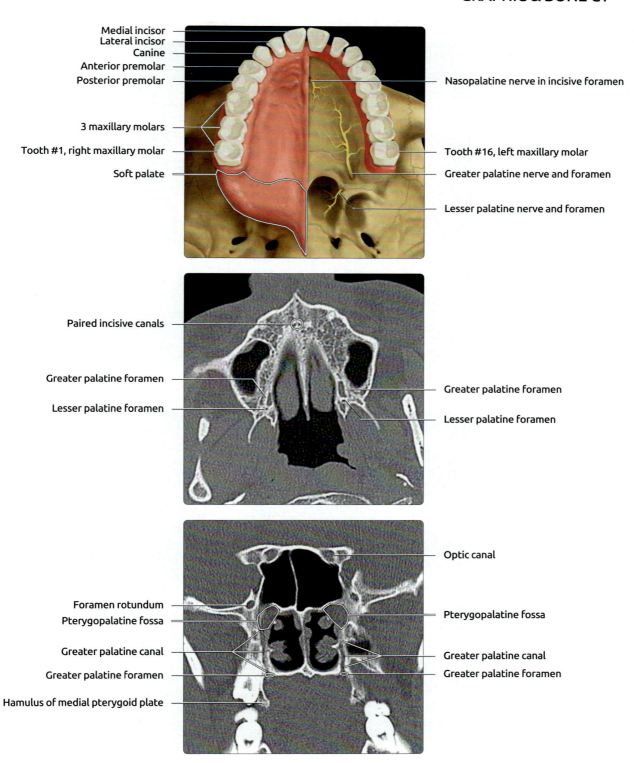

(Top) Axial graphic of the hard palate viewed from below with mucosa removed on the right side is shown. Hard palate sensory innervation is shown on the right with the anterior 1/3 of the hard palate supplied by the nasopalatine nerve and the posterior 2/3 of the hard palate supplied by the greater palatine nerve. Notice there are 16 adult teeth, numbered beginning at the right 3rd molar from 1-16. (Middle) Axial bone CT depicts foramina carrying nerves to the hard palate. Anterior paired incisive canals lead to more inferior incisive foramen (not shown). Greater and lesser palatine foramina transmit greater and lesser palatine nerves, respectively. (Bottom) Coronal bone CT through the vertical aspect of the greater palatine canal shows this canal connecting the pterygopalatine fossa above with the greater palatine foramen below. Greater palatine nerve uses the greater palatine canal to access the palate.

Mandible and Maxilla

AXIAL BONE CT

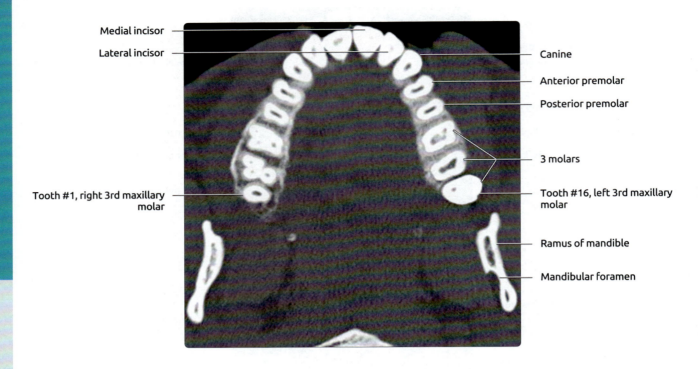

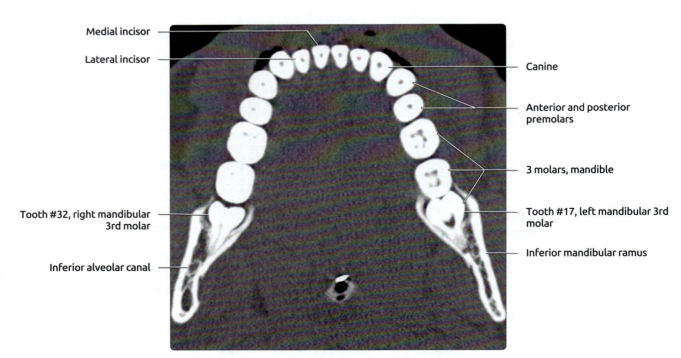

(Top) *Axial bone CT at the level of the maxillary ridge delineates the 16 upper teeth. Numbering convention begins with tooth #1 (upper posterior right molar tooth) extending from there across to the opposite left posterior maxillary molar, which is as designated tooth #16. Note there are 2 each of medial and lateral incisors, canine, anterior and posterior premolars, and 3 molar teeth.* **(Bottom)** *Axial bone CT of the 16 mandibular teeth is shown. Continuing the numbering convention for the mandibular teeth, the left 3rd molar is considered tooth #17 with numbering moving across to the opposite right 3rd mandibular molar designated as tooth #32. Note again there are paired medial and lateral incisors, canines, anterior and posterior premolars, and 3 molar teeth in the mandible.*

Mandible and Maxilla

3D CT OF MANDIBLE

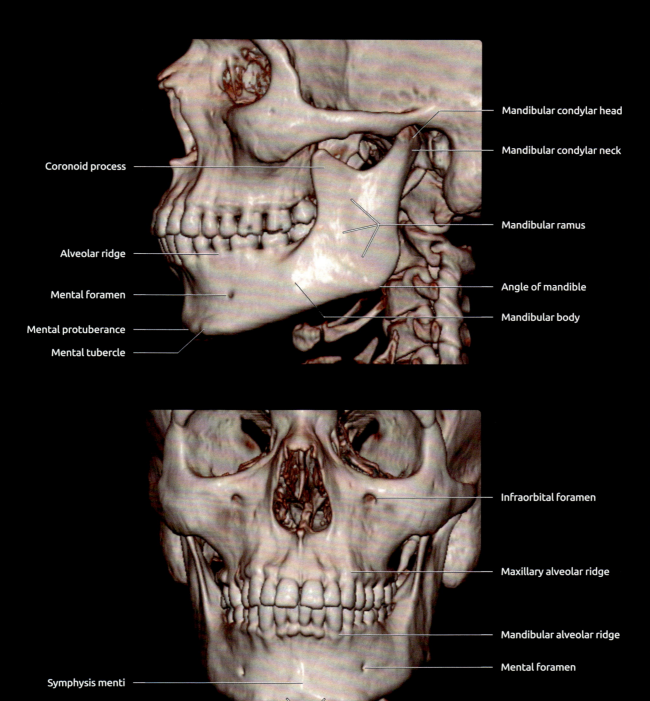

(Top) Lateral view of a 3D reconstruction of the facial bones is shown. The mandible can be divided into condyle, neck, ramus, coronoid process, body, and alveolar ridge. The mental foramen is seen in the anterior body and transmits the mental nerve, a sensory nerve to the chin. (Bottom) Frontal view of a 3D reconstruction of the facial bones is shown. The mandible anterior body is best delineated with the paired mental foramina evident. The infraorbital nerves are transmitted via the paired infraorbital foramina.

SECTION 7
Spine

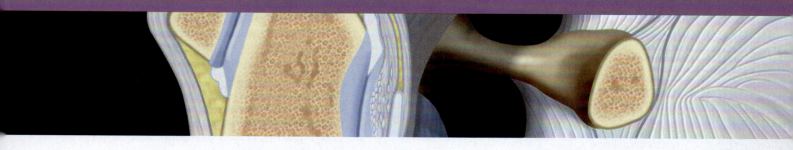

Craniocervical Junction	**498**
Cervical Spine	**514**
Brachial Plexus	**532**

Craniocervical Junction

TERMINOLOGY

Definitions

- Craniocervical junction (CCJ): C1, C2, and articulation with skull base

GROSS ANATOMY

Overview

- CCJ comprises occiput, atlas, axis, their articulations, ligaments

Components

- **Bones**
  - **Occipital bone**
    - Occipital condyles are paired, oval-shaped, inferior prominences of lateral exoccipital portion of occipital bone
    - Articular facet projects laterally
  - **C1 (atlas)**
    - Composed of anterior and posterior arches; no body
    - Paired lateral masses with their superior and inferior articular facets
    - Large transverse processes with transverse foramen
  - **C2 (axis)**
    - Large body and superiorly projecting odontoid process
    - Superior articulating facet surface is convex and directed laterally
    - Inferior articular process + facet surface typical of lower cervical vertebrae
    - Superior facet positioned relatively anteriorly; inferior facet posterior with elongated pars interarticularis
- **Joints**
  - **Atlantooccipital joints**
    - Inferior articular facet of occipital condyle: Oval, convex surface; projects laterally
    - Superior articular facet of C1: Oval, concave anteroposteriorly; projects medially
  - **Median atlantoaxial joints**
    - Pivot-type joint between dens + ring formed by anterior arch + transverse ligament of C1
    - Synovial cavities between transverse ligament/odontoid and atlas/odontoid articulations
  - **Lateral atlantoaxial joints**
    - Inferior articular facet of C1: Concave mediolaterally; projects medially in coronal plane
    - Superior articular facet of C2: Convex surface; projects laterally
- **Ligaments (from anterior to posterior)**
  - **Anterior atlantooccipital membrane**: Connects anterior arch C1 with anterior margin foramen magnum
  - **Odontoid ligaments**
    - Apical ligament: Small fibrous band extending from dens tip to basion
    - Alar ligaments: Thick, horizontally directed ligaments extending from lateral surface of dens tip to anteromedial occipital condyles
  - **Cruciate ligament**
    - Transverse ligament: Strong horizontal component between lateral masses of C1, passes behind dens
    - Craniocaudal component: Fibrous band running from transverse ligament superiorly to foramen magnum and inferiorly to C2
  - **Tectorial membrane**: Continuation of posterior longitudinal ligament; attaches to anterior rim foramen magnum (posterior clivus)
  - **Posterior atlantooccipital membrane**
    - Posterior arch C1 to margin of foramen magnum
    - Deficit laterally where vertebral artery enters on superior surface of C1
- **Biomechanics**
  - Atlantooccipital joint: 50% cervical flexion/extension and limited lateral motion
  - Atlantoaxial joint: 50% cervical rotation

IMAGING ANATOMY

Overview

- **Lateral assessment of CCJ**
  - **C1-2 interspinous space**
    - ≤ 10 mm
  - **Atlantodental interval**
    - Adults < 3 mm, children < 5 mm in flexion
  - **Pseudosubluxation**
    - Physiologic anterior displacement seen in 40% at C2-3 level and 14% at C3-4 level to age 8
    - Anterior displacement of C2 on C3 up to 4 mm
  - **Posterior cervical line**: Line drawn from anterior aspect of C1-3 spinous processes → anterior C2 spinous process should be within 2 mm of this line
  - **Wackenheim line**
    - Posterior surface of clivus → posterior odontoid tip should lie immediately inferior
    - Relationship does not change in flexion/extension
  - **Welcher basal angle**
    - Angle between lines drawn along plane of sphenoid bone and posterior clivus
    - Normal < 140°, average 132°
  - **Chamberlain line**
    - Between hard palate and opisthion
    - Odontoid tip ≥ 5 mm above line abnormal
  - **McGregor line**
    - Between hard palate to base of occipital bone
    - Odontoid tip ≥ 7 mm above line abnormal
  - **Clivus canal angle**
    - Junction of Wackenheim line and posterior vertebral body line
    - 180° extension, 150° flexion, < 150° abnormal
  - **McRae line**
    - Drawn between basion and opisthion
    - Normal 35 mm diameter
- **Frontal assessment of CCJ**
  - Lateral masses of C1 and C2 should align
    - Overlapping lateral masses can be normal variant in children
  - **Atlantooccipital joint angle**
    - Angle formed at junction of lines traversing joints
    - 125-130° normal, < 124° may reflect condyle hypoplasia

Craniocervical Junction

GRAPHICS

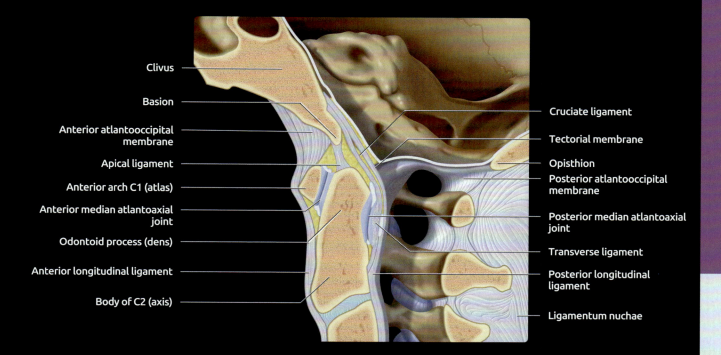

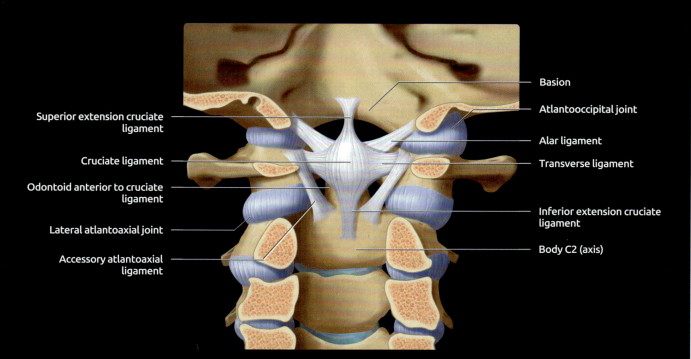

(Top) Sagittal midline graphic of the craniocervical junction (CCJ) is shown. The complex articulations and ligamentous attachments are highlighted. The midline atlantoaxial articulations consist of anterior and posterior median atlantoaxial joints. The anterior joint is between the posterior aspect of the anterior C1 arch and the ventral aspect of odontoid process. The posterior joint is between the dorsal aspect of the odontoid process and the cruciate ligament. The midline view shows a series of ligamentous connection to the skull base, including the anterior atlantooccipital membrane, apical ligament, superior component of cruciate ligament, tectorial membrane, and posterior atlantooccipital membrane. (Bottom) Posterior view shows the CCJ with posterior elements cut away to define the components of the cruciate ligament and alar ligaments.

Craniocervical Junction

C1 GRAPHICS

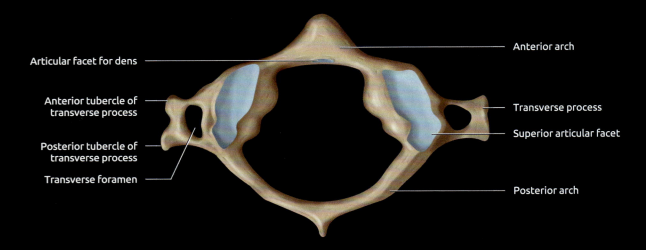

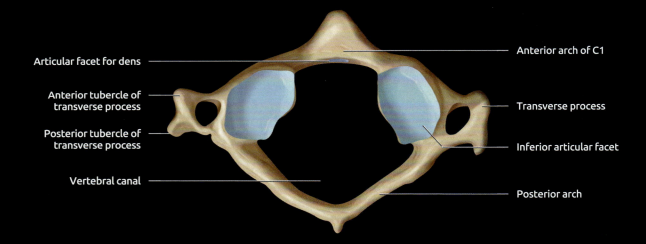

(Top) Axial graphic shows atlas viewed from above. The characteristic ring shape is shown, composed of anterior and posterior arches and paired large lateral masses. The superior articular facet is concave anteroposteriorly and projects medially for articulation with the convex surface of the occipital condyle at the atlantooccipital joint. The anterior arch articulates with the odontoid process at the anterior median atlantoaxial joint. (Bottom) Axial graphic shows the atlas viewed from below. The large inferior facet surface is concave mediolaterally and projects medially for articulation with the convex surface of the superior articular facet of C2. The canal of the atlas is ~ 3 cm in AP diameter. Spinal cord, odontoid process, and free space for cord are each about 1 cm in diameter. The size of the anterior midline tubercle of the anterior arch and the spinous process of the posterior arch are quite variable.

Craniocervical Junction

C2 GRAPHICS

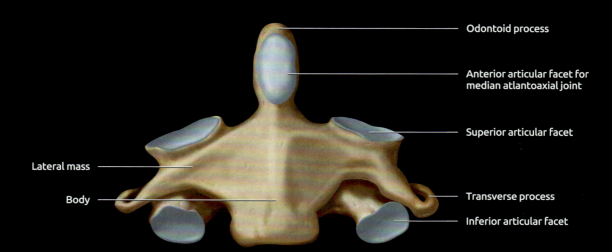

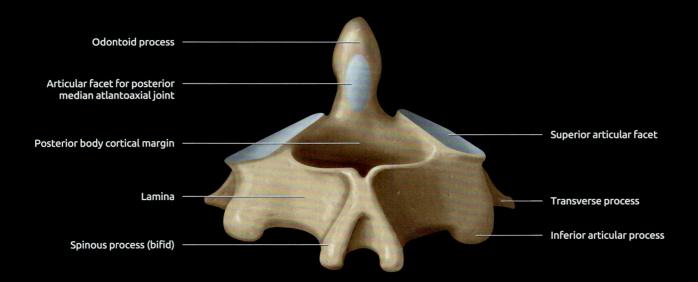

(Top) Axis viewed from the anterior perspective is shown. The odontoid process is the "purloined" embryologic centrum of C1, which is incorporated into C2, giving C2 its unique morphology. The C2 body laterally is defined by large lateral masses for articulation with the inferior facet of C1. The elongated pars interarticularis of C2 ends with the inferior articular process for articulation with the superior articular facet of C3. (Bottom) Axis viewed from the posterior perspective is shown. The odontoid process has anterior and posterior joints for articulation with C1. The anterior median joint articulates with the C1 arch, while the posterior median joint (shown here) involves the transverse ligament.

Craniocervical Junction

CRANIOMETRY GRAPHICS

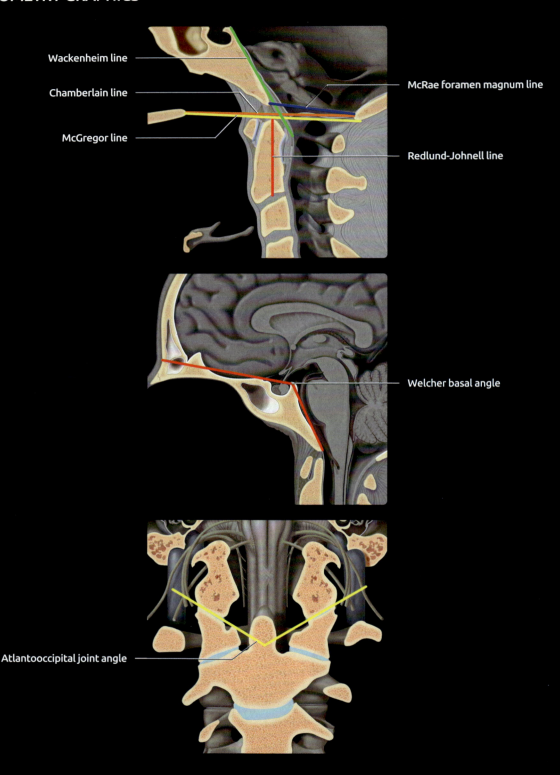

(Top) *Sagittal graphic shows important skull base craniometry. The Chamberlain line (orange) is drawn between the hard palate and the opisthion. The McGregor line (yellow) is drawn from the hard palate to the caudal point (base) of the occipital bone. The Wackenheim line (green) is drawn along the posterior surface of the clivus. The McRae foramen magnum line (blue) is drawn between the basion and the opisthion. The Redlund-Johnell line (red) is drawn from the base of C2 to the McGregor line.* (Middle) *Sagittal midline graphic shows the Welcher basal angle, which is the angle between the lines drawn along the plane of the sphenoid bone and along the clivus (nasion to sella, sella along posterior clivus to basion). Normal is < 140°; platybasia if > 140°.* (Bottom) *Coronal graphic of the CCJ shows lines drawn along the atlantooccipital joints to measure the atlantooccipital joint angle. Normal is 125-130°; < 124° may reflect condyle hypoplasia.*

Craniocervical Junction

BONE CT & T1 MR CRANIOMETRY

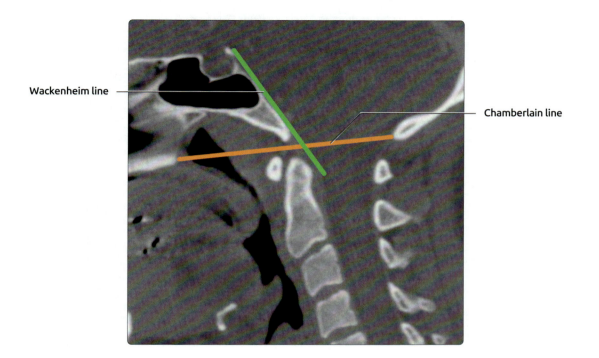

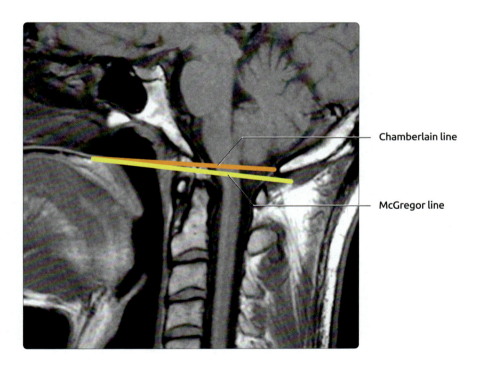

(Top) *Sagittal CT reformat in the midline is shown. The Chamberlain line is shown in orange extending from the hard palate to the opisthion. Projection of up to 1/3 of the dens (5 mm) above this line is normal. The Wackenheim line is shown in green along the clivus. The dens should lie immediately inferior to this line, and any intersection is considered abnormal.* **(Bottom)** *Sagittal T1 MR shows the Chamberlain line in orange. The odontoid tip ≥ 5 mm above the line defines the basilar impression. The McGregor line is shown in yellow. This line has the same significance as the Chamberlain line, with the odontoid tip ≥ 7 mm above the line, defining the basilar impression.*

Craniocervical Junction

LATERAL RADIOGRAPHY CRANIOMETRY

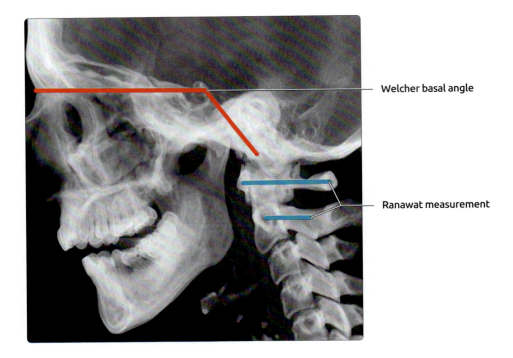

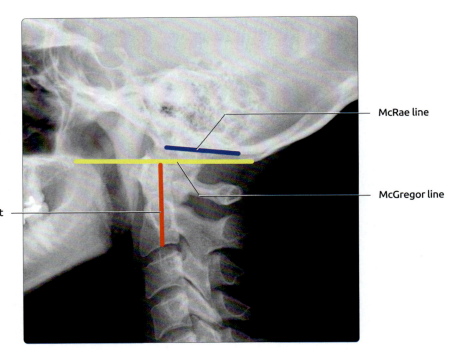

(Top) In this lateral plain film radiograph, the Welcher basal angle is shown in red. The platybasia exists if the angle is > 140° (normal is < 140°). The Ranawat measurement is shown in blue and is used to assess collapse at the C1-2 articulation. Measurement is taken from the center of C2 pedicle to the line connecting the anterior and posterior arches of C1. Normal is ~ 14 mm in men and ~ 13 mm in women (< 13 mm is consistent with impaction). **(Bottom)** In this lateral plain film radiograph, the McRae line is shown in blue. Normal is ~ 35 mm diameter. The normal odontoid process does not extend above this line. The Redlund-Johnell measurement is shown in red. This measurement is from the base of the C2 body to the McGregor line (shown in yellow). Normal is ~ 34 mm in men and ~ 28 mm in women.

Craniocervical Junction

LATERAL RADIOGRAPHY

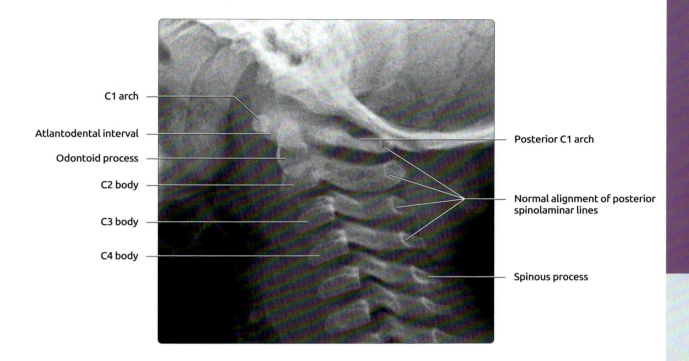

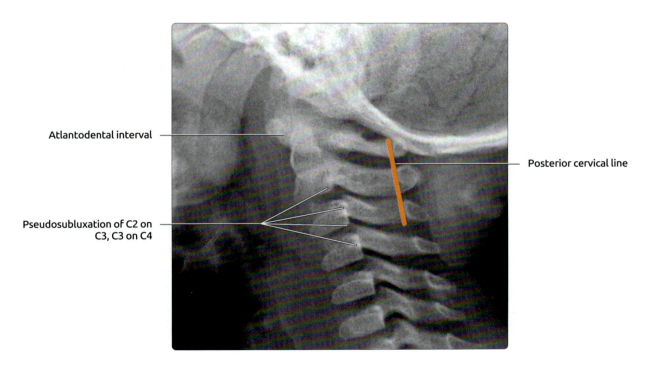

(Top) *Lateral plain film radiograph of the cervical spine in a child shows physiologic anterior displacement of C2 with respect to C3, and C3 with respect to C4, the so-called pseudosubluxation. Physiologic subluxation is differentiated from pathologic anterior displacement by the absence of prevertebral soft tissue swelling, reduction on extension, and assessment of the posterior cervical line.* (Bottom) *Posterior cervical line is drawn along the anterior aspect of the C1-3 spinous processes. The anterior C2 spinous process should be within 2 mm of this line in flexion and extension. The atlantodental interval is < 3.5 mm in children and < 3 mm in adults.*

Craniocervical Junction

RADIOGRAPHY

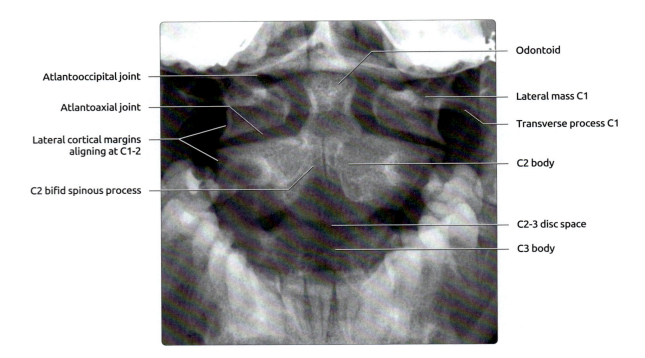

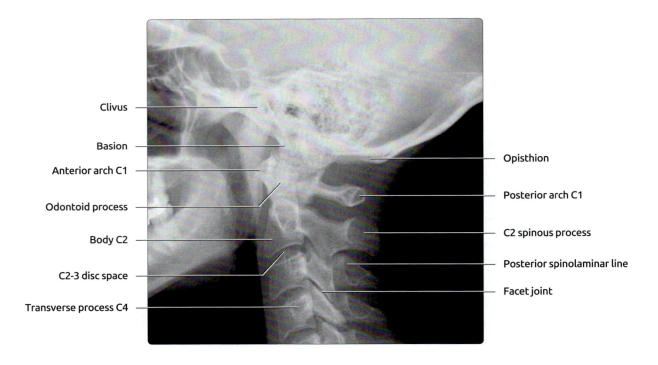

(Top) AP open-mouth view shows the odontoid process. With proper positioning, the odontoid process is visualized in the midline with symmetrically placed lateral C1 masses on either side. The medial space between the odontoid and C1 lateral masses should be symmetric as well. The lateral cortical margins of the C1 and C2 lateral masses should align. The atlantoaxial joints are visible bilaterally with smooth cortical margins. The bifid C2 process should not be confused for fracture. *(Bottom)* Lateral radiograph shows the CCJ. There is smooth anatomic alignment of the posterior vertebral body margins and the posterior spinolaminar line of the posterior elements. The anterior arch of C1 should assume a well-defined oval appearance with sharp margination between the anterior C1 arch and the odontoid process.

Craniocervical Junction

CORONAL BONE CT

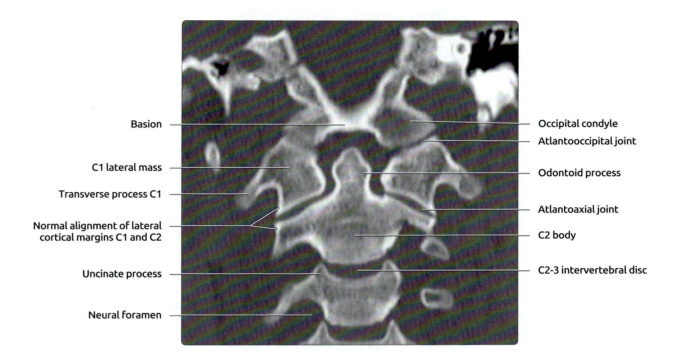

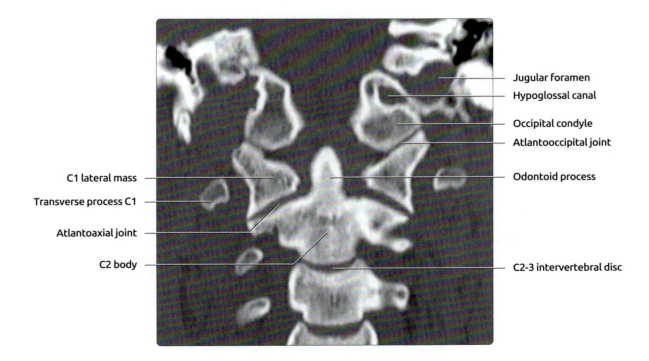

(Top) First of 2 coronal bone CT reconstructions of the CCJ presented from anterior to posterior is shown. The odontoid process is visualized in the midline as a sharply corticated, bony peg with symmetrically placed lateral C1 masses on either side. The lateral cortical margins of the C1 lateral masses and the C2 lateral masses should align. The atlantooccipital and atatlantaxial joints are visible bilaterally with even joint margins and sharp cortical margins. (Bottom) More posterior view of the CCJ is shown. Both atlantooccipital joints are now well-defined with smooth cortical margins sloping superolateral to inferomedial. The atlantoaxial joints are smoothly sloping inferolateral to superomedial.

Craniocervical Junction

AXIAL BONE CT

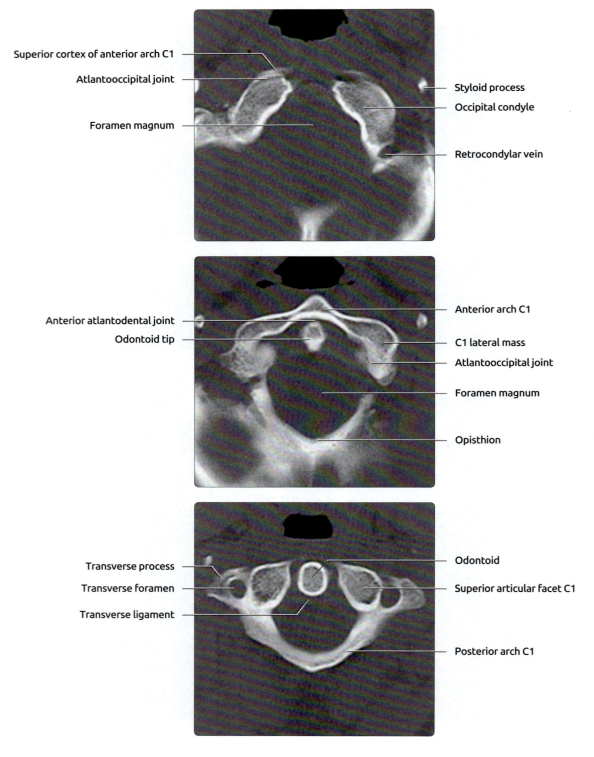

(Top) First of 6 axial bone CT images through the CCJ presented from superior to inferior is shown. The anterolateral margin of the foramen magnum is formed by the prominent occipital condyles, which articulate with the superior articular facets of the C1 lateral masses. (Middle) More inferior image of the CCJ is shown. The anterior arch of C1 is now well defined with the odontoid process of C2 coming into plane. The atlantooccipital joint is seen in oblique section and therefore has poorly defined margins. The odontoid is tightly applied to the posterior margin of the C1 arch, held in place by the strong transverse component of the cruciate ligament. (Bottom) Image at the level of the atlas is shown. The unique morphology of the C1 body is defined with its large transverse process with transverse foramen and ring shape.

Craniocervical Junction

AXIAL BONE CT

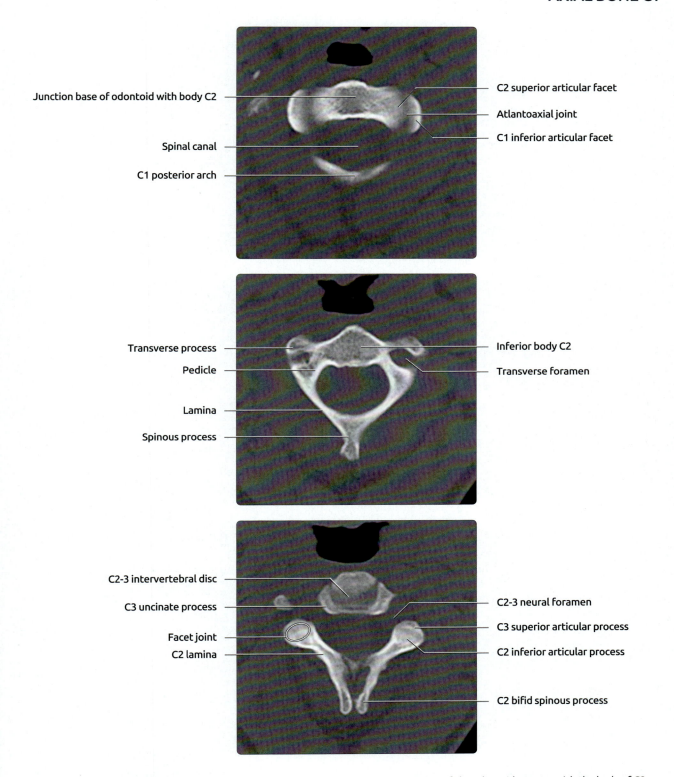

(Top) Image through lateral atlantoaxial joints is shown. This section defines the junction of the odontoid process with the body of C2. The obliquely oriented atlantoaxial joints are partially seen with the C1 component lateral to the joint space and the C2 component medial. (Middle) Image through inferior C2 body level shows large C2 vertebral body and vertebral arch formed by gracile pedicles and laminae. (Bottom) Image through C2-3 intervertebral disc level is shown. The C2-3 neural foramen is well defined with the posterior margin formed by the superior articular process of C3. The spinous process of C2 is large and typically bifid. The C2-3 disc assumes the characteristic cervical cup-shaped morphology bounded by uncinate processes.

Craniocervical Junction

3D-VRT NECT

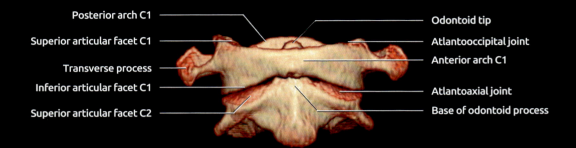

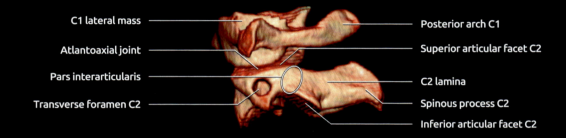

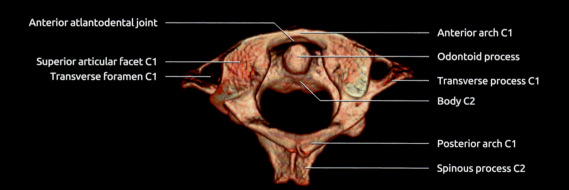

(Top) Anterior view shows a 3D-VRT NECT examination. The unique ability of the C1-2 articulation to provide rotation is apparent in this projection with the bony peg of the odontoid process forming the pivot point for the C1 ring. (Middle) Lateral view shows a 3D-VRT NECT examination. The complex lateral components of C1 and C2 bodies are highlighted in this projection. The superior facet of C2 is anteriorly positioned to articulate with the inferior articular facet of C1, while the inferior articular facet of C2 is more posterior, forming the top of the cervical articular "pillar." The articular facets are separated by the elongated pars interarticularis. (Bottom) Superior view shows a 3D-VRT NECT examination depicting the relationship of the C1 ring with underlying C2 odontoid and lateral masses.

Craniocervical Junction

SAGITTAL T1 MR

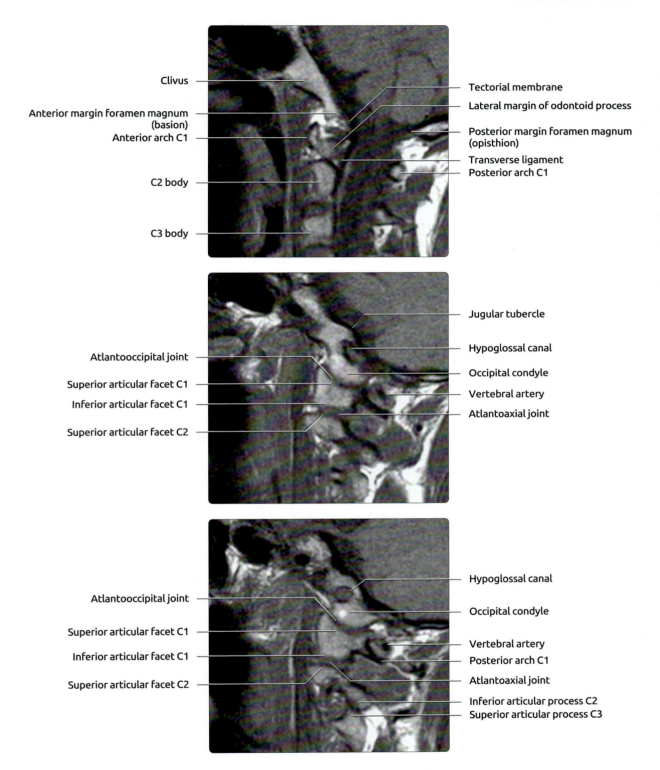

(Top) First of 3 parasagittal T1 MR images from medial to lateral through the atlantooccipital joint is shown. This image extends through the lateral cortical margin of the odontoid, which is incompletely visualized. The anterior arch of C1 is obliquely visualized as it curves posterolaterally. The lateral extension of the cruciate ligament, the transverse ligament, is prominent. (Middle) The relationship of the occipital condyle, C1 lateral mass, and atlantoaxial joint is highlighted in this image. The articular surface of the occipital condyle is convex and the superior facet of C1 is concave, allowing for flexion/extension. (Bottom) More lateral image of the CCJ is shown. The atlantooccipital joint and atlantoaxial joints are visible with sharp, smooth cortical margins.

Craniocervical Junction

SAGITTAL CT & MR

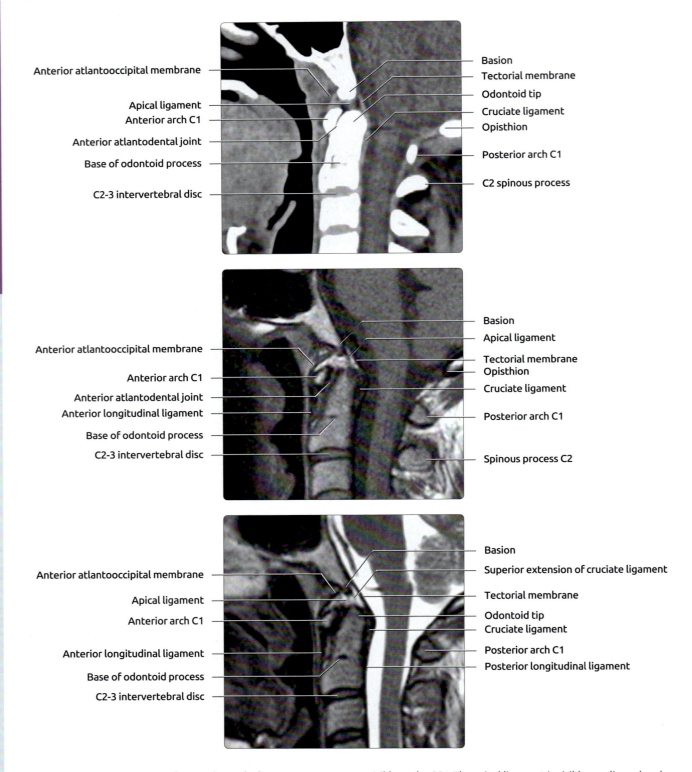

(Top) Sagittal midline CT reformat shows the ligamentous structures visible at the CCJ. The apical ligament is visible as a linear band between the odontoid tip and clivus. The tectorial membrane is the superior extension of the posterior longitudinal ligament. The anterior atlantooccipital membrane is the extension of the anterior longitudinal ligament. (Middle) Sagittal T1 MR midline image of the CCJ is shown. The atlantodental interval is well defined by the adjacent low-signal cortical margins of the C1 anterior arch and the odontoid process. The cruciate ligament is a low-signal band dorsal to the odontoid. (Bottom) Sagittal T2 MR of the CCJ is shown. The tectorial membrane, superior extension of cruciate ligament, apical ligament, and anterior atlantooccipital membranes are evident.

Craniocervical Junction

AXIAL T2 MR

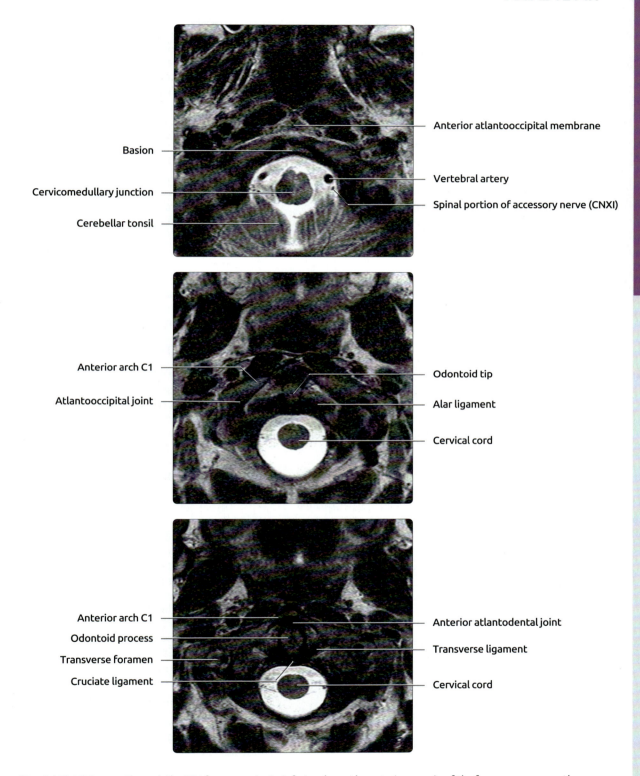

(Top) First of 3 axial T2 MR images through the CCJ from superior to inferior shows the anterior margin of the foramen magnum, the cervicomedullary junction, and adjacent vertebral artery flow voids. (Middle) Image at level of C1 anterior arch is shown. The odontoid tip is seen as rounded, intermediate signal in the midline, ventral to the cervical cord. The anterior arch of C1 is visible with its well-defined cortical margins. The alar ligaments are identified as low signal intensity bands extending laterally from the lateral margins of the odontoid process toward the occipital condyles. (Bottom) More inferior image through the atlantodental joint is shown. The anterior atlantodental joint is seen along the ventral margin of the odontoid process. The cruciate ligament (transverse component) is seen as low-signal bands curving over the dorsal margin of odontoid.

513

Cervical Spine

TERMINOLOGY

Definitions

- Cervical spine consists of 7 uppermost spinal bones, including atlas (C1) and axis (C2); subaxial cervical spine = C3-C7

GROSS ANATOMY

Overview

- Consists of 7 vertebrae (C1-C7)
  - **Craniocervical junction (CCJ)**: C1, C2, and articulation with skull base constitutes CCJ
  - **Subaxial spine**: C3-C7
    - C3-C6 typical cervical vertebrae
    - C7 has features that differ slightly from C3-C6

Components of Subaxial Cervical Spine

- **Bones C3-C7**
  - **Body**
    - Small, broader transversely than in AP dimension
    - Posterolateral edges of superior surface are turned upward = uncinate processes
  - **Vertebral arch**
    - Pedicle: Delicate, projects posterolaterally
    - Lamina: Thin and narrow
    - Vertebral foramen: Large, triangular-shaped
  - **Transverse process**
    - Project laterally and contain foramen for vertebral artery
    - Anterior and posterior tubercles are separated by superolateral groove (lateral neural recess) for exiting spinal nerve
  - **Articular processes**
    - Superior and inferior articular processes with articular facets oriented ~ 45° superiorly from transverse plane
    - Form paired osseous shafts posterolateral to vertebral bodies = articular pillars
  - Spinous process: Short and bifid
  - **C7 unique features**
    - Spinous process: Long, prominent
    - Transverse process: Short and project inferolaterally compare with T1 spinous processes, which are long and project superolaterally
- **Intervertebral foramen**
  - Oriented anterolaterally below pedicles at ~ 45° to sagittal plane
- **Joints**
  - Intervertebral disc
    - Narrowest in cervical region
    - Thinner posteriorly than anteriorly
    - Do not extend to lateral margins of vertebral bodies in cervical spine → joints of Luschka
  - **Uncovertebral joint** (joints of Luschka)
    - Oblique, cleft-like cavities between superior surfaces of uncinate processes and lateral lips of inferior articular surface of next superior vertebrae
    - Lined by cartilaginous endplate of vertebral body
    - No true synovial lining present; contains serum, simulating synovial fluid

- Uncinate process develops during childhood with uncovertebral joint forming by fibrillation and fissuring in fibers of annulus fibrosus
  - **Facet (zygapophyseal) joints**
    - Facet joints oriented ~ 45° superiorly from transverse plane in upper cervical spine; assume more vertical orientation toward C7
    - Formed by articulation between superior and inferior articular processes = articular pillars
    - Forms 2 sides of flexible tripod of bone (vertebral bodies, right and left articular pillars) for support of cranium
- **Ligaments**
  - Anterior and posterior longitudinal, ligamentum flavum, interspinous and supraspinous ligaments
  - Additional ligaments of CCJ include apical, alar, and cruciate ligaments
- **Biomechanics**
  - Subaxial cervical spine shows free motion range relative to remainder of presacral spine
    - Cervical extension checked by anterior longitudinal ligament and musculature
    - Cervical flexion checked by articular pillars and intertransverse ligaments

IMAGING ANATOMY

Lateral Assessment of Subaxial Spine

- Principles apply equally to radiography, CT or MR
- **Prevertebral soft tissues**: Distance between air column and anterior aspect of vertebral body
  - Adults: < 7 mm at C2 and < 22 mm at C6
  - Child: < 14 mm at C6
- Bony alignment
  - **Anterior vertebral line**: Smooth curve paralleling anterior vertebral cortex
    - Less important than posterior cortical line
  - **Posterior vertebral line**: Smooth curve paralleling posterior vertebral cortex
    - Translation > 3.5 mm is abnormal
    - Flexion and extension allow physiological offset < 3 mm of posterior cortical margin of successive vertebral bodies
  - **Spinolaminar line**: Smooth curve from opisthion to C7 formed by junction of laminae with spinous processes
  - **Spinous process angulation**: Cervical spinous processes should converge toward common point posteriorly
    - Widening is present when distance is > 1.5x interspinous distance of adjacent spinal segments

Frontal Assessment of Subaxial Spine

- Lateral masses: Bilateral smooth undulating margins
- Spinous processes: Midline
  - Lateral rotation of 1 spinous process with respect to others is abnormal
- Interspinous distance: Symmetric throughout
  - Interspinous distance 1.5x distance of level above or below is abnormal

Cervical Spine

GRAPHICS

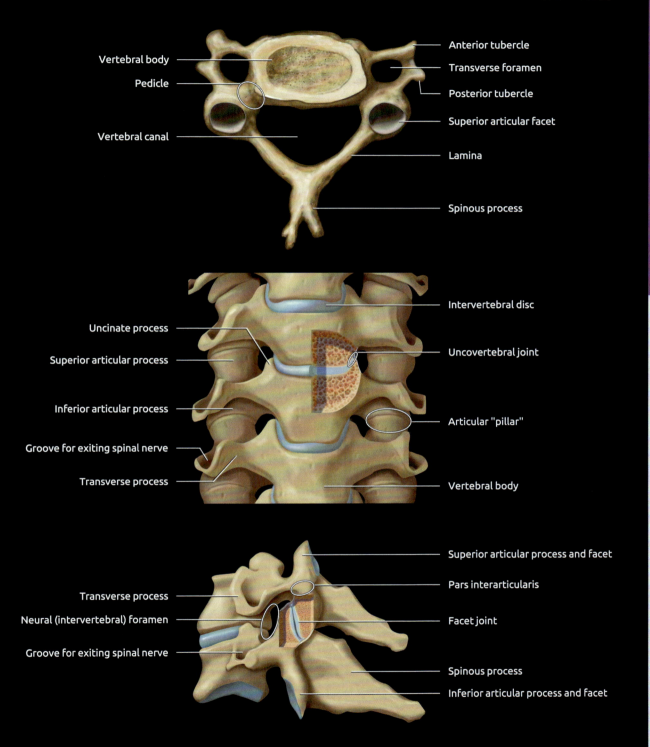

(Top) Graphic of a typical cervical vertebra viewed from above demonstrates important morphology. Vertebral body is broader transversely than in AP dimension, central vertebral canal is large and triangular in shape, pedicles are directed posterolaterally, and laminae are delicate and give rise to a spinous process with a bifid tip. Lateral masses contain the vertebral foramen for passage of vertebral artery and veins. (Middle) Frontal graphic of subaxial cervical spine with cutout shows intervertebral disc and uncovertebral joints. Paired lateral articular "pillars" are formed by articulation between superior and inferior articular processes. (Bottom) Lateral graphic of 2 consecutive typical cervical vertebrae with cutout shows facet (zygapophyseal) joint detail. Note also the prominent groove on the superior surface of the transverse process for exiting spinal nerves.

Cervical Spine

GRAPHICS

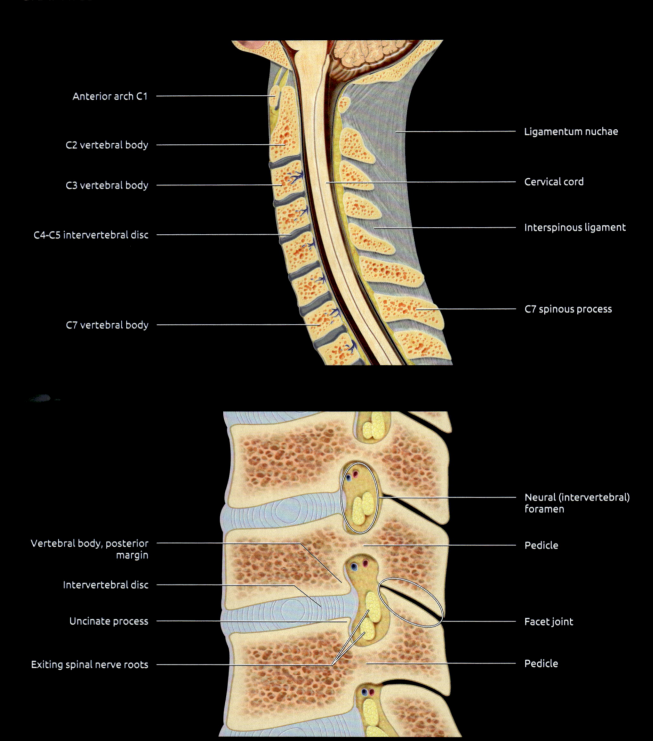

(Top) Sagittal midline graphic of the cervical spine and cord shows a gentle lordotic curve and smooth alignment of the adjacent vertebrae. C1, C2, and their articulation with the skull base constitutes the craniocervical junction. C3-C7 constitutes the subaxial cervical spine. C3-C6 are regarded as typical cervical vertebrae, whereas C7 has features that differ slightly from C3-C6, including a long, prominent spinous process. (Bottom) Sagittal graphic through the cervical neural foramen shows position of exiting spinal nerves within the lower part of the neural foramen. Neural foramina are oriented anterolaterally (compare with thoracic and lumbar regions). Anterior boundary of the neural foramen include the uncinate process, intervertebral disc, and vertebral body from inferior to superior. Pedicles form superior and inferior boundaries. Posterior boundary is the facet joint complex.

Cervical Spine

GRAPHIC & 3D-VRT NECT

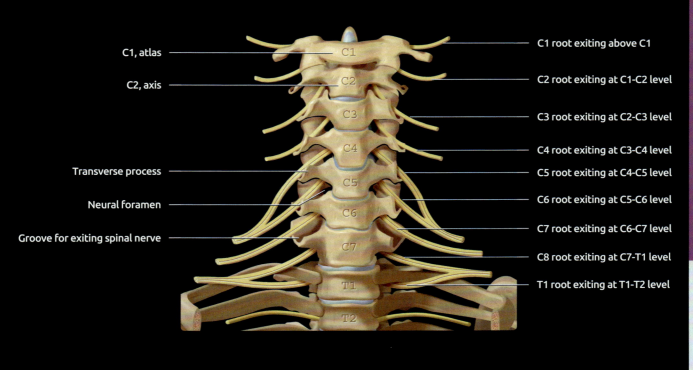

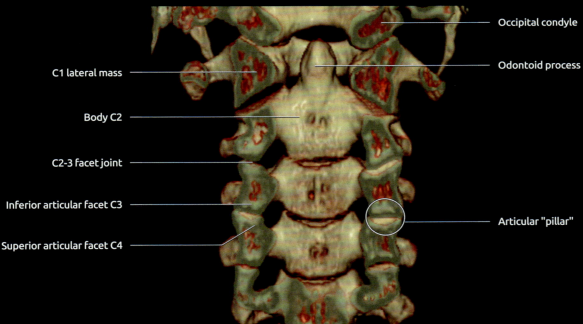

(Top) Coronal graphic of the cervical spine shows vertebrae and corresponding cervical nerves. The vertebra are numbered and are shown with their exiting nerves. There are 8 cervical nerves with C1 nerve exiting above the C1 body and C2 nerve exiting at the C1-C2 level. The C8 nerve exits at C7-T1. Below this level, the thoracic roots exit below their respective numbered vertebra. The roots exit inferiorly within the neural foramen, along the bony groove in the transverse process. (Bottom) Coronal 3D-VRT examination of the cervical spine, viewed posteriorly with the dorsal elements partially removed to show the dorsal vertebral body surface, is shown. The concept of the cervical articular pillars is well shown in this view with the facets forming paired columns of bone with superior and inferior articulating facets.

Cervical Spine

GRAPHIC & LATERAL RADIOGRAPH

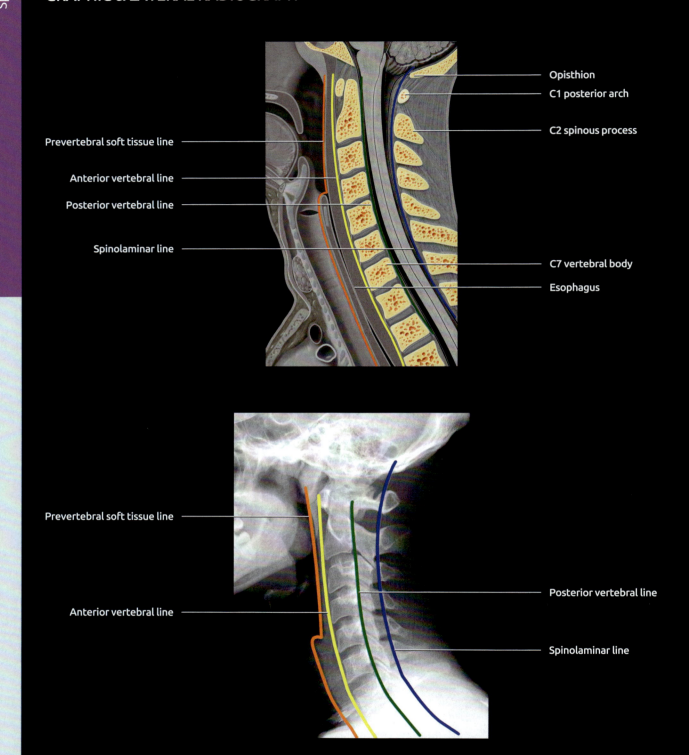

(Top) Sagittal midline graphic of the cervical spine is shown. The normal cervical spine shows a smooth lordotic curve with smooth alignment of a series of lines going from ventral to dorsal, including prevertebral soft tissues (orange), anterior vertebral body cortical margins (yellow), posterior vertebral body margins (green), and posterior spinolaminar line (blue). In adults, the prevertebral soft tissues measure < 7 mm at C2 and < 22 mm at C6. In children, they measure < 14 mm at C6. (Bottom) Lateral radiograph of the cervical spine shows normal alignment. A series of gently curving lines make up the normal cervical curvature, extending from prevertebral soft tissues to the posterior spinolaminar line. In addition, the cervical spinous processes should all converge toward a common point posteriorly.

Cervical Spine

RADIOGRAPHY

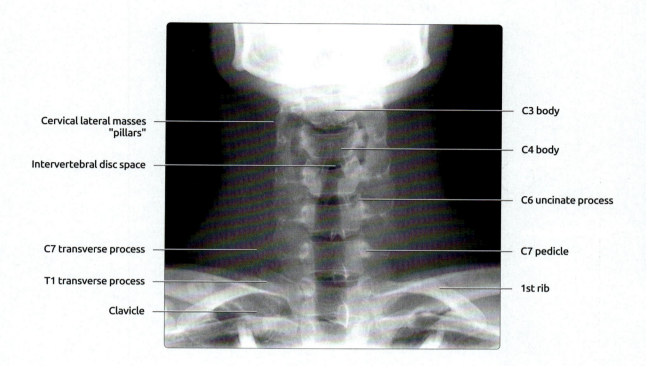

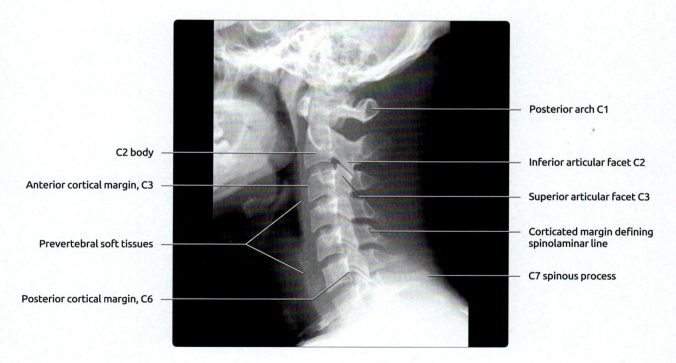

(Top) AP plain film view of the cervical spine is shown. The articular facets are viewed obliquely in this projection and therefore not defined, giving the appearance of smoothly undulating lateral columns of bone. The superior and inferior vertebral endplate margins are sharp with regular spacing of the intervertebral discs. The spinous processes are midline. C7 transverse process is directed inferolaterally compared with T1, which is directed superolaterally. (Bottom) Lateral radiograph of cervical spine is shown. The prevertebral soft tissues should form a defined, abrupt "shelf" at ~ C4/C5 where the hypopharynx/esophagus begins, hence thickening the prevertebral soft tissues. The bony cervical spine is aligned from anteriorly to posteriorly with the anterior vertebral body margins, the posterior vertebral body margins, and ventral margins of the spinous processes (spinolaminar line).

Cervical Spine

RADIOGRAPHY & 3D-VRT NECT

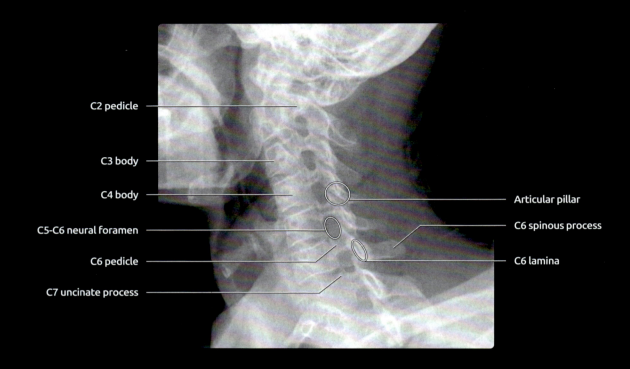

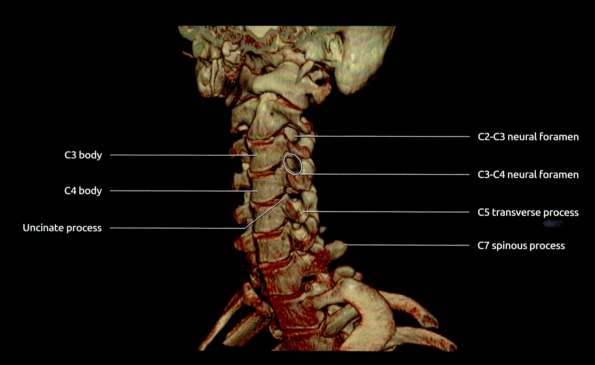

(Top) Oblique radiograph of the cervical spine best demonstrates the neural foramina, as these are oriented obliquely at ~ 45° from the sagittal plane. With the patient rotated to the left, the radiograph demonstrates the right-sided foramina. The anterior boundary of the neural foramina includes the uncinate process, intervertebral disc, and vertebral body. The posterior boundary is the facet joint complex. The articular pillar facet joints are viewed obliquely and hence are not well defined. The lamina are seen end on and hence sharply corticated. (Bottom) Oblique 3D-VRT examination of the cervical spine shows the neural foramina end on. The groove on the superior surface of the transverse processes for the exiting spinal nerves is well shown.

Cervical Spine

3D-VRT NECT

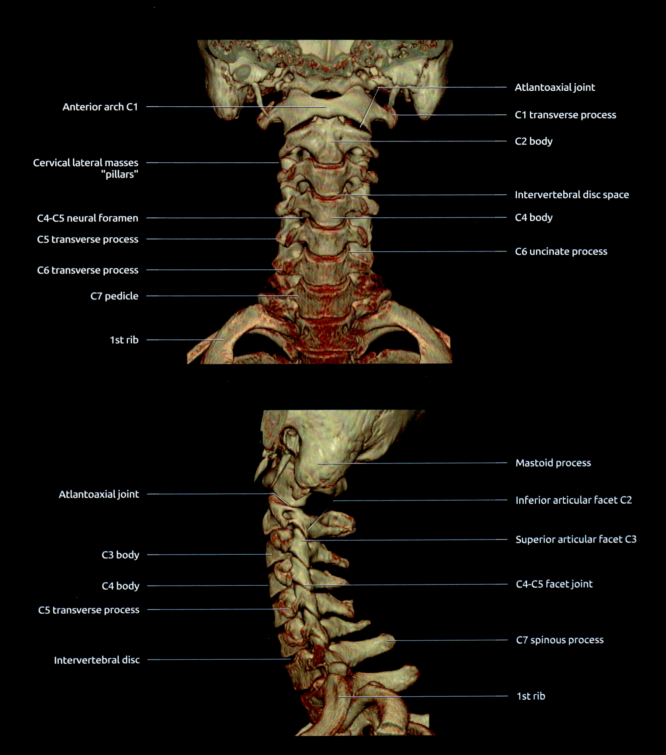

(Top) Anterior view of 3D-VRT NECT examination of the cervical spine is shown. The wide neural foramina with the groove or sulcus on the superior surface of the transverse processes for the exiting nerves are well seen. The transverse processes with the tubercles for muscle attachments are well identified from C3-C7 levels. The uncinate processes are acquired, superior bony projections along the posterolateral margins of the vertebral bodies and form the uncovertebral joints with the adjacent superior vertebral body. (Bottom) Lateral view of 3D-VRT NECT examination of the cervical spine is shown. The facet joints are seen in profile angled ~ 45° superiorly from the transverse plane. They align in a smooth interlocking fashion with the superior articular facets directed posteriorly and the inferior articular facets directed anteriorly.

Cervical Spine

AXIAL BONE CT

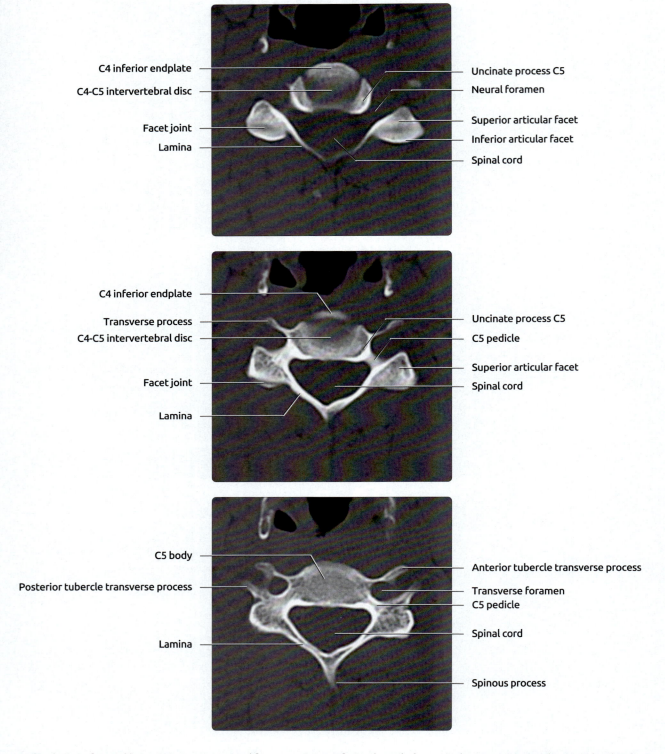

(Top) First of 6 axial bone CT images presented from superior to inferior through the cervical spine starting at the C4-C5 level is shown. The cup-shaped intervertebral disc of the cervical region is seen centrally, bounded along the posterolateral margin by the uncinate processes. The uncinate process defines the joint of Luschka between adjacent vertebral segments. The neural foramina exit at around 45° in an anterolateral direction, bounded posteriorly by the superior articular process. **(Middle)** Image through inferior margin of intervertebral disc is shown. The gracile pedicles arise obliquely from the posterolateral margins of the vertebral bodies. The bony canal is large relative to the posterior elements and assumes a triangular configuration. **(Bottom)** Image through C5 body level is shown. The transverse process contains the transverse foramen for the vertebral artery.

Cervical Spine

AXIAL BONE CT

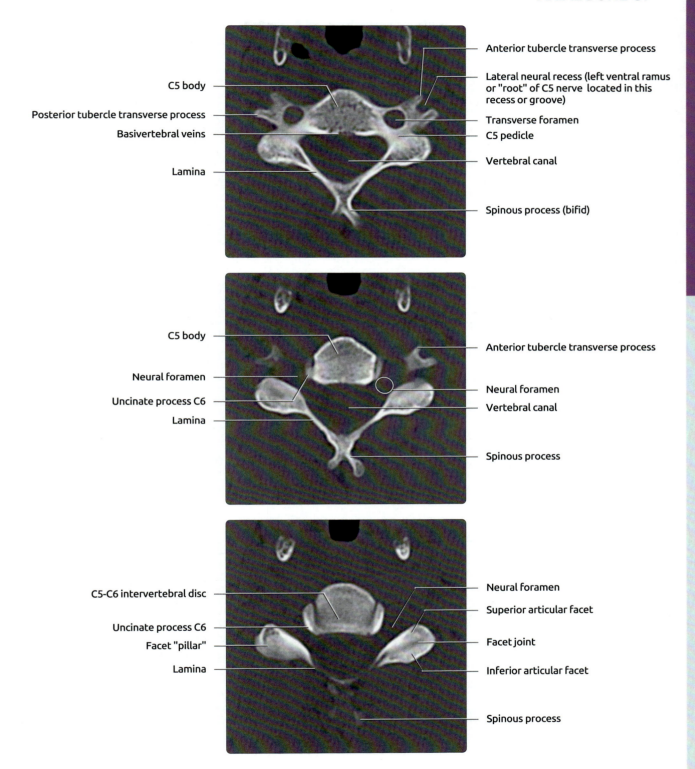

(Top) Image through mid-C5 body at the pedicle level is shown. The transverse foramina are prominent at this level with the round, sharply marginated transverse foramen encompassing the vertical course of the vertebral artery. The anterior and posterior tubercles give rise to muscle attachments in the neck. The vertebral body is interrupted along the posterior cortical margin for the passage of the basivertebral venous complex. (Middle) Image at the inferior C5 body level is shown. The uncinate process arising off of the next inferior vertebral body is coming into view. The inferior margins of the transverse processes are incompletely visualized. The spinous process is well seen, joining with the thin lamina. (Bottom) View at the C5-C6 level shows the next neural foraminal level bounded by the uncovertebral joint anteriorly and facet posteriorly.

Cervical Spine

CORONAL CT MYELOGRAM

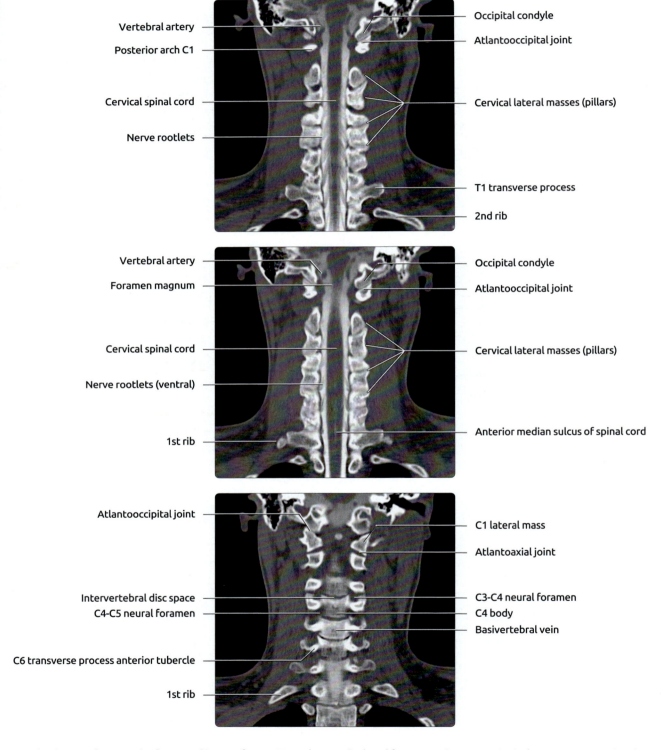

(Top) First of 3 coronal reformatted images from a CT myelogram displayed from posterior to anterior is shown. Most posterior view shows the spinal cord with exiting nerve rootlets at each segmental level traversing in a craniocaudal direction within the thecal sac. T1 transverse process is prominent and directed superolaterally. **(Middle)** More anterior view shows the ventral margin of the cervical spinal cord with the anterior median sulcus, which would contain the anterior spinal artery. The ventral nerve rootlets are also visible. The articular pillars of the facet joints are well shown, giving a view similar to an AP radiograph of the undulating lateral margin of the cervical pillars. **(Bottom)** More anterior view shows transverse processes with adjacent neural foramina. The posterior margins of the vertebral bodies show the midline basivertebral veins.

Cervical Spine

SAGITTAL CT MYELOGRAM

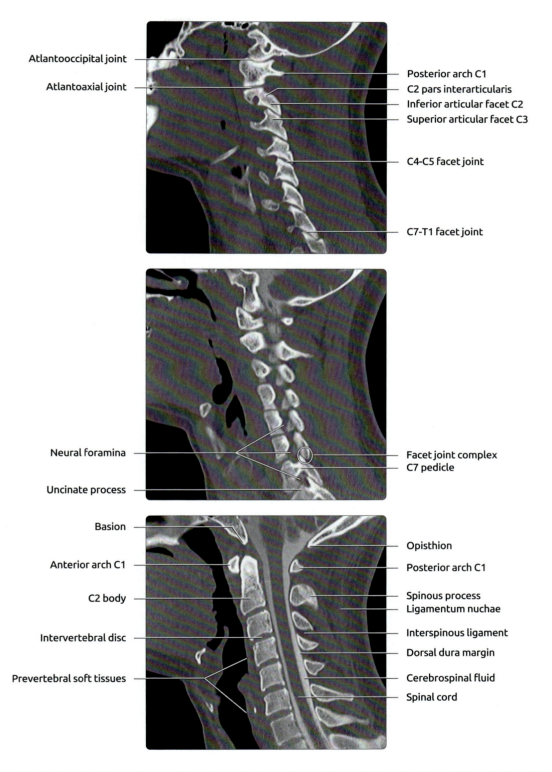

(Top) First of 3 sagittal reformatted images from a CT myelogram is shown. Paramedian sagittal section through the articular pillar shows the facet joints in profile. Superior articular facets are directed posteriorly, while inferior facets are directed anteriorly. The curvilinear shape of the atlantooccipital joint is visible, allowing for flexion/extension. (Middle) More medial section through obliquely oriented neural foramina, which are bounded above and below by pedicles, anteriorly by uncovertebral joint, disc and vertebral body, and posteriorly by facet joint complex, is shown. (Bottom) Midline section shows the spinal cord outlined by the high attenuation of the contrast within the cerebrospinal fluid. Vertebral alignment is normal and prevertebral soft tissues demonstrate an abrupt "shelf" at ~ the C4-C5 level where the esophagus begins.

Cervical Spine

SAGITTAL T1 MR

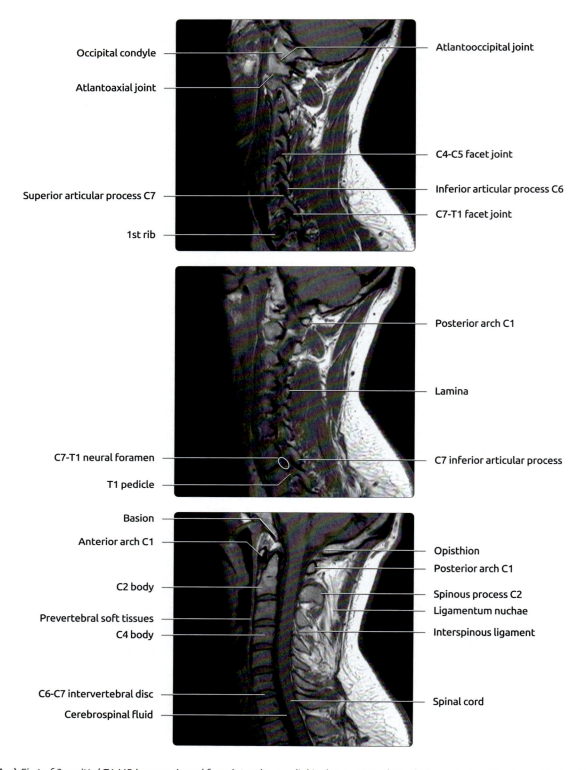

(Top) First of 3 sagittal T1 MR images viewed from lateral to medial is shown. View through the articular pillar shows the facet joints in profile. Margins of the facet joints are well corticated and seen as thin hypointense lines. (Middle) More medial section through obliquely oriented neural foramina is shown. (Bottom) Midline image shows the well-defined, low-signal cortical margins of the vertebral bodies, which merge along their anterior and posterior margins with the hypointense anterior and posterior longitudinal ligaments, respectively. Vertebral marrow signal is hyperintense relative to intervening discs on T1 MR. Cerebrospinal fluid is hypointense.

Cervical Spine

SAGITTAL T2 MR

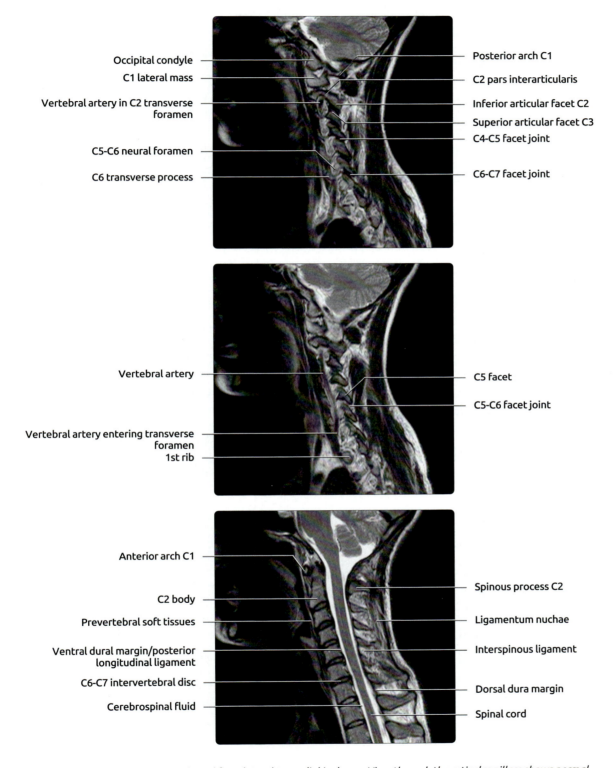

(Top) First of 3 sagittal T2 MR images viewed from lateral to medial is shown. View through the articular pillars shows normal alignment of the facet joints. The rhomboidal configuration of the cervical facets is noted with their complementary superior and inferior articular facets. The exiting spinal nerves run in the groove along the superior aspect of transverse processes. (Middle) More medial section shows the overlapping facets at each level and the flow void of the vertebral artery within the transverse foramen. (Bottom) Midline image shows the relationship of the cervical cord, vertebral bodies, and spinous processes with smooth straight margins and alignment. The posterior dural margin merges with the low signal of the ligamentum flavum and spinous process cortex. The anterior dural margin merges with the posterior body cortex and posterior longitudinal ligament.

Cervical Spine

AXIAL GRE MR

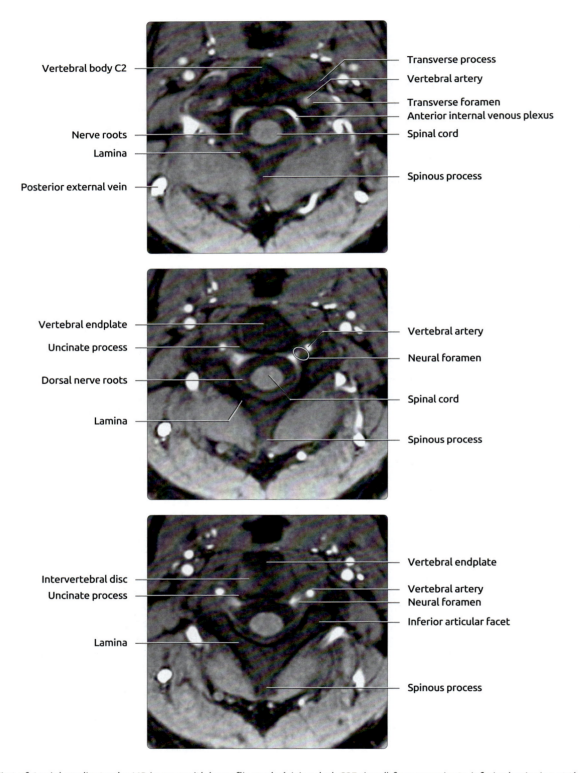

(Top) First of 6 axial gradient-echo MR images with large flip angle (giving dark CSF signal) from superior to inferior beginning at the inferior C2 body level is shown. The prominent transverse foramen with the vertebral artery is apparent. Flow-related enhancement is also visible in the cervical dorsal veins as well as the epidural veins (anterior internal venous plexus). (Middle) Image at the inferior endplate of C2 is shown. The neural foramina are directed at 45° anterolaterally and show flow-related enhancement in epidural/foraminal venous plexus and the ascending vertebral arteries. The spinal cord and dural margins are well defined and smooth. The dorsal nerve rootlets are barely visible within the dorsal thecal sac. (Bottom) Image at the C2-C3 disc level is shown. The inferior articular facet of C2 and the prominent C2 spinous process are visible.

Cervical Spine

AXIAL GRE MR

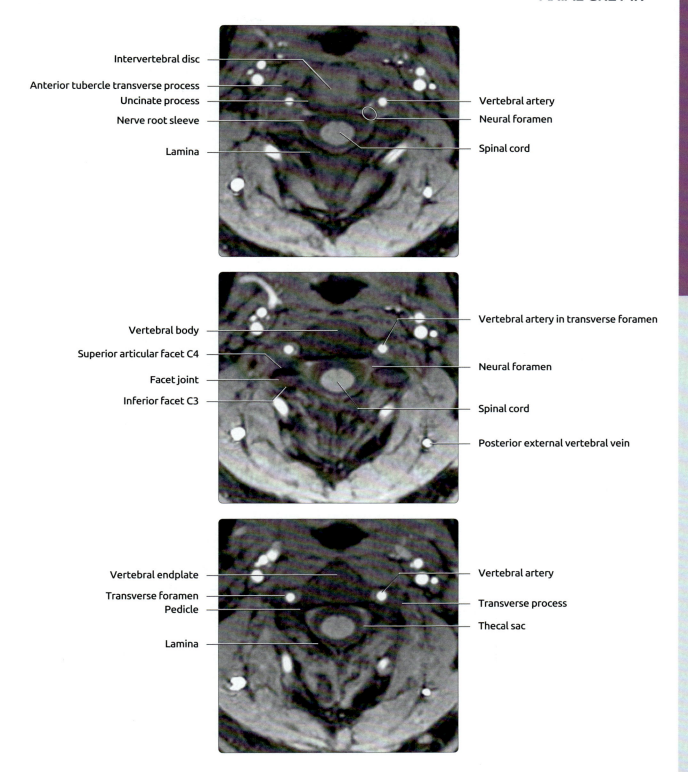

(Top) Image through C2-C3 intervertebral disc is shown. The intermediate signal, square-shaped intervertebral disc is evident with the bounding lower signal uncinate processes. The low-signal, CSF-containing, triangular-shaped root sleeves are seen extending anterolaterally into the neural foramina. (Middle) Image through superior C3 vertebral body shows the C3-C4 facet joint with the anterior low-signal superior facet of C4, the intermediate-signal linear joint space, and the dorsal-positioned low-signal inferior facet of C3. (Bottom) Image through the C3 pedicles, which project posterolaterally from the vertebral body, is shown. The delicate laminae complete the triangular-shaped vertebral foramen containing the thecal sac and contents. The transverse foramina containing the vertebral arteries are prominent within the transverse processes.

Cervical Spine

AXIAL T2 MR

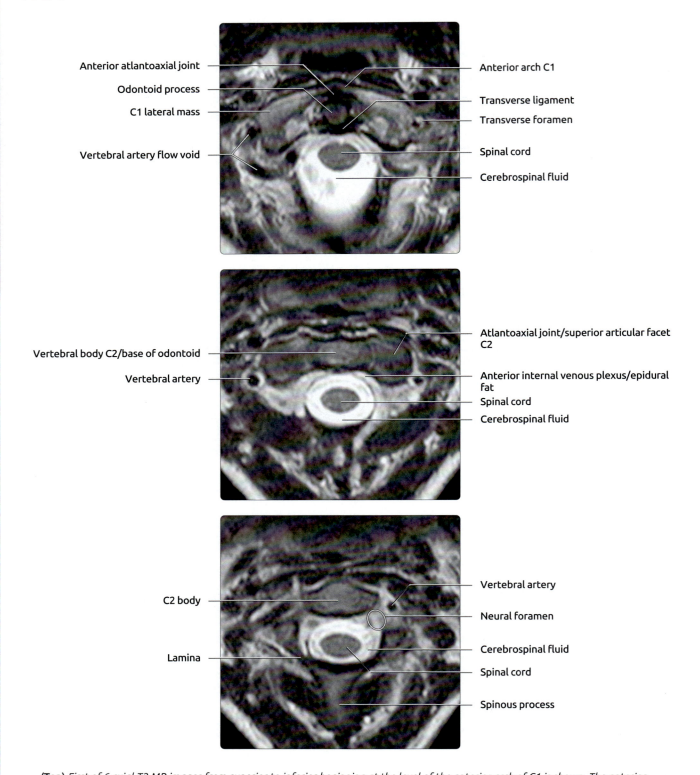

(Top) First of 6 axial T2 MR images from superior to inferior beginning at the level of the anterior arch of C1 is shown. The anterior atlantodental joint is well identified, bounded by the low-signal cortical margins of the anterior odontoid and anterior arch of C1. Posterior to the odontoid is the low-signal transverse ligament complex. (Middle) Image at odontoid/C2 body level is shown. The base of the odontoid is at the level of the lateral atlantoaxial articulation. This joint is sloped, being more superior at the medial margin. The vertebral arteries are identified by their flow voids, located just lateral to the lateral masses, passing superiorly toward the C1 transverse foramen. (Bottom) Image at C2 body level is shown. The relationship of the vertically oriented vertebral artery to the neural foramen is highlighted in this section.

Cervical Spine

AXIAL T2 MR

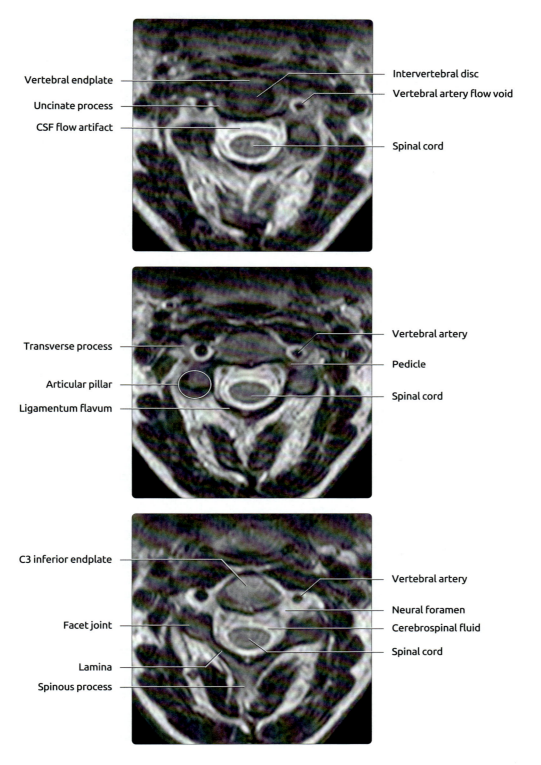

(Top) Image at C2-C3 disc level is shown. The intervertebral disc is fully visualized as low signal with the bounding posterior lateral uncovertebral joints. (Middle) Image through the pedicles of C3 is shown. Pedicles are delicate and are directed posterolaterally from the vertebral body. The articular pillars are formed by the superior and inferior articular processes and intervening facet joints. Prominent vertebral artery flow voids are seen within the transverse foramina of the transverse processes. (Bottom) Image through the neural foramina of C3, which are oriented ~ 45° anterolaterally, is shown. The posterior margin of the neural foramen is the facet joint; the ventral margin is the disc and uncinate process.

Brachial Plexus

TERMINOLOGY

Abbreviations

- Brachial plexus (BP)

Definitions

- Collection of interconnecting nerves of lower cervical spine (C5-8) and 1st thoracic nerve (T1) that provide cutaneous and motor innervation of upper extremity

GROSS ANATOMY

Overview

- **Cervical cord**
  - Internally, cervical spinal cord is arranged so that white matter tracts are positioned in periphery of cord
  - Gray matter is formed by neuronal cell bodies arranged in vertical columns that are centrally located within cord
  - Gray matter columns form H-shaped arrangement in axial plane (in cross section) where lateral, sagittally oriented components are referred to as horns and transverse coronal components are referred to as gray commissures
  - Ventral (anterior) horns of H are thicker, shorter, and contain multipolar motor neurons
  - Dorsal (posterior) horns are thinner, longer, and contain cell bodies that receive sensory axons from dorsal root ganglions (DRGs)
- **Cervical nerve rootlets, nerve roots, and proximal nerves**
  - At each cervical level, ventral horns give rise to motor axons that exit ipsilateral ventrolateral sulci of cervical cord as several tiny (< 1-mm) **nerve rootlets**
  - Ventral nerve rootlets at each level coalesce within few millimeters of cord to form an ipsilateral **ventral root** (~ 1 mm)
  - Similarly, dorsal horns receive multiple tiny nerve rootlets at posterolateral sulcus of cord
  - Dorsal nerve rootlets also coalesce within few millimeters of cord to form **dorsal root**
  - Dorsal root extends laterally from cord and merges with **DRG** within neural foramen (NF)
  - Within lateral aspect of cervical NF, DRG fuses with ventral root to become **spinal nerve proper**
  - Immediately after proper spinal nerve is formed, small, posteriorly oriented **dorsal ramus** is given off, supplying motor and sensory innervation to posterior paraspinous muscles and cervical soft tissues
  - Larger remaining segment of spinal nerve represents **ventral ramus**
    - Since ventral ramus is typically main part of spinal nerve in cervical region, it is often referred to as simply spinal nerve itself
    - These large ventral rami of nerves C5-T1 are also referred to as roots of BP
  - **1st cervical nerve** exits spinal canal between occiput and C1; that is, C1 nerve exits above C1 vertebra (atlas)
    - C2 nerve exits between C1 and C2 vertebrae and so forth
    - C8 nerve exits between C7 and T1 vertebrae
- **Cervical plexus**
  - Formed from ventral rami of C1-4 ± minor branch of C5

  - Has ascending superficial, descending superficial, deep branches
  - Supplies nuchal muscles, diaphragm, cutaneous head/neck tissues
- **Brachial Plexus (BP)**
  - Formed from **ventral rami of C5-T1** ± minor branches from C4 and T2
  - BP divided into anatomic segments moving from medial to lateral: Rami/roots, trunks, divisions, cords, terminal branches
    - Relationships of these segments with adjacent anatomic structures is variable
  - **Ventral rami/roots of BP**
    - Originate from spinal cord levels C5 to T1
    - Roots of BP represent ventral rami of nerves C5-T1
    - Term "root" in this context is not to be confused with nerve roots discussed previously, which represent small nerves within spinal canal and within proximal NF
    - Some nerves arise directly from roots: Dorsal scapular nerve (C5), phrenic (mainly C5), long thoracic nerve (C5, 6, and 7)
  - **Trunks**
    - Within interscalene triangle, upper roots of BP (C5-6) fuse to form **superior (upper) trunk**
    - Lower roots (C8-T1) fuse to form **inferior (lower) trunk**
    - C7 root continues laterally as **middle trunk**
    - Minor nerves arising directly from upper trunk: Suprascapular nerve, nerve to subclavius muscle
  - **Divisions**
    - As BP passes laterally beyond interscalene triangle over lateral margin of 1st rib and begins to descend toward axilla, each trunk divides into 2 main nerve branches: **Anterior and posterior divisions**
    - Subsequently, each BP contains total of 6 divisions: 3 anterior and 3 posterior
    - Anterior divisions innervate anterior (flexor) muscles
    - Posterior divisions innervate posterior (extensor) muscles
    - No named minor nerves arising directly from divisions
    - Divisions are located at level of clavicle and above junction of subclavian and axillary arteries
  - **Cords**
    - As BP passes into axilla, divisions fuse again to form **cords**
    - Cords are intimately associated with axillary artery and are named by their relationship to artery itself
    - **Lateral cord** (anterior divisions of superior, middle trunks) innervates anterior (flexor) muscles
    - **Medial cord** (anterior division of inferior trunk) innervates anterior (flexor) muscles
    - **Posterior cord** (posterior divisions of all 3 trunks) innervates posterior (extensor) muscles
  - **Branches (terminal)**
    - Cords form terminal **branches** of BP at approximately level of lateral margin of pectoralis minor muscle
    - **Musculocutaneous nerve** (C5-6) arises from lateral cord
    - Medial cord gives rise to **ulnar nerve** (C8-T1)

Brachial Plexus

- □ Medial cord also gives rise to medial pectoral nerve, medial cutaneous nerve of arm, medial cutaneous nerve of forearm
- – Axillary nerve (C5-6), radial nerve (C5-T1), thoracodorsal nerve (C6-8), upper (C6-7) and lower (C5-6) subscapular nerves all arise from posterior cord
- – **Median nerve** (C5-T1) formed by confluence of contributions from both medial and lateral cords

Anatomy Relationships

- **NF**
  - C5 nerve passes through NF at C4-5
    - – C6 nerve passes through NF at C5-6
    - – C7 nerve through C6-7 NF
    - – C8 nerve passes through NF at C7-T1
    - – T1 nerve passes through NF at T1-2
  - Within NF, most conspicuous neural structure is DRG, bulbous enlargement of dorsal root
  - Within NF, nerves of C5, 6, and 7 are positioned immediately posterior to vertebral artery
- **Lateral neural sulcus**
  - Transverse processes of C3-6 have similar anatomic appearance with transverse foramen that transmits vertebral artery and lateral neural sulcus (superolateral groove of transverse process), where corresponding cervical nerve is positioned
    - – e.g., after exiting NF at C4-5, C5 nerve descends and passes laterally to lateral neural sulcus of transverse process of C5 vertebra
  - When vertebrae of C3-6 are viewed in axial plane through transverse process, vertebral artery is separated from proximal ventral ramus by small bony bar that separates transverse foramen from lateral neural sulcus
- **Interscalene triangle**
  - Anterior scalene muscle arises from anterior tubercles of transverse processes of 3rd through 6th cervical vertebrae and inserts on superior surface of 1st rib anteriorly
  - Middle scalene muscle arises from posterior tubercles of transverse processes of 2nd through 7th vertebrae and attaches to 1st rib laterally
  - Borders of interscalene triangle
    - – Anterior border: Posterior margin of anterior scalene muscle
    - – Posterior border: Anterior edge of middle scalene muscle
    - – Inferior border (base): Superior margin of 1st rib, between separate attachments for 2 muscles
    - – Interscalene triangle can also be considered 3-dimensional space with both lateral and medial borders as well
    - – Medial border is represented by plane extending from medial margins of anterior and middle scalene muscles and lateral border as plane between lateral margins of both muscles
  - Widest portion of triangle is at base, along 1st rib
    - – Distance between attachments of anterior and middle scalene muscles to ribs is ~ 1 cm (range: 1.0-2.5 cm)
  - Interscalene triangle contains variable amounts of fat
    - – Interscalene fat is most conspicuous in lower aspect of triangle

- – More superiorly, anterior and middle scalene muscles are closely approximated and distinct fat separating muscles may be minimal or absent
- – Presence of fat, particularly perineural fat, is useful for identifying proximal components of BP within interscalene triangle on MR and CT scans
  - BP roots of C5-7 are located within upper aspect of interscalene triangle and begin to form upper and middle trunks as they pass through triangle itself
  - BP roots of C8-T1 are actually medial to triangle initially and begin to form lower trunk as they enter medial margin of interscalene triangle
  - Interscalene triangle is considered to contain upper, middle, and lower trunks of BP
- **Subclavian artery**
  - Subclavian artery gives off vertebral artery and internal thoracic artery before entering interscalene triangle
  - Subclavian artery passes through base of interscalene triangle, passing just over superior margin of 1st rib
  - Within triangle, subclavian artery is intimately associated with proximal BP
  - C5-7 roots are located superior to artery; C8 and T1 roots are often more posterior to artery
  - Subclavian artery and BP are separated from subclavian vein by anterior scalene muscle itself
  - Subclavian artery transitions to axillary artery at lateral margin of 1st rib
- **Axillary artery**
  - As subclavian artery passes 1st rib, it becomes axillary artery
  - Components of BP above proximal axillary artery generally consists of anterior and posterior divisions
  - Divisions then form cords that are intimately associated with axillary artery and are named by their relationship to artery itself
  - Cords are generally formed prior to reaching sagittal plane that passes through coracoid process of scapula
- **Phrenic nerve**
  - Arises primarily as branch from C4 ventral ramus with variable contributions from C5, and occasionally, C3
  - Passes around lateral margin of anterior scalene muscle and descends in neck along anterior surface of anterior scalene
  - Near base of anterior scalene muscle, phrenic nerve passes between subclavian vein and subclavian artery before passing anterior to internal thoracic artery and entering mediastinum
  - Supplies motor and sensory innervation to diaphragm

IMAGING ANATOMY

Overview

- Knowledge of normal BP anatomy and relationship of BP components to surrounding structures critical for evaluating BP
- Multiplanar high-resolution MR using surface coil is single best method for imaging BP
- Components of BP are complex and difficult to identify and fully evaluate with single MR sequence or in single plane
- Surrounding perineural fat often provides excellent visualization of nerves on T1WI and allows them to be distinguished from adjacent soft tissues

Brachial Plexus

- Corresponding T2WI, STIR sequences are best for evaluating intrinsic signal and architecture of nerves
- Characteristics of normal nerve on MR
  - In cross section, nerve appears as well-defined oval structure
  - Discrete fascicles can be identified with high-resolution imaging
    - Fascicles are uniform in size, shape
  - Isointense to adjacent muscle tissue on T1WI
  - Slightly hyperintense to adjacent muscle on fat-saturated T2WI, STIR
  - Normal nerves should be similar in signal intensity compared to adjacent normal nerves and contralateral normal nerves
  - While DRG enhances with intravenous gadolinium, major components of BP should not enhance normally

ANATOMY IMAGING ISSUES

Imaging Recommendations

- Multiplanar high-resolution MR peripheral nerve imaging using surface coil is **single best** method for imaging BP
- MR of cervical spine can be useful primary examination to evaluate for spinal cord pathology as well as common degenerative findings, including spinal stenosis and NF stenosis, that create BP symptoms
- CECT of neck or chest may be useful for evaluation of neck masses or apical pulmonary masses (Pancoast tumor) that involve BP
- CT myelography can be effective tool at evaluating for traumatic nerve root avulsion and associated traumatic pseudomeningoceles
- CT of cervical spine with bone windows preferred for cervical spine fracture
- CTA neck can demonstrate relationship of proximal BP masses with vertebral arteries
- USG is alternative imaging technique to visualize small component of BP
  - Excellent spatial resolution provided by high-frequency transducer
  - Seen as long, tubular, hypoechoic structures against background of echogenic fat on longitudinal scan
  - Several small ovoid/round hypoechoic nodules in lower posterior triangle between scalenus anterior and scalenus medius muscles on transverse scan
  - Lack of flow distinguishes them from vascular structures

Imaging Approaches

- Preferred coil: Multipurpose flexible phase array surface coil
- Alternative coil: Neurovascular phase array coil
- Best imaging planes: Coronal and oblique sagittal planes from C3 (rostral) through T2 (caudal), nerve roots (medial) through axilla (lateral)
- Best imaging sequences: Coronal T1, coronal STIR, oblique sagittal T1, and oblique sagittal STIR
- Optional sequences
  - Oblique sagittal and coronal contrast-enhanced fat-saturated T1WI (for cases of known or suspected neoplasm, scar, or infection)
  - Coronal technique with larger field of view (FOV) can include contralateral BP for comparison

Imaging Pitfalls

- Too-large FOV reduces spatial resolution, compromises visualization of internal BP architecture
- Technically simpler to evaluate supraclavicular plexus than infraclavicular plexus
- STIR provides more reliable fat suppression than chemical fat-saturated T2WI
- Motion artifact (especially respiratory motion of chest) can degrade image quality
- Subclavian and axillary vessels (especially venous structures) can demonstrate linear high signal on fast spin-echo or inversion recovery sequences and can be difficult to separate from BP
  - Saturation bands can help decrease vascular signal
- Enhancing vascular structures and normal perineural venous plexus can mimic pathologically enhancing BP components

CLINICAL IMPLICATIONS

Clinical Importance

- Variety of pathologies can affect BP, including idiopathic inflammation, traumatic injuries, neoplasm, and compression syndromes
- Due to complex anatomy of BP and variable pathologies, clinical symptoms may range from focal neurologic symptoms involving distal branch to more extensive brachial plexopathy involving multiple nerves
- Combination of neurologic evaluation and MR is key to identifying and localizing lesion as well as treatment planning

Brachial Plexus

GRAPHICS: OVERVIEW

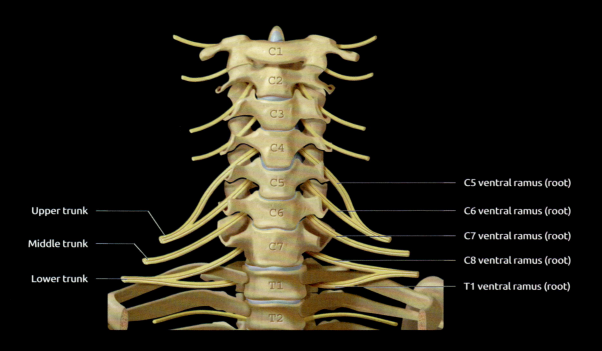

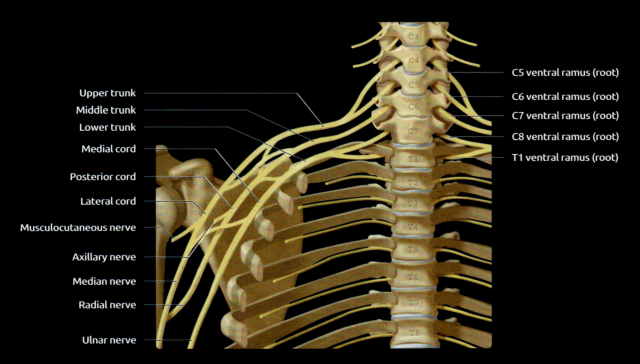

(Top) *Coronal graphic demonstrates an overview of the cervical spine and supraclavicular brachial plexus. This shows the basic arrangement of the cervical ventral primary rami combining to form the brachial plexus. The C1-7 cervical nerves exit above the same numbered pedicle, C8 nerve exits above the T1 pedicle, and more caudal roots exit below their numbered pedicle.* (Bottom) *Coronal graphic of the brachial plexus demonstrates an overview of the more distal plexus elements extending into the axilla. The trunks recombine into posterior and anterior divisions that form the cords. The posterior cord forms the radial and axillary nerves. The medial cord forms the ulnar nerve, while the lateral cord forms the musculocutaneous nerve. The median nerve is formed from branches of both the lateral and medial cords.*

Brachial Plexus

GRAPHIC: BRACHIAL PLEXUS

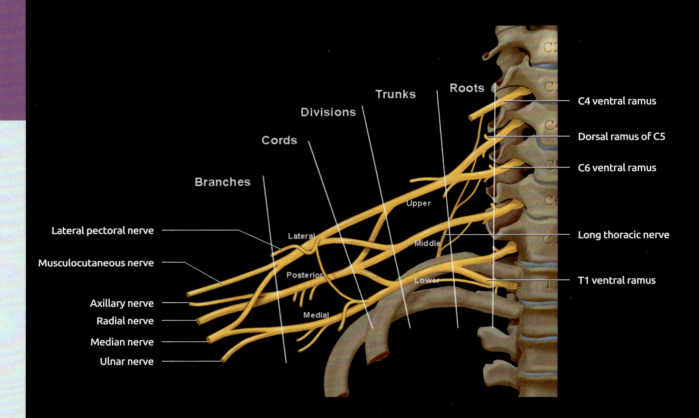

Graphic schematically demonstrates the components of the brachial plexus. The exiting nerves quickly divide into small dorsal rami and larger ventral rami. The ventral rami (roots) of C5-T1 pass into the scalene triangle and merge into trunks. The upper trunk is formed by C5 and C6 ventral rami or roots. The middle trunk is formed by continuation of the C7 root. The lower trunk is formed by the coalescence of C8 and T1 roots. Each trunk divides into a ventral and dorsal division. The 3 dorsal divisions merge into the posterior cord. Ventral divisions of the upper and middle trunks unite to form the lateral cord. The ventral division of the lower trunk merges and forms the medial cord. The cords ultimately give rise to the terminal branches of the upper extremity.

Brachial Plexus

CORONAL RELATIONSHIPS OF BRACHIAL PLEXUS

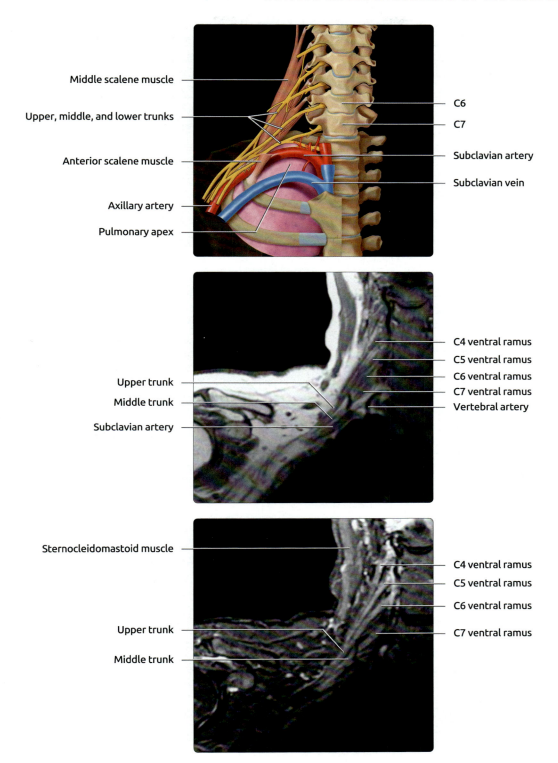

(Top) Graphic demonstrates the relationship of the proximal brachial plexus to the vertebral bodies, middle scalene muscle, subclavian artery, & pulmonary apex. The anterior scalene has been removed to expose the scalene triangle, the region between the scalene muscles. Note the subclavian vein passes anterior to the inferior attachment of the anterior scalene muscle & the subclavian artery passes posterior to this attachment. The subclavian artery can serve as a marker to find the brachial plexus elements on imaging. Note that if an apical lung tumor invades superiorly, it often involves the subclavian artery before it involves the brachial plexus. (Middle) Slightly more anterior image demonstrates the proximal cervical roots/ventral primary ramus (VPR) combining to form the upper & middle trunks of the brachial plexus. Normal nerve is slightly isointense to muscle on T1 MR imaging. Note the close anatomic proximity of the brachial plexus elements to the subclavian artery. (Bottom) Image shows the proximal cervical ventral rami "roots" combining to form the upper & middle trunks of the brachial plexus. Normal nerve is slightly hyperintense to muscle on STIR & FS T2 MR imaging.

AXIAL ANATOMY: PROXIMAL CERVICAL NERVES

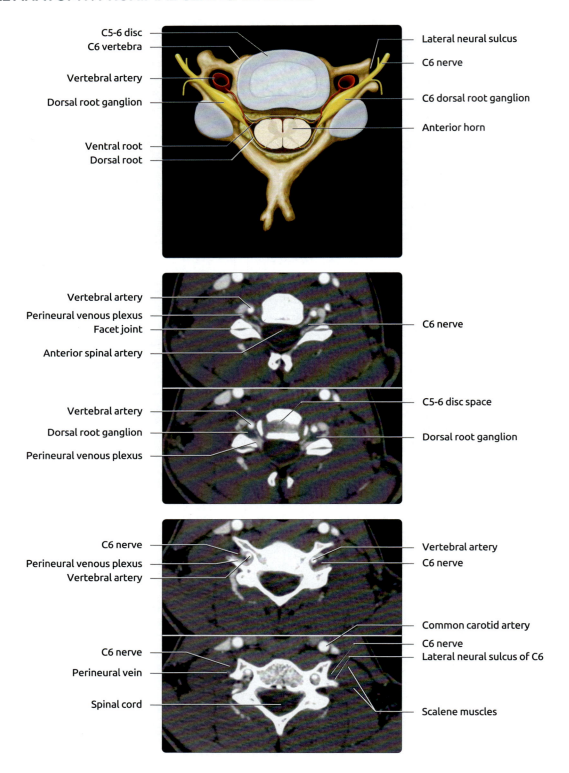

(Top) Graphic demonstrates ventral & dorsal roots of C6 nerve merging in upper medial neural foramen (NF). Localized expansion of the dorsal nerve is the dorsal root ganglion (DRG). Note the intimate relationship of the DRG to the vertebral artery as it passes through NF. The extraforaminal nerve descends slightly toward the lateral neural sulcus that cradles the nerve before it extends into the scalene triangle. When the nerve is within lateral neural sulcus, it is separated from the vertebral artery within transverse foramen by thin bony bridge of the lateral process. (Middle) Axial CTA images descending through C5-6 disc space show there is prominent enhancement of epidural & perineural venous plexus that surround exiting nerves. (Bottom) Axial images continue to descend from disc space at C5-6 into C6 vertebrae. As the nerve begins to exit NF, it moves inferiorly & laterally & begins to separate from vertebral artery. The extraforaminal nerve will pass lateral to the transverse process within a shallow groove know as lateral neural sulcus, which is a reliable landmark for cervical nerves C3-6. In many patients, it is difficult to fully distinguish separate scalene muscles on imaging.

Brachial Plexus

CORONAL STIR MR

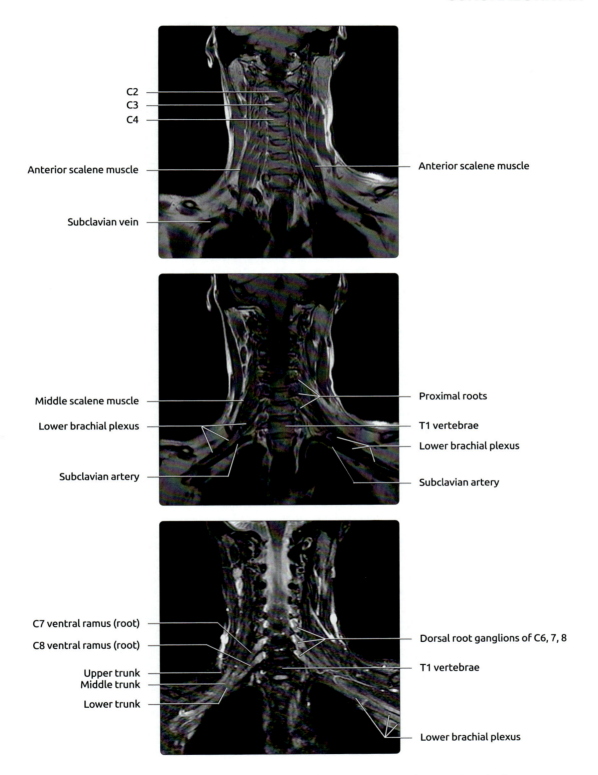

(Top) Coronal T1 MR shows vertebral bodies (upper) & anterior scalene muscles (lower). Anterior scalene muscles arise from transverse processes of the cervical vertebrae & attach to the 1st rib laterally. Subclavian vein passes anteriorly to attachment of anterior scalene. **(Middle)** Coronal T1 MR reveals the difficulty in distinguishing normal nerve tissue from adjacent muscle. Oblique bands of hypointense tissue traverse the ventral face of middle scalene muscle, but the nerves are difficult to separate from oblique tendinous attachments of the muscle itself. There is minimal interscalene fat to provide satisfactory contrast. Subclavian artery is a useful landmark for determining the best plane for proximal components of the brachial plexus, particularly the trunks. The trunks will pass above the subclavian artery as it passes over the 1st rib. **(Bottom)** Coronal STIR MR shows relative hyperintensity of normal nerves to muscle. Fat has been suppressed to enhance contrast resolution of nerves. Note DRGs are easily identified as focal enlargements of proximal nerves within NF. Given complex curvature of components, it is difficult to obtain a full view of the brachial plexus in a single slice.

Brachial Plexus

AXIAL STIR MR

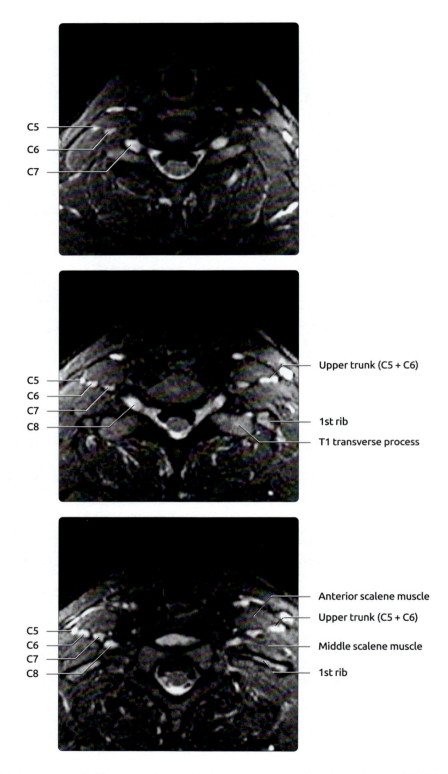

(Top) First of 3 axial STIR MR images presented from rostral to caudal shows the upper brachial plexus elements (C5-7 VPR) traveling between the anterior and middle scalene muscles in preparation to form the brachial plexus. *(Middle)* Image at the C7/T1 level depicts the linear alignment of the C5 through C8 VPR. C5 and C6 are closely approximated and form the left upper trunk. *(Bottom)* Imaging more caudal at C7/T1 level depicts the upper trunk on the left. Note that the brachial plexus elements exit the neck between the anterior and middle scalene muscles.

Brachial Plexus

OBLIQUE SAGITTAL STIR MR

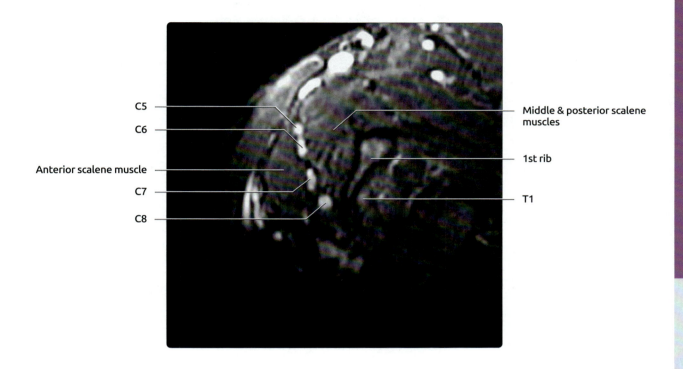

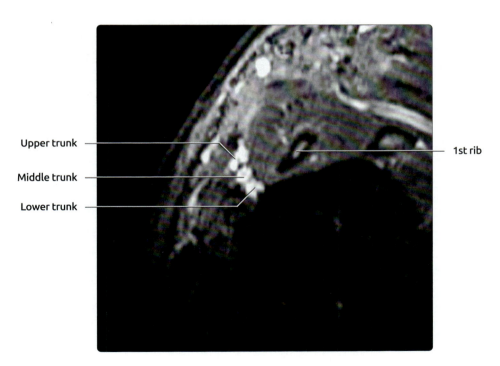

(Top) First of 4 oblique sagittal STIR MR images presented from medial to lateral demonstrates the ventral primary rami of C5 through T1 proximal to the trunks. C8 exits above the 1st rib while T1 exits below. The brachial plexus is normally sandwiched between the anterior and middle scalene muscles. (Bottom) A slightly more lateral slice demonstrates the formation of the upper, middle, and lower trunks arranged in a vertical line between the scalene muscles. The C5 and C6 VPR can be still resolved as distinct elements within the upper trunk at this level.

Brachial Plexus

OBLIQUE SAGITTAL STIR MR

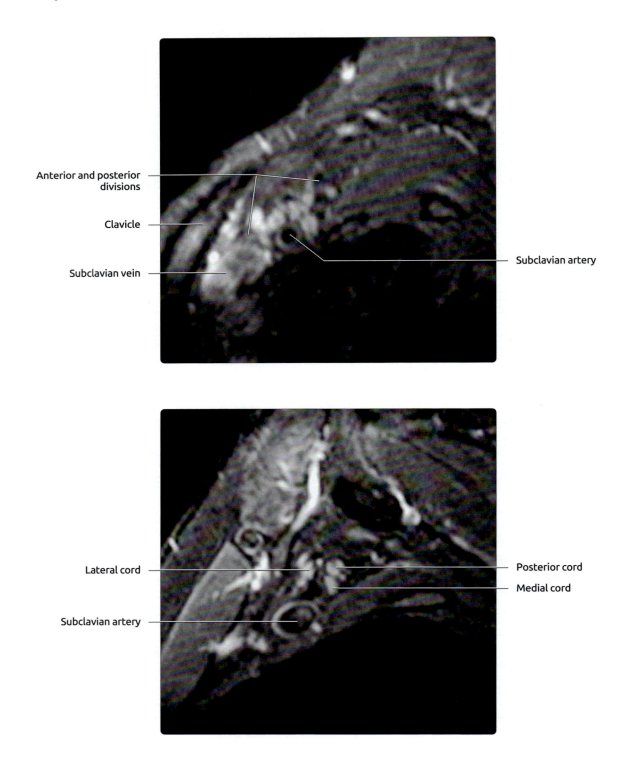

(Top) Image at the division level shows mixing and matching of the trunks into anterior and posterior divisions. Note that the divisions are retroclavicular. The posterior divisions will form the posterior cord, and the anterior divisions will form the lateral and medial cords. It is generally not possible to follow individual branches of the divisions from trunk to cord. (Bottom) Image demonstrates the formation of the 3 cords (lateral, medial, and posterior). The most important terminal branch of the lateral cord is the musculocutaneous nerve. The posterior cord forms the axillary and radial nerve terminal branches. The medial cord terminates as the ulnar nerve.

Brachial Plexus

ANATOMIC-PATHOLOGIC CORRELATION

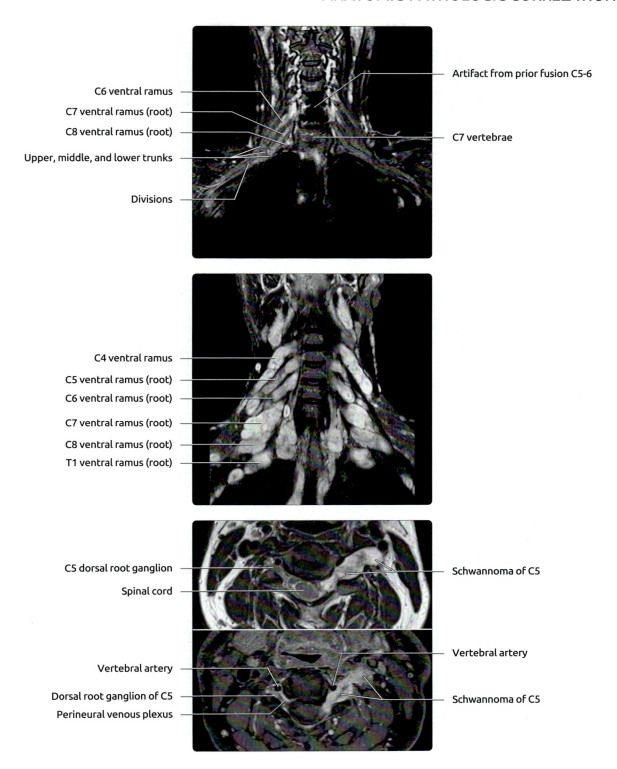

(Top) Coronal T2 FS MR demonstrates mild relative hyperintensity in the brachial plexus diffusely in the right side of this patient with idiopathic plexitis. *(Middle)* Coronal STIR MR depicts massive enlargement of all of the proximal cervical nerves and supraclavicular components of the brachial plexus in this patient with neurofibromatosis type 1. In this case, essentially all the nerves have given rise to neurofibromas. *(Bottom)* Axial T2 and FS contrast-enhanced T1 MR images through the C4-5 NF demonstrate a solitary enlarged, fusiform enhancing mass along the proximal C5 nerve on the patient's left. Notice the lesion's relationship to the left vertebral artery; the lesion pushes the vertebral artery anteriorly. Notice the DRG on the unaffected side enhances normally.

Brachial Plexus

TRANSVERSE AND LONGITUDINAL ULTRASOUND

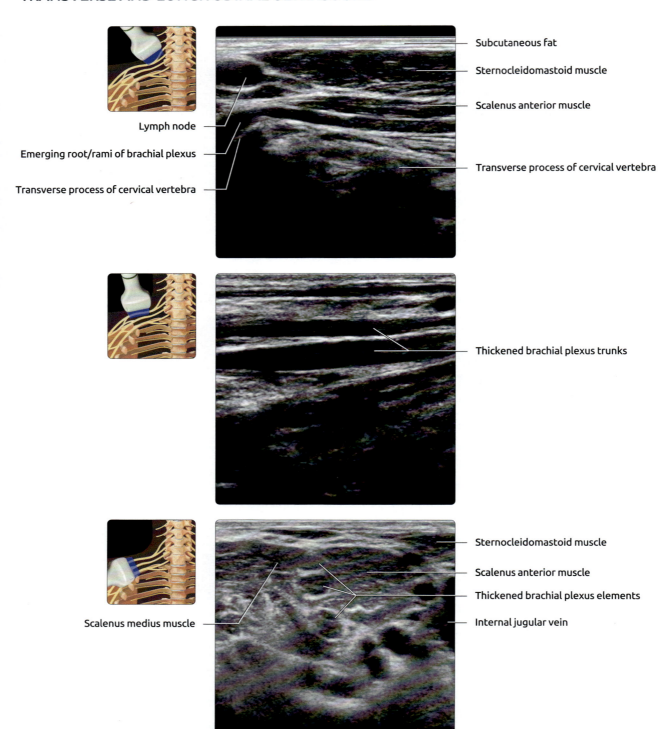

(Top) Longitudinal grayscale ultrasound of the posterior triangle of the neck shows the root and trunk of the brachial plexus, which appears as a thin, tubular, hypoechoic structure related superficially to the scalenus anterior muscle and deeply to the cervical vertebrae. (Middle) Longitudinal grayscale ultrasound of right posterior triangle/supraclavicular fossa confirms the elongated linear, hypoechoic, thickened elements of the brachial plexus. The patient had past history of neck irradiation for metastatic neck nodes, and the nerve thickening is likely secondary to postradiation change. (Bottom) Transverse grayscale ultrasound of right lower posterior triangle/supraclavicular fossa shows round smooth hypoechoic "nodules" between the scalenus anterior and medius muscles representing thickened brachial plexus elements viewed in cross section. If there is a question, rotate the transducer to elongate the nerve.

Brachial Plexus

TRANSVERSE AND LONGITUDINAL ULTRASOUND

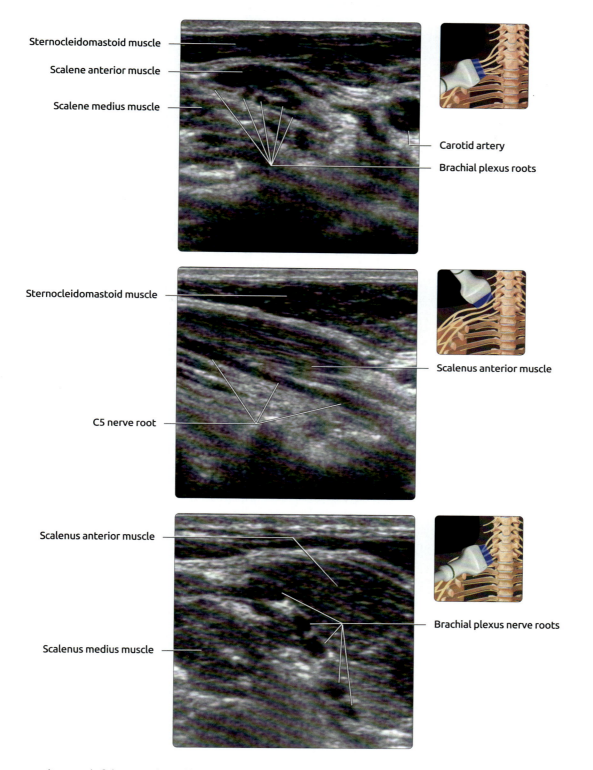

(Top) Transverse ultrasound of the anterolateral lower neck shows the hypoechoic roots of the brachial plexus as they exit the neural foramina and move to the scalene triangle. (Middle) Longitudinal ultrasound shows the longitudinal section of the hypoechoic C5 nerve root as it exits from the foramen and descends to the intrascalene area. (Bottom) Transverse ultrasound at the entry into the interscalene triangle shows 5 hypoechoic roots of the brachial plexus between the scalenus anterior and medius muscles. The hypoechoic roots are clearly seen against the adjacent hyperechoic intermuscular fat.

INDEX

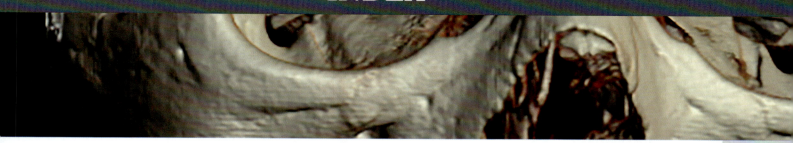

A

Abdomen, vagus to, **190**
Abducens nerve (CNVI), **17, 31, 37, 52, 95, 96, 99, 116, 117, 118, 119, 123, 154, 157, 160, 161, 164–167, 179, 207, 211, 216, 217, 226–227, 228, 229, 233, 234**
 - axial T2 and T1 C+ MR, **166**
 - within basilar venous plexus, **166**
 - in Dorello canal, **99, 158, 228**
 - graphics, **165**
 - lateral rectus, **165**
 - left, **166**
 - neuropathy, **166**
 - piercing dura, **124, 165, 167**
     entering Dorello canal, **123**
 - in prepontine cistern, **167**
 - right, **166**
 - sagittal T2 MR, **166**
 - sulcus, **156**
 - traverses superior orbital fissure, **165**
Abducens nucleus, **52, 164, 165, 167, 169**
Abscess, retropharyngeal space, **344**
Accessory atlantoaxial ligament, **499**
Accessory nerve (CNXI), **41, 116, 117, 119, 183, 184, 189, 191, 194–197, 199, 333, 334, 356, 357, 358**
 - ascending portion, **41**
 - axial bone CT & T2 MR, **197**
 - function dysfunction, **194**
 - graphics, **195**
     intracranial & extracranial, **196**
 - spinal portion, **513**
Accessory parotid tissue, **474, 478**
Acoustic meatus
 - external, **6**
 - internal, **5, 40**
Adenoids, **36, 285, 304, 306, 309**
 - of nasopharyngeal mucosal space, **36**
Aditus ad antrum, **50, 54, 68, 75, 78**
AEA. *See* Anterior ethmoid artery.
AEF. *See* Aryepiglottic fold.
Aerated pterygoid plate, **258**
Afferent lymphatic vessels, **428**
Agger nasi cell, **238, 243, 245, 248, 251, 261, 262, 263, 266, 267**
 - above, **261**
 - inadequate removal of, **261**
 - not abutting, **261**
 - right and left, **268**
AICA. *See* Anterior inferior cerebellar artery.

Air
 - in cervical esophagus
     artifact from, **425**
     shadowing from, **424**
 - in retropharyngeal space, **347**
Alar fascia, **272, 275, 340, 341, 342, 347, 366, 435**
Alar ligament, **499, 513**
Alar nasalis, **441, 443, 445**
Alisphenoid, **32**
Alveolar nerve, **163**
 - inferior, **31**
Alveolar ridge, **495**
Ambient cistern, **125, 150**
Amygdala, **129**
AN. *See* Agger nasi cell.
Angle of mandible, **110, 111, 319, 459, 491, 495**
Angle of mouth, muscles inserting at, **442**
Angular artery, **441**
Angular veins, **441**
Annular tendon, **221**
Annulus of Zinn, **149, 207, 212**
Annulus tendineus (annulus of Zinn), **133, 136, 142**
Anomalous nasi, **441, 443, 446**
Ansa cervicalis, **198**
 - inferior root, **333, 337**
 - lower root, **200**
 - superior root, **333, 337**
 - upper root, **200**
Anterior atlantoaxial joint, **530**
Anterior atlantodental joint, **508, 510, 512, 513**
Anterior band of disc, **109, 112, 113**
Anterior cerebral artery, **125, 138, 234**
 - left, **231, 233**
 - right, **147, 231, 232**
Anterior cervical space, **275, 279, 280, 283, 333, 366, 367, 368, 422, 423**
Anterior chamber, **211**
Anterior choroidal artery, **127**
Anterior commissure, **135, 373, 375, 380, 381, 387, 389, 397, 400**
 - fibers crossing in, **129**
Anterior communicating artery, **232**
Anterior compartment, thrombosis, **235**
Anterior cranial fossa, **240**
Anterior division, trigeminal nerve, **155**
Anterior ethmoid artery, **17, 246, 260, 261**
 - and canal, **17, 242**
Anterior ethmoid complex, **240, 249, 250**
Anterior ethmoid ostia, **249**
Anterior ethmoidal canal, **260, 261**
 - left, **269**
 - right, **269**

i

INDEX

Anterior ethmoidal notch (foramen), **260, 265**
- left, **268, 269**
- right, **268, 269**
Anterior ethmoids, **251**
Anterior horn, **538**
Anterior inferior cerebellar artery (AICA), **102, 106, 107, 122, 123, 126, 145, 151, 166, 179, 180, 187, 193**
- loop, **102, 106, 123**
Anterior intercavernous sinus, **230**
Anterior internal venous plexus, **528, 530**
Anterior lacrimal crest, **214, 215**
Anterior median sulcus, spinal cord, **524**
Anterior mediastinum, with thymic remnant, **413**
Anterior parotid space, **273, 292, 311**
Anterior perforated substance, **129**
Anterior premolar, **492, 493, 494**
Anterior recess, inferior compartment, **109, 112, 113**
Anterior scalene muscle, **280, 281, 283, 284, 345, 346, 349, 352, 353, 354, 355, 360, 361, 368, 432, 537, 539, 540, 541**
- posterolateral border of, oblique line along posterior border of, **432**
Anterior skull base, **4, 14–29, 31**
- axial bone CT, **19–21**
  development, **24**
- bony landmarks of, **14**
- coronal bone CT, **22–23**
  development, **25**
- coronal T2 MR development, **26–27**
- development of, **15**
- foramina and fissures of, **14–15**
- graphics, **16–18**
- sagittal T1 MR development, **28–29**
Anterior spinal artery, **538**
Anterior tonsillar pillar, **300, 453, 455, 461, 487**
Anterior tubercle, **515**
Anterior tympanic segment, facial nerve, **170, 173**
Anterior vertebral line, **518**
Anterior wall fascia, retropharyngeal space, **340**
Antihelix, **74**
 - crura of, **74**
Antitragus, **74**
Aortic arch, **369, 407, 432**
Apical ligament, **499, 512**
Arachnoid, **228**
Arcuate eminence, **50, 51, 58, 59, 65, 71, 90, 172, 173**
 - superior semicircular canal and, **97**
Arnold nerve, **188**
Artery, **428**
Articular disc, **109**
Articular eminence, **109, 110, 111, 112, 113**
Articular pillar, **517, 520, 531**
Articular processes, **514**
Aryepiglottic fold (AEF), **300, 301, 303, 372, 374, 377, 378, 380, 382, 383, 384, 386, 387, 392, 394, 396, 398, 399**
 - displaced medially, **401**
Aryepiglottic muscle, **378**
Arytenoid cartilage, **303, 372, 375, 376, 377, 380, 382, 384, 387, 388, 389, 396, 400, 427**
 - superior tip of, **389**
Arytenoid prominence, **388**

Arytenoid superior process, **374, 396**
Ascending aorta, **413**
Atlantoaxial joint, **506, 507, 509, 510, 511, 521, 524, 525, 526, 530**
 - anterior median, **499**
 - posterior median, **499**
Atlantoaxial ligament, accessory, **499**
Atlantodental interval, **505**
Atlantooccipital joint, **46, 49, 499, 506, 507, 508, 511, 513, 524, 525, 526**
 - angle, **502**
Atlantooccipital membrane
 - anterior, **499, 512, 513**
 - posterior, **499**
Auricular branch, vagus nerve, **188**
Auriculotemporal nerve, **152, 155, 310**
Axillary apex, **361**
Axillary artery, **533, 537**
Axillary nerve, **535, 536**
Axillary nodes, **427**

B

Barium esophagram, **393**
Barium swallow, **417**
Basal vein, **137, 151**
Base of tongue, **398, 480**
 - sensory & taste from, **185**
Basilar artery, **99, 122, 123, 137, 143, 145, 151, 154, 157, 193, 229, 230, 258**
Basilar membrane, **88**
Basilar plexus, **230**
Basilar venous plexus, **166**
Basilar venous sinus, thrombosis, **235**
Basiocciput, **10, 12, 28, 29, 32, 39, 40, 44, 45, 47, 48, 49, 57**
Basion, **499, 506, 507, 512, 513, 525, 526**
Basisphenoid, **8, 12, 98, 232, 233, 241, 273, 292, 299, 309**
Basivertebral veins, **523, 524**
Bilaminar zone, **112, 113**
Bolgerization, **261**
Bony labyrinth, **50, 86**
Bony orbit, **206, 209**
 - and foramina, **216–219**
Bony vestibular aqueduct, **70**
Bony-cartilaginous junction, **74**
BP. *See* Brachial plexus.
Brachial plexus (BP), **191, 348, 532–545**
 - anatomic-pathologic correlation, **543**
 - anterior division, **542**
 - axial stir MR, **540**
 - in axillary apex, **361**
 - branches, **532–533, 536**
 - cords, **532, 536**
 - coronal relationship, **537**
 - divisions, **532, 536, 543**
 - elements, **362**
 - emerging root/rami, **544**

INDEX

- lower, **539**
- oblique sagittal stir MR, **541–542**
- overview, **535**
- in posterior cervical space, **361**
- posterior division, **542**
- preaxillary, **356**
- transverse and longitudinal ultrasound, **544–545**

Brachial plexus roots, **281, 283, 284, 349, 352, 354, 355, 357, 360, 532, 536, 545**
- location, **280**
- in neural foramen, **355**
- in perivertebral space, **361**

Brachial plexus trunks, **355, 532, 536**
- lower, **535**
- middle, **535, 537**
- thickened, **544**
- upper, **535, 537**

Brachiocephalic artery, **338, 407**
Brachiocephalic (innominate) vein, **432**
Brachium pontis, **157, 180, 324**
Branchial pouch
- 3rd, **412**
- 4th, **412**
BS. *See* Buccal space.
Buccal artery, **447, 474, 476, 478**
Buccal branch
- abducens nerve, **169**
- facial nerve, **322, 474**
- mandibular nerve, **474**
Buccal fat, **476**
- deep projection, **477**
Buccal fat pad, **441, 447, 448, 474, 476, 478**
Buccal mucosa, **461, 476**
Buccal nodes, **474**
Buccal space (BS), **274, 277, 282, 284, 293, 295, 296, 304, 306, 311, 313, 315, 316, 317, 318, 320, 325, 474–479**
- anatomic-pathologic correlation squamous cell carcinoma, **479**
- axial CT, **476**
- axial MR, **478**
- coronal CT, **477**
- graphics, **475**
Buccal space fat, **476**
Buccal submucosal fat pad, **448**
Buccinator muscle, **277, 282, 284, 293, 296, 301, 305, 307, 316, 318, 320, 325, 328, 394, 444, 448, 453, 457, 461, 474, 475, 476, 477, 478, 482, 483, 484, 487, 488, 489**
Buccinator node, **429**
Buccopharyngeal fascia, **392**
Bulbar fibers, accessory nerve, **195, 196**
Bulbar (cranial) motor fibers, **194**
Bulbar portion, accessory nerve, **193, 197**
Bulbopontine sulcus, **167**
Bulla ethmoidalis, **238, 260, 266, 267**

C

C1 (atlas), **498, 500, 517**
- anterior arch, **47, 277, 499, 500, 506, 508, 510, 511, 512, 513, 516, 521, 525, 526, 527, 530**
  - superior cortex, **508**
- arch, **505**
- inferior articular facet, **509, 510, 511**
- lateral mass, **46, 47, 49, 202, 203, 506, 507, 508, 510, 517, 524, 527, 530**
- posterior arch, **500, 505, 506, 508, 509, 510, 511, 512, 518, 519, 524, 525, 526**
- superior articular facet, **508, 510, 511**
- transverse process, **506, 507, 510, 521**
- vertebral body, **435**
  - posterior ring, **195**
C2 (axis), **498, 501, 517, 539**
- body, **499, 501, 505, 506, 507, 510, 511, 519, 521, 525, 526, 527, 530**
- inferior articular facet, **509, 510, 511, 519, 521, 525**
- inferior body, **509**
- lamina, **510**
- lateral mass, **501**
- pars interarticularis, **525**
- pedicle, **520**
- spinous process, **506, 509, 510, 512, 525, 527**
- superior articular facet, **509, 510, 511, 530**
- transverse foramen, **510**
  - vertebral artery, **527**
- vertebral body, **516, 528, 530**
C3, **539**
- anterior cortical margin, **519**
- body, **505, 506, 511, 519, 520, 521**
- inferior articular facet, **517**
- inferior endplate, **531**
- inferior facet, **529**
- superior articular facet, **519, 521, 525**
- superior articular process, **509, 511**
- uncinate process, **509**
- vertebral body, **516**
C4, **539**
- body, **505, 519, 520, 521, 524**
- inferior articular facet, **517**
- inferior endplate, **522**
- superior articular facet, **529**
- transverse process, **506**
- ventral ramus, **536, 537, 543**
C5, **540, 541**
- body, **522, 523**
- dorsal root ganglion, **543**
- facet, **527**
- nerve root, **545**
- pedicle, **522, 523**
- schwannoma, **543**
- transverse process, **520, 521**
- uncinate process, **522**
- ventral ramus, **535, 537, 543**
- vertebral body, **355**

iii

INDEX

C6, **537, 538, 540, 541**
- dorsal root ganglion, **538, 539**
- inferior articular facet, **526**
- lamina, **520**
- lateral neural sulcus, **538**
- nerve, **538**
- pedicle, **520**
- posterior cortical margin, **519**
- spinous process, **520**
- transverse process, **521**
    - anterior tubercle, **524**
- uncinate process, **519, 521, 523**
- ventral ramus, **535, 537, 543**
C7, **514, 537, 540, 541, 542**
- dorsal root ganglion, **539**
- inferior articular process, **526**
- pedicle, **519, 521, 525**
- spinous process, **516, 519, 520, 521**
- superior articular facet, **525**
- transverse process, **519**
- uncinate process, **520**
- ventral ramus, **535, 537, 539, 543**
- vertebral body, **516**
C8, **540, 541**
- dorsal root ganglion, **539**
- ventral ramus, **535, 539, 543**
Canalicular segment, optic nerve, **220**
Canaliculus innominatus, **30**
Canine tooth, **492, 493, 494**
Capsule, **428**
Caroticotympanic artery, **53**
Carotid artery, **545**
Carotid bifurcation, **335**
Carotid body, **185**
Carotid bulb, **53**
Carotid canal, **30, 75, 96, 273, 292**
- entrance, **44**
- floor of, **120**
- horizontal segment, **120, 121**
- sympathetic plexus, **120**
- temporal bone, **11**
- vertical segment, **6, 98, 120**
    - opening, **184**
Carotid sheath, **275, 332, 333, 357**
- with deep cervical fascia, **184, 191**
- from multiple fascial contributions, **291**
- tricolor, **341, 343**
Carotid sinus branch, vagus nerve, **188**
Carotid sinus nerve, **182**
Carotid space, **6, 188, 272, 273, 274, 275, 277, 279, 280, 281, 282, 283, 284, 291, 292, 293, 294, 295, 296, 297, 299, 300, 304, 306, 308, 312, 313, 320, 321, 323, 325, 326, 327, 328, 329, 332–339, 333, 334, 336, 337, 341, 342, 343, 344, 345, 346, 347, 349, 350, 352, 353, 357, 359, 360, 361, 366, 367, 368, 419, 420, 421, 422, 423, 435**. *See also* Parapharyngeal space.
- axial CECT, **336–337**
- component, hypoglossal nerve, **198**
- fascia of, **332**
- graphics, **333–334**
- mass, **334**

- nasopharyngeal, **45, 48**
- superior margin, **47**
- vessels, CECT & MRA of, **335**
Carotid sulcus, anterior, **8**
Cartilage, of external auditory canal, **74**
Cavernous carotid artery, **246**
Cavernous segment
- abducens nerve, **164, 166**
- oculomotor nerve, **141**
- trochlear nerve, **148**
Cavernous sinus, **37, 42, 95, 118, 142, 143, 146, 154, 158, 159, 160, 226–235, 259**
- anatomy relationship, **226**
- anterior wall, **226**
- area (CNIII, IV, VI, V1, and V2), **121**
- CNIII, **142**
- inferolateral wall, maxillary nerve, **162**
- internal contents, **227**
- lateral wall, **226, 227, 231, 235**
- medial wall, **226**
- osseous relationships, **226**
- posterior wall, **226–227**
- roof, **226**
- wall of, trochlear nerve, **149**
Central caudal nucleus, **140**
Central nucleus, **140**
Central retinal artery, **134, 207, 220, 221**
Central retinal vein, **134, 220, 221**
Central skull base, **4, 16, 30–39**
- axial bone CT, **33–35**
- axial T1 C+ MR, **37–38**
- bony landmarks of, **30**
- coronal bone CT, **36**
- development of, **30**
- foramina and fissures of, **30**
- graphics, **31–32**
- sagittal T1 & T2 MR development, **39**
- variant anatomy of, **30**
Cephalad clivus, **156**
Cephalad 4th ventricle, **124**
Cephalad nasal cavity, **120**
Cerebellar hemisphere, **105, 175**
Cerebellar tonsil, **48, 180, 513**
Cerebellopontine angle (CPA), **100, 101, 102, 106**
- cistern, **52, 62, 106, 126, 180, 181**
    - facial nerve, **169**
    - other structures in, **102**
- CSF in, **93**
Cerebellopontine angle-internal auditory canal anatomy, **102–107**
- axial bone CT, **104**
- axial T2 MR, **106**
- coronal T2 MR, **107**
- graphics, **103**
- sagittal T2 MR, **105**
Cerebellum, **181**
Cerebral aqueduct, **125, 144**
Cerebral peduncle, **125, 126, 135, 144, 145, 150**
Cerebrospinal fluid, **525, 527, 530, 531**
Cervical branch
- abducens nerve, **169**

INDEX

- facial nerve, **322**
Cervical cord, **513, 516, 532**
Cervical esophageal cancer, **427**
Cervical esophagus, **301, 338, 364–365, 375, 394, 397, 405, 406, 411, 416–425**
- air-contrast barium swallow, **416**
- anatomy relationships, **416**
- axial CECT, **420–421**
- blood supply, **416**
- embryology, **416**
- fascia, **416**
- generic mass, graphic and CECT, **423**
- graphics, **419**
    - muscles and spaces, **418**
- junction of, **417, 420**
- longitudinal ultrasound and CT, **425**
- lymphatic drainage, **416**
- mass, **423**
- mucosa, **416**
- transverse ultrasound, **424**
Cervical lateral masses, **519, 521, 523, 524**
Cervical lymph nodes, **426–439**
- axial CECT, **433**
- axial CT, **430–432**
- axial T1 & T2 MR, **434**
- classifications, **426**
    - image based, **426**
- graphics, **429**
    - anatomy and histology, **428**
- grayscale ultrasound, **436, 438**
- nomenclature, **426**
- normal, **437**
- power Doppler ultrasound, **437, 439**
Cervical nerve rootlets, **532**
Cervical plexus, **532**
Cervical spinal cord, **361, 524**
Cervical spine, **514–531**
- 3D-VRT NECT, **517, 521**
- axial bone CT, **522–523**
- axial GRE MR, **528–529**
- axial T2 MR, **530–531**
- coronal CT myelogram, **524**
- lateral radiograph, **518**
- radiography, **519**
    - 3D-VRT NECT, **520**
- sagittal CT myelogram, **525**
- sagittal T1 MR, **526**
- sagittal T2 MR, **527**
- vertebral body, **515**
Cervical trachea, **364, 416–425**
- anatomy relationships, **416**
- axial CECT, **420–421**
- blood supply, **416**
- cartilage anatomy, **416**
- embryology, **416**
- fascia, **416**
- generic mass, graphic and CECT, **422**
- graphics, **419**
    - muscles and spaces, **418**
- longitudinal ultrasound and CT, **425**
- lymphatic drainage, **416**

- mucosa, **416**
- multislice CT, **416**
- transverse ultrasound, **424**
Cervical vertebra, **409, 415, 425**
- tip of transverse process of, **362**
- transverse process, **544**
Cervicomedullary junction, **513**
Chamberlain line, **498, 502, 503**
Chaotic peripheral and central intranodal vessel, **439**
Chewing, weakness in, **152**
Chiasm, **133**
Chiasmatic sulcus, **14, 16**
Chief cells, **403**
Chondrocranium, **29**
- anterior skull base, **28**
- unossified, **18**
Chorda tympani, **81**
- canal, **68**
- nerve, **57, 68, 155, 168, 169, 312, 322**
Choroid, **134, 139, 211, 224, 225**
Choroid plexus, **102**
Ciliary body, **211, 224, 225**
Ciliary ganglion, **142, 155**
Circumferential squamous cell carcinoma, **401**
Circumvallate papilla, **453, 461, 481**
Cistern, oculomotor nerve and, **146**
Cisternal abducens nerve, **118, 169**
Cisternal (preganglionic) segment, **31**
- abducens nerve, **164, 165, 166**
- accessory nerve, **194**
- facial nerve, **168**
- glossopharyngeal nerve, **182**
- hypoglossal nerve, **198, 199**
- optic nerve, **220**
- trigeminal nerve, **107, 117, 118, 124, 126, 152, 153, 155, 157, 158, 159, 162**
- trochlear nerve, **148, 149**
- vagus nerve, **188**
Clavicle, **357, 359, 361, 369, 432, 519, 542**
Clinoid process
- anterior, **5, 7, 14, 16, 17, 19, 22, 33, 36, 121, 135, 138, 159, 161, 206, 210, 214, 215, 219, 230, 232, 234**
- posterior, **5, 7, 33, 99**
Clival venous plexus, **99, 229**
Clivus, **10, 13, 43, 98, 99, 100, 120, 123, 154, 156, 158, 162, 167, 186, 192, 197, 201, 304, 306, 499, 506, 511**
- basiocciput part of, **34**
- basisphenoid part of, **8, 34, 37**
- canal angle, **498**
- occipital bone, **11**
CNI. *See* Olfactory nerve.
CNII. *See* Optic nerve.
CN3. *See* Oculomotor nerve.
CNIII. *See* Oculomotor nerve.
CNIV. *See* Trochlear nerve.
CNV. *See* Trigeminal nerve.
CNV1. *See* Ophthalmic nerve.
CNV2. *See* Maxillary nerve.
CNV3. *See* Mandibular nerve.
CN6. *See* Abducens nerve.
CNVI. *See* Abducens nerve.

INDEX

CN7. *See* Facial nerve.
CNVII. *See* Facial nerve.
CN8. *See* Vestibulocochlear nerve.
CNVIII. *See* Vestibulocochlear nerve.
CN9. *See* Glossopharyngeal nerve.
CNIX. *See* Glossopharyngeal nerve.
CNIX-XI, **122**
CNX. *See* Vagus nerve.
CN11. *See* Accessory nerve.
CNXI. *See* Accessory nerve.
CNXII. *See* Hypoglossal nerve.
Cochlea, **8, 50, 60, 69, 71, 80, 86–87, 93, 98, 106, 121, 126, 170, 173, 179**
 - 2nd turn of, **60, 61, 64, 65, 88, 89, 92**
 - apical 1/2 turn of, **88, 89**
 - axial view of, **90**
 - basal (1st) turn of, **56, 57, 59, 60, 61, 62, 64, 65, 69, 88, 89, 90, 92, 107, 171, 172, 173, 175, 178, 181**
   apical, **63**
   cephalad aspect of, **55**
   distal, **92**
   proximal, **90, 92**
 - middle turn of, **107**
 - with pathologic calcification, **93**
Cochlea duct (scala media), **53**
Cochlear aperture, **176, 177, 178**
Cochlear aqueduct, **46, 56, 57, 64, 92, 105, 171, 202**
Cochlear duct, **88**
Cochlear foramen, **177**
Cochlear modiolus, **104, 177**
Cochlear nerve, **52, 62, 88, 89, 103, 105, 106, 107, 123, 174, 175, 176, 177, 179, 180, 181**
 - canal, **55, 56, 60, 71, 87, 88, 89, 92, 102, 103, 104, 106**
 - injury, **102**
Cochlear nuclei (CNVIII), **119**
Cochlear promontory, **59, 71, 79, 85**
Cochleariform process, **56, 60, 61, 80, 82, 85, 92, 173**
Cochleovestibular and facial nerves, **96**
Collapsed lateral pharyngeal recess, **304, 306**
Combined mucosa, of postcricoid and posterior wall mucosa, **401**
Common carotid artery, **191, 279, 280, 283, 284, 288, 289, 333, 335, 337, 338, 339, 345, 346, 360, 361, 367, 368, 399, 404, 405, 406, 407, 408, 411, 421, 422, 431, 432, 436, 437, 438, 538**
 - at aortic arch, **335**
 - displaced, **423**
 - edge of, **339**
 - right, **371**
 - ultrasound, **338**
Complete cervical MR with gadolinium and fat-saturation, perivertebral space, **348**
Complex CNIX-XI neuropathies (Vernet syndrome), **182**
Compressor narium minor, **442, 443, 444, 445**
Concha bullosa, **238, 248, 250, 251, 266**
Concha cavum, **74**
Concha cymba, **74**
Conchae, **238**
Condylar canal, **6**
 - posterior, **40**

Condylar fossa, **47, 57**
 - of temporomandibular joint, **60, 312**
Condylar head, **109, 110, 111, 112, 113**
Condylar neck, **109, 110, 111, 112, 113**
Constrictor muscle, **294, 296**
Conus elasticus, **373, 377**
Cornea, **225**
Corniculate cartilage, **372, 376**
Coronoid process, **109, 110, 111, 490, 491, 492**
 - of mandible, **285, 293, 315**
Corrugator supercilii (CS), **441, 443, 445, 446**
Cortex, lymph node, **426**
Cortical hypertrophy, **436**
CPA. *See* Cerebellopontine angle.
Cranial fossa
 - anterior, **7**
 - middle, **7, 8, 20, 33**
 - posterior, **7, 8**
Cranial nerves, **52**
 - axial bone CT, **120, 121**
 - axial T2 MR, **122, 123, 124, 125**
 - coronal T2 MR, **126, 127**
 - global, graphics, **117**
 - lower, graphics, **119**
 - overview of, **116–127**
 - upper, graphics, **118**
Craniocervical junction (CCJ), **498–513, 514**
 - 3D-VRT NECT, **510**
 - axial bone CT, **508–509**
 - axial T2 MR, **513**
 - coronal bone CT, **507**
 - craniometry, **502**
   bone CT & T1 MR, **503**
   lateral radiography, **504**
 - lateral radiography, **505**
 - radiography, **506**
 - sagittal CT & MR, **512**
 - sagittal T1 MR, **511**
Craniopharyngeal canal, **32**
 - persistent, **30**
Cribriform plate, **5, 14, 17, 21, 25, 26, 27, 28, 29, 130, 243**
 - CNI, **117, 120**
 - ethmoid bone, **11, 12, 16, 23, 25**
 - foramina, **15, 178**
 - site, **25**
Cricoarytenoid joint, **390, 400, 401**
Cricoid cartilage, **280, 284, 337, 358, 368, 372, 375, 377, 380, 381, 382, 383, 384, 385, 387, 388, 391, 397, 400, 401, 404, 418, 419, 425, 429**
 - anterior ring, **376**
 - plane, **429**
 - posterior ring, **376**
 - superior margin, **389, 427**
Cricopharyngeus muscle, **301, 392, 395, 417, 418, 425**
 - indentation, **303, 417**
 - location, **418**
Cricothyroid joint, **375, 381, 387, 397, 420**
Cricothyroid membrane, **375, 376, 381, 387, 397**
Cricothyroid muscle, **373, 378, 418**
 - superior laryngeal nerve, **190**
Cricothyroid space, **375, 381, 397**

INDEX

Crista falciformis, **52, 60, 62, 65, 71, 102, 107, 126, 175, 177, 178**
- horizontal crest, **103, 105**

Crista galli, **5, 8, 9, 11, 12, 13, 14, 16, 19, 20, 21, 24, 25, 26, 27, 28, 29, 120, 121, 129, 130, 242, 243, 246**
- area, **24**
- base, **21**
- ethmoid bone, **23**
- site, **18, 25**

Cruciate ligament, **498, 499, 512, 513**
- inferior extension, **499**
- odontoid anterior to, **499**
- superior extension, **499, 512**

Crus communis, **53, 54, 63, 70, 71, 88, 90, 91**

CS. *See* Carotid space.

Cuneiform cartilage, **372**

D

Danger space (DS), **272, 275, 276, 300, 333, 340, 341, 342, 347, 349, 350, 366, 418, 419, 435**

Decompression, postsurgical changes of, **215**

Deep cervical fascia, **332**

Deep lamina propria, **373**

Deep layer, deep cervical fascia, **272, 275, 276, 291, 333, 341, 342, 347, 348, 349, 350, 351, 352, 357, 366, 418, 419, 435**

Deep parotid space, **454**

Delphian (prelaryngeal/precricoid) node, **427**

Demineralization of otic capsule, **93**

Dens, **49, 195, 203**

Dental anatomy, **490**

Dentin, **490**

Depressor angularis oris, **444**

Depressor anguli oris (DAO), **442, 443, 448, 449**

Depressor labii inferioris (DLI), **442, 443, 444, 449**

Depressor septi nasi, **441, 443, 444, 445**

Depressor supercilii (DS), **441, 443, 445, 446**

Deviated nasal septum with spurring, **248**

Diaphragma sella, **118, 154, 228**

Differentiated thyroid carcinoma primary tumor, **410**

Digastric muscle
- anterior belly of, **283, 284, 286, 287, 312, 430, 433, 454, 456, 458, 459, 467, 470, 472, 473, 475, 477, 482, 485**
- posterior belly of, **275, 278, 282, 287, 288, 291, 294, 296, 297, 320, 321, 322, 325, 326, 327, 328, 330, 331, 336, 346, 430, 457, 458, 466, 469, 472, 484, 485**

Digastric notch, of digastric muscle, **327**

Dilator naris anterior (DNA), **441, 443, 444, 445**

Dilator naris vestibularis (DNV), **441, 443, 444, 445**

Displaced hilar vascularity, **439**

Distal internal maxillary artery, **253**

DL-DCF. *See* Deep layer, deep cervical fascia.

Dorello canal, **95, 97, 99, 165, 226–227**
- abducens nerve (CNVI) in, **99, 158, 228**
- classic, **164**

Dorsal cochlear nuclei, **176, 177**

Dorsal dura margin, **525, 527**

Dorsal gray column, **195**

Dorsal median sulcus, **122**

Dorsal nerve roots, **528**

Dorsal root, **538**

Dorsal root ganglion, **538**

Dorsal scapular nerve, **356, 357**

Dorsal vagal nucleus, **119, 188, 189, 190**

Dorsolateral nucleus, **140**

Dorsomedial nuclei, **140**

Dorsum sella, **7, 8, 11, 12, 13, 16, 19, 28, 29, 33, 37, 39, 41, 43, 121, 230**

DS. *See* Danger space.

Dura, **18**

Dural sheath, CNII, **134**

E

EB. *See* Bulla ethmoidalis; Ethmoid bulla.

ECA. *See* External carotid artery.

Echogenic fatty hilum, **331**

Echogenic hilum, preserved, **436**

Ectopic parathyroid adenoma, **413, 414**

Edinger-Westphal nucleus (EWn), **140**

Efferent lymphatic vessel, **428**

Eight cranial nerve. *See* Vestibulocochlear nerve.

11th CN. *See* Accessory nerve.

Enamel, **490**

Endolymph, **50, 86**

Endolymphatic duct (ELD), **53, 86, 87, 88**

Endolymphatic sac (ELS), **86, 87**
- intradural component, **53**
- intraosseous component, **53**

Endolymphatic spaces, membranous labyrinth, **50**

EOM. *See* Extraocular muscle.

Epidural extension, **352**

Epidural fat, **530**

Epidural tumor, **352**
- compressing spinal cord, **351**

Epiglottic area taste fibers, **190**

Epiglottic free margin, **346**

Epiglottis, **285, 301, 337, 364, 370, 372, 374, 377, 378, 383, 384, 385, 394, 399, 404, 410, 417, 425, 483, 485**
- fixed portion, **385, 388, 396**
- free edge, **377, 379, 396, 398**
- free margin, **278, 303, 376, 385, 386, 388, 419**
- petiole (stem) of, **376**

Epitympanic cavity, of middle ear, **178**

Epitympanic cog, **55, 82**

Epitympanic recess
- anterior, **75, 78, 82**
- lateral, **82, 84**

Epitympanum, **50, 51, 54, 60, 61, 68, 78, 80, 82, 84, 90, 91, 104**

Esophageal carcinoma, **423**

Esophageal lumen, air and fluid, **424**

Esophageal malignancy, **423**

Esophageal mass, **370**

vii

INDEX

Esophageal verge, **392**
Esophagopharyngeal diverticulum (Zenker), **393, 395**
Esophagus, **276, 280, 283, 342, 344, 354, 366, 368, 370, 408, 411, 414, 415, 518**
- circular muscle of, **395**
- circumferential lesion proximal, **371**
Esophagus junction, **381**
Ethmoid, cribriform plate, **238, 242**
Ethmoid air cells, **8, 214, 215, 257**
- anterior, **19, 20, 21, 24, 25, 239, 242, 243, 244, 245, 246, 248**
- posterior, **19, 20, 21, 24, 33, 34, 37, 244, 245, 246**
Ethmoid artery foramen and canal, anterior, **8**
Ethmoid bone, **5, 18, 24, 209, 216, 217, 218, 219**
- cribriform, **27**
- cribriform plate of, **9, 11, 12, 16, 23, 25**
- perpendicular plate of, **14, 21, 23, 25, 26, 27**
Ethmoid bulla, **238, 239, 242, 243, 244, 245, 248, 249, 250, 251, 264, 266, 267**
Ethmoid drainage, posterior, **239**
Ethmoid infundibulum, **242**
- bilateral frontal recesses draining into corresponding, **266**
Ethmoid medial foramen
- anterior, **16**
- posterior, **16**
Ethmoid nerves, anterior and posterior, **31, 155**
Ethmoid roof, **14, 17**
Ethmoid sinus, **9, 136, 156, 214, 215, 218, 238**
- anterior, **10, 13, 27, 130**
- developing, **26**
- posterior, **10, 12, 13**
Ethmoidal artery foramen, canal, and sulcus
- anterior, **14–15**
- posterior, **15**
Ethmoidal foramen
- anterior, **20**
- posterior, **20**
Ethmoidal sulcus, **260**
- left, **269**
- right, **269**
Eustachian tube (ET), **68, 81, 94, 98, 99, 101**
- bony, **35, 98**
- cartilaginous, **75, 98**
   portion, **101**
- entrance to, **75**
- opening, **293, 299, 301, 304, 306, 309, 394**
EWn. *See* Edinger-Westphal nucleus.
EWncp (centrally projecting components), **140**
EWnp (parasympathetic component), **140**
Exocciput, **32**
External auditory canal (EAC), **50, 56, 58, 59, 72, 76, 104, 110, 111, 171, 312, 321, 324**
- anatomy, **72–77**
   axial CT, **75**
   normal, **74**
   sagittal CT, **76**
   sagittal MR, **77**
- anterior wall of, **75**
- bony component of, **51, 74, 75, 76, 77**
- bony-cartilaginous junction of, **51**

- cartilaginous component of, **51, 74, 75, 76, 77**
- fibrocartilaginous roof of, **77**
- floor of, **74, 75, 76, 77**
- lateral cartilaginous component of, **72**
- lumen of, **77**
- meatus of, **74**
- medial bony component of, **72**
- roof of, **74, 75, 76**
- tympanic bone of, **110**
External carotid artery, **53, 277, 278, 282, 288, 320, 321, 322, 325, 326, 330, 331, 335, 336, 404, 433**
- branches of, **288**
External ear, **51, 327**
- arterial supply to, **72–73**
- nodal drainage, **73**
- sensory innervation to, **72**
External jugular vein, **279, 280, 283, 284, 337, 357, 359, 371**
- tributaries, **362**
Extraconal fat, **246**
Extracranial branches
- glossopharyngeal nerve, **182**
- vagus nerve, **188**
Extracranial segment
- abducens nerve, **164**
- accessory nerve, **194**
- facial nerve, **168, 169**
- glossopharyngeal nerve, **182**
- hypoglossal nerve, **198**
- trochlear nerve, **148**
- vagus nerve, **188**
Extralaryngeal extension, of tumor, **389**
Extramural paranasal air cells, **238**
"Extranodal" mass in SHN or IHN, **340**
Extraocular muscle (EOM), **140, 206, 212**
Extrinsic muscles, **373**
Extrinsic tongue muscles, **291**
Eye
- anterior segment, **223**
- vitreous chamber, **223**

F

Facet joint, **352, 506, 509, 514, 515, 516, 521, 523, 529, 531, 538**
- C2-3, **517**
- C4-C5, **521, 525, 526**
- C7-T1, **525, 526**
- complex, **525**
Facet "pillar," **523**
Facial artery, **287, 441, 447, 471, 473, 474, 476**
Facial colliculus, **164, 165, 169**
Facial expression, muscle of, **477**
Facial hiatus, **97**
Facial muscles, **440–449**
- axial T1 MR, **446–449**
- coronal T1 MR, **449**
- coronal T2 MR, **445**

INDEX

- graphic
  - mimic, **443**
  - origin, **444**
Facial nerve (CNVII), **41, 52, 62, 63, 64, 65, 89, 102, 103, 105, 106, 107, 116, 117, 118, 119, 123, 126, 165, 168–175, 177, 179, 180, 321, 440**
- anterior cerebellopontine cistern, **181**
- anterior tympanic segment, **60, 61, 63, 178**
- anterosuperior, in internal auditory canal, **181**
- axial bone CT, **170–171**
- axial T2 & T1 MR, **174**
- coronal bone CT, **172–173**
- extracranial, **320**
- geniculate ganglion, **81, 96**
- graphics, **169**
- internal auditory canal fundus, **175**
- intratemporal, **50**
- labyrinthine segment, **52, 54, 60, 61, 63, 177, 178**
- mastoid segment, **56, 57, 58, 81, 178**
- motor nucleus, **52, 168, 169**
- oblique sagittal T2 MR, **175**
- porus acusticus, **175**
- process, **83**
- recess, **55, 56, 170, 171**
- root exit zone, **52**
- stylomastoid foramen, **174, 327**
- tympanic segment, **51, 52, 59, 60, 90, 92, 168, 169, 170, 172, 173, 324**
Facial nerve canal, **81**
- anterior tympanic segment, **71, 84, 85**
- cephalad mastoid segment, **121**
- geniculate ganglion, **82, 85**
- labyrinthine segment, **55, 69, 71, 80, 82, 121**
- mastoid segment, **68, 83, 121, 202**
- tympanic segment, **55, 68, 69, 70, 71, 79, 80, 84**
Facial nerve nucleus, **165**
Facial nerve paralysis, **168**
Facial nodal group, **427**
Facial vein, **278, 282, 283, 284, 285, 288, 441, 447, 448, 455, 456, 458, 459, 468, 470, 471, 472, 473, 474, 475, 476, 477, 478, 479**
Facial vessels, **447**
Falciform crest, **176, 180, 181**
False vocal cord (FVC), **300, 372, 374, 377, 378, 380, 384, 387, 390, 396, 400, 419**
Falx cerebri, **131**
Fascial "trap door," **276, 342**
Fat
- density pterygopalatine fossa, normal, **259**
- within PFF, **252**
- in posterior cervical space, **356, 363**
FBC. *See* Frontal bullar cell.
Fila olfactoria, **128**
- through cribriform plate, **129**
1st cranial nerve. *See* Olfactory nerve.
1st rib, **281, 541**
Fissural segment, oculomotor nerve, **141**
Fissures of Santorini, **51, 72, 73, 74**

Flocculus, **157**
- of cerebellum, **65, 102, 106, 107, 123, 126, 174, 179, 180**
Floor of mouth (FOM), **480**
FN recess, **78**
FO. *See* Foramen ovale.
Follicular cells, **402**
Fonticulus frontalis, **18, 28**
Foramen cecum, **5, 14, 16, 18, 28, 403, 404, 410**
- area, **24**
- remnant, **8, 9, 16, 18**
- remnant pit, **20, 24, 29**
Foramen lacerum, **5, 6, 9, 11, 30, 31, 35, 36, 44, 69, 75, 94, 96, 98, 99, 101, 273, 292, 299, 309**
- floor of carotid canal, **120**
Foramen magnum, **5, 6, 9, 10, 11, 40, 41, 44, 46, 194, 201, 508, 524**
- anterior margin, **511**
Foramen of Luschka, **122**
Foramen of Vesalius, **30**
Foramen ovale, **30, 31, 35, 36, 45, 57, 75, 96, 98, 101, 111, 117, 154, 156, 160, 171, 201, 216, 217, 241, 255, 292, 299, 314, 319**
- CNV3 in, **5, 6, 9, 10, 11, 120, 162, 273, 292, 311, 312**
- enlarged, **314**
Foramen rotundum, **5, 10, 11, 30, 31, 34, 36, 38, 96, 97, 99, 111, 117, 156, 158, 216, 217, 218, 219, 241, 252, 254, 255, 256, 258, 259, 493**
- maxillary nerve (CNV2), **22, 31, 120, 161, 162**
Foramen spinosum, **17, 30, 31, 35, 45, 57, 75, 96, 98, 111, 117, 120, 156, 171, 201, 255, 273, 292, 312, 317**
- middle meningeal artery, **5, 6, 10, 11, 13, 38, 120, 162**
4th cranial nerve. *See* Trochlear nerve.
4th ventricle, **106, 122, 123, 124, 150, 157, 166, 174, 179, 187, 193, 199**
- inferior, **122**
- superior recess, **125**
Fovea, **91, 224**
- of endolymphatic sac, **70**
- intradural endolymphatic sac, **90, 91**
Fovea ethmoidalis, **19, 23, 25, 26, 27, 28, 130, 238, 242, 243, 265, 268**
- frontal bone, **25, 27**
FR. *See* Frontal recess.
Frontal beak (nasofrontal process), **260, 262, 264, 266**
Frontal bone, **5, 6, 7, 8, 11, 12, 16, 18, 19, 23, 24, 28, 29, 209, 216, 217, 218, 219, 245**
- orbital plate, **96, 130**
Frontal bullar cell, **260, 264, 266, 267**
- right, **268**
Frontal crest, **7, 14, 19, 23**
Frontal infundibulum, **260, 262, 266**
- above and frontal recess below, narrowed, **266, 267**
- below, frontal sinus with, **264**
Frontal lobe, **18, 19, 212**
- orbital gyri of, **17**
Frontal nerve, **17, 31, 155**
- branch, **153**
Frontal recess, **218, 248, 251, 262, 263, 264, 266, 268**
- air gap of, **268**

ix

INDEX

- inverted funnel, **262**
- narrowed, **267**
- related air cells and, **260–269**
    coronal, axial, and sagittal bone CT, **268–269**
    coronal and sagittal graphics of suprabellar cells and bullar cells, **264**
    coronal and sagittal graphics of type 1 and 2 Kuhn cells, **262**
    coronal and sagittal graphics of type 3 and 4 Kuhn cells, **263**
    coronal graphics, **265**
    sagittal and coronal bone CT, **266**
    sagittal bone CT, **267**
Frontal sinus, **7, 8, 9, 12, 16, 19, 23, 24, 28, 219, 238, 239, 240, 243, 244, 248, 251, 260, 262, 263, 266, 268**
- air gap of, **268**
- forming anterior wall of Type 4 Kuhn cell, anterior table of, **267**
- with frontal infundibulum below, **264**
- frontal recess, **245**
- ostium, **260, 262, 264, 266**
Frontalis, **443, 445, 446**
FVC. *See* False vocal cord.

G

Galea aponeurotica, **443**
Gas within larynx, **288**
- supraglottic, **288, 289**
Gasserian ganglion, **232, 254**
Generic posterior cervical space mass, **359**
Geniculate fossa, **91, 97, 170**
- geniculate ganglion in, **173**
Geniculate ganglion, **52, 55, 61, 65, 68, 168, 169, 322, 324**
- in geniculate fossa, **173**
Genioglossus muscle, **200, 286, 287, 398, 454, 455, 456, 457, 458, 459, 463, 464, 465, 466, 472, 480, 481, 482, 483, 484, 485**
Geniohyoid muscle, **198, 200, 283, 287, 453, 461, 464, 467, 482, 483, 491**
Gingiva, **487**
Global cranial nerves, graphics, **117**
Globe, **135, 139, 206, 210, 211, 213, 214, 215, 224–225**
- anterior segment, **224**
- chambers, **224**
- posterior segment, **224**
Glossoepiglottic fold, **300, 303, 374, 379, 386, 396**
Glossoepiglottic ligament, **378, 481**
Glossopharyngeal nerve (CNIX), **41, 116, 117, 119, 122, 182–187, 189, 191, 193, 195, 196, 199, 333, 334, 454, 461, 462, 464**
- axial bone CT, **186**
- axial T2 MR, **187**
- graphics, **183**
    extracranial, **184–185**
Glossopharyngeal neuralgia, **182**
Glottic larynx, **419**

Glottis, **364, 400**
- of endolarynx, **372–373**
Gracile nucleus, **119**
Greater palatine canal (pterygopalatine canal), **253, 256, 257**
Greater palatine foramen, **6, 22, 242, 244, 255, 256, 257, 492, 493**
Greater palatine nerve, **31, 155, 252, 254, 490, 493**
Greater superficial petrosal nerve, **52, 81, 95, 96, 168, 169, 322**
- facial hiatus, **170**
Gum line, **448**
Gyrus rectus, **13, 16, 17, 19, 20, 27, 129, 131**

H

Haller cell, **238, 248, 250**
Hamulus, **36, 241**
- of medial pterygoid plate, **277, 305, 306, 307**
Hard palate, **242, 257, 295, 306**
- mucosa, **461**
Head of malleus, **93, 170**
Hearing event, process, **87**
Helix, **74**
- crus of, **74**
Hering nerve, **188**
Hiatus semilunaris, **238, 239, 244, 245, 249, 250, 251**
High jugular bulb, **104**
Hilar vascularity within normal lymph node, **437**
Horizontal crest, **177**
Horizontal petrous carotid, **99**
- canal, **197**
Horizontal segment, petrous internal auditory canal, **173**
HP. *See* Hypopharynx.
Hyoepiglottic ligament, **374, 377, 379, 396**
Hyoglossus muscle, **163, 200, 282, 285, 287, 301, 394, 454, 455, 456, 457, 458, 459, 461, 463, 464, 465, 466, 467, 469, 471, 472, 473, 480, 481, 482, 483, 484, 485**
Hyoglossus-styloglossus muscles, **484**
Hyoid bone, **276, 279, 284, 303, 334, 335, 336, 337, 342, 350, 353, 366, 367, 370, 374, 376, 377, 379, 383, 384, 385, 386, 388, 391, 396, 398, 399, 400, 404, 407, 410, 414, 417, 418, 419, 425, 431, 453, 456, 458, 483, 491**
- body, **399**
- greater cornu, **398**
- inferior margin, **431**
- plane, **429**
- tip of, **395**
Hypertrophic levator scapulae muscle, **348**
Hypodense parathyroid adenoma, **414**
Hypoglossal canal, **5, 10, 40, 41, 45, 46, 49, 57, 58, 117, 120, 122, 171, 172, 198, 201, 202, 203, 507, 511**
- external opening, **47**
- inferior margin, **45**
Hypoglossal cisternal rootlets, **199**
Hypoglossal eminence, **199**
Hypoglossal intraaxial axons, **199**

INDEX

Hypoglossal nerve (CNXII), **41, 48, 49, 116, 117, 119, 122, 183, 184, 189, 191, 195, 198–203, 333, 334, 454, 461, 462, 464, 480**
- root, **201**

Hypoglossal nucleus, **119, 198, 199, 200**
- location, **201**

Hypoglossal rootlet, **201**

Hypoglossal trigone, **122**

Hypopharyngeal airway, **400**

Hypopharyngeal mucosal space, **301, 394**

Hypopharyngeal-esophageal junction, **345, 406**

Hypopharynx (HP), **303, 342, 344, 345, 364, 366, 370, 378, 380, 381, 392–401, 417, 418, 420, 425**
- axial CECT, **398–401**
- blood supply, **392**
- graphics, **394–397**
- internal contents, **392**
- junction of, **417, 420**
- layers, **392**
- muscles, **392**
- nerve supply, **392**
- posterior wall, **375, 379, 380, 382, 385, 387, 388, 392, 397, 399**
  - tumor evaluation, **393**

Hypophysis, **228**

Hypothalamus, tuber cinereum, **228**

Hypotympanum, **50, 51, 60, 61, 78, 80, 84**

I

IAC. *See* Internal auditory canal.

IHN. *See* Infrahyoid neck.

Incisive canals, paired, **493**

Incisive foramen, **6, 492**
- nasopalatine nerve, **493**

Incisive nerve, **490, 491**

Incudal ligament, posterior, **80**

Incudostapedial articulation, **56, 70, 80, 83**

Incus (anvil), **78, 81**
- body, **55, 60, 61, 68, 80, 82, 84, 85**
- lenticular process, **56, 60, 80, 83, 84**
- long process, **56, 70, 80, 83, 84**
- short process, **55, 59, 60, 68, 80, 82, 84, 90, 170**
- superior ligament, **81**

Inferior alveolar artery, **491**

Inferior alveolar canal, **494**

Inferior alveolar nerve, **155, 163, 285, 312, 314, 318, 319, 453, 459, 464, 470, 471, 472, 473, 489, 490, 491**
- branch, **310**
- mandibular foramen, **163**

Inferior articular facet, **500, 501, 522, 523, 528**

Inferior articular process, **515**

Inferior cavernous sinus, **99**

Inferior cerebellar peduncle, **122, 123, 187**

Inferior colliculi, **125, 150, 151**

Inferior compartment, **109, 113**

Inferior cricoid cartilage, **420**

Inferior extension cruciate ligament, **499**

Inferior hyoid bone, **379**

Inferior joint compartment, **108**

Inferior jugular foramen, **201**
- CNIX-XI, **120**

Inferior mandibular ramus, **494**

Inferior meatus, **238, 242, 243, 247, 249, 250, 251**
- anterior recess, **243, 244**

Inferior oblique muscle, **134, 207, 211, 212, 213**

Inferior olivary nucleus, **199**
- area, **193**

Inferior ophthalmic vein (IOV), **134, 207, 212, 213, 221, 222, 229**

Inferior orbital fissure, **9, 10, 21, 22, 30, 34, 38, 120, 156, 209, 216, 217, 218, 219, 241, 242, 246, 252, 253, 255, 256, 257, 258, 317**

Inferior orbital nerve, **252**

Inferior paraglottic space fat, **401**

Inferior parapharyngeal space, **285**

Inferior petrosal sinus, **99, 100, 192**
- and clival plexus, **99**
- groove for, **97**

Inferior pharyngeal constrictor muscle, **300, 301, 395, 396, 397, 401, 418**
- circular cricopharyngeus part, **394**
- oblique thyropharyngeus part, **394**

Inferior portion, bilaminar zone, **109**

Inferior rectus muscle, **134, 136, 139, 206, 211, 212, 213, 214, 215**

Inferior salivatory nucleus, **119, 182, 183, 185**

Inferior thyroid arteries, **402, 403, 405, 408, 409, 415**

Inferior thyroid vein, **405**

Inferior turbinate, **240, 241, 242, 243, 244, 245, 247, 249, 250, 251, 266**
- attachment, **239**

Inferior tympanic canaliculus, **182**

Inferior vestibular nerve (IVN), **102, 103, 105, 106, 116, 174, 175, 177, 179, 181**

Inferior vestibular nucleus, **177**

Infiltrating thyroid neoplasm, **371**

Infracricoid nodes, **426**

Infraglottic (subglottic) space, **384**

Infrahyoid neck (IHN), **272, 276, 334, 350**
- axial CECT, **279–280**
- carotid space, **332**
  - adjacent spaces, **332**
  - lesion in, **332**
- retropharyngeal space, **340**
  - axial, generic mass, **344**
  - lesion, **340**

Infrahyoid strap muscles, **279, 280, 281, 283, 284, 367, 405, 406, 411**

Infraorbital canal, **219**

Infraorbital ethmoid cells, **238**

Infraorbital foramen, **209, 216, 217, 495**

Infraorbital nerve, **13, 31, 34, 136, 155, 162, 211, 212, 217, 223, 240, 242, 243, 246, 253, 254, 258, 447**
- branch, **153**
  - of CNV2, **134**
- entering inferior orbital fissure, **259**

Infraorbital node, **429**

INDEX

Infraorbital vessels, **447**
Infratemporal fossa, **9**
Infrazygomatic masticator space, **273, 274, 285, 292, 311, 319**
Infundibular recess, **146**
Infundibulum, **13, 124, 138, 160, 230, 231, 233**
Inner cortical table of mandible, **458**
Inner ear (IE)
- anatomy, **86–93**
  anatomic-pathologic correlation, **93**
  axial bone CT, **91–92**
  axial T2 MR, **89**
  graphics, **88**
  longitudinal and transverse CT reformations, **90**
- components, **50**
- nerves, **87**
Inner true capsule, **402**
Intact bulla technique, **261**
Interarytenoid notch, **400**
Interclinoid fold, **226**
Interdural segment
- abducens nerve, **164**
- trigeminal nerve, **152**
Interfrontal sinus septal cell, **261, 268**
Intermediate lamina propria, **373**
Intermediate olfactory stria, **129**
Intermediate zone of disc, **109**
Intermuscular fat plane, **362**
Intermuscular transverse ligament (ITL), **208**
Internal acoustic canal
- fundus of, **103, 104, 107**
- labyrinthine segment of CNVII exit from, **104**
Internal auditory canal (IAC), **8, 13, 43, 47, 52, 54, 55, 58, 63, 65, 71, 82, 91, 93, 95, 96, 97, 102, 107, 117, 159, 166, 172, 173, 178, 202, 203**
- anterior margin, **175**
- anteroinferior quadrant, **176**
- cistern, other structures in, **102**
- CNVII and VIII, **121**
- facial nerve, **168, 169, 170**
  anterosuperior in, **181**
- floor, **92**
- fundus of, **88, 92, 106, 170, 175**
  vertical crest (Bill bar) in, **91**
Internal carotid artery (ICA), **48, 81, 94, 96, 100, 101, 138, 143, 144, 146, 150, 184, 191, 201, 214, 215, 223, 227, 228, 229, 230, 231, 277, 278, 282, 284, 288, 293, 294, 295, 296, 297, 326, 327, 333, 334, 335, 336, 346, 347, 369, 404, 414, 430, 431, 433, 435**
- canal, distal horizontal, **11**
- in carotid canal, **334, 335**
- cavernous, **13, 19, 34, 37, 53, 97, 118, 138, 154, 158, 159, 160, 166, 232, 233, 234, 235, 258**
  left, **231, 232**
  posterior, **233**
  proximal, **97**
- cervical, **53**
- clinoid segment, **235**
- horizontal segment, **111**
- lacerum, **53, 69, 97, 98, 99, 100, 121**

- left, **371**
- nasopharyngeal, **122**
- ophthalmic segment, **235**
- supraclinoid, **13, 138**
  left, **233**
  right, **232**
- thrombosis of, **235**
Internal jugular chain node, **434**
Internal jugular lymph nodes, **429**
- high, **429, 433, 434**
- low, **429**
- middle, **429**
Internal jugular nodal chain, **410**
Internal jugular vein, **42, 48, 49, 57, 184, 191, 203, 277, 278, 279, 280, 281, 282, 283, 284, 288, 289, 293, 294, 295, 296, 326, 327, 333, 334, 336, 337, 338, 339, 345, 346, 358, 360, 361, 367, 368, 369, 371, 406, 407, 408, 411, 421, 422, 423, 424, 430, 431, 432, 433, 435, 436, 437, 438, 544**
- exits jugular foramen, **335**
- infrahyoid, **335**
- left, **371**
- right, **371, 432**
- suprahyoid, **335**
Internal maxillary artery, **247, 254, 315, 317, 319**
- in pterygopalatine fossa, **162**
Interpeduncular cistern, **125, 126, 144, 145, 147, 150, 159, 230**
Interpeduncular cisternal segment, **140**
Interpeduncular fossa, **144**
Interscalar septum(a), **88, 89**
Interscalene triangle, **533**
Intersphenoidal suture, **32**
Intersphenoidal synchondrosis, **32, 39**
Interspinous ligament, **516, 525, 526, 527**
Intervertebral disc, **514, 515, 521, 525, 528, 529, 531**
- C4-C5, **516, 522**
- C5-C6, **523**
- C6-C7, **527**
Intervertebral disc space, **519, 521, 524**
Intervertebral foramen, **514**
Intraaxial axons, hypoglossal, **199**
Intraaxial segment
- abducens nerve, **164**
  fibers, **165**
- accessory nerve, **194**
- facial nerve, **168**
- glossopharyngeal nerve, **182**
- trigeminal nerve, **152**
- vagus nerve, **188**
Intracanalicular segment (CNII), **132, 133, 135, 139**
Intracavernous CNVI, **118, 165**
Intracranial olfactory bulb and tract, **128**
- central pathways, **128**
Intracranial segment (CNII), **132, 133, 135, 138**
Intracranial tumor, **314**
Intradural endolymphatic sac, **88**
Intramesencephalic segment, **140**
- trochlear nerve, **148**
Intranodal cystic necrosis, **438**
Intranodal necrosis, **439**

INDEX

Intraocular segment (CNII), **132, 133, 134**
Intraorbital nerves, **207**
Intraorbital segment
- abducens nerve, **164**
  innervating lateral rectus muscle, **165**
- optic nerve, **132, 134, 135, 139, 220**
  in dural sheath, **133**
Intraosseous endolymphatic sac, **88**
Intraparotid duct, **331**
Intraparotid facial nerve, **321, 322, 327**
- course, **328**
Intraparotid lymph nodes, **320, 322, 331**
Intraparotid malignancy, **324**
Intraparotid nodes, **430**
Intratemporal segment, facial nerve, **168**
Intrinsic muscles, **373, 390, 391, 481**
Intrinsic tongue muscles, **200, 291, 452, 454, 457, 463, 464**
Iris, **211, 224, 225**
Isthmus, **75**
- tumor extension to, **371**
IVN. *See* Inferior vestibular nerve.

J

Jacobson nerve, **182, 185**
Joint capsule, **109**
Jugular bulb, **8, 42, 43, 48, 49, 56, 92, 203, 324**
- apex, **56**
- within jugular foramen, **48**
- roof, **8, 43, 121**
Jugular foramen, **57, 58, 75, 90, 95, 96, 107, 117, 122, 156, 172, 187, 192, 199, 202, 203, 292, 321, 335, 507**
- CNIX-XI, **5, 6, 13, 40, 41, 44, 46, 47, 120, 273**
- pars nervosa (CNIX), **120, 121**
- pars vascularis (CNX-XI), **120, 121**
Jugular fossa, **184**
Jugular spine, **41, 43, 57, 120, 121, 183, 186, 192**
Jugular tubercle, **9, 11, 40, 41, 44, 46, 47, 49, 58, 107, 121, 186, 192, 202, 203, 511**
- diverticulum, **58**
Jugulodigastric (sentinel) node, **278, 288, 427, 429, 433, 458, 472**
Jugulodigastric reactive node, **471**
Jugulo-omohyoid node, **427**
Junction cavernous sinus with petrosal sinuses, **99**

K

Kerckring ossicle, **40**
Keros classification, **238**
Killian dehiscence (or Killian triangle), **393**
- location of, **394**
- region of, **395**
Körner septum, **50, 54, 55, 82**

Kuhn cells, **238, 243, 261**
- coronal and sagittal graphics of type 1 and 2, **262**
- coronal and sagittal graphics of type 3 and 4, **263**
- modified, **261**
- type 1, **262, 266**
- type 2, **262, 267**
  left, **268**
- type 3, **263, 267**
  left, **268**
  right, **268**
- type 4, **263, 267, 268**

L

Labyrinthine segment, facial nerve, **104, 168, 169, 170, 173**
- canal, **69, 71, 90, 91**
Lacrimal artery, **134**
Lacrimal bone, **209, 216, 217, 218, 219**
Lacrimal duct, **214, 215**
Lacrimal gland, **139, 208, 213, 214, 222**
Lacrimal nerve, **31, 134, 155**
Lacrimal sac, **214, 215**
Lamina, **501, 509, 515, 522, 523, 526, 528, 529, 530, 531**
Lamina papyracea, **8, 9, 20, 23, 240, 242, 243, 246, 260**
- right uncinate process inserting on, **266**
Laryngeal aperture, **372**
Laryngeal ventricles, **372, 377, 378, 384, 385, 388, 418, 419**
- anterior portion of, **389**
- leading to saccule, **385**
- saccule of, **389**
Laryngeal vestibule, **372, 384**
Larynx, **344, 364, 366, 370, 372–391, 417, 425**
- axial CECT cords abducted
    apart, **379–381**
    together, **382**
- axial T1 MR, **386–387**
- cartilages, **372**
- clinical correlates, **389**
- coronal NECT, **383–384**
- embryology, **373**
- graphics, **374–377**
    reformatted CT and, **378**
- innervation, **373**
- longitudinal ultrasound, **391**
- muscles, **373**
- sagittal NECT, **385**
- sagittal T1 MR, **388**
- transverse ultrasound, **390**
Lateral canthal ligament, **208**
Lateral cord, **535, 542**
Lateral cricoarytenoid muscle, **373, 378**
Lateral geniculate body, **133, 135**
Lateral incisor, **492, 493, 494**
Lateral lamella, **21, 23, 25, 27, 130, 238, 242**
- of cribriform plate, **268**
Lateral lobes, **402**

xiii

INDEX

Lateral mesencephalic vein, **151**
Lateral neural recess, **523**
Lateral neural sulcus, **533, 538**
Lateral olfactory stria(e), **128, 129**
Lateral pectoral nerve, **536**
Lateral pharyngeal recess, **302, 306, 309**
Lateral plain film, perivertebral space, **348**
Lateral pons, **162**
Lateral pterygoid muscle, **109, 155, 160, 163, 258, 277, 285, 293, 295, 297, 304, 306, 310, 311, 312, 315, 317, 318, 319, 323**
 - inferior head, **319**
 - small superior head, **315**
 - superior head, **319**
Lateral pterygoid plate, **241, 247, 255, 256, 258, 293, 312, 315**
Lateral rectus muscle, **133, 134, 135, 136, 139, 206, 210, 211, 212, 213, 214, 215, 223**
 - abducens nerve, **165**
Lateral retropharyngeal node, **341, 347**
Lateral retropharyngeal space, **295, 296, 333, 336**
 - mass, **343**
Lateral thyrohyoid ligament, **376**
Lateral vestibular nucleus, **177**
Lateralized middle turbinate, **261**
Left abducens nerve, **166**
Left foramen ovale, **233**
Lens, **210, 211, 214, 215, 223, 225**
Lesser palatine foramen, **255, 492, 493**
Lesser palatine nerve, **31, 253, 490, 493**
Lesser superficial petrosal nerve, **96**
Levator anguli oris (LAO), **442, 443, 444, 447, 448**
Levator aponeurosis, **211**
Levator labii superioris (LLS), **442, 443, 444, 445, 447**
Levator labii superioris alaeque asir (LLSAN), **442, 443, 444, 445**
Levator palatini muscle, **295**
Levator palpebrae muscle, **17, 134, 142, 149, 212, 213**
Levator palpebrae superioris muscle, **136, 139, 206, 207, 211, 212, 213, 215**
Levator scapulae muscle, **279, 280, 281, 283, 284, 349, 353, 354, 358, 360, 361, 362, 363**
Levator veli palatini muscle, **297, 299, 301, 302, 304, 306, 394**
Ligamentum flavum, **531**
Ligamentum nuchae, **349, 360, 499, 516, 525, 526, 527**
Liliequist membrane, **146**
Lingual artery, **454, 461, 462, 463, 464, 465, 466, 467, 473, 480**
 - branch of, **286, 287**
Lingual branch, glossopharyngeal nerve, **182**
Lingual nerve, **31, 155, 163, 310, 312, 452, 453, 454, 461, 462, 464, 491**
 - location, **316**
Lingual septum, **454, 455, 457, 458, 464, 465, 466, 467, 481, 483, 484, 485**
 - cephalad aspect, **457**
Lingual thyroid, **403**

Lingual tonsil, **285, 291, 300, 301, 303, 305, 308, 345, 346, 385, 394, 404, 417, 434, 455, 457, 461, 465, 481, 483**
 - tongue base, **388**
Lingual tonsillar tissue, **398**
Lingual vein, **462, 465, 480**
Lingula, **492**
Lip mucosa, **461**
Lobule, **74**
Lockwood ligament, **208**
Long ciliary nerve, **155**
Long thoracic nerve, **536**
Longissimus capitis muscle, **349**
Longitudinal esophageal muscle, **418**
Longitudinal ligament
 - anterior, **499, 512**
 - posterior, **499**
Longus capitis muscle, **375, 488**
Longus capitus muscle, **99**
Longus colli muscle, **288, 349, 408, 409, 488**
Loose areolar plane, **446, 449**
Low internal jugular lymph node (level IV), **369, 410, 426, 432**
Low palatine tonsil, **465**
Lower alveolar ridge mucosa, **461**
Lower cranial nerves, graphics, **119**
Lower lip, muscles inserting at, **442**
Lower trunk, **541**
LP. *See* Lateral pterygoid.
Lung apex, **281**
Lymph node, **289, 329, 339, 426, 544**
 - hilar vascularity in, **339**
Lymphatic system, **426**
Lymphoid follicles, **426**
Lymphomatous lymph node, **438**
Lymphovascular malformation, **363**
Lytic lesion vertebral body, **352**

M

Macula, **224**
Macula cribrosa, **59, 91, 102, 104**
 - foramen, **178**
Main motor nucleus, **153**
Main sensory nucleus CNV, **152, 153, 157**
Major foramina, **216**
Malar fat pad, **440, 447, 448**
Malar node, **429**
Malaris muscle, **441**
Malignant otitis externa, **73**
Malignant retropharyngeal node, **343**
Malleal ligament
 - anterior, **82**
 - lateral, **80, 85**
 - superior, **80, 85**
Malleoincudal articulation, **68, 80, 82**
Malleus (hammer), **78, 173**
 - anterior process, **80**

INDEX

- head, **55, 61, 68, 80, 81, 82, 85**
    in epitympanum, **54**
- lateral process, **80, 85**
- manubrium, **56, 57, 60, 61, 70, 80, 81, 83, 85**
- neck, **56, 80, 82, 85**
- umbo, **60, 80, 83, 84**
Mammillary body, **125, 137, 144, 150**
Mandible, **430, 449, 475, 490–495**
- 3D CT, **495**
- mylohyoid ridge of, **467, 470**
Mandibular alveolar ridge, **495**
Mandibular alveolus buccal margin, **448**
Mandibular body, **110, 490, 495**
Mandibular branch
- abducens nerve, **169**
- facial nerve, **322**
Mandibular canal, **490**
Mandibular condyle, **10, 45, 57, 75, 76, 77, 108, 109, 111, 113, 163, 171, 293, 297, 315, 317, 318, 324, 327**
- erosion, **313**
- head, **492, 495**
- lateral, **76**
- neck, **492, 495**
Mandibular coronoid process, **318, 319**
Mandibular cortex, **473**
Mandibular foramen, **241, 277, 318, 319, 489, 490, 491, 492, 494**
- inferior alveolar nerve, **163**
    location, **316**
Mandibular fossa, **75, 108, 109, 110, 111, 112, 113**
Mandibular head, **47**
Mandibular nerve (CNV3), **31, 38, 117, 118, 152, 153, 154, 155, 158, 159, 160, 163, 227, 228, 230, 233, 299, 310, 311, 313, 314, 317, 319, 453, 491**
- anterior division, **312**
- exiting foramen ovale, **31**
- in foramen ovale, **13, 38, 162, 292, 311, 312, 317**
- main trunk, **312**
- perineural tumor on, **314**
- posterior division, **312**
- surrounded by bright trigeminal fat pad, **317**
Mandibular node, **429**
Mandibular notch, **109, 110**
Mandibular ramus, **109, 110, 111, 163, 282, 284, 293, 294, 315, 316, 318, 319, 488, 490, 494, 495**
Mandibular teeth, **489**
Manubrium, **432**
Marginal supraglottis, **300**
"Marionette lines," **442**
Masseter muscle, **155, 163, 277, 278, 282, 284, 285, 293, 294, 295, 296, 297, 310, 311, 312, 315, 316, 318, 319, 325, 326, 327, 328, 329, 330, 353, 448, 449, 457, 469, 470, 473, 475, 477, 478, 479, 483, 488**
- new, **476**
Masticator motor nerve branches, **310**

Masticator space, **6, 22, 184, 240, 272, 273, 274, 275, 277, 278, 282, 284, 285, 291, 292, 293, 294, 295, 296, 297, 299, 300, 302, 304, 305, 306, 307, 310–319, 311, 312, 313, 315, 316, 317, 318, 321, 322, 323, 325, 326, 327, 328, 329, 334, 341, 343, 448, 454, 463, 469, 473**
- axial CECT, **315–316**
- axial T1 MR, **317–318**
- chondrosarcoma, **313**
- continuation of fat into, **476**
- coronal T1 MR, **319**
- graphics, **311–312**
- infrazygomatic, **310**
- malignancy, **314**
- mass, generic, **313**
- perineural CNV3 malignancy, **314**
- suprazygomatic, **310**
Mastoid air cells, **7, 8, 43, 46, 54, 63, 68, 74, 75, 76, 97, 111, 121, 202, 324**
- pneumatized, **77**
- superolateral, **74**
Mastoid antrum, **50, 54, 55, 58, 59, 68, 82, 104, 170, 172, 178**
Mastoid canaliculus, **188**
Mastoid emissary vein, **48**
Mastoid foramen, **40**
Mastoid node, **429**
Mastoid process, **6, 11, 46, 110, 111, 521**
- tip of, **330**
Mastoid segment
- facial nerve, **46, 168, 170, 171, 172, 324**
    canal, **68**
- temporal bone, **96**
Mastoid sinuses, **174**
Mastoid tip, **10, 45, 57, 58, 65, 76, 77, 96, 171, 172, 202, 277, 282, 321, 322, 325, 327, 329, 357, 359, 361**
Matted tuberculous lymph nodes, **438**
Maxilla, **6, 96, 209, 216, 217, 218, 219, 475, 478, 490–495**
- frontal process, **209**
- palatine process, **11, 12, 492**
Maxillary alveolar ridge, **476, 488, 489, 495**
Maxillary alveolus buccal margin, **448**
Maxillary artery, **310, 311, 325**
- internal, **38, 53**
Maxillary (ethmoid) infundibulum, **242, 244, 248, 249, 250**
Maxillary nerve (CNV2), **31, 38, 117, 118, 123, 152, 153, 154, 155, 158, 159, 160, 161, 227, 228, 229, 234, 246, 252, 254**
- in cavernous sinus, **162**
- in foramen rotundum, **162**
- in superior pterygopalatine fossa, **162**
Maxillary ostium, **249**
Maxillary ridge, **277, 295**
Maxillary sinus, **13, 22, 38, 136, 156, 162, 217, 238, 239, 240, 242, 243, 244, 246, 247, 248, 249, 250, 254, 255, 257, 258, 259, 317**
Maxillary tuberosity, **488**
McGregor line, **498, 502, 503, 504**
McRae foramen magnum line, **502**
McRae line, **498, 504**

INDEX

Meckel cave, **13, 37, 38, 63, 94–95, 99, 100, 106, 123, 127, 137, 138, 146, 152, 155, 157, 158, 160, 162, 166, 227, 228, 229, 231, 232, 233, 258, 259, 312, 319**
- anterior/inferior, **100**
- dural margin, **159**
- lateral dural margin, **157**
- lateral margin of, **259**
- lateral wall, **99**
- location, **97**
- trigeminal fascicles, **157, 162, 231**
- with trigeminal ganglion, **153**
Medial canthal ligament, **208**
Medial canthal tendon, **446**
Medial cord, **535, 542**
Medial fascial slip, **310**
Medial forebrain bundle, **128**
Medial geniculate body, **133**
Medial incisor, **492, 493, 494**
Medial longitudinal fasciculus (MLF), **140**
Medial olfactory stria(e), **128, 129**
Medial palpebral ligament, **214, 215**
Medial pterygoid muscle, **155, 160, 163, 277, 278, 282, 284, 285, 294, 295, 296, 297, 306, 310, 311, 312, 315, 316, 318, 319, 320, 323, 325, 326, 327, 328, 353, 457, 459, 466, 469, 472, 476**
Medial pterygoid plate, **241, 246, 255, 256, 293, 312, 315**
- hamulus, **316, 318, 476, 487, 488, 493**
Medial rectus muscle, **133, 134, 135, 136, 139, 206, 212, 213, 214, 215, 223, 246**
Medial retropharyngeal node, **341**
Medial temporal lobe, **100**
Medial vestibular nucleus, **177**
Median atlantoaxial joint, anterior, **501**
Median nerve, **535, 536**
Median raphe, **347**
- retropharyngeal space, **340**
Median sulcus, **481**
Medulla, **122, 126, 167, 203**
- lymph node, **426**
Medulla oblongata, **48, 151, 180**
Medullary pyramid, **193, 197, 201**
Medullary region, lymph node, **428**
"Melomental folds," **442**
Membranous labyrinth, **53, 86**
- endolymphatic spaces, **50**
Meningeal artery, middle, in foramen spinosum, **53**
Meningeal branch, hypoglossal nerve, **200**
Meningioma, optic nerve, **215**
Mental foramen, **110, 163, 472, 490, 491, 495**
Mental nerve, **490, 491**
Mental protuberance, **495**
Mental tubercle, **495**
Mentalis, **442, 443, 444, 449**
Mesencephalic nucleus (CNV), **119, 152**
Mesotympanum, **50, 51, 57, 58, 61, 78, 80, 85, 104**
- anterior, **68**
Metastatic lymph nodes, **438, 439**
- level IV, **371**
Midbrain, **125, 144, 150, 151**
Middle cerebellar peduncle, **106, 123, 124, 151, 162, 179**

Middle cerebral artery
- genu, **232**
- M1 segment, **127, 138**
- right, **147, 231**
Middle cerebral peduncle, left, **147**
Middle cranial fossa, **240, 255**
Middle ear, **51**
Middle ear-mastoid, **50**
- anatomy, **78–85**
    axial bone CT, **82–83**
    coronal bone CT, **84–85**
    coronal graphics, **80**
    medial and lateral walls, **81**
Middle layer, deep cervical fascia, **272, 273, 274, 275, 276, 291, 292, 298, 299, 300, 309, 333, 341, 342, 349, 350, 366, 402, 403, 405, 418, 419, 421, 435**
Middle meatus, **238, 242, 246, 247, 248, 249, 250, 251, 260**
- right frontal recess draining directly into, **266**
Middle meningeal artery, **120, 273, 312, 317**
- in foramen spinosum, **158, 162**
Middle pharyngeal constrictor muscle, **301, 308, 394, 395, 396, 399**
Middle scalene muscle, **280, 281, 283, 284, 349, 352, 353, 354, 355, 360, 361, 537, 539, 540, 541**
Middle trunk, **541**
Middle turbinate, **241, 242, 243, 245, 246, 247, 249, 250, 251, 260, 262, 266**
- attachment, **239**
- attachment, basal lamella of, **267**
    dividing anterior from posterior ethmoid air cell, **266**
- left uncinate process inserting on, **266**
- middle and posterior portions of basal lamella of, **260**
- vertical portion forming medial boundary of frontal recess, **266**
Mid IAC facial nerve, **175**
Mid internal auditory canal, **106**
Mid internal jugular chain nodes (level III), **426, 431**
Midline pharyngeal raphe, **395**
Midpoint vestibular aqueduct, **90**
Minor salivary glands, **298**
ML-DCF. *See* Middle layer, deep cervical fascia.
MLF. *See* Medial longitudinal fasciculus.
Modiolus, **56, 64, 86, 88, 89, 90, 92, 103, 106, 177**
- muscles inserting at, **442**
Motor fibers, **182, 188**
Motor nerve, to stylopharyngeus, **185**
Motor nucleus
- CNV, **152, 153, 157**
- facial nerve, **168, 169**
Mouth mucosal surface, floor of, **461**
MP. *See* Medial pterygoid.
MS. *See* Masticator space.
Mucosa, **309, 364**
- hypopharynx, **392**
Mucosa inferior turbinate, **212**
Mucosal component, of supraglottic carcinoma, **389**
Mucosal tumor, **389**
Müller muscle, **208, 211**
Multifidus muscle, **349**

INDEX

Muscular branch, hypoglossal nerve, **198**
Muscular layer, **364**
- hypopharynx, **392**
Musculocutaneous nerve, **535, 536**
Mylohyoid muscle, **155, 163, 282, 286, 287, 291, 292, 294, 312, 326, 430, 452, 453, 454, 455, 456, 457, 458, 459, 461, 462, 463, 464, 465, 466, 467, 469, 470, 471, 472, 475, 481, 482, 483, 484, 485, 491**
- attaching to mylohyoid ridge, **457**
- cleft, **452, 456, 458, 469, 472, 485**
    with vessel, **465, 471**
- posterior margin, **294, 465**
Mylohyoid nerve, **152, 312, 453, 491**
- branch, **310**
Mylohyoid ridge, **464, 471, 490, 491**
- of mandible, **453, 459, 467**

N

Nasal airway, **285**
Nasal bone, **12, 13, 16, 18, 23, 28, 29, 209, 216, 217, 218**
- fat, **246**
Nasal capsule, cartilage of developing, **18**
Nasal cartilage, **18**
Nasal cavity, **161, 238, 245**
- posterior, **247**
- roof of, **120**
Nasal epithelium, **128**
Nasal meati, **238**
Nasal pyriform aperture, **238**
Nasal septum, **130, 238, 240, 242, 243, 247**
Nasal turbinates, **238**
Nasociliary nerve, **134**
Nasolacrimal apparatus, **208**
Nasolacrimal duct, **218, 219, 239, 240, 243, 244, 246, 247**
Nasolacrimal sac, **243**
Nasomaxillary suture, **218**
Nasopalatine nerve, **490**
Nasopharyngeal airway, **36, 160, 247, 285**
Nasopharyngeal carotid space, **182, 184, 200, 333**
- injury to, **332**
Nasopharyngeal mucosal space, **273, 274, 292, 301, 309, 394**
Nasopharyngeal/adenoidal tissue, **233**
Nasopharynx, **95, 228, 241**
Neck of mandible, **325**
Necrotic adenopathy, **401**
Necrotic level IV node, **371**
Nerve root, **528, 532**
- sleeves, **529**
Nerve rootlets, **524**
Neural foramen, **507, 515, 517, 522, 523, 525, 528, 529, 530, 531, 533**
- C2-C3, **520**
- C3-C4, **520, 524**
- C4-C5, **521**
- C5-C6, **520**
- C7-T1, **526**

Neuropore, anterior, **18, 24**
9th cranial nerve. *See* Glossopharyngeal nerve.
Normal contralateral CNIII, **147**
Normal jugular lymph node with echogenic hilum, **436**
Nose, muscles inserting at, **441–442**
Nuclei, facial nerve, **168**
Nucleus ambiguus, **119, 182, 183, 185, 188, 189, 190, 194, 195, 196**
Nucleus area, CNIII, **144**
Nucleus of Perlia, **140**

O

Oblique arytenoid, **373, 378**
Occipital bone, **5, 6, 7, 9, 10, 11, 40, 44, 96, 498**
- basilar portion, **40, 45**
- basiocciput, **299**
- clival, **38, 44, 45, 47, 48, 49**
- condylar, **40, 44, 45, 46, 57**
- squamous part, **40, 43, 44**
Occipital condyle, **6, 10, 11, 45, 46, 49, 58, 202, 203, 282, 507, 508, 511, 517, 524, 526, 527**
Occipital crest, internal, **41, 43**
Occipital node, **429**
Occipital protuberance, internal, **44**
Occipital triangle, **356**
Occipitofrontalis, frontal belly of, **441, 443**
Occipitomastoid suture, **7, 8, 9, 41, 43, 44, 57**
Oculomotor cistern, **143, 146**
- CNIII in, **124**
Oculomotor nerve (CNIII), **17, 37, 116, 117, 118, 119, 124, 125, 126, 127, 137, 138, 140–147, 143, 144, 145, 146, 149, 151, 154, 159, 160, 161, 165, 167, 207, 211, 216, 217, 227, 228, 232, 233, 234**
- axial T2 & T1 MR, **144**
- axial T2 MR, **143**
- cistern, **142**
- clinical correlation, **147**
- complex, **140**
- coronal T2 MR, **145, 146**
- enlarged & enhancing right, **147**
- graphics, **142**
- in oculomotor cistern, **127, 146**
- rootlets, **145**
Oculomotor nuclear complex (ONC), **140**
Oculomotor nucleus, **142**
Oculomotor triangle, **226**
Odontoid ligaments, **498**
Odontoid process (C2), **46, 499, 501, 505, 506, 507, 510, 513, 517, 530**
- base, **512, 530**
- body, **49**
- lateral margin, **511**
- posterior margin, **511**
Odontoid tip, **508, 510, 512, 513**
Olfactory bulb, **16, 17, 128, 129, 131**
- area, **130**
Olfactory cortex, **128**

INDEX

Olfactory mucosa, **130**
- in olfactory recess, **21, 23**
Olfactory nerve (CNI), **16, 116, 117, 128–131**
- coronal NECT, **130**
- coronal T2 MR, **131**
- graphics, **129**
Olfactory recess, **26, 242, 243**
- with olfactory mucosa, **25**
Olfactory sulcus, **129, 131**
Olfactory tract, **128, 129, 131**
Olfactory trigone, **129**
Olivary eminence, **32**
Olive, **122, 187**
Omohyoid muscle, **200, 338, 357, 408, 432**
- anterior belly, **200**
- inferior belly, **357**
- posterior belly, **200**
OMS. *See* Oral mucosal space.
ONC. *See* Oculomotor nuclear complex.
Operculum, **90**
Ophthalmic artery (OphA), **134, 136, 139, 207, 212, 214, 215, 220, 222, 230**
Ophthalmic nerve (CNV1), **31, 117, 118, 152, 153, 154, 155, 161, 227, 228, 234**
Ophthalmic veins, **207**
Opisthion, **499, 506, 508, 512, 518, 525, 526**
Optic canals, **5, 7, 8, 11, 15, 17, 19, 22, 30, 31, 33, 117, 121, 216, 217, 218, 219, 220, 241, 256, 493**
- with optic nerve and ophthalmic artery, **17**
Optic chiasm, **125, 127, 132, 133, 135, 138, 146, 159, 210, 220, 221, 223, 230, 231, 232, 233, 234**
Optic disc, **135**
Optic fissure, **224**
Optic nerve (CNII), **13, 16, 31, 116, 117, 118, 125, 132–139, 206, 207, 210, 211, 212, 214, 215, 216, 217, 220, 221, 222, 223, 225, 230, 232, 234, 246**
- axial & sagittal T1 MR, **139**
- axial stir MR, **135**
- band, **211**
- canal, **209, 210, 214, 215**
- chiasm and tract, **117**
- coronal T1 MR, **136**
- coronal T2 MR, **137, 138**
- graphics, **133, 134**
- head, **210**
- intracanalicular segment, **210**
- sheath, **210, 211**
Optic nerve meningioma, **215**
Optic nerve/sheath complex, **220–223**
Optic neuritis, **220**
Optic radiation, **132, 133**
Optic recess, **146**
Optic sheath, **220, 221, 222, 225**
Optic strut, **7, 17, 22, 209, 210, 214, 215, 217, 218, 219, 221, 222**
- base of, **8**
Optic tract, **125, 127, 132, 133, 135, 137, 144, 146, 150, 154, 167, 210, 220, 221, 223, 228, 231**
Ora serrata, **224**

Oral cavity (OC), **309**
- axial CECT, **455–456**
- axial T2 MR, **457–458**
- coronal T1 MR, **459**
- fascia, **452**
- graphics, **453–454**
- oral mucosal space/surface (OMS), **452**
- oral tongue, **452**
- overview, **452–459**
- root of tongue (ROT), **452**
- sublingual space (SLS), **452**
- submandibular space (SMS), **452**
Oral mucosa, **477**
Oral mucosal space (OMS), **452, 454, 460–461, 464, 470**
Oral tongue, **285, 305, 308, 435, 453, 480, 489**
Oral tongue mucosa, **461**
Oral tongue mucosal surface, **461**
Oral-cutaneous fistula, **479**
Orbicularis oculi (OOc), **441, 445, 448**
- lacrimal portion, **441, 444**
- orbital portion, **441, 443, 444**
- palpebral portion, **441, 443, 444**
Orbicularis oris (OOr), **442, 443, 444, 448**
Orbit, **19**
- bones, **216**
- CNIII, **142**
- muscles inserting at, **441**
- overview, **206–215**
Orbit periosteum (periorbita), **133, 134**
Orbital apex, **21**
- enhancing tumor in, **147**
Orbital branch, **155**
Orbital fascia, **207**
Orbital fat, **207**
Orbital gyrus, **131**
Orbital roof, **7, 17, 19**
- frontal bone, **23, 25**
Orbital segment, oculomotor nerve, **141**
Orbital septum, **208, 211**
Orbitosphenoid, **32**
Organ of Corti, **88, 103, 177**
Oropharyngeal airway, **347**
Oropharyngeal mucosal space, **273, 274, 292, 301, 309, 394, 469**
Oropharynx, **303, 378, 417, 434, 455**
Osseous spiral lamina, **86, 88, 89**
Ossicles, **78–79**
Ossification, **389**
Ostiomeatal unit, **248–251**
Otic ganglion, **155, 163**
- location, **317**
Outer false capsule, **402**
Oval window, **55, 59, 70, 82, 92, 172, 173**
- niche, **79**

P

Palatine bone, **6, 209, 216, 217**
- horizontal plate, **11, 492**

INDEX

Palatine canal, greater, **493**
Palatine nerves, **253, 254, 258**
Palatine tonsil, **278, 285, 293, 294, 297, 300, 301, 302, 305, 307, 308, 309, 345, 346, 394, 457, 459, 461, 466, 473, 481, 484, 487, 489**
- normal, **430**
Palatoglossus muscle, **198, 200, 300, 453, 461, 480, 481, 482, 484, 485**
Palatopharyngeus muscle, **395**
Palatovaginal (palatinovaginal) canal, **253, 256**
Paracortex, lymph node, **426, 428**
Paradoxical middle turbinate, **248, 250**
Paraglottic fat, **399, 400**
- anterior margin of tumor in, **401**
Paraglottic space, **372, 374, 377, 379, 380, 382, 384, 386, 387, 390, 391, 396, 398**
- fat, **389, 401**
    submucosal tumor invading, **389**
    tumor obliterates, **389**
- with fat density, **389**
Parahippocampal gyrus, **129**
Paranasal air cells, extramural, **238**
Parapharyngeal fat, **476, 478**
Parapharyngeal space, **272, 273, 274, 275, 277, 278, 282, 284, 285, 290–297, 291, 292, 293, 294, 295, 296, 297, 299, 300, 302, 304, 305, 306, 307, 308, 309, 311, 312, 313, 315, 316, 318, 319, 320, 322, 325, 326, 327, 328, 329, 333, 334, 336, 341, 342, 343, 347, 435, 455, 457, 459, 473**
- abuts skull base, **274**
- axial CECT, **293–294**
- axial T1 MR, **295–296**
- coronal T1 MR, **297**
- fascial of, **290**
- fat, **323, 448**
- graphics, **291–292**
- masticator space mass enters, **313**
Paraspinal component, perivertebral space, **348, 349, 350, 353, 354, 357, 359, 360**
Paraspinal muscles, **279, 280, 281, 283, 284, 349, 353, 357, 360, 361**
Parasympathetic fibers, **168, 182, 188, 252**
Parathyroid adenoma, **411, 414, 415**
- ectopic, **413**
Parathyroid gland (PTG), **191, 365, 366, 403, 405, 419, 422, 423**
- anatomy, **402–415**
- arterial supply, **403**
- axial CECT, **406**
- coronal CECT, **407**
- embryology, **403**
    graphics of, **412**
- fascia, **403**
- graphics, **404–405**
- inferior, **405, 410, 412**
    locations of, **403**
- internal contents, **403**
- longitudinal ultrasound, **409**
- superior, **405, 410, 412**
    locations of, **403**

- transverse ultrasound, **408**
- ultrasound, **415**
Paratracheal lymph node, **191, 366, 405, 419**
- level VI, **369, 410**
Parietal bone, **5, 6**
Parotid deep lobe, **327**
Parotid duct (Stensen duct), **277, 282, 284, 320, 325, 327, 328, 448, 475, 476, 477, 478, 479**
- anterior, **477**
- distal, **474**
- exits parotid, **320**
- midportion, **477**
- penetrates buccinator muscle, **320**
Parotid gland, **51, 74, 77, 163, 174, 282, 293, 318, 320, 414, 430, 448, 449, 475, 476, 477, 478, 479**
- accessory, **282, 316, 320, 327**
- deep lobe, **293, 295, 296, 297, 322, 325, 326, 329**
    mass, **323**
    space mass, **323**
- superficial lobe, **295, 297, 323, 325, 330, 331**
- tail, **471**
Parotid malignant tumor, **324**
Parotid nodal group, **427**
Parotid nodes, **51, 429, 433**
Parotid space, **6, 272, 273, 274, 275, 277, 278, 282, 284, 285, 291, 292, 293, 294, 295, 296, 297, 311, 312, 313, 315, 316, 318, 320–331, 321, 325, 326, 327, 328, 329, 334, 343, 360**
- axial CECT, **325–326**
- axial T1 MR, **327–328**
- axial T2 FS MR, **329**
- fascia of, **320**
- generic parotid space mass, **323**
- graphics, **321–322**
- longitudinal ultrasound, **331**
- perineural parotid space malignancy, **324**
- transverse ultrasound, **330**
Parotid tail, **282, 324, 326**
Parotid tissue, **77**
- medial, **77**
- region of, **76**
Parotideomasseteric fascia, **441, 447, 449**
Pars interarticularis, **511, 515**
Pars nervosa, **182, 192, 199**
- jugular foramen, **8, 40, 41, 42, 43, 44, 57, 183, 186, 197**
Pars vascularis, **188, 192, 199**
- jugular foramen, **8, 9, 40, 41, 42, 43, 44, 57, 186, 197**
Party wall, **421**
PCS. *See* Posterior cervical space.
Pedicle, cervical spine, **509, 515, 516, 529, 531**
Periaqueductal gray matter, **144**
Perilymph, **50, 86**
Perilymphatic labyrinth, **86**
Perilymphatic spaces, **50**
Perineural malignancy on mastoid CNVII, **324**
Perineural tumor
- along CNIII, **147**
- on mandibular nerve, **314**
Perineural tumor spread (PNTS), **253**
Perineural vein, **538**
Perineural venous plexus, **538, 543**

xix

INDEX

Perioptic cerebrospinal fluid, **210, 221**
Periorbita, **134, 207**
Peripheral capsule, **426**
Peripheral facial neuropathy, **102**
Perivertebral space (PVS), **272, 276, 278, 291, 333, 334, 337, 348–355, 364, 392**
- axial CECT, **353–354**
- axial T2 FS and coronal stir MR, **355**
- CECT, **348**
- graphics, **349–350**
- paraspinal component, **274, 275, 276, 278, 279, 280, 281, 283, 284**
- prevertebral component, **274, 275, 276, 278, 279, 280, 281, 282, 283, 284, 302, 304, 305, 306, 307, 308**
- suprahyoid mass, **351–352**
Petroclinoid fold, **226**
- posterior, **226**
Petroclinoid ligament, **142**
Petroclinoid segment, oculomotor nerve, **141**
Petrolingual ligament (PLL), **95, 227**
- sphenoid lingula for, **97**
Petrooccipital fissure (POF), **6, 8, 9, 34, 35, 41, 44, 47, 75, 94, 96, 98, 101, 186, 192**
- cephalad aspect (CNVI), **121**
- chondrosarcoma, **101**
Petrosal sinus
- inferior, **9, 42, 48**
- superior, **42**
Petrosphenoid junction, **98**
Petrosphenoid suture, **75**
Petrosphenoidal fissure, **98**
Petrosquamous suture, **96**
Petrotympanic fissure, **76**
Petrous apex (PA), **7, 8, 34, 43, 44, 50, 54, 61, 63, 91, 104, 121, 186, 192, 197**
- air cells, **111**
- anatomic-pathologic correlation: POF chondrosarcoma, **101**
- anatomy, **94–101**
- asymmetric, **40**
- bone, **94**
- marrow, **13, 55, 94, 98, 162**
  space, **55**
- normal, **96**
  axial CT, **97–98**
  contrast-enhanced CT, **99**
  T1-weighted MR, **100**
- pneumatization of, **94**
- pneumatized air cells of, **97**
- superior cortex, **100**
- with suppressed fat signal, **101**
- trabecular bone, **99**
Petrous bone, **99**
Petrous carotid canal, **94, 98**
Petrous internal carotid artery, **50, 53, 93, 100, 158, 233**
- horizontal, **8, 38, 43, 44, 53, 57, 61, 69, 162**
  anterior genu of, **38**
  canal, **9, 34, 47, 186, 192, 255**

- vertical, **9, 13, 53, 57, 60, 69, 156, 163, 171, 173, 186, 192, 324**
  canal, **35, 44**
Petrous ridge, **5, 11, 31, 32, 34, 96**
Pharyngeal artery, ascending, **53**
Pharyngeal branches
- glossopharyngeal nerve, **182**
- vagus nerve, **188**
Pharyngeal constrictor muscle, **374, 375, 484, 485**
Pharyngeal mucosal space, **272, 277, 278, 292, 294, 295, 296, 297, 298–309, 299, 300, 305, 307, 308, 318, 341, 342, 345, 346, 347**
- abuts basisphenoid, **309**
- axial T1 MR, **304–305**
- axial T2 MR, **306–308**
- barium swallow, **302, 303**
- fascia of, **298**
- graphics, **299–301**
  coronal T1 C+ MR and, **309**
- hypopharynx, **283**
- lymphatic ring, **298**
- mass, **302**
  generic, **302**
- muscles, **298**
- surface, **6, 273, 274, 275, 277, 282, 284, 285, 291, 293, 294, 299, 312**
- tumor
  invades basisphenoid, **302**
  pushing from medial to lateral, **302**
Pharyngeal plexus, **190**
- vagus nerve, **188**
Pharyngobasilar fascia, **298, 301, 364, 392, 394, 395**
Pharyngoepiglottic fold, **301, 374, 386, 394, 396, 398**
Pharyngotympanic groove, **6**
Pharynx, sensory from, **185**
Phrenic nerve, **349, 533**
- location, **353**
Pinna (auricle), **72, 74**
- meatus of, **74**
Piriform area, **129**
Pituitary gland, **28, 37, 118, 124, 127, 138, 154, 160, 230, 233, 234**
- normal, **235**
Pituitary infundibulum, **125, 133, 144, 146, 221**
Planum sphenoidale, **5, 7, 11, 14, 16, 17, 22, 28, 29, 39**
Platysma muscle, **278, 279, 280, 283, 284, 285, 286, 287, 288, 297, 326, 330, 333, 436, 437, 442, 443, 444, 449, 454, 456, 458, 459, 467, 469, 470, 471, 472, 473, 481, 482, 483**
PMS. *See* Pharyngeal mucosal space.
Pneumatized anterior clinoid, **241**
Pneumatized petrous apex, **98**
Pneumatized pterygoid wing, **247**
Pons, **49, 106, 123, 124, 126, 143, 145, 157, 158, 166, 167, 180, 203**
- anterior belly of, **107**
- ventral belly of, **126**
Pontine belly, **127, 137**
Pontine sensory nucleus (CNV), **119**
Pontomedullary junction, **126, 174, 180**

INDEX

Porus acusticus, **41, 43, 47, 59, 65, 102, 104, 106, 107, 123, 126, 178, 180, 181**
- facial nerve, **175**
- of internal auditory canal, **54**
- posterior margin, **46**

Porus trigeminus, **95, 153, 157, 162**
- inferior bony margin of, **121**
- inferior margin, **57**
- trigeminal nerve in, **127, 158**

Pöschl view, **66**

Postcricoid hypopharynx, **301, 303, 375, 387, 394, 397, 417**
- mucosa, **394**
- wall, **381**

Postcricoid region, **392**
- of hypopharynx, **405**
- tumor evaluation, **393**
- of visceral space, **364**

Posterior auricular branch
- abducens nerve, **169**
- facial nerve, **322**

Posterior band of disc, **109, 112, 113**

Posterior body cortical margin, **501**

Posterior cerebral artery, **124, 126, 137, 142, 143, 144, 145, 147, 149, 150, 151, 154, 167**

Posterior cervical line, **498, 505**

Posterior cervical space (PCS), **272, 275, 278, 279, 280, 281, 282, 283, 284, 294, 326, 328, 336, 337, 349, 353, 354, 356–363**
- axial CECT, **360**
- coronal T1 MR, **361**
- fascia of, **356**
- generic mass in, **359**
- graphics, **357**
- longitudinal and transverse ultrasound, **363**
- lymphatic malformation, **359**
- nodal stations/diseases, **358**
- nodes of, **426–427**
    level VA, **431**
    level VB, **432**
- surgical triangles, **356**
- transverse ultrasound, **362**

Posterior chamber, **211**

Posterior choana, **238**

Posterior clinoid, **99**

Posterior commissure, **373, 380, 389**

Posterior communicating artery, **124, 127, 143, 146**
- aneurysm, left, **147**

Posterior cord, **535, 542**

Posterior cribriform plate, **20**

Posterior cricoarytenoid muscle, **373, 375, 378, 381, 387, 395, 397, 401**

Posterior division, trigeminal nerve, **155**

Posterior elements, vertebrae, **349**

Posterior ethmoid complex, **240**

Posterior ethmoidal artery, **17**
- and canal, **17**

Posterior ethmoids, **251**

Posterior external vein, **528**

Posterior genu, facial nerve, **52, 55, 58, 169, 170, 172, 324**
- canal, **68, 82**

Posterior hypopharyngeal wall, **396, 400**

Posterior inferior cerebellar artery, **122, 187, 197**

Posterior intercavernous sinus, **230**

Posterior lacrimal crest, **214, 215**

Posterior mandible, inferior portion attaches to, **109**

Posterior median atlantoaxial joint, **499**

Posterior middle meatus, **242**

Posterior nasal cavity, **301, 394**

Posterior oropharyngeal wall, lower margin, **396**

Posterior pharyngeal wall, **374**

Posterior premolar, **492, 493, 494**

Posterior recess, inferior compartment, **109, 112, 113**

Posterior scalene muscle, **280, 281, 283, 349, 352, 354, 360, 541**

Posterior skull base, **4, 31, 40–49**
- axial bone CT, **43–45**
- axial T1 C+ FS MR, **48**
- bony landmarks, **40**
- coronal bone CT, **46–47**
- coronal T1 C+ MR, **49**
- development of, **40**
- foramina and fissures of, **40**
- graphics, **41**
    and MR venogram, **42**
- variant anatomy of, **40**

Posterior spinolaminar lines, **505, 506**

Posterior temporal artery, **151**

Posterior tonsillar pillar, **300**

Posterior triangle, **356**
- lymph node in, **363**

Posterior tubercle, **515**

Posterior vertebral line, **518**

Posterior wall, of visceral space, **364**

Posterior wall fascia, retropharyngeal space, **340**

Posterior wall hypopharynx, **300, 303, 347, 417**

Postganglionic fibers, sympathetic from, **252**

Postolivary sulcus, **122, 182, 187, 188, 193, 197**

Postsphenoid, **32, 39**

Poststyloid PPS. *See* Parapharyngeal space.

PPF. *See* Pterygopalatine fossa.

PPG. *See* Pterygopalatine ganglion.

PPS. *See* Parapharyngeal space.

Preepiglottic fat, **378, 399**

Preepiglottic space, **372, 374, 377, 379, 384, 385, 388, 390, 391, 396, 398**

Preganglionic segment. *See* Cisternal (preganglionic) segment.

Premaxilla, **490, 492**

Prenasal space, **18**

Preolivary sulcus, **119, 122, 193, 197, 198, 201**

Prepontine cistern, **124, 143, 146, 147, 157, 230**
- abducens nerve, **167**

Prepontine segment, CNV, **126**

Preseptal soft tissue, **210**

Presphenoid, **32, 39**

Prestyloid PPS. *See* Parapharyngeal space.

Pretectal nucleus, **133**
- area of, **135**

INDEX

Prevertebral component, perivertebral space, **341, 342, 343, 345, 346, 347, 348, 349, 350, 351, 352, 353, 354, 355, 357, 359, 360, 366, 367, 368**
- extension to, **352**
Prevertebral muscles, **279, 281, 282, 293, 294, 295, 304, 306, 308, 344, 345, 346, 347, 349, 351, 352, 353, 354, 367, 368, 420, 421, 435**
- anteriorly displaced, **351, 352**
- strap, **279**
Prevertebral soft tissues, **519, 525**
- line, **518**
Prevertebral-perivertebral space tumor, **351**
Primary follicles, **428**
Primary vitreous, **224**
Procerus, **441, 443, 444, 445, 446**
Projected CNVII course, **325**
Proximal carotid canal, **75**
Proximal cavernous CNVI, **166**
Proximal cervical nerves, **538**
Proximal intraparotid facial nerve, **327**
Proximal nerves, **532**
Proximal preganglionic segment, CNV, **126**
Proximal roots, **539**
Prussak space, **50, 54, 55, 60, 72, 75, 78, 80, 82, 84**
PS. *See* Parotid space.
Pseudosubluxation, **498**
Pterygoid muscle
- lateral, **77**
- medial, **484, 485, 488, 489**
Pterygoid nerve and artery, **156**
Pterygoid plate
- hamulus of medial, **488, 489**
- lateral, **36**
- medial, **36**
Pterygoid process, **477**
- marrow, **163**
Pterygoid venous plexus, **295, 310, 315, 319**
Pterygomandibular gap, **455**
Pterygomandibular raphe, **296, 301, 305, 307, 316, 394, 452, 453, 461, 475, 476, 477, 486, 487, 488**
- cephalad attachment, **488, 489**
- inferior attachment, **487**
- region of, **479**
- site of, **478**
- superior attachment, **487**
Pterygomaxillary fissure, **10, 22, 34, 35, 240, 241, 242, 253, 255, 256, 258, 259, 315, 317**
Pterygopalatine fossa, **10, 13, 22, 34, 35, 37, 38, 99, 100, 101, 156, 163, 216, 217, 218, 240, 242, 244, 247, 252–259, 315, 317, 477, 493**
- abnormal, **259**
- anatomic-radiologic correlation, **259**
- axial bone CT, **255**
- axial T1 MR, **258**
- cephalad aspect of, **162**
- coronal bone CT, **256**
- enhancing tumor within, **259**
- graphics, **254**
- internal maxillary artery in, **162**
- sagittal bone CT, **257**

Pterygopalatine ganglion, **31, 155, 252, 254, 258**
Pterygovaginal artery, **253**
PTG. *See* Parathyroid gland.
Pulmonary apex, **537**
Pulp, **490**
PVS. *See* Perivertebral space.
Pyramid, **122, 187**
Pyramidal eminence, **55, 58, 78, 80, 83, 170, 171, 172**
Pyramidal lobe, thyroid gland, **402, 406**
Pyriform sinuses (PS), **300, 301, 303, 347, 364, 367, 369, 374, 378, 379, 380, 382, 383, 384, 386, 387, 392, 394, 396, 398, 399**
- apex, **375, 378, 383, 392, 397, 400**
- left, **407**
- residual asymmetric, lumen, **401**
- superior margin, **398**
- tumor, **401**
    evaluation, **393**

Q

Quadrangular membrane, **372, 377**
Quadrigeminal plate cistern, **150**

R

Radial nerve, **535, 536**
Ramus of mandible, **330, 331**
- with posterior acoustic shadowing, **331**
- and posterior body, **310**
Ranawat measurement, **504**
Reactive nodes, **363**
Recessus terminalis, **248, 260, 266**
Recurrent laryngeal nerve (RLN), **188, 190, 191, 333, 365, 366, 373, 375, 378, 397, 405, 411, 419**
- location of, **280, 381**
- right, **405**
Red nucleus, **142**
Redlund-Johnell line, **502**
Redlund-Johnell measurement, **504**
Referred otalgia (ear pain), **73, 393**
Retained medialized uncinate process, **261**
Retaining ligaments, **441**
Retina, **134, 211, 224, 225**
Retinal artery, **134**
Retinal vein, **134**
Retrobulbar fat, **139**
Retrobullar recess, **260**
Retrocondylar vein, **508**
Retromandibular vein, **277, 282, 284, 293, 316, 320, 321, 322, 325, 326, 327, 328, 330, 331, 336**
Retromaxillary extension, **479**
Retromaxillary fat pad, **240, 247, 258, 274, 277, 293, 447**
Retromolar triangle, **318**
Retromolar trigone (RMT), **316, 452, 453, 486–489**
- axial T1 MR, **489**

INDEX

- axial T2 MR, **488**
- location, **487**
- mucosa, **461, 487**
- region, **476**

Retroolivary sulcus, **201**
Retroorbital fat, **212, 214, 215**
Retropharyngeal fat, loss of, **401**
Retropharyngeal nodal group, **427**
Retropharyngeal nodes, **429, 435**
- lateral, **435**
- malignant, **435**
- medial, **435**

Retropharyngeal space (RPS), **272, 273, 274, 275, 276, 278, 282, 283, 284, 291, 292, 296, 299, 300, 305, 307, 308, 333, 337, 340–347, 349, 350, 351, 353, 354, 360, 366, 367, 368, 370, 392, 399, 406, 418, 419, 420, 421, 425, 435**
- axial bone CT and T2 MR, **347**
- axial CECT, **345**
- axial T1 MR, **346**
- fascia, **340**
- fat, **278, 279, 401**
- graphics, **341–342**
- minimal fat in, **399**

Retrotympanum, **78**
Retrozygomatic node, **429**
Right abducens nerve, **166**
Right jugulodigastric node (level IIA), **358, 430, 431**
Right petrous carotid artery, **232**
Right subclavian artery, **407**
Right vagus nerve, **405**
Right vertebral artery flow void, **435**
Rima glottidis, **377, 384**
Rima vestibuli, **377, 384**
Risorius, **442, 443, 444, 448**
RLN. *See* Recurrent laryngeal nerve.
RMT. *See* Retromolar trigone.
Root entry zone, **31, 153, 155, 157, 158, 162**
- CNV, **119, 124**

Root exit zone, **168**
Root of tongue (ROT), **452, 454, 459, 461, 464, 470, 480, 483**
Rotundum notch, **256**
Round window, **56, 90**
- membrane, **69, 70, 83, 92**
- niche, **56, 59, 70, 79, 83, 90, 92, 98, 172**

Rouvière node, **427**
RPS. *See* Retropharyngeal space.

S

Sagittal sinus, superior, **42**
SBC. *See* Suprabullar cells.
Scala media, **86–87, 88, 103, 177**
Scala tympani, **64, 87, 88, 89, 103, 177**
Scala vestibuli, **64, 87, 88, 89, 103, 177**
Scalene medius muscle, **545**
Scalene muscles, **538**

Scalenus anterior muscle, **279, 288, 339, 362, 544, 545**
Scalenus medius muscle, **362, 545**
Scalp, muscles inserting at, **441**
Scaphoid fossa, **74**
Schwannoma, **259**
Sclera, **134, 139, 210, 211, 221, 224, 225**
Scutum, **51, 56, 59, 60, 70, 72, 74, 79, 80, 82, 83, 84, 90, 173**
- anterior, **61**

2nd cranial nerve. *See* Optic nerve.
2nd rib, **281**
Secondary follicles
- enlarged, **428**
- in superficial cortex region of node, **428**

Sella, **7, 19, 97**
- floor of, **33**

Sella turcica, **12, 33, 39, 218**
Semicircular canal, **87**
- anterior crus, **97**
- lateral, **7, 54, 58, 59, 63, 65, 68, 69, 79, 81, 82, 84, 89, 90, 91, 93, 97, 169, 172, 173, 178, 202, 322**
  bone island of, **91**
  calcified, **93**
- posterior, **54, 55, 58, 63, 64, 89, 91, 92, 93, 172, 178**
  ampulla of, **92**
- superior, **7, 54, 58, 59, 60, 63, 65, 68, 69, 71, 90, 91, 173, 178, 180, 181**
  anterior crus of, **97**
  arcuate eminence and, **97**

Semicircular duct
- lateral, **53, 88**
- posterior, **53, 88**
- superior, **53, 88**

Semispinalis muscle, **349**
Sensorineural hearing loss (SNHL), **102, 176**
Sensory branch superior laryngeal nerve, **190**
Sensory fibers, **182, 185, 188**
Septum, **210**
Sheath mass (possible meningioma), **220**
SHN. *See* Suprahyoid neck.
Short ciliary nerve, **155**
Short process of incus, **93**
Sigmoid plate, **43, 54, 57, 186**
Sigmoid sinus, **8, 9, 42, 43, 44, 48, 54, 55, 56, 99, 104, 186, 192, 324, 335**
- groove for, **40**

Signal (Virchow) node, **427**
Singular canal, **55, 104, 178**
Singular nerve, **52, 103, 177**
- canal, **92**

Sinonasal overview, **238–247**
Sinus confluence (torcular Herophili), **42**
Sinus tympani, **55, 58, 78, 83, 170, 171, 172**
Sinusitis, **235**
6th cranial nerve. *See* Abducens nerve.
Skin, face, **440**
Skull base, **260**
- osteomyelitis, **73**
- overview, **4–13**
  3D-VRT bone CT, **11**
  axial bone CT, **7–10**

xxiii

INDEX

axial T1 MR, **13**
graphics, **5–6**
sagittal bone CT & T1 MR, **12**
- right uncinate process inserting at, **266**
Skull base segment
- accessory nerve, **194**
- glossopharyngeal nerve, **182**
- hypoglossal nerve, **198**
- vagus nerve, **188**
SL-DCF. *See* Superficial layer, deep cervical fascia.
SLS. *See* Sublingual space.
SMAS. *See* Superficial musculoaponeurotic system.
SMS. *See* Submandibular space.
SOEC. *See* Supraorbital ethmoid cells.
SOF. *See* Superior orbital fissure.
Soft palate, **295, 301, 305, 307, 309, 394, 483**
- sensory from, **185**
Soft tissue, **400**
Solitarius tract nucleus, **168**
Solitary tract nucleus, **52, 119, 169, 182, 183, 185, 188, 189, 190**
Space-occupying lesion, **344**
Sphenoethmoidal cells, **238**
Sphenoethmoidal recess, **239, 242, 251**
Sphenoid bone, **6, 18, 36, 39, 45, 96, 209, 216, 217, 218, 234, 299, 317**
- body of, **10, 28, 29, 33, 38, 259**
- greater wing of, **5, 8, 9, 19, 20, 31, 33, 34, 36, 37, 101, 121, 216, 217, 218**
- lateral process, **100**
- lesser wing of, **5, 7, 11, 14, 16, 17, 22, 31, 206, 215, 216, 217, 218**
- pterygoid process of, **11, 38**
pneumatized, **13**
- pterygoid wing, **285**
Sphenoid lingula, **99**
Sphenoid ostia, **239**
Sphenoid sinus, **7, 8, 9, 13, 16, 19, 20, 21, 22, 24, 28, 29, 33, 34, 35, 37, 38, 39, 97, 98, 100, 118, 154, 156, 158, 161, 162, 201, 210, 214, 215, 219, 221, 228, 229, 235, 238, 239, 240, 241, 242, 244, 245, 246, 251, 255, 256, 257, 258, 285**
- extensive pneumatization of, **30**
- imaginary lateral recess of, **256**
- lateral recess of, **256**
- ostium, **21**
- secretions, **99**
- sinusitis of right, **259**
- in sphenoid body, **33**
Sphenooccipital synchondrosis, **9, 10, 21, 28, 29, 30, 32, 34, 35, 39, 43, 44, 156, 186, 192, 201**
- area, **39**
Sphenopalatine foramen, **22, 35, 239, 241, 247, 253, 255, 256, 258, 259**
Sphenotemporal suture, **218**
Sphenozygomatic suture, **218**
Sphincteric cricopharyngeus, **393**
Spinal accessory lymph nodes, **429, 433**
- high, **429**
- level V, **369, 410**
- level VA, **358**
- low, **429**
Spinal accessory nodal (SAN) chain, **356, 357, 410**
- above cricoid level, **358**
- below cricoid level, **358**
Spinal canal, **509**
Spinal cord, **522, 525, 526, 527, 528, 529, 530, 531, 538, 543**
- anterior median sulcus, **524**
Spinal fibers, accessory nerve, **195**
Spinal motor fibers, **194**
Spinal nerve, **515, 517**
Spinal nucleus
- accessory nerve, **119, 194, 195, 196**
- CNV, **119, 152, 153, 182, 183, 185, 189, 190**
Spinal portion, accessory nerve, **197**
Spinal root of accessory nerve, **122, 195**
Spinal rootlets, accessory nerve, **195**
Spinal tract, CNV, **119**
Spinolaminar line, **518**
- cortical margin, **519**
Spinous process, **505, 509, 515, 522, 523, 525, 528, 530, 531**
Spiral ganglia, **86, 88, 103, 176, 177**
- distal axon from, **103, 177**
Splenius capitis muscle, **349**
Squamous cell carcinoma (SCCa), **479**
- nodal staging, **427**
Squamous epithelium, **373**
Squamous portion, temporal bone, **7, 54, 96, 111**
Stapedius muscle, **50, 56, 78, 80, 81, 83, 171**
- head, **83**
- in pyramidal eminence, **56**
Stapedius nerve, **168, 169, 322**
Stapedius tendon, **79, 80, 81**
Stapes (stirrup), **60, 78–79, 81**
- crura, **59**
anterior, **69, 80, 83, 84**
posterior, **69, 80, 83**
- footplate/oval window, **80, 83, 84**
- head, **59, 80, 84**
- hub, **80**
- posterior crus, **56, 70**
- superstructure, **79**
Stenver view, **66**
Sternocleidomastoid muscle, **278, 279, 280, 282, 283, 284, 288, 289, 291, 294, 325, 326, 328, 330, 337, 338, 339, 353, 354, 357, 359, 360, 361, 362, 363, 371, 406, 407, 408, 409, 411, 424, 430, 431, 433, 436, 437, 438, 537, 544, 545**
- lateral, **432**
insertion, **432**
- medial, **432**
insertion, **432**
- oblique line along posterior border of, **432**
- transverse line along posterior, **431**
edge, **430, 431**
margin, **430, 431**
Sternohyoid muscle, **200, 289, 338, 366, 408, 409, 424**
Sternomastoid muscle, accessory nerve, **194, 196**
Sternothyroid muscle, **200, 289, 338, 366, 409, 424**

INDEX

Straight sinus, **42**
Strap muscles, **368, 371, 380, 382, 386, 390, 391, 408, 415, 420, 421, 422, 424, 425**
- medial edge of, **391**
Styloglossus muscle, **200, 294, 296, 301, 394, 480, 484**
Stylohyoid ligament, **301, 394**
Stylohyoid muscle, **482**
Styloid process, **6, 45, 58, 109, 110, 277, 293, 294, 295, 321, 322, 325, 333, 334, 336, 343, 508**
- inferior tip, **336**
Stylomandibular gap, **323**
Stylomastoid foramen, **57, 58, 68, 168, 169, 171, 172, 202, 292, 321, 324, 325**
- CNVII, **6, 10, 40, 45, 46, 111, 120, 174, 273**
mastoid segment, **9**
temporal bone, **11**
- fat, **322**
- malignancy enters, **324**
Stylopharyngeus branch, glossopharyngeal nerve, **182**
Stylopharyngeus muscle, **185, 294, 296, 301, 394, 395, 482, 484**
Subarachnoid space, **135, 136**
- CNII, **134**
Subaxial spine, **514**
Subcallosal gyrus area, **129**
Subcapsular/peripheral nodal vascularity, **439**
Subclavian artery, **281, 338, 361, 405, 533, 537, 540, 542**
Subclavian triangle, **356**
Subclavian vein, **537, 539, 542**
Subcutaneous fat, **478, 544**
- face, **440**
Subcutaneous tissue, **279, 286, 287, 288, 330, 331, 338, 339, 362, 390, 391, 408, 409, 424, 425, 436, 437**
- in suprasternal notch, **424**
Subfrenular sublingual space isthmus, **457**
Subfrontal cistern (olfactory bulb here), **121**
Subglottic larynx, **419**
Subglottis, **346, 364, 368**
- of endolarynx, **373**
Sublingual gland, **286, 287, 453, 456, 457, 461, 462, 463, 464, 465, 466, 467, 472, 491**
Sublingual space (SLS), **273, 452, 454, 455, 459, 462–467, 469, 470, 480, 483**
- axial CECT, **465**
- axial T2 FS MR, **466**
- coronal T1 MR, **464, 467**
- graphic & axial CECT, **463**
- isthmus, **455**
connecting, **466**
- lateral compartment, **462, 466**
- medial compartment, **462, 466**
Submandibular (Wharton) duct, **461, 462, 463, 464, 472, 491**
Submandibular ganglion, **462**
Submandibular gland, **163, 278, 283, 284, 285, 287, 288, 294, 297, 319, 326, 336, 337, 353, 367, 413, 414, 430, 431, 433, 434, 454, 455, 456, 458, 459, 465, 468, 471, 472, 473, 485, 491**
- anterior margin of, **473**
- deep portion, **453, 458, 462, 463, 465, 466, 469, 472**

- deep "process" of, **287**
- duct, **453, 454**
- hilum, **472**
- superficial portion, **453, 458, 463, 465, 466, 469, 470, 471, 472**
- transverse line along posterior, **430**
edge, **430**
margin, **430**
Submandibular node, **454, 456, 458, 469, 470, 471**
- high, **471**
- level IB, **426, 429, 430, 433, 434, 468**
Submandibular space (SMS), **273, 274, 275, 276, 279, 283, 284, 285, 291, 292, 294, 297, 311, 326, 367, 452, 454, 455, 456, 461, 463, 464, 468–473, 477**
- axial CECT, **471**
- axial T2 MR, **472**
- coronal T1 MR, **473**
- graphic & coronal T1 MR, **470**
- graphic and axial T2 MR, **469**
- parapharyngeal space communicates with, **285**
- vertical horseshoe, **452, 459**
"Submaxillary space." *See* Submandibular space.
Submental (level IA) nodes, **426, 429, 430, 431, 433, 468**
Submucosa, **364**
- hypopharynx, **392**
Submucosal fat, **476, 477, 478, 479**
- of posterior wall mucosa, **401**
Suborbicularis oculi fat pad, **440**
Substantia nigra, **142**
Superficial facial muscles, **441**
Superficial fascia, **477**
Superficial investing fascia, **477**
Superficial lamina propria, **373**
Superficial layer, deep cervical fascia, **272, 273, 274, 275, 276, 291, 292, 309, 310, 311, 312, 321, 322, 333, 334, 341, 342, 349, 350, 357, 366, 418, 419**
- lateral slip, **310**
Superficial musculoaponeurotic system (SMAS), **440–449**
- merging with orbicularis oculi anteriorly and temporoparietal fascia (superficial fascia) superiorly, **447**
Superficial space, **367, 368**
Superficial temporal artery and vein branches, **77**
Superior air cells, **76**
Superior articular facet, **500, 501, 515, 522, 523**
Superior articular process, **515**
Superior auricular muscle, **440**
Superior cerebellar artery, **124, 126, 127, 137, 142, 143, 145, 149, 151, 154, 167**
Superior cerebellar peduncle, **124, 125**
Superior colliculus, **133, 135, 144**
Superior compartment, **109, 112, 113**
Superior constrictor muscle, **297, 302, 475, 476, 478**
Superior extension cruciate ligament, **499**
Superior joint compartment, **108**
Superior laryngeal branch, **404**
Superior laryngeal nerve, **188, 190, 373, 378**
- external branch of, **378**
- internal branch of, **378**
aperture for, **376, 377**

INDEX

Superior margin of high jugular bulb, **104**
Superior meatus, **238**
Superior mediastinal (level VII) nodes, **369, 410, 427, 429, 432**
Superior mediastinum, **407**
Superior medullary velum, **125, 150**
- CNIV decussation, **149**
Superior nasal turbinate, **130**
Superior oblique muscle, **134, 136, 139, 149, 206–207, 211, 212, 213, 214, 215**
- trochlea of, **446**
Superior ophthalmic vein (SOV), **134, 136, 139, 207, 211, 212, 213, 214, 215, 221, 222**
- thrombosis, **235**
Superior orbital fissure (SOF), **5, 8, 9, 15, 17, 19, 20, 22, 30, 31, 33, 34, 37, 97, 117, 121, 140, 156, 158, 209, 214, 215, 216, 217, 218, 219, 230, 241, 256, 257**
- abducens nerve, **165**
- CNIII, IV, VI and V1, **121**
- ophthalmic division of CNV (CNV1) exiting, **31**
- perineural tumor extending through, **147**
Superior petrosal sinus, **230, 235**
- groove for, **97**
Superior pharyngeal constrictor muscle, **299, 300, 301, 305, 307, 394, 395, 396, 453, 457, 487, 488, 489**
Superior portion, bilaminar zone, **109**
Superior pterygopalatine fossa, maxillary nerve in, **162**
Superior rectus muscle, **134, 136, 139, 142, 206, 211, 212, 213, 215, 223**
- distal attachment, **214, 215**
- proximal, **206, 214**
Superior salivatory nucleus, **52, 168, 169**
Superior thyroid arteries, **402, 403, 404, 405, 409**
Superior thyroid cornua, **404**
Superior thyroid gland, **420**
Superior transverse ligament, **208**
Superior turbinate, **249**
- attachment, **239**
Superior vagal (jugular) ganglion, **188**
Superior vena cava, **432**
Superior vestibular nerve (SVN), **69, 89, 90, 102, 103, 105, 106, 174, 175, 177, 179, 181**
- canal, **91, 104**
Superior vestibular nucleus, **177**
Suprabullar cells, **260, 264, 267**
- left, **269**
Suprabullar recess, **260**
Supraclavicular nodes, **427, 432**
Supraclinoid carotid artery, left, **231**
Supraclinoid internal cerebral artery, left, **231, 232**
Supraglottic larynx, **367, 419**
- gas in, **436**
Supraglottis, **300, 364**
- of endolarynx, **372**
Suprahyoid and infrahyoid neck overview, **272–289**
- axial CECT, **277–280**
    cervicothoracic junction, **281**
- axial T1 MR, **282–283**
- axial T2 MR, **284**
- coronal T1 MR, **285**

- graphics, **273–276**
- power Doppler ultrasound and transverse ultrasounds, **287**
- spaces of, **272**
- transverse ultrasound, **286, 288–289**
Suprahyoid neck (SHN), **272, 276, 334, 350**
- axial CECT, **277–278**
- carotid space, **332**
    adjacent spaces, **332**
    lesion in, **332**
- retropharyngeal space, **340**
    axial, generic mass, **343**
    lesion, **340**
- spaces surrounding PPS, **272**
Suprahyoid nodes, **426**
Supraorbital ethmoid cells, **238, 260, 265, 268**
Supraorbital foramen, **209, 216, 217**
Supraorbital nerve, **31, 155, 212**
- branch of CNV1, **134**
Supraorbital notch, **17, 209, 212**
Suprasellar cistern, **138, 230, 231, 232**
Supratrochlear vein, **214, 215**
Suprazygomatic masticator space, **273, 274, 285, 311, 317, 319**
SVN. *See* Superior vestibular nerve.
Sympathetic chain, **191, 337, 349**
- location, **279**
Sympathetic plexus, **332**
Sympathetic schwannoma, **332**
Sympathetic trunk, **333**
Symphysis menti, **492, 495**
Symptomatic right posterior communicating artery aneurysm, **147**

T

T1, **541**
- pedicle, **526**
- transverse process, **519, 524, 540**
- ventral ramus, **535, 536, 543**
- vertebrae, **539**
T3, vertebral body, **276, 342**
Tarsal plate, **208, 211**
Taste fibers, **182, 185, 188**
- epiglottic area, **190**
Tc-99m sestamibi scan, delayed, parathyroid adenoma, **414**
Tectorial membrane, **498, 499, 511, 512**
Teeth, **490**
TEG. *See* Tracheoesophageal groove.
Tegmen mastoideum, **50, 58**
Tegmen tympani, **47, 51, 60, 61, 65, 70, 78, 80, 84, 85, 90, 172, 173**
Temporal bone, **5, 6, 8, 9, 209, 217**
- anatomy, **50–65**
    axial bone CT, **54–57**
    axial T2 MR, **63–64**
    coronal bone CT, **58–61**

xxvi

INDEX

coronal T2 MR, **65**
graphics, **51–53**
sagittal T1 MR, **62**
- oblique reformation anatomy, **66–71**
longitudinal & transverse oblique reformations, **67**
longitudinal oblique reformations, **68–69**
transverse oblique reformations, **70–71**
- petrous ridge of, **40, 41**
Temporal branch
- abducens nerve, **169**
- facial nerve, **322**
Temporal horn of lateral ventricle, **105**
Temporal lobe, **37, 65, 105, 175, 181, 324**
Temporalis fascia, **441, 446, 449**
Temporalis muscle, **155, 162, 163, 277, 282, 285, 295, 297, 310, 311, 312, 315, 317, 318, 319, 449, 477, 488**
Temporalis tendon, **315, 316, 317, 318, 319, 489**
Temporomandibular joint (TMJ), **44, 75, 76, 108–113**
- 3D-VRT bone CT, **110**
- articular disc of, **108**
- articular surfaces of, **108**
- articular tubercle, **77**
- bone CT, **111**
- capsule & ligaments, **108**
- compartments, **108**
- condylar fossa of, **60**
- graphics, **109**
- meniscus, **77**
- sagittal T1 MR, **112**
- sagittal T2 MR, **113**
Temporoparietal fascia, **440, 446, 449**
Temporoparietal muscle, **440**
Tenon capsule, **207–208**
Tensor palatini muscle, **295**
Tensor tympani muscle, **50, 56, 57, 61, 71, 78, 80, 81, 83, 93, 98, 171**
- tendon, **56, 61, 79, 80, 81, 85, 173**
Tensor veli palatini muscle, **163, 299, 301, 304, 306, 317, 318, 394**
- palatal component, **305**
Tentorial segment, trochlear nerve, **148**
Tentorium cerebelli, **126**
- cut margin of, **119**
Terminal motor branches, facial nerve, **168**
Thalamus, **135**
Thecal sac, **529**
3rd cranial nerve. *See* Oculomotor nerve.
3rd mandibular molar, **487, 488, 489, 492**
3rd ventricle, **126, 127, 137, 138, 145, 146**
Thorax, vagus to, **190**
Thymopharyngeal duct, **410, 412**
- origin of, **410, 412**
- tract, **410, 412**
Thymus, **410, 412**
Thyroarytenoid gap, **375, 380, 387, 397**
Thyroarytenoid muscles (TAMs), **373, 375, 377, 378, 389, 397**
Thyrocervical trunk, **405**
Thyroepiglottic ligament, **380, 382**
Thyroepiglottic muscle, **373, 378**

Thyroglossal duct, **403**
- cyst, **403, 410**
- tract, **404, 410**
Thyrohyoid ligament, **391**
Thyrohyoid membrane, **376, 377, 378, 383, 398, 418**
Thyroid cancer, **427**
Thyroid capsule, **404, 408, 415**
Thyroid cartilage, **279, 280, 337, 367, 368, 369, 370, 372, 374, 375, 377, 379, 380, 381, 382, 383, 385, 386, 387, 388, 389, 391, 396, 397, 400, 401, 404, 407, 418, 419, 425, 427**
- anterior lamina, **376**
- inferior cornu, **368, 375, 376, 381, 387, 397, 420**
- isthmus of, **391**
- marrow fat within, **389**
- normal ossified, **389**
- superior cornu, **376**
- superior horn, **398**
- superior margin, **399**
Thyroid follicles, **402**
Thyroid gland, **280, 281, 301, 333, 337, 338, 345, 346, 353, 365, 366, 368, 369, 375, 381, 383, 384, 394, 397, 419, 420, 421, 422, 423, 432**
- anatomy, **402–415**
- arterial supply to, **402**
- axial CECT, **406**
- coronal CECT, **407**
- embryology, **403**
- fascia, **402**
- graphics, **369, 404–405**
- inferior pole of, **409**
- isthmus, **404, 405, 406, 407, 408, 410, 411, 421, 422, 424**
- left lobes, **371, 402, 405, 406, 407, 413, 414, 424, 425**
superior pole, **404**
- lobe, **404, 406**
- longitudinal ultrasound, **409**
- lymphatic drainage, **402**
- right, lower pole of, **408**
- right lobe, **338, 339, 371, 402, 405, 407, 408, 413, 415, 424**
inferior, **414**
- superior pole of, **409**
right, **289**
- transverse ultrasound, **408**
- venous drainage from, **402**
- in visceral space, **283, 284**
Thyroid lamina, **289, 390**
Thyroid lesion, graphics, **410**
Thyroid mass, **370**
- graphic & coronal CECT, **369**
Thyroid neoplasm, **369**
Thyroid notch, **376, 379, 380, 382, 386**
Thyroid tissue remnants, **403**
Thyroidea ima, **402**
Tic douloureux (trigeminal neuralgia), **152**
TMJ. *See* Temporomandibular joint.
Tongue, **480–485**
- axial T2 MR, **484–485**
- intrinsic muscle, **200, 482, 483**

INDEX

- sagittal and coronal T1 MR, **483**
Tonsillar pillar, anterior, **481**
Torus lateralis, **248**
Torus tubarius, **36, 161, 293, 299, 301, 302, 304, 306, 309, 394**
Trabecular bone and marrow space, **97**
Trachea, **276, 303, 345, 361, 366, 368, 369, 370, 378, 383, 385, 404, 406, 407, 408, 411, 415**
 - tumor, **371**
 - in visceral space, **283**
Tracheal invasion, **423**
Tracheal ring, **408, 425**
 - 1st, **376, 418, 419**
 - 2nd, **419**
 - of cartilage, **424**
Tracheal wall, **423**
 - malignancy, **422**
 - mass, **370, 422**
Tracheoesophageal groove, **188, 191, 280, 368, 371, 405, 406, 415, 420, 421, 422, 423**
 - generic mass, **411**
 - mass, **368**
 - normal fat plane of right, **371**
 - tumor, **371, 422**
Tracheoesophageal lymph node, **368**
Tragus, **74**
Transethmoidal segment, **128**
Transspatial component, hypoglossal nerve, **198**
Transverse arytenoid muscle, **373, 378**
Transverse cervical nodes, **429**
Transverse foramen, **500, 508, 509, 513, 515, 522, 523, 528, 529, 530**
 - vertebral artery, **529**
Transverse intrinsic muscle, shadow, **455**
Transverse ligament, **499, 508, 511**
Transverse nasalis, **441, 443**
 - insertion, **445**
 - origin, **445**
Transverse process, **288, 349, 500, 501, 508, 509, 510, 514, 515, 517, 522, 529, 531**
 - anterior tubercle, **500, 522, 523, 529**
 - of cervical vertebra, **279, 339**
 - posterior tubercle, **500, 522, 523**
 - tips of, **363**
Transverse sinus, **42, 428**
Transversus menti muscle, **442**
Trapezius muscle, **278, 279, 280, 281, 283, 349, 353, 354, 357, 359, 360, 361, 362**
 - accessory nerve, **194, 196**
Triangular fossa, **74**
Trigeminal fascicles, **159**
 - Meckel cave with, **157, 162, 231**
Trigeminal ganglion, **17, 31, 37, 142, 153, 155, 158, 159, 160, 211, 231, 312, 319**
 - within Meckel cave, **153, 228, 229**
Trigeminal groove, **8, 156**
Trigeminal impression, **95, 97, 99**

Trigeminal nerve (CNV), **94–95, 96, 100, 116, 119, 127, 137, 142, 145, 151, 152–163, 165, 180, 207, 211, 216, 217, 229, 491**
 - axial bone CT, **156**
 - axial T1 C+MR, **158**
 - axial T1 MR, **162, 163**
 - axial T2 MR, **157**
 - coronal T1 C+MR, **160–161**
 - coronal T2 MR, **159**
 - entering Meckel cave, **124, 137**
 - graphics, **153–155**
 - in porus trigeminus, **127, 158**
 - preganglionic segment, **65, 137**
 - rootlets in Meckel cave, **127, 154**
 - sagittal T2, **162**
Trigonal segment, oculomotor nerve, **141**
Trochlea, **211, 212**
Trochlear nerve (CNIV), **17, 31, 116, 117, 118, 119, 142, 148–151, 154, 160, 161, 165, 207, 211, 216, 227, 228, 233, 234**
 - axial T2 MR, **150**
 - coronal T2 MR, **151**
 - decussation, in superior medullary velum, **149**
 - graphics, **149**
 - neuropathy, **148**
 - in wall of cavernous sinus, **149**
Trochlear nuclei, **148, 149**
True retropharyngeal space, **342, 347**
True vocal cord (TVC), **368, 373, 374, 377, 378, 380, 382, 384, 387, 390, 396, 400, 401, 419**
 - inferior margin of, **400**
 - level, **303**
 - medial margin of, **389**
 - medialized margin of left, **389**
 - undersurface of, **375, 381, 397, 407**
Tuber cinereum, **137**
Tuberculum sellae, **16, 19, 30, 31, 33**
Tunica fibrosa, **224**
Tunica interna, **224**
Tunica vasculosa, **224**
TVC. *See* True vocal cord.
Tympanic annulus, **51, 59, 60, 70, 72, 74, 79, 80, 84, 85, 172, 173**
 - anterior, **61**
Tympanic artery, inferior, in inferior tympanic canaliculus, **53**
Tympanic branch, glossopharyngeal nerve, **182**
Tympanic membrane (TM), **51, 57, 59, 61, 70, 72, 74, 75, 79, 90, 173**

U

Ulcerated squamous cell carcinoma, buccal mucosa, **479**
Ulnar nerve, **535, 536**
Uncinate process, **242, 244, 248, 249, 250, 507, 515, 516, 520, 525, 528, 529, 531**
Uncovertebral joint, **514, 515**
Uncus, **129, 137, 143, 145, 150**

INDEX

Unilateral-nodal SHN mass, **340**
Upper alveolar ridge mucosa, **461**
Upper clivus, **166, 186, 192**
Upper cranial nerves, graphics, **118**
Upper internal jugular chain nodes (level II), **426**
 - level IIB, **358, 430, 431**
Upper lip, muscles inserting at, **442**
Upper trunk, **541**
Uvea, **224**
Uvula, **285, 297, 301, 302, 309, 394, 483**

V

Vagal nerve dysfunction, **188**
Vagal neuropathy, **188**
Vagus nerve (CNX), **41, 116, 117, 119, 122, 183, 184, 187, 188–193, 195, 196, 199, 288, 289, 333, 334, 339**
 - areas of, **337**
 - axial bone CT, **192**
 - axial T2 MR, **193**
 - branch, to carotid branch of CNIX, **190**
 - entering jugular foramen, **193**
 - graphics
    extracranial, **190, 191**
    proximal, **189**
 - injury, **332**
 - location, **279**
 - trunk, **191**
 - ultrasound, **339**
Vallecula, **278, 285, 300, 303, 374, 378, 379, 384, 385, 386, 388, 396, 398, 417, 456**
Vein, cervical lymph node, **428**
Vein of Labb, **42**
Venous communications, **226**
Venous plexus
 - clival, **42**
 - suboccipital, **42**
 - in vidian canal, **161**
Ventral cochlear nuclei, **176, 177**
Ventral gray column, **195**
Ventral nucleus, **140**
Ventral ramus, **532**
Ventral root, **538**
Ventral wall of petrous apex, **96**
Ventrolateral sulcus, **198**
Vertebral arch, **514**
Vertebral artery, **41, 48, 49, 107, 122, 126, 127, 167, 180, 197, 201, 203, 279, 281, 282, 283, 284, 335, 349, 351, 352, 353, 354, 361, 435, 511, 513, 524, 527, 528, 529, 530, 531, 538, 543**
 - encasement of, **352**
 - loop, **335, 336**
Vertebral body, **349, 514, 515, 529**
 - destruction, **351, 352**
 - enhancing mass, **352**
 - posterior margin, **516**
Vertebral canal, **500, 515, 523**
Vertebral endplate, **528, 529, 531**

Vertebral vein, **279, 281, 349, 351, 352, 354**
Vertical crest (Bill bar), **52, 55, 69, 90, 102, 103, 104, 176, 177**
Vertical plate, ethmoid bone, **24**
Vestibular aqueduct, **91**
 - axial view of, **90**
 - bony, **54, 58**
    fovea of, **54, 55**
Vestibular folds, **372**
Vestibular (Reissner) membrane, **88**
Vestibular nerve, **176**
 - inferior, **52, 62, 64**
 - superior, **52, 62, 63**
Vestibular nuclear complex, **176**
Vestibular nuclei (CNVIII), **119**
Vestibule, **53, 54, 55, 58, 59, 63, 64, 65, 69, 70, 82, 86, 87, 88, 89, 90, 91, 97, 104, 170, 178, 180, 202**
 - with calcification, **93**
Vestibulocochlear nerve (CNVIII), **41, 62, 64, 65, 102, 105, 106, 107, 116, 117, 118, 119, 123, 126, 165, 174, 175, 176–181, 177**
 - axial & coronal bone CT, **178**
 - axial T2 MR, **179**
 - coronal T2 MR, **180**
 - graphics, **177**
 - oblique sagittal T2 MR, **181**
Vidian canal, **10, 13, 30, 35, 36, 38, 45, 98, 100, 101, 120, 156, 161, 216, 219, 234, 241, 252, 255, 256, 257, 258, 259**
 - secondary to perineural tumor spread, **259**
 - vidian nerve, **31, 155, 162**
Vidian nerve, **161, 252, 254**
 - in vidian canal, **31, 155, 162**
Visceral nodes, **427, 429, 432**
Visceral space (VS), **272, 275, 276, 279, 280, 281, 283, 334, 337, 345, 346, 350, 353, 364–371, 419, 420, 421, 422, 423**
 - axial CECT, **367–368**
 - fascia, **365**
 - graphics, **366**
 - lymph nodes, **365**
 - mass graphic & sagittal anatomy, **370**
 - radiologic correlation, **371**
 - thyroid mass graphic & coronal CECT, **369**
Visual cortex, **132**
 - calcarine, **133**
Vitreous, **211, 225**
 - chamber, **224**
 - primary, **224**
Vocal ligament, **375, 377, 378, 397**
Vocal process, arytenoid cartilage, **375, 378, 380, 397**
Vocalis muscle, **375, 377, 378, 397**
Vomer, **6, 12**
VS. *See* Visceral space.

xxix

INDEX

W

Wackenheim line, **498, 502, 503**
Welcher basal angle, **498, 502, 504**
Whitnall ligament, **208**
Wrinkles on face, **442**

Z

Zonule fibers, **211, 225**
Zuckerkandl tubercle, **402, 406**
Zygoma, **76, 447**
Zygomatic arch, **10, 11, 13, 76, 109, 110, 111, 273, 274, 285, 311, 312, 315, 317, 318, 319, 447, 449, 477**
 - base of, **77**
Zygomatic bone, **6, 11, 209, 216, 217, 218, 219**
Zygomatic branch
 - abducens nerve, **169**
 - facial nerve, **322**
Zygomaticomaxillary suture, **219**
Zygomaticus major (ZMj), **442, 443, 444, 447, 448, 475, 476, 478**
Zygomaticus minor (ZMi), **442, 443, 444, 447**
Zygomaticus muscle, **476, 479**
 - proximal, **477**